Current Vascular Surgery: 2013

Current Vascular Surgery: 2013

Mark K. Eskandari, MD

James S.T. Yao, MD, PhD
Professor of Education in Vascular Surgery
Professor of Radiology and Cardiology
Chief, Division of Vascular Surgery
Department of Surgery
Northwestern University
Feinberg School of Medicine
Chicago, Illinois

William H. Pearce, MD

Violet R. and Charles A. Baldwin
Professor of Vascular Surgery
Division of Vascular Surgery
Department of Surgery
Northwestern University
Feinberg School of Medicine
Chicago, Illinois

James S.T. Yao, MD, PhD

Professor Emeritus
Division of Vascular Surgery
Department of Surgery
Northwestern University
Feinberg School of Medicine
Chicago, Illinois

2014
PEOPLE'S MEDICAL PUBLISHING HOUSE—USA
SHELTON, CONNECTICUT

People's Medical Publishing House-USA
2 Enterprise Drive, Suite 509
Shelton, CT 06484
Tel: 203-402-0646
Fax: 203-402-0854
E-mail: info@pmph-usa.com

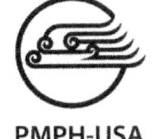

PMPH-USA

14 15 16 17/King/9 8 7 6 5 4 3 2 1

ISBN-13   978-1-60795-184-1
ISBN-10   1-60795-184-3
eISBN-13 978-1-60795-260-2

Printed in the United States of America by King Printing Company, Inc.
Editor: Linda H. Mehta; Copyeditor/Typesetter: diacriTech; Cover designer: Mary McKeon

Library of Congress Cataloging-in-Publication Data

Annual Northwestern University Vascular Symposium (38th : 2013 : Chicago, Ill.), author.
  Current vascular surgery 2013 / [edited by] Mark K. Eskandari, William H. Pearce, James S.T. Yao.
    p. ; cm.
  Includes bibliographical references and index.
  ISBN-13: 978-1-60795-184-1
  ISBN-10: 1-60795-184-3
  ISBN-13: 978-1-60795-260-2 (eISBN)
  I. Eskandari, Mark K., editor of compilation. II. Pearce, William H., editor of compilation.
III. Yao, James S. T., editor of compilation. IV. Title.
  [DNLM: 1. Vascular Diseases—surgery—Congresses. 2. Vascular Surgical Procedures—methods—Congresses. WG 170]
  RD598.5

617.4'13—dc23

2013044311

Sales and Distribution

Canada
Login Canada
300 Saulteaux Cr., Winnipeg, MB, R3J 3T2
Phone: 1.800.665.1148
Fax: 1.800.665.0103
www.lb.ca

Foreign Rights
John Scott & Company
International Publisher's Agency
P.O. Box 878
Kimberton, PA 19442,
USA
Tel: 610-827-1640
Fax: 610-827-1671

United Kingdom, Europe, Middle East, Africa
Eurospan Limited
3, Henrietta Street,
Covent Garden,
London WC2E 8LU,
UK
Within the UK: 0800 526830
Outside the UK: +44 (0)20 7845 0868
http://www.eurospanbookstore.com

Singapore, Thailand, Philippines,
Indonesia,Vietnam, Pacific Rim, Korea
McGraw-Hill Education
60 Tuas Basin Link
Singapore 638775
Tel: 65-6863-1580
Fax: 65-6862-3354
www.mcgraw-hill.com.sg

Australia, New Zealand
Elsevier Australia
Locked Bag 7500
Chatswood DC NSW 2067
Australia
Tel: 161 (2) 9422-8500
Fax: 161 (2) 9422-8562
www.elsevier.com.au

Brazil
SuperPedido Tecmedd
Beatriz Alves, Foreign Trade Department
R. Sansao Alves dos Santos, 102 | 7th floor
Brooklin Novo
Sao Pãolo 04571-090,
Brazil
Tel: 55-16-3512-5539
www.superpedidotecmedd.com.br

India, Bangladesh, Pakistan, Sri Lanka,
Malaysia
CBS Publishers
4819/X1 Prahlad Street 24
Ansari Road, Darya Ganj,
New Delhi-110002,
India
Tel: 91-11-23266861/67
Fax: 91-11-23266818
Email: cbspubs@vsnl.com

People's Republic of China
People's Medical Publishing House
International Trade Department
No. 19, Pan Jia Yuan Nan Li
Chaoyang District
Beijing 100021, P.R.
China
Tel: 8610-67653342
Fax: 8610-67691034
www.pmph.com/en/

Acknowledgments

We thank our esteemed authors who have thoughtfully contributed to this year's book. Their willingness to share their personal expertise and knowledge is what makes our book a success to other practitioners. Special thanks to Sara Minton, administrative coordinator, for her hard work in assembling and proofing the chapters and for keeping us on track with the deadlines of the symposium. Without her, the symposium and book would not have been possible. We would also like to thank W.L. Gore & Associates, Incorporated for their continued generous educational grant that helps support the Symposium and printing of the book.

Mark K. Eskandari, MD
William H. Pearce, MD
James S.T. Yao, MD, PhD

Contents

SECTION VIII Complex Arterial and Venous Diseases 407

SECTION IX Abdominal Aortic Diseases 465

Contributors

Omar Al-Nouri, DO, MS
Loyola University Medical Center
Maywood, IL

Peter Angelos, MD, PhD
University of Chicago
Chicago, IL

Efthimios Avgerinos, MD
University of Pittsburgh School of
    Medicine
Pittsburgh, PA

Abdulhameed Aziz, MD
Washington University
St. Louis, MO

Aaron C. Baker, MS, MD
University of California @ Davis
Sacramento, CA

Joseph E. Bavaria, MD
University of Pennsylvania
Philadelphia, PA

Adam W. Beck, MD
University of Florida College of Medicine
Gainesville, FL

Megan Brenner, MD, MS
University of Maryland
Baltimore, MD

Thomas C. Bower, MD
Mayo Clinic College of Medicine
Rochester, MN

Kellie R. Brown, MD
Medical College of Wisconsin
Milwaukee, WI

O. William Brown, MD, JD
Oakland University William Beaumont
    School of Medicine
Royal Oak, MI

Neal S. Cayne, MD
NYU Medical Center
New York, NY

Rabih A. Chaer, MD
University of Pittsburgh Medical Center
Pittsburgh, PA

Claudia Chavez-Munoz, MD, PhD
Northwestern University Feinberg School
    of Medicine
Chicago, IL

Jae S. Cho, MD
Loyola University Stritch School of
    Medicine
Maywood, IL

W. Darrin Clouse, MD
University of California @ Davis
Sacramento, CA

Mark F. Conrad, MD, MMSc
Harvard Medical School
Boston, MA

Paul R. Crisostomo, MD
Loyola University Stritch School of
    Medicine
Maywood, IL

Caroline Cusack, BS
Creighton University School of Medicine
Omaha, NE

Katherine Cusack, BS
Creighton University School of Medicine
Omaha, NE

Michael C. Dalsing, MD
Indiana University School of Medicine
Indianapolis, IN

Courtney M. Daly, MD
Northwestern University Feinberg School
    of Medicine
Chicago, IL

R. Clement Darling III, MD
Albany Medical College
Albany, NY

B.G. DeRubertis, MD
David Geffen School of Medicine @ UCLA
Los Angeles, CA

Elizabeth L. Detschelt, MD
Albany Medical College
Albany, NY

Gregory A. Dumanian, MD
Northwestern University Feinberg School
    of Medicine
Chicago, IL

Audra A. Duncan, MD
Mayo Clinic College of Medicine
Rochester, MN

Grant T. Fankhauser, MD
Mayo Clinic Arizona
Phoenix, AZ

Erin C. Farlow, MD
Indiana University School of Medicine
Indianapolis, IN

Cindy Felty, RN
Mayo Clinic College of Medicine
Rochester, MN

Sunny Fink, MD
Northwestern University Feinberg School
    of Medicine
Chicago, IL

Julie Freischlag, MD
Johns Hopkins Hospital
Baltimore, MD

Robert D. Galiano, MD
Northwestern University Feinberg School
    of Medicine
Chicago, IL

Patrick J. Geraghty, MD
Washington University Medical School
St. Louis, MO

Bruce L. Gewertz, MD
Cedars-Sinai Medical Center
Los Angeles, CA

Heather L. Gill, MD
Columbia University College of Physicians
    and Surgeons
New York, NY

Natalia Glebova, MD, PhD
Johns Hopkins Hospital
Baltimore, MD

Roger T. Gregory, MD
Eastern Virginia Medical School (Retired)
Norfolk, VA

Robert I. Hacker, MD
University of Pittsburgh Medical Center
Pittsburgh, PA

Eric S. Hager, MD
University of Pittsburgh Medical Center
Pittsburgh, PA

Andrew W. Hoel, MD
Northwestern University Feinberg School
    of Medicine
Chicago, IL

Thomas S. Huber, MD, PhD
University of Florida College of Medicine
Gainesville, FL

G. Chad Hughes, MD
Duke University Medical Center
Durham, NC

Glenn Jacobowitz, MD
NYU Medical Center
New York, NY

Mila H. Ju, MD
Northwestern University Feinberg School
    of Medicine
Chicago, IL

Ravi Kapadia, MD
Monmouth Medical Center
Long Branch, NJ

William D.T. Kent, MD, MSc
University of Calgary
Calgary, Alberta
Canada

S.C. Kiang, MD
David Geffen School of Medicine at UCLA
Los Angeles, CA

Melina R. Kibbe, MD
Northwestern University Feinberg School
    of Medicine
Chicago, IL

Hari R. Kumar, MD
Northwestern University Feinberg School
    of Medicine
Chicago, IL

Brajesh K. Lal, MD
University of Maryland School of
    Medicine
Baltimore, MD

Frank A. Lederle, MD
Minneapolis VA Medical Center
University of Minnesota
Minneapolis, MN

S. Chris Malaisrie, MD
Northwestern University Feinberg School
    of Medicine
Chicago, IL

Neel A. Mansukhani, MD
Northwestern University Feinberg School
    of Medicine
Chicago, IL

R. Scott McClure, MD, SM
Queen's University
Kingston, Ontario
Canada

Robert B. McLafferty, MD
Oregon Health Sciences University
Portland, OR

George H. Meier III, MD
University of Cincinnati College of
    Medicine
Cincinnati, OH

Mark H. Meissner, MD
University of Washington School of
    Medicine
Seattle, Washington, DC

Monish Merchant, MD
Advocate Illinois Masonic Medical
    Center
Chicago, IL

Ross, Milner, MD
University of Chicago Pritzker School of
    Medicine
Chicago, IL

Nicholas J. Morrissey, MD
Columbia University College of Physicians
    and Surgeons
New York, NY

Mark R. Nehler, MD
University of Colorado Denver School of
    Medicine
Aurora, CO

Richard F. Neville, MD
George Washington University
Washington, DC

William Frank Oppat, MD
Wayne State University School of Medicine
Detroit, MI

Philip S.K. Paty, MD
Albany Medical College
Albany, NY

William H. Pearce, MD
Northwestern University Feinberg School
    of Medicine
Chicago, IL

Bruce A. Perler, MD
Johns Hopkins University School of
    Medicine
Baltimore, MD

Todd E. Rasmussen, MD
The Uniformed Services University of
    Health Sciences
Bethesda, MD

Scott Resnick, MD
Northwestern University Feinberg School
    of Medicine
Chicago, IL

Norman M. Rich, MD
Uniformed Services University of Health
    Sciences
Bethesda, MD

Sean P. Roddy, MD
Albany Medical College
Albany, NY

Heron E. Rodriguez, MD
Northwestern University Feinberg School
    of Medicine
Chicago, IL

Thom W. Rooke, MD
Mayo Clinic
Rochester, MN

Salvatore T. Scali, MD
University of Florida College of
    Medicine
Gainesville, FL

Andres Schanzer, MD
University of Massachusetts Medical
    School
Worcester, MA

Dhiraj M. Shah, MD
Albany Medical College
Albany, NY

Sherene Shalhub, MD, MPH
University of Washington
Seattle, WA

Anton Skaro, MD, PhD
Northwestern University Feinberg School
    of Medicine
Chicago, IL

H. Bob Smouse, MD
University of Illinois College of Medicine
Peoria, IL

William M. Stone, MD
Mayo Clinic Arizona
Phoenix. AZ

Jason M. Souza, MD
Northwestern University Feinberg School
  of Medicine
Chicago, IL

Nigel Tai, MS
Royal London Hospital
Birmingham, UK

Patrick Thompson, BS
University of Massachusetts Medical
  School
Worcester, MA

Vivian Marie Torres, MD
Wayne State University School of Medicine
Detroit, MI

R. James Valentine, MD
University of Texas Southwestern Medical
  Center
Dallas, TX

Ashley K. Vavra, MD
Northwestern University Feinberg School
  of Medicine
Chicago, IL

Robert L. Vogelzang, MD
Northwestern University Feinberg School
  of Medicine
Chicago, IL

Alyson L. Waterman, MD
University of Florida
Gainesville, FL

Judson B. Williams, MD, MHS
Duke University Medical Center
Durham, NC

Abby Wochinski, MD
Medical College of Wisconsin
Milwaukee, WI

James S.T. Yao, MD, PhD
Emeritus
Northwestern University Feinberg School
  of Medicine
Chicago, IL

Preface

Welcome to our 38th Annual Vascular Symposium sponsored by the Division of Vascular Surgery, Feinberg School of Medicine, Northwestern University. Originally developed by Drs. Bergan and Yao, who currently reside in Chicago, our annual symposium has hosted renowned leaders in vascular surgery who have provided thought-provoking and spirited discussions centered on the evolution of vascular and endovascular surgery. Over the years, the program has morphed from a topic-oriented program to a more comprehensive overview as developed by Dr. Pearce. This year we have brought together 50 national experts for our two and a half day annual meeting to address contemporary topics and controversies in vascular and endovascular surgery. As has been the tradition, presentations cover the full spectrum of vascular surgery including changes in management of extracranial cerebrovascular disease, new treatment options for lower extremity arterial occlusive disease, hemodialysis, novel techniques for complex venous disease, and recent cutting-edge developments in aortic stent graft repair in the chest and abdomen. In conjunction with the presentations are corresponding chapters found in this hardcover book with more in-depth details and "pearls" from the experts. Over the past three decades, our symposium has been held at iconic hotels in the heart of Chicago including the Drake and Fairmont. This year we have again chosen the InterContinental Hotel as the venue for our December Symposium, given its prime location in the heart of Chicago along the Magnificent Mile. It is our sincere hope that you will find the contributions in this book valuable to your practice of vascular and endovascular surgery. We thank you for your interest and support of our annual meeting.

Mark K. Eskandari, MD
William H. Pearce, MD
James S.T. Yao, MD, PhD

Interviews with Pioneers of Vascular Surgery: Observations and Lessons Learned

Roger T. Gregory, MD; James S. T. Yao, MD, PhD; Norman M. Rich, MD; and the History Project Work Group of the Society for Vascular Surgery

INTRODUCTION

The audiovisual recording of interviews by Society for Vascular Surgery (SVS) began with the 50th anniversary celebration of SVS. As president of SVS in 1991, Calvin B. Ernst appointed a 50th Anniversary Committee consisting of Calvin Ernst (co-chair), James Yao (co-chair), Jesse Thompson, Allan Callow, James DeWeese, Wiley Barker, and Harris B. Shumacker, Jr. The committee decided to have audiovisual videotape recordings made on the two surviving founders, Harris B. Shumacker, Jr and Michael E. DeBakey. The recordings were produced by the AV service of Northwestern Memorial Hospital under the supervision of James Yao. Dr. DeBakey was interviewed by William Blaisdell and Dr. Shumacker by Calvin Ernst. Part of the interview with DeBakey has been published in the special June issue of *Journal of Vascular Surgery*.[1] These videotapes were shown at the special anniversary celebration meeting on June 11, 1996, and were well received. Because of this success, Calvin Ernst suggested to extend the interviews to other past presidents. Unfortunately, because of lack of funds available, the project faded into history.

Fifteen years later, in September 2011, under the leadership of Richard Cambria (president 2011–2012) and Peter Gloviczki (president 2012–2013), SVS revived this original initiative with an audiovisual program to interview contributors or leaders of vascular surgery to preserve the history of SVS and vascular surgery as a surgical specialty. A committee called the History Project Work Group was formed, chaired by James Yao with Norman Rich and Roger Gregory as members and Calvin Ernst as a consultant. Because of the workload, the committee was expanded to include younger members, as reported previously. The methodology and the program of Interviews with Pioneers of Vascular Surgery have been reported in detail recently.[2,3] Since the first recording of the new series of interviews was initiated with Dr. Denton Cooley in September 2011, 67 interviews have been completed. In November 2012, we were instructed by the leadership of SVS that honorary members of SVS should also be included. These foreign surgeons will give us information on the current status of US vascular surgery in the eyes of others.

Since the interview program is soon coming to an end, perhaps it is time for us to review what we have observed and learned from these interviews. Although the primary goal of the program is to preserve history, there may be educational value from the experience of these 67 leading surgeons. As Dale said in his first oral history book on vascular surgery, *The Band of Brothers*, "We will know what they have contributed but we (also) want to know how this happened."[4] It is often said, "Those who cannot learn from history are doomed to repeat it." The 67 interviews from this group of leaders and contributors provide a unique historical experience for others to follow and learn from.

In this chapter, we would like, first, to examine the adequacy of the selection criteria and the academic productivity of these candidates; second, to briefly review historical events of SVS as told firsthand by the interviewees; and, finally, to consider personal opinions from the interviewed subjects on issues such as leadership, mentorship, time management, women in surgery, life balance, and advice to young surgeons.

SELECTION CRITERIA

The selection criteria for members of this interview program have been described in detail previously.[2,3] In essence, all past presidents of the Society for Vascular Surgery (SVS) and American Association for Vascular Surgery (AAVS; formerly ISCVS-NA) as well as recipients of the Lifetime Achievement Award or the Innovation Award will be interviewed automatically. The Work Group has selected several other surgeons who have made unique contributions in our specialty. Since vascular surgery is a technically demanding surgical discipline, we selected George Noon and Jimmy Howell for their clinical and operative skills. We also selected Ken Mattox for his vast experience with vascular trauma. Denton Cooley, America's best technical surgeon, was our first surgeon to be interviewed by Roger Gregory. All these surgeons were trained by Michael DeBakey at the Mecca of vascular surgery, Houston, Texas. George Noon participated in many surgical procedures with DeBakey on foreign dignitaries such as President Boris Yeltsin of Russia and Dr. Mstislav Keldysh of the USSR Academy of Sciences. The type of surgical event of an American surgeon operating on the Russian President, a political adversary, will probably never take place again. Jimmy Howell distinguished himself as the best surgeon in Houston with a beyond-belief operative case record. In a span of 40 years, he performed 27,500 cardiac and vascular procedures with follow-up.[5] Ken Mattox's teaching in vascular trauma, especially thoracic aortic injury, is legendary.

The other group of individuals we have selected are surgeons who later became CEOs, presidents, or deans of their institutions. Richard Dean became president of Wake Forest University. While serving at the American Board of Surgery, Dean was the first to suggest the sub-board structure for vascular surgery. Larry Hollier was the first president of Mount Sinai Hospital and later chancellor of Louisiana State University. Jock Wheeler became dean of the Eastern Virginia Medical School and

TABLE 1. NAME AND COUNTRY OF ORIGIN OF THE 11 HONORARY MEMBERS INTERVIEWED

Roger Greenhalgh	United Kingdom
Jean-Baptiste Ricco	France
Stephen Cheng	Hong Kong, China
John Harris	Australia
James May	Australia
Anatoly Pokrovsky	Russia
Jonathan D. Beard	United Kingdom
José Fernandes e Fernandes	Portugal
Jan Brunkwall	Germany
Jan Blankensteijn	The Netherlands
Frans Moll	The Netherlands

Anthony Whittemore became chief medical officer of Brigham and Women's Hospital, while Tom O'Donnell served as CEO of Tufts Medical Center. All these individuals offer valuable information on how vascular surgeons should position themselves in the changing world of health-care delivery.

Since the first interview with Dr. Denton Cooley in September 2011, we have completed 67 interviews. Of these, 11 were honorary members. Table 1 shows the names and countries of origin of these 11 honorary members.

Of the past presidents, it is of interest to review their academic productivity. Judgment of an academic surgeon's academic productivity is often placed on his or her publication record. The old saying "publish or perish" remains true. Another consideration is membership in prestigious surgical societies such as American Surgical Association or Society of University Surgeons and, of course, in vascular surgery, the Society for Vascular Surgery. Although there is no strict number of publications needed to be considered a contributor, all would agree that only peer-reviewed articles would be counted. In this review only 38 subjects had submitted a complete publication record. Of these 38 subjects to be interviewed, the number of articles published in peer-reviewed journals is generally in the range of 100–250. A publication record of more than 300 was rare, and there are only a handful with over 400 publications (see Table 2). Denton Cooley, Ben Eiseman, and Larry Hollier were not past presidents but all have an impressive publication record (Cooley – 1379, Eiseman – 455, and Hollier – 363). Although these are impressive numbers, no one can top Dr. DeBakey, who has published 1478 peer-reviewed articles (DeBakey L. Personal communication. June 9, 2013). This 1478 number will probably never be repeated. Obviously, a number is just a quantitative measurement. Perhaps quality of the publication is more important, and an article with great impact on clinical practice or scientific discovery is more important than just the numbers of publications.

Another consideration in the publication record is book chapters and books authored by or edited or co-edited by an author. Most members have no more than five books with the exception of John Bergan – 31, Jack Cronenwett – 13, Denton Cooley – 12, Ted Diethrich – 10, Ben Eiseman – 27, Wesley Moore – 19, William Pearce – 19, Ron Stoney – 9, Anthony Whittemore – 12, and, top of the list, James Yao who co-edited 59 books. The submission of numbers of book chapters written by some members is haphazard and difficult to count. Nevertheless, Frank Vieth is on top of the list with 339 book chapters.

TABLE 2. PAST PRESIDENTS WITH PUBLICATION RECORDS
EXCEEDING 300 PEER-REVIEWED ARTICLES

DeBakey	1478
Veith	779
Bergan	703
Stanley	649
Mattox	608
Miller	536
Wiseman	455
Greenfield	404
Yao	319
Moore	303
Sicard	300

LESSONS LEARNED FROM THE INTERVIEWS

The unique feature of the current interview program is the opportunity to inquire of those who were involved firsthand in the particular historical events. Table 3 shows the historical events of SVS and vascular surgery. The decade of the 1950s is the breakthrough decade with introduction of three signature operations: carotid surgery, femoropopliteal vein bypass, and aortic homograft for aortic aneurysm. The era of direct arterial surgery began with various types of reconstructive arterial surgery. In this era, several vascular societies were established, including the International Society for Cardiovascular Surgery-North American Chapter in the 1950s, the five regional vascular societies in 1977, and the establishment of the American Venous Forum in 1988. The ISCVS-NA became the sister society of SVS and the two societies had a joint council to manage the business and later a professional management firm, Professional Relation Research Institute (PRRI) under Mr. William Maloney, was hired to manage the business affairs of both societies.

In 1996, SVS celebrated its 50th anniversary with two audiovisual interview recordings: William Blaisdell on Dr. DeBakey and Calvin Ernest on Dr. Shumacker. Dr. DeBakey, one of the two survivors of the 31 founders of SVS, stated clearly why the SVS was formed. As DeBakey said, "It was due to the experience of high amputation rate at World War II." DeBakey further emphasized the importance of recognizing vascular surgery as a surgical specialty. In the interview with Harry Shumacker, he told the humorous story of the business transaction of the first meeting.

Another interview highlights the quest of vascular surgical training by a one year fellowship proposed by E.J. Wylie as told by Ron Stoney, a close colleague of Dr. Wylie. The importance of vascular training promoted by the DeWeese committee was described in the interview with Jim Adams. Both these former presidents have changed the training of vascular surgeons forever. The interview with Tom Fogarty on his invention of the catheter embolectomy device is of great interest and, subsequently, the use of the closed endarterectomy device by Cannon and Barker represents the early stage of endovascular technique to treat vascular disease.

In the decade of the 1970s, many vascular surgeons were interested in noninvasive diagnostic tests. Led by the Strandness group from University of Washington

TABLE 3. CHRONOLOGICAL ORDER OF MAJOR EVENTS OF SVS AND VASCULAR SURGERY AFTER THE FOUNDING OF SVS

Year	Event
1946	SVS founded
1947	Thromboendarterectomy by Cid dos Santos
1949	Femoropopliteal vein bypass graft Kunlin
1950s	Establishment of the International Society for Cardiovascular Surgery-North American Chapter
1950–53	Korean War—Arterial repair—Spencer
1952	Renal artery endarterectomy—Freeman Vinyon N prosthetic graft—Voorhees
1953	Aortic homograft for AAA—Dubost Carotid endarterectomy—DeBakey Dacron/Dacron-velour graft—DeBakey
1954	Carotid artery reconstruction—Eastcott, Rob
1955	Endoarterial stripper—Cannon, Barker
1960	Segmental distribution of atherosclerosis—DeBakey
1963	Catheter embolectomy—Fogarty Extra-anatomical bypass—Blaisdell Femoral-tibial-peroneal bypass—Mannick
1967–1970	Doppler flow velocity detector—Strandness *Hemodynamics for Surgeons*—Sumner Ankle systolic pressure and ABI—Yao Fee for service vascular diagnostic laboratory—Darling, Raines, Yao Duplex scan—Strandness
1970	Training and certification in vascular surgery—Wylie, DeWeese
1973	Formation of regional vascular societies begins—Linton, Darling
1977	*Vascular Surgery*—Rutherford
1978	Thoracoabdominal aneurysm—Crawford
1982	Lifeline Foundation—Callow
1983	Certificate of competence in general vascular surgery—Wylie, DeWeese
1984	*Journal of Vascular Surgery*—DeBakey, Ochsner
1988	Research Initiatives meeting—Strandness Critical Issue Forum—Crawford, Ernst American Venous Forum—Bergan
1990	Contribution from von Liebig Foundation in partnership with NHLBI/NIH for K-08 and K-23 awards—Mannick, Clowes, Yao Endovascular graft—Parodi
1996	50th anniversary celebration of SVS—Ernst, Yao
1997	The American Board of Vascular Surgery—Stanley, Veith
2002	Political Action Committee (PAC)—Zwolak
2003	Merger of SVS-AAVS to become SVS—Cronenwett, Riles Electronic media for communication: SVS website (www.vascularweb.org)—Pearce, Johnston Official newspaper (*Vascular Specialist*)—Andros Official newsletter (*Pulse*)

Year	Event
2005	Vascular Surgery Board 0–5 integrated program approved by ACGME SAAAVE Act passed
2010	Collaboration between SVS and Elsevier to publish Rutherford's *Vascular Surgery*, 7th edition, and Rich's *Vascular Trauma*
2011	Vascular Quality Initiative launched SVS PSO (Patient Safety Organization) established Interviews with Pioneers of Vascular Surgery Project—History Project Work Group
2013	New quarterly journal with AVF—*JVS: Venous and Lymphatic Disorders* published in January 2013

Seattle, James Yao of Chicago, and Darling and Raines of Boston, the fee-for-service noninvasive diagnostic laboratory became an important diagnostic service in many hospitals in the United States. Further development of duplex ultrasound by the Seattle group has replaced plethysmography as an important diagnostic tool for many vascular disorders. As a result, the noninvasive technology group has now changed their name to the Society of Vascular Ultrasound. Noninvasive diagnostic testing was invented and developed solely by vascular surgeons.

One of the breakthroughs in operative surgery was the repair of thoracoabdominal aortic aneurysm by Crawford. We regretted that he died before the interview program began. We have interviewed participants of all the important historical events of the 1980s up to the present time. How William Blasdell conceived the idea for the first extra-anatomical bypass was told vividly by Wesley Moore, who participated in the first operation. The accidental discovery of the Gore-Tex graft as told by Ben Eiseman and the first implantation in America of the graft by Roger Gregory were indeed magical moments in vascular surgery.[6–8] In the 1970s, regional surgical societies began to form—New England Society for Vascular Surgery (1973), Southern Association for Vascular Surgery (1976), and Midwestern Vascular Surgical Society (1977) followed by Eastern Vascular Society and Western Vascular Society in 1986. In the decade of the 1980s, the Research Initiatives meeting was founded with NHLBI/NIH and, in 1988, 20 members of SVS founded the American Venous Forum.

The interview with Juan Parodi on the development of the endovascular graft is revealing. It took him nearly 20 years before it became reality. Parodi submitted his report of five patients with endovascular graft to repair the abdominal aneurysm to *Journal of Vascular Surgery (JVS)* and it was rejected (as told by Greg Sicard in his interview). It was John Bergan who recognized the potential of the new technique. Bergan convinced Ramon Buerger, editor of *Annals of Vascular Surgery*, to publish the work by Parodi.[8] The article appeared in *Annals* with a commentary by Bergan and caught the attention of many surgeons, thus starting the endovascular explosion.[9] The endovascular grafting technique changed the training and practice of vascular surgery. Another significant event of this era is the birth of *JVS*. The idea was from Michael DeBakey and John Ochsner, who was the chair of the committee to oversee the negotiation for the journal, gave us an accurate account of the history of the birth of *JVS* in his interview.

In the decades of the 1980s and later, SVS has taken on many duties in addition to the annual meeting. We were able to interview Allen Callow on the formation of the Lifeline Foundation to support research and Julius Jacobson about microvascular surgery as well as philanthropy and support of the research initiatives meeting. John Mannick, James Yao, and Alec Clowes recalled how Lifeline Foundation developed a partnership with the von Liebig Foundation and with NHLBI/NIH. Jack Cronenwett and Tom Riles gave a detailed description of how they shepherded one of our most significant events—the merger of SVS and AAVS.

One of the most contentious issues in the history of SVS is the pursuit of an independent board, the American Board of Vascular Surgery. Interviews with those leaders involved are of great historical interest. There are two views on the specialty board certification. The first one is to work within the ABS in a sub-board structure. This was first suggested by Richard Dean while he served as a director at ABS. The other view is to pursue a new Board of Vascular Surgery within the American Board of Medical Specialties (ABMS). As Jon Towne said, there has been great passion and zeal for each of these plans.[10] For the first time, the cooperative and congenial working relationship within SVS was replaced by combative and argumentative behavior. If you did not agree with those who were for an independent board, you were called a traitor. SVS spent a great deal of resources to pursue the independent board including the hiring of a consultant and renting of an office. On October 6, 1996, the leadership of SVS and ISCVS-NA notified governing agencies of our incorporation of the American Board of Vascular Surgery and our intention to file an application to the Liaison Committee to become a specialty board of the ABMS.[11] Interviews with Frank Veith, Jim Stanley, Pat Clagett, Richard Green, Jack Cronenwett, and Jerry Goldstone provide interesting statements about this endeavor. On June 20, 2001, in a letter to William Pearce and Tom O'Donnell from Wallace P. Ritchie, Executive Director of ABS, it was stated that, after a thorough discussion, the directors voted unanimously *not* to support the development of a separate American Board of Vascular Surgery. Despite this setback, ABS and ABMS made some concessions. First, the Vascular Surgery Board was instituted under the umbrella of ABS with full control, including training and education requirements, by vascular surgeons. Second, the requirements of the general surgery certificate as a requirement to sit for the vascular examination was waived and a 0–5 integrated vascular training program was approved by ABMS and ACGME. Vascular surgery is on its own to train vascular surgeons and to regulate the practice of vascular surgery. Although the application of an independent board failed, the movement for an independent board certainly made an impact on the ABS to make the desired changes. The emergence of the endovascular technique helped the separation of vascular surgery from general surgery as the complexity of endovascular techniques has made it impossible for general surgeons to do the occasional vascular cases.

In recent years, the Political Action Committee (PAC) for lobbying in Washington became an important function of SVS. The PAC deals with government agencies regarding reimbursement and the passage of the laws relating to vascular disease. Recently, the Society has established the Vascular Quality Initiative (VQI), which includes the SVS PSO (Patient Safety Organization) to improve care of patients.

SVS is keeping pace with electronic media for communication. Both Pearce and Johnston helped to install the website. At present, the *Vascular Specialist* is the official newspaper managed by George Andros and the newsletter *Pulse* provides instant electronic communications. The current program on Interviews with Pioneers of Vascular Surgery is an audiovisual recording of interviews to preserve the history of SVS as well as vascular surgery as a specialty. These interviews will be accessible via the website. We will also produce hard copies of DVDs for distribution.

EDUCATIONAL VALUE OF THE INTERVIEWS

The interviews are not to glorify anyone's position but to learn how he or she rose to the position. In our interviews, we ask questions such as mentorship, time management, life balance, issues of women in surgery, how to cope with failures, and, finally, advice for young surgeons. Answers from these 67 accomplished surgeons on these questions are educational and helpful. Nearly everyone agrees there is nothing more important than mentorship even for surgeons like Dr. DeBakey, who often respectfully cited Dr. Alton Ochsner as his mentor. Mentorship is not limited only to teaching surgical skills, it should provide a role model for the younger generation to follow. Quite often young students choose a specialty depending on the conduct of a mentor. As Craig Kent said in his interview, nearly half of the students at University of Wisconsin chose their career based on one mentor. Other often discussed subjects that are equally important are leadership, time management, and the future of vascular surgery—especially the impact of endovascular surgery on training and the practice of vascular surgery.

With the decline in the numbers of open vascular surgery, the concern by most program directors of vascular fellowship training programs is the lack of training for direct open surgery. On the other hand, technology is always getting better and the future may be all endovascular surgery. Dr. Juan Parodi submitted his prediction recently in an article on the 20th anniversary of the endovascular graft for abdominal aortic aneurysm that it is not too far-fetched to envision in the near future a purely percutaneous device that can replace the aortic valve and recreate the entire aorta—from the valve to the iliac bifurcation with branches to critical supra-aortic trunk and visceral arterial structures. Parodi concluded that it is up to the younger generation surgeons to think with no boundaries.[12]

SUMMARY

Vascular surgery began in the 15th century with Ambroise Paré who focused his attention simply on control of bleeding. Since then, vascular surgery has evolved into three distinct eras. The first was the era of INDIRECT SURGERY, which primarily involved vessel ligation and sympathectomy. The second era, DIRECT SURGERY, was a period of reconstructive surgery that was capable of treating most forms of vascular disease, although open exposure was required. In 1990, vascular surgery took a giant step forward with the dawning of the third era, ENDOVASCULAR SURGERY. This minimally invasive catheter-based technology provides new challenges for the younger generation of vascular surgeons. We are in the midst of a technological explosion of endovascular techniques and young surgeons need to lead this revolution and to maintain the position of the vascular surgeon as the icon for treatment of vascular disease.

ACKNOWLEDGMENT

We thank Janet Goldstein for her expert editorial assistance in the preparation of this manuscript.

REFERENCES

1. DeBakey ME, Blaisdell FW. The Society for Vascular Surgery: As I remember—An interview with Dr. Michael E. DeBakey. *J Vasc Surg*. 1996;23:1031–1034.
2. Yao JST, Gregory RT, Rich NM. Interviews with pioneers of vascular surgery. *J Vasc Surg*. 2012;56:e52–57.
3. Yao JST, Gregory RT, Rich NM, et al. Interviews of leaders and contributors in vascular surgery. In: Eskandari MK, Pearce WH, Yao JST, eds. *Current Vascular Surgery 2012*. Shelton, CT: People's Medical Publishing House—USA; 2013:1–8.
4. Dale WA. *Band of Brothers: Creators of Modern Vascular Surgery*. George Johnson and James DeWeese; 1996.
5. Howell JF. Four decades of clinical experience. *Methodist DeBakey Cardiovasc J*. 2011;7:4–18.
6. Yao JST, Eskandari MK. Accidental discovery: The polytetrafluoroethylene graft. *Surgery*. 2011;151:126–128.
7. Gregory RT, Yao JST. The first Gore-Tex femoral-popliteal bypass. *J Vasc Surg*. 2013;58:266–269.
8. Chandler JG. Magical moments in vascular surgery. Presented at the Rocky Mountain Vascular Surgical Society 31st Annual Meeting; July 28–August 1, 2010; Squaw Valley, CA.
9. Parodi JC, Palmaz JC, Barone HD. Transfemoral intraluminal graft implantation for abdominal aortic aneurysms. *Ann Vasc Surg*. 1991;5:491–499.
10. Towne JB. Vascular surgery and the American Board of Surgery: Political reality. *J Vasc Surg*. 2001;33:899–901.
11. Special communication. The American Board of Vascular Surgery: Rationale for its formation. *J Vasc Surg*. 1997;25:411–413
12. Yao JS, Eskandari MK. Transfemoral intraluminal graft implantation for abdominal aortic aneurysms: Two decades later. *Ann Vasc Surg*. 2012;26:895–905.

Cerebrovascular and Supra-Aortic Trunk Disease

1

Cervical Carotid Dissections—Treatment and Outcomes

Rabih A. Chaer, MD

Carotid artery dissection is a relatively uncommon entity that results from either traumatic injury or can be spontaneous without a clear etiology. The incidence in community series ranges from about 2.5 to 3 per 100,000.[1,2] Although carotid dissection accounts for only a small fraction of all cerebrovascular events, it represents a major cause of stroke in young and middle-aged patients, encompassing about 10%–25% of ischemic cerebral events in this subset.[3–6]

Arterial dissection occurs when disruption of the intima allows blood to extravasate between layers of the vessel wall. The resulting intramural hematoma usually extends distally and can lead to acute stenosis or occlusion, and later to aneurysmal change with an associated risk for thromboembolic events. Patients can present with a range of symptoms from being completely asymptomatic to having facial/neck pain, headaches, tinnitus, Horner's syndrome, retinal ischemic events, or even cerebral ischemic symptoms (transient ischemic attacks and stroke).[4,7]

Dissection of the carotid artery is spontaneous or has a precipitating mechanical event (traumatic or iatrogenic). Although each type of dissection is relatively uncommon, both are important clinically because they can be a source of stroke and occur particularly in young people. The purpose of this chapter is to review the pathophysiology of spontaneous and traumatic carotid dissections and the current therapeutic strategies.

SPONTANEOUS CAROTID ARTERY DISSECTION

Spontaneous cervical carotid artery dissection occurs most frequently in the third through the fifth decades of life, and the mean age at diagnosis is 45 years. There is no gender predilection for spontaneous dissection, but women are affected at an average of 5 years younger than men.[4,8]

Spontaneous dissection can occur in any artery but is more likely to occur in the extracranial carotid and vertebral arteries than in other vessels of similar size.

A history of minor trauma is often elicited, but the course is often distinctly different from the clinical events.[8] Chiropractic manipulation has been implicated as an etiology of "spontaneous" dissection of the carotid and vertebral arteries, but a true relationship has not been clearly established.

Atherosclerosis and other known risk factors for peripheral vascular disease are typically absent in patients with spontaneous dissection. These patients do, however, have a higher incidence of hypertension.[9,10] A recent study suggested hypertension and hypercholesterolemia as risk factors in spontaneous carotid dissection, speaking for vascular wall abnormalities as potential contributors to its pathophysiology.

Carotid can present with a variety of symptoms, with a mean time to presentation from onset of symptoms of 7 days, ranging from 0 to 45 days.

The most common initial symptom in patients with spontaneous dissection of the carotid artery is headache, existing in 70% of cervical dissections. Although carotid dissections typically cause ipsilateral, frontotemporal headaches—commonly described as gradual and pulsating—any pattern of headache can occur.[11,12]

Other symptoms can include neck pain, amaurosis fugax, anisocoria, pulsatile tinnitus, and cranial nerve palsy.[4,11] The classic clinical description of patients with spontaneous carotid dissection of ipsilateral head or neck pain, ipsilateral partial Horner's syndrome, and cerebral or retinal ischemia is uncommon.

TRAUMATIC CAROTID ARTERY DISSECTION

Traumatic carotid artery dissection in patients seeking medical care after blunt traumatic injury is rare, but the incidence is higher in patients with specific patterns of injury.[13] After blunt head and neck trauma, the incidence of internal carotid dissection is 0.86%,[14] and patients with head and neck injury and an altered level of consciousness have a reported incidence of carotid injury of up to 3.2%.[15]

Improved imaging modalities and increased awareness of cervical carotid arterial injury may have contributed to an apparent rise in incidence over the past decade. Despite that, it is suggested that cervical carotid artery dissection is underdiagnosed, specifically in patients with severe head and cervical spine injuries.[15,16]

Traumatic cervical carotid artery dissection can occur after blunt or penetrating trauma, and both direct and indirect forces contribute to injury. The most common mechanism of injury is extreme cervical hyperextension or lateral hyperflexion associated with severe blunt head and neck trauma caused by a motor vehicle collision.[13,14]

The clinical manifestations are similar to those seen with spontaneous dissection and can range from no symptoms to lateralizing symptoms appearing either acutely or in delayed fashion.[13,15] Symptoms include head and neck pain, hemiparesis, hemiplegia, dysphasia, aphasia, Horner's syndrome, transient ischemic attack, and stroke, and these have all been described as initial symptoms of traumatic cervical carotid artery dissection.

DIAGNOSTIC MODALITIES

The diagnosis is frequently made with a definitive imaging study: duplex (Fig. 1-1), magnetic resonance angiography (MRA), computed tomography angiography (CTA), or angiography (Fig. 1-2).

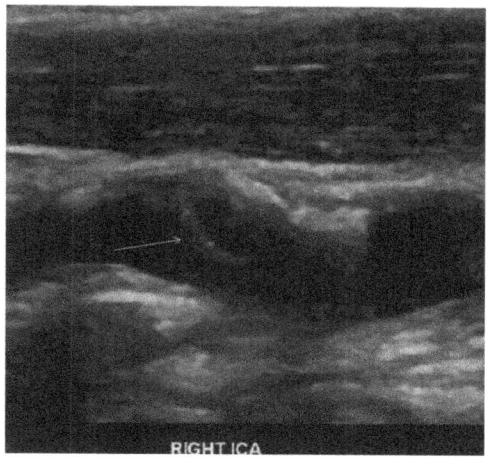

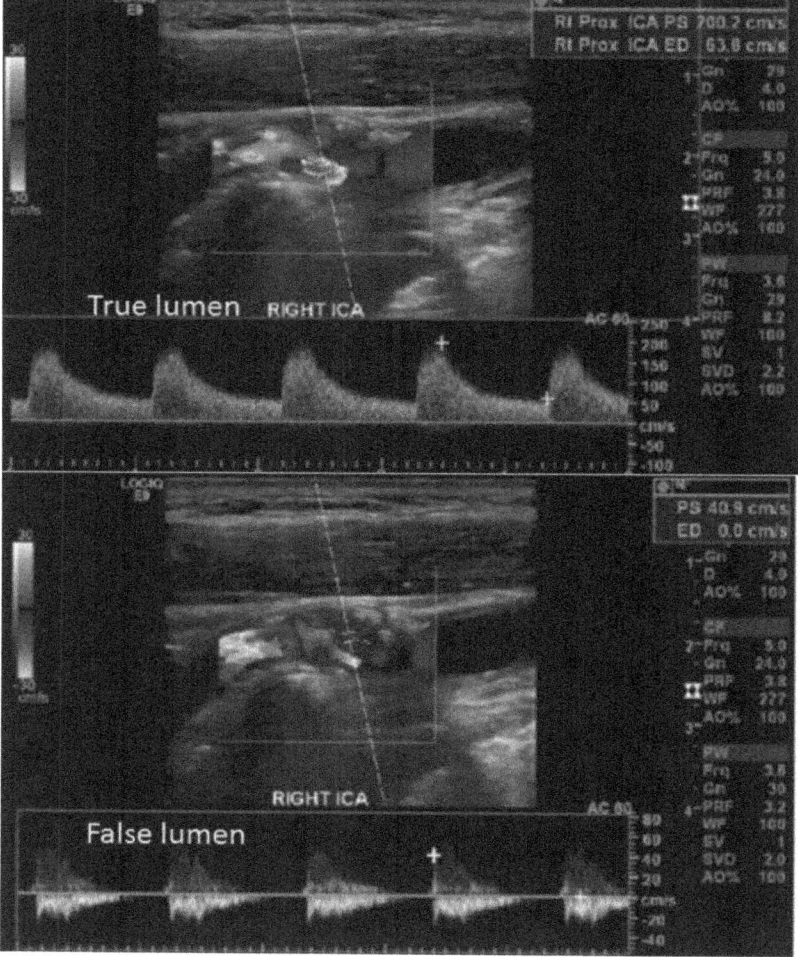

Figure 1-1. *A*, B mode duplex image of the right ICA showing a dissection flap (arrow). *B*, Color flow duplex imaging showing a moderate stenosis resulting from the dissection flap in the true lumen.

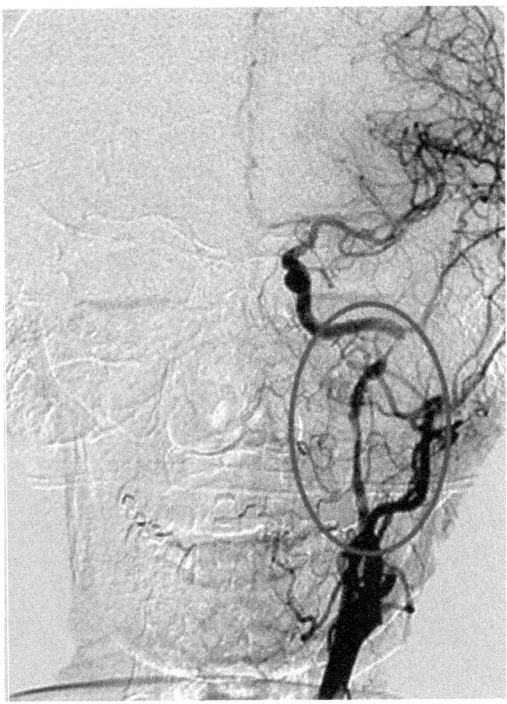

Figure 1-2. Selective carotid angiogram showing a dissection of the internal carotid artery beyond its origin. The classic long tapered stenosis of the extracranial portion of the ICA is noted, with restoration of a normal flow channel distally.

CTA and MRA are particularly attractive for diagnosis because their resolution approaches that of conventional angiography in detecting direct signs of vascular injury, such as irregular vessel margins, filling defects, changes in caliber, extravasation of contrast material, and occlusion,[17] and they are superior to angiography for evaluation of intramural hematoma and injury to surrounding structures. Recent studies show 97.7% sensitivity and 100% specificity for 16-slice CTA in the diagnosis of blunt carotid and vertebral artery injuries.[18] These results suggest that CTA is a reliable, safe, fast, and cost-effective means of diagnosing cerebral artery dissections.

Although MRA and duplex ultrasound can also be utilized to make the diagnosis of carotid dissection, they have few limitations.

Disadvantages of MRA are lack of availability, longer time required for imaging, and interference from extrinsic structures such as external cervical fixation devices. Ultrasound has several disadvantages as well, which have to be weighed against some of its advantages such as accessibility, convenience, and the ability to monitor disease progression and resolution over time. Limitations include operator dependence and the inability to reliably visualize the distal internal carotid and the extent of the dissection.

NATURAL HISTORY

It is important to understand the natural history of carotid dissection, as this may impact decision making and management. Cerebral infarction is documented in 42% of spontaneous carotid dissections, and 58% of patients have persistent neurologic deficits.[11]

The prognosis is worse for traumatic carotid dissection, and studies of blunt traumatic carotid injury report mortality rates of up to 30%. Patients with traumatic dissection are more likely to develop aneurysms and progress to occlusion and are less likely to show improvement or resolution of aneurysms and stenoses than are patients with spontaneous dissection.[19,20] In addition, the prognosis after stroke caused by dissection is worse than the prognosis after stroke caused by atherosclerosis. Dissection patients seem to have more global middle cerebral artery involvement and severe clinical impairment.

In addition, in patients with spontaneous dissection managed medically, the incidence of recurrent dissection is 0.3%–1.4%, and recurrent dissection is more frequent in the first month and more common in patients with connective tissue disease or with a family history of cervical carotid artery dissection. The annual risk of recurrent stroke ranges from 0.3% to 3.4%.[19,20]

Although dissection is the most common cause of extracranial internal carotid aneurysm, two thirds of carotid aneurysms resolve, and complications related to aneurysm are rare.[19,20]

THE UPMC EXPERIENCE

In a recent series of 29 patients with carotid dissection (75% spontaneous), complete luminal recovery was seen in 10 patients (53%), 10% residual stenosis in 5 patients (26%), partial recanalization in 3 patients (16%), and only 1 patient with persistent occlusion. In all, 15 (79%) patients demonstrated either complete luminal recovery or minimal persistent stenosis (Fig. 1-3). Of the four patients with persistent significant stenosis on follow-up imaging, three had near complete resolution of symptoms, while the fourth patient had progression of stenosis and developed recurrent stroke-like symptoms. The mean time to complete or near-complete anatomic resolution was 11.2 months. Two patients developed asymptomatic aneurysms that were conservatively managed.[21]

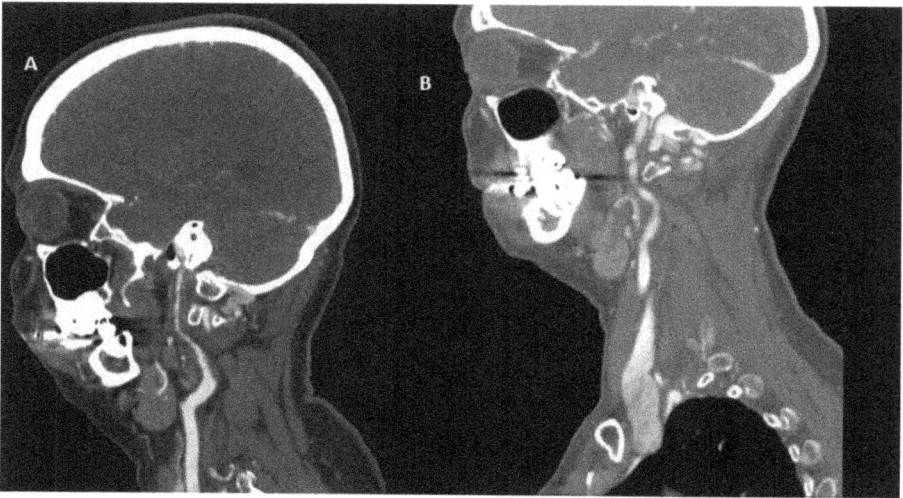

Figure 1-3. *A*, CT scan of a 48-year-old healthy female who presented with a four day history of left-sided headache. A classic tapering stenosis of the left cervical ICA with restoration of normal flow lumen in the intracranial portion of the artery is noted. *B*, Six-month follow-up CT demonstrates complete resolution of the dissection/stenosis with restoration of a normal flow channel with anticoagulation therapy.

Our data confirm that most cervical carotid dissections can safely be conservatively managed, with the majority achieving anatomic and symptomatic resolution, with low rates of recurrence over long-term follow-up. These findings seem to suggest that a conservative approach in warranted for at least one year prior to addressing any persistent asymptomatic carotid stenosis as a result of a dissection.

TREATMENT

Medical Therapy

Carotid artery dissection is thought to cause stroke as a result of flow limitation or embolism from the site of the intimal tear. Microemboli have been detected acutely after dissection and correlate with the presence of stroke in patients with spontaneous and traumatic dissections. Because of these factors, antithrombotic therapy has become the mainstay of medical treatment of carotid artery dissection. Concerns regarding anticoagulation include possible worsening of intramural bleeding at the site of dissection, bleeding from associated injuries in the case of trauma, and bleeding from unrelated sources. A Cochrane Database Systematic Review in 2003 unfortunately found no randomized trials that compared antiplatelet drugs with anticoagulants or either type of agent with controls for the treatment of dissection. Although nonrandomized studies do not show a difference in mortality between patients receiving antiplatelet medications and patients receiving anticoagulation, the intracranial hemorrhage rate of anticoagulated patients is 0.5%, as opposed to 0% in those receiving antiplatelet medications alone.[22]

More recently, the Cervical Artery Dissection in Stroke Study (CADISS) trial was designed to be a prospective multicenter randomized-controlled trial in acute (within seven days of onset) carotid and vertebral artery dissection. Intracerebral artery dissection was excluded. Patients were randomized to antiplatelet therapy (aspirin, dipyridamole, or clopidogrel alone or in dual combination) or anticoagulation therapy (heparin followed by warfarin aiming for an international normalized ratio ranging from 2 to 3) for at least three months. The primary endpoint was ipsilateral stroke or death within three months of randomization, and secondary endpoints included any transient ischemic attack or stroke, major bleeding, and residual stenosis.[23]

The results of the nonrandomized arm of the CADISS-NR trial, along with a meta-analysis of these results with previously published studies comparing the two therapeutic strategies, were published recently. A total of 88 patients from 22 centers with extracranial carotid and vertebral dissection were recruited within 1 month of symptom onset.[24] At the primary endpoint of three months, three (5.08%) patients treated with antiplatelet had recurrent transient ischemic attack (TIA), compared with none in the anticoagulation group. For meta-analysis, there were data from 40 nonrandomized studies including 1636 patients. There was no significant difference between the two treatments in recurrent stroke risk or risk of death. These data suggested no superiority of anticoagulation or antiplatelet therapy in prevention of stoke after carotid and vertebral artery dissection.

Surgical Treatment

Acute indications for surgical treatment of acute carotid artery dissection are fluctuating or deteriorating clinical neurologic symptoms despite medical treatment, compromised cerebral blood flow, contraindications to antithrombotic therapy, and a symptomatic or expanding aneurysm.[7,12] Delayed indications for surgery after initial medical treatment are persistent high-grade stenosis and a new or persistent carotid aneurysm. Aneurysms rarely enlarge or rupture but may be a source of distal thromboembolization.[25]

Exposure of the internal carotid artery for treatment of dissection is more difficult than exposure for atherosclerotic disease because lesions are more distal. Once exposure is obtained, surgical options include carotid ligation, interposition saphenous vein graft to a cervical or intracranial segment, and patch angioplasty.

Postoperative complications are common after surgery for carotid dissection and include death, ipsilateral stroke in 8%, carotid occlusion, and cranial nerve dysfunction.[25]

Endovascular Therapy

Two trials have compared intravenous thrombolysis and stent-assisted intraarterial thrombolysis for symptomatic middle cerebral artery occlusion secondary to carotid dissection. The larger series ($N = 18$) showed no difference between the groups at three months, and the smaller series ($N = 10$) showed a better outcome at three months with endovascular treatment.[26,27] The authors of both papers agree that larger randomized controlled trials are needed.

Endovascular treatment is increasingly being applied to a number of acute cerebrovascular conditions, including stroke secondary to atherosclerosis or dissection.[27] Endovascular treatment of spontaneous and traumatic cervical carotid artery dissection has been addressed by multiple case reports, documenting encouraging outcomes in a handful of patients with stenting.[28,29]

Given the morbidity and mortality associated with surgical repair, endovascular treatment of carotid dissection seems appropriate if indicated in the setting of failure of medical therapy. A recent systematic review confirmed the safety and technical feasibility of stenting of carotid dissection in the setting of failed medical management, stroke, hemodynamic instability, or pseudoaneurysm formation. No distal protection devices were used in any of the studies reviewed. The technical success rate was 99%, with a 1.3% procedural complication rate.[30]

However, given the high rate of spontaneous clinical and angiographic resolution with medical management alone,[21] prospective randomized trials comparing stenting with medical management are needed to further elucidate the role and indications for stenting.

Treatment Selection

While the best treatment modality remains to be elucidated by large randomized trials, most patients can be safely treated with either anticoagulation or antiplatelet therapy and have good clinical and anatomic outcomes over long-term follow-up.

Surgical outcomes, including carotid ligation, have been inferior to conservative management with unacceptably high rates of stroke and cranial nerve injury.[25] Thus, surgery should be limited to those cases with progression of symptoms in anatomically accessible lesions.

Endovascular interventions represent an attractive minimally invasive alternative, with potentially less cranial nerve injury compared with surgery. Although early data suggest that they are indeed safe,[30] they also pose potential hazards, including stroke and perforation in these thin-walled acutely dissected arteries, with unproven long-term benefit.

Thus, larger series and longer term follow-up are needed to determine whether such interventions provide low risk-to-benefit ratio compared with conservative medical management alone.

REFERENCES

1. Schievink WI, Mokri B, Whisnant JP. Internal carotid artery dissection in a community: Rochester, Minnesota, 1987–1992. *Stroke*. 1993;24:1678–1680.
2. Giroud M, Fayolle H, Andre N, et al. Incidence of internal carotid artery dissections in the community of Dijon. *J Neurol Neurosurg Psychiatry*. 1994;330:393–397.
3. Mokri B, Sundt TM Jr, Houser OW. Spontaneous internal carotid dissection, hemicrania, and Horner's syndrome. *Arch Neurol*. 1979;36:677–680.
4. Schievink WI. Spontaneous dissection of the carotid and vertebral arteries. *N Engl J Med*. 2001;344:898–906.
5. Rouhart F, Zagnoli F, Goas JY, Mocquard Y. [Cerebral ischemic arterial accidents in young adults. 40 cases]. *Rev Neurol (Paris)*. 1993;149:547–553.
6. Leys D, Bandu L, Hénon H, et al. Clinical outcome in 287 consecutive young adults (15 to 45 years) with ischemic stroke. *Neurology*. 2002;59:26–33.
7. Debette S, Leys D. Cervical-artery dissections: predisposing factors, diagnosis, and outcomes. *Lancet Neurol*. 2009;8:668–678.
8. Schievink WI, Mokri B, O'Fallon WM. Recurrent spontaneous cervical-artery dissection. *N Engl J Med*. 1994;330:393–397.
9. Pezzini A, Caso V, Zanferrari C, et al. Arterial hypertension as risk factor for spontaneous cervical artery dissection. A case-control study. *J Neurol Neurosurg Psychiatry*. 2006;77:95–97.
10. Mokri B, Piepgras DG, Wiebers DO, Houser OW. Familial occurrence of spontaneous dissection of the internal carotid artery. *Stroke*. 1987;18:246–251.
11. Chandra A, Suliman A, Angle N. Spontaneous dissection of the carotid and vertebral arteries: the 10-year UCSD experience. *Ann Vasc Surg*. 2007;21:178–185.
12. Baumgartner RW, Bogousslavsky J. Clinical manifestations of carotid dissection. *Front Neurol Neurosci*. 2005;20:70–76.
13. Laitt RD, Lewis TT, Bradshaw JR. Blunt carotid arterial trauma. *Clin Radiol*. 1996;51:117–122.
14. Nedeltchev K, Baumgartner RW. Traumatic cervical artery dissection. *Front Neurol Neurosci*. 2005;20:54–63.
15. Hughes KM, Collier B, Greene KA, Kurek S. Traumatic carotid artery dissection: a significant incidental finding. *Am Surg*. 2000;66:1023–1027.
16. Rommel O, Niedeggen A, Tegenthoff M, et al. Carotid and vertebral artery injury following severe head or cervical spine trauma. *Cerebrovasc Dis*. 1999;9:202–209.
17. Stallmeyer MJ, Morales RE, Flanders AE. Imaging of traumatic neurovascular injury. *Radiol Clin North Am*. 2006;44:13–39, vii.
18. Eastman AL, Chason DP, Perez CL, et al. Computed tomographic angiography for the diagnosis of blunt cervical vascular injury: is it ready for primetime? *J Trauma*. 2006;60:925–929; discussion 929.
19. Touze E, Gauvrit JY, Meder JF, Mas JL. Prognosis of cervical artery dissection. *Front Neurol Neurosci*. 2005;20:129–139.
20. Mokri B. Traumatic and spontaneous extracranial internal carotid artery dissections. *J Neurol*. 1990;237:356–361.
21. Rao AS, Makaroun MS, Marone LK, et al. Long-term outcomes of internal carotid artery dissection. *J Vasc Surg*. 2011;54(2):370–374; discussion 375.
22. Lyrer P, Engelter S. Antithrombotic drugs for carotid artery dissection. *Cochrane Database Syst Rev*. 2003;000255.

23. Cervical Artery Dissection in Stroke Study Trial Investigators. Antiplatelet therapy vs. anticoagulation in cervical artery dissection: rationale and design of the Cervical Artery Dissection in Stroke Study (CADISS). *Int J Stroke*. 2007;2:292–296.
24. Kennedy F, Lanfranconi S, Hicks C, et al. Antiplatelets vs anticoagulation for dissection: CADISS nonrandomized arm and meta-analysis. *Neurology*. 2012;79(7):686–689.
25. Schievink WI, Piepgras DG, McCaffrey TV, Mokri B. Surgical treatment of extracranial internal carotid artery dissecting aneurysms. *Neurosurgery*. 1994;35:809–815; discussion 815–816.
26. Lavallee PC, Mazighi M, Saint-Maurice JP, et al. Stent-assisted endovascular thrombolysis versus intravenous thrombolysis in internal carotid artery dissection with tandem internal carotid and middle cerebral artery occlusion. *Stroke*. 2007;38:2270–2274.
27. Nikas D, Reimers B, Elisabetta M, et al. Percutaneous interventions in patients with acute ischemic stroke related to obstructive atherosclerotic disease or dissection of the extracranial carotid artery. *J Endovasc Ther*. 2007;14:279–288.
28. Lin PH, Bush RL, Lumsden AB. Endovascular treatment for symptomatic carotid artery dissection. *J Vasc Surg*. 2005;41:555.
29. Chaer RA, DeRubertis B, Kent KC, McKinsey JF. Endovascular treatment of traumatic carotid pseudoaneurysm with stenting and coil embolization. *Ann Vasc Surg*. 2008;22(4):564–567.
30. Malek AM, Higashida RT, Phatouros CC, et al. Endovascular management of extracranial carotid artery dissection achieved using stent angioplasty. *AJNR Am J Neuroradiol*. 2000;21:1280–1292.

2

Anatomic Risk Factors for Carotid Stenting

Courtney M. Daly, MD and Melina R. Kibbe, MD

INTRODUCTION

Stroke is the fourth leading cause of death in the United States.[1] It is also the number one cause of longer term disability. Eighty-seven percent of these strokes are ischemic in nature, and 13%–32% of these are attributable to large vessel atherosclerosis and stenosis.[2,3] Carotid artery stenting has been shown to reduce the risk of stroke from carotid artery disease. However, the perioperative risk of stroke associated with carotid artery stenting remains a challenge. Determining risk factors for procedure-related stroke may help identify patients who are better suited for carotid artery stenting. The purpose of this chapter is to review the literature regarding the association between patient anatomy, plaque characterics, age, and sex and the risk of stroke following carotid artery stenting. We also describe the relationship between these factors and the risk of stroke in our patient population. Knowledge of how these anatomic variables effect stroke risk following intervention may have implications for patient selection and the evolution of carotid artery stenting technology in the future.

ARCH ANATOMY

Arch Type

Aortic arch type is defined by the location of the target vessel along the aortic arch (Figure 2-1). A type I arch is defined by the target vessel arising from the superior or cranial aspect of the outer curvature of the aortic arch. A type II arch is defined as the target vessel arising between the parallel lines tangent to the outer and inner curvature of the arch. A type III arch is defined as the target vessel arising inferior or caudal to the lesser curvature of the arch. Higher arch types theoretically are more difficult due to the angle of take-off of the target artery from the arch and may involve additional catheter manipulation to cannulate the target vessel.

In our review of the literature (Table 2-1), there were two studies that found arch type to be a risk factor for stroke. Wimmer et al., using the Stenting and Angioplasty With Protection in Patients at High-Risk for Endarterectomy (SAPPHIRE) patient population, found the presence of type II or type III arches to be predictors of stroke with carotid stenting.[4] Werner et al. showed that bovine arch is associated with higher stroke and transient ischemic attack (TIA).[5] However, three other studies did not find arch type to be a risk factor for perioperative stroke.[6–8]

Arch Calcification

Manipulation of catheters in a calcified aortic arch has the potential to dislodge micro- or macroparticles potentially embolizing to any arch vessel, creating a theoretical risk for bilateral stroke during target vessel cannulation. Surprisingly, none of the studies in our literature review demonstrated an increased risk of stroke or TIA with increasing arch calcification. Figure 2-2 demonstrates aortic arch calcification ranging from mild to severe.

Ostial Lesions

Ostial lesions involve disease at the take-off of the target artery from the aortic arch and again would be expected to increase the risk of stroke through manipulation of wires or catheters during cannulation of the target vessel. Sayeed et al. did demonstrate an increased risk of stroke in patients with ostial centered lesions,[8] but no other studies found this to be a risk factor.

Sidedness

Right- and left-sided cannulations can carry different risks. To cannulate the right carotid artery requires passing an angled catheter past both the left carotid and subclavian arteries, potentially increasing the risk of a contralateral stroke. It also involves additional manipulation of the innominate artery to gain access to the right common carotid artery. To further address this concern, Naggara et al. demonstrated an increased risk of stroke with left-sided interventions, while Wimmer et al. demonstrated an increased risk of stroke with right-sided lesions.[4,6,7]

CAROTID ARTERY ANATOMY

Common Carotid Artery Tortuosity

Passing a wire along a tortuous common carotid artery may be more likely to contact the wall and increase the risk of embolization (Figure 2-3A). Faggioli et al. demonstrated that a tortuous common carotid artery leads to an increased risk of stroke defined by diffusion-weighted magnetic resonance imaging (MRI) following carotid artery stenting.[7] Wimmer et al. and Werner et al. also demonstrated that a tortuous common carotid arterial system was associated with an increased risk of stroke or TIA.[4,5]

Internal Carotid Artery/Common Carotid Artery Angulation

Greater angulation of the internal carotid artery from the common carotid artery may increase the difficulty of passing a wire and catheter across the lesion (Figure 2-3B).

Naggara et al. demonstrated an increased risk of stroke with internal/common carotid artery angulation >60°,[6] and Werner et al. demonstrated an increased risk of stroke with an angulated distal internal carotid artery.[5]

Internal Carotid Artery Stenosis

Lesions with a higher degree of stenosis would be expected to contribute to perioperative stroke risk because there is less space between which to pass the wire and distal protection device, increasing the odds for embolization. However, surprisingly, none of the published studies mentioned found an association between degree of stenosis and perioperative risk of stroke.

Lesion Length

Longer carotid lesions may require additional angioplasty and stent placement to fully treat and cover the lesion. Longer lesions also involve additional surface area to traverse with wires and catheters and can increase difficulty of placing a distal filter in the event of a particularly long lesion. Naggara et al. demonstrated an increased risk of stroke with lesions >1 cm,[6] and Sayeed et al. demonstrated an increased risk with lesions >15 mm.[8]

External Carotid Artery Stenosis

While passing a wire into a stenotic external carotid artery for stabilization could theoretically increase the risk of stroke by dislodging emboli, none of the studies reviewed found external carotid artery stenosis to be a risk factor for perioperative stroke risk.

Plaque Characteristics

An ulcerated plaque with a soft necrotic core may lead to increased embolization while crossing the lesion and placing a stent. Kastrup et al. demonstrated that an ulcerated plaque was an independent risk factor for new diffusion-weighted MRI lesions following carotid artery stenting.[9]

AGE

Several studies have evaluated anatomic risk factors as it relates to age, and whether these risk factors increase stroke rates in older patients.[10,11] Bazan et al. demonstrated that patients older than 75 years had more arch calcification as well as increased number of type II versus type I aortic arches.[12] Werner et al. demonstrated that octogenarians had a four times higher risk of stroke and death with carotid artery stenting.[5] Kastrup et al. demonstrated that octogenarians had a higher incidence of severe arch calcification and ulcerated stenosis.[9] However, there was no difference in arch elongation, common carotid artery or internal carotid artery tortuosity, degree of stenosis, or lesion length. They found that octogenarians had an increased number of lesions on diffusion-weighted MRI, both within the vascular territory of the carotid artery stenosis and the total number of lesions. Ulcerated lesions were associated with increased diffusion-weighted MRI lesions in the same vascular territory, and severe arch calcification tended to be associated with new lesions outside of the vascular territory of the treated artery.[9]

SEX

Differences between men and women with respect to carotid artery disease have been demonstrated in multiple studies. Li et al. demonstrated a difference in carotid plaques by B-mode ultrasonography, where men had increased acoustic shadowing suggesting a more complex atherosclerotic plaque than women.[13] de Weerd et al. demonstrated that men presented with increased severity of carotid artery stenosis at older ages compared with women.[14] den Hartog et al. demonstrated that women had smaller carotid arteries with increased rates of restenosis following intervention.[15]

With respect to carotid artery intervention outcomes, comparisons between men and women have yielded mixed results. In the asymptomatic carotid artery stenosis (ACAS), women were found to have higher perioperative complications compared to men. Both the ACAS and Asymptomatic Carotid Surgery Trial (ACST) demonstrated less risk reduction with carotid artery intervention in women compared to men.[16–18] In addition, Ballotta et al. demonstrated higher rates of late occlusive events in women, but these were not clinically significant.[19] With respect to carotid artery stenting, the Carotid Revascularization Endarterectomy versus Stenting Trial (CREST) lead-in phase demonstrated similar rates of 30-day stroke and death between men

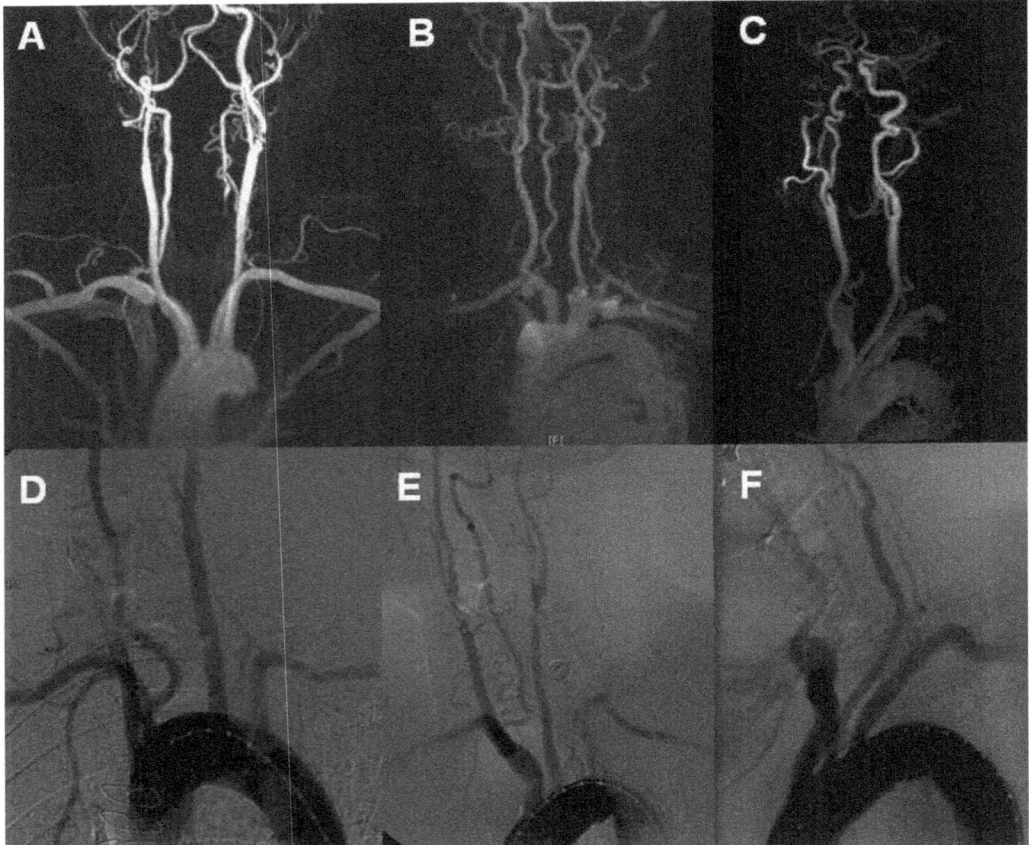

Figure 2-1. Images of the aortic arch from MRA (top row) and digital subtraction angiography (bottom row). *A* and *D*, Type I arch, *B* and *E*, type II arch, and *C* and *F*, type III arch.

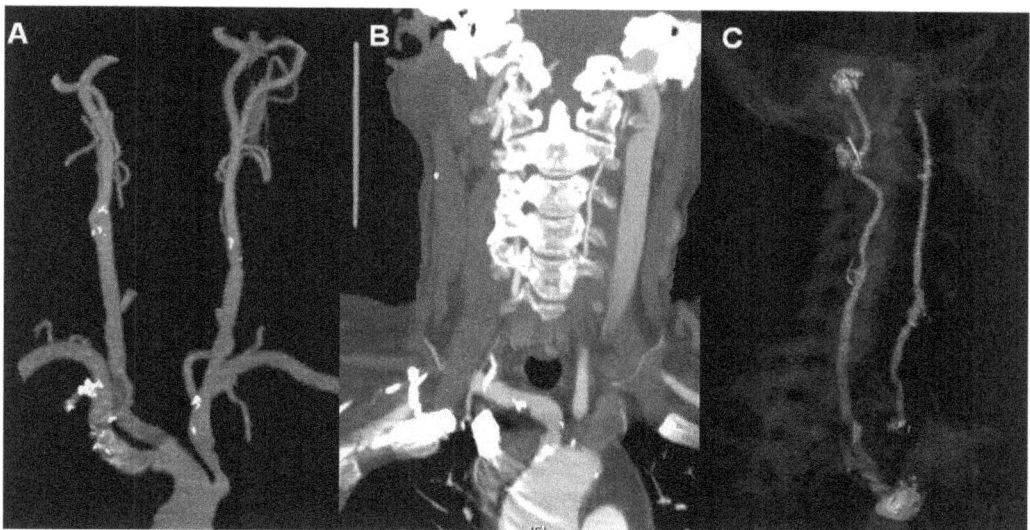

Figure 2-2. Images of the aortic arch from CTA. *A*, Mild arch calcification; *B*, moderate arch calcification; and *C*, severe arch calcification.

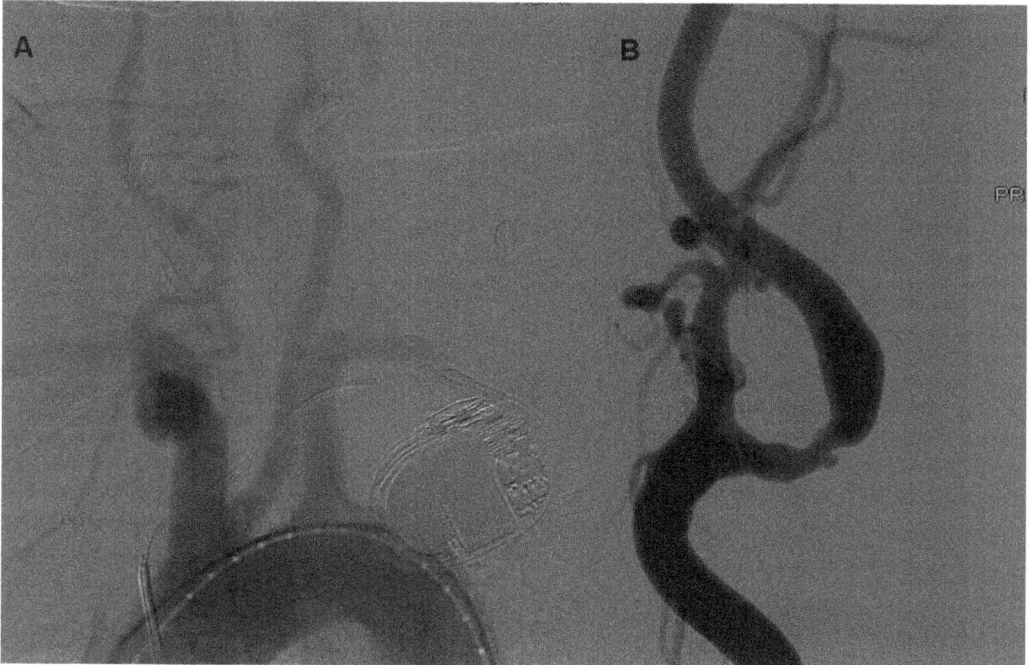

Figure 2-3. Images the common and internal carotid artery by digital subtraction angiography. *A*, Tortuous common carotid artery; *B*, severe internal carotid artery to common carotid artery angulation.

and women,[20] and Goldstein et al. demonstrated similar perioperative stroke and death, stroke-free survival, and restenosis between the sexes, although women tended toward a larger internal-to-common carotid artery diameter ratio, and had more plaques isolated to the common carotid artery.[21]

TABLE 2-1. SUMMARY OF THE LITERATURE ON ANATOMIC RISK FACTORS

Study	Patient Population	Anatomic Risk Factors
Naggara et al.[6]	EVA3S Symptomatic	ICA/CCA angulation >60 Length >1 cm Left-sided lesions
Faggioli et al.[7]	Asymptomatic, lesions detected by diffusion-weighted MRI	Complicated aortic plaque CCA tortuosity
Wimmer et al.[4]	SAPPHIRE (symptomatic or asymptomatic with one high-risk variable)	Right-sided lesions, longer carotid plaque, type II or type III arch, tortuous carotid arterial system
Werner et al.[5]	All comers	Bovine arch, tortuous CCA, angulated distal ICA
Sayeed et al.[8]	All comers	Lesion >15 mm, ostial centered lesions

Abbreviations: ICA, internal carotid artery; CCA, common carotid artery; MRI, magnetic resonance imaging; EVA3S, Endarterectomy Versus Angioplasty in Patients With Symptomatic Severe Carotid Stenosis Trial; SAPPHIRE, Stenting and Angioplasty With Protection in Patients at High-Risk for Endarterectomy.

OUR DATA

We recently conducted a retrospective review of a prospectively maintained database of our patients undergoing carotid artery stenting. Our goal was to determine whether anatomic characteristics, including arch type (I, II, and III), aortic arch calcification, ostial lesions, common carotid artery tortuosity, internal-to-common carotid artery angulation, external carotid artery stenosis, degree of internal carotid artery stenosis, tandem lesions, and contralateral internal carotid artery occlusion, or plaque characteristics, predicted perioperative outcomes. Our primary outcome was defined as 30-day stroke or TIA, and secondary outcome was defined as 30-day death, myocardial infarction (MI), or any stent fracture or in stent restenosis. We also compared anatomic characteristics to age and sex. In our patient population of 375 patients with 381 carotid arteries studies, we found that a higher degree of internal carotid artery stenosis was associated with an increased risk of perioperative stroke or TIA, and that patients with these events trended toward an increase in aortic arch calcification. We also found that patients who died within 30 days trended toward an increase in common carotid artery tortuosity, and patients who developed subsequent in-stent restenosis had a decreased internal-to-carotid artery angulation compared with patients who had no restenosis. Surprisingly, we found that arch type, ostial involvement, tandem lesions, and plaque calcification did not correlate with primary outcomes. When comparing anatomic characteristics to sex, we found that women had an increased common carotid artery tortuosity compared with men, and had a trend towards both increased plaque calcification as well as increased aortic arch calcification compared with men. When comparing anatomic characteristic with age, we found that octogenarians had a trend toward increased common carotid artery tortuosity as well as a decreased internal-to-common carotid artery angulation compared with younger patients. Regarding the secondary outcome, there was a trend towards decreased plaque ulceration in patients with in-stent restenosis. Together, our data suggest that degree of internal carotid artery stenosis and aortic arch calcification may be associated with an increased perioperative neurologic risk during carotid stenting, but surprisingly, arch type is not.

SUMMARY/CONCLUSION

These studies demonstrate that anatomic variables likely do contribute to stroke risk associated with carotid stenting. Although there is not a clear trend from the published literature, many of the studies suffer from small numbers, and more significant data may become apparent with larger studies. Risk factors consistent across several studies included tortuosity of the carotid artery, angulation between the internal and common carotid artery, and longer lesions. In short, anatomic risk factors should be a consideration when planning a carotid intervention for each patient.

REFERENCES

1. Minino AM, Murphy SL, Xu J, Kochanek KD. Deaths: final data for 2008. *Natl Vital Stat Rep.* 2011;59(10):1–127. cdc.gov
2. Petty GW, Brown RD, Whisnant JP, et al. Ischemic stroke subtypes: a population-based study of incidence and risk factors. *Stroke.* 1999;30:2513–2516.
3. Kirshner HS. Differentiating ischemic stroke subtypes: risk factors and secondary prevention. *J Neurol Sci.* 2009;279:1–8.
4. Wimmer NJ, Yeh RW, Cutlip DE, Mauri L. Risk prediction for adverse events after carotid artery stenting in higher risk surgical patients. *Stroke.* 2012;43(12):3218–3224.
5. Werner M, Bausback Y, Braunlich S, et al. Anatomic variables contributing to higher peri-procedural incidence of stroke and TIA in carotid artery stenting: single center experience of 833 consecutive cases. *Catheter Cardiovasc Interv.* 2012;80(2):321–328.
6. Naggara O, Touze E, Beyssen B, et al. Anatomical and technical factors associated with stroke or death during carotid angioplasty and stenting: results from the Endarterectomy Versus Angioplasty in patients with symptomatic severe carotid stenosis (EVA-3S) Trial and systematic review. *Stroke.* 2011;42:380–388.
7. Faggoli G, Ferri M, Rapezzi C, et al. Atherosclerotic aortic lesions increase the risk of cerebral embolism during carotid stenting in patients with complex aortic arch anatomy. *J Vasc Surg.* 2009;49:80–85.
8. Sayeed S, Stanziale SF, Wholey MH, Makaroun MS. Angiographic lesion characteristics can predict adverse outcomes after carotid artery stenting. *J Vasc Surg.* 2008;47(1):81–87.
9. Kastrup A, Groschel K, Schnaudigel S, et al. Target lesion ulceration and arch calcification are associated with increased incidence of carotid stenting-associated ischemic lesions in octogenarians. *J Vasc Surg.* 2008;47(1):88–95.
10. Hobson RW II, Howard VJ, Roubin GS, et al. Carotid artery stenting is associated with increased complications in octogenarians: 30 day stroke and death rates in the CREST lead-in phase. *J Vasc Surg.* 2004;40:1106–1111.
11. van Lammeren GW, Reichman BL, Moll FL, et al. Atherosclerotic plaque vulnerability as an explanation for the increased risk of stroke in elderly patients undergoing carotid artery stenting. *Stroke.* 2011;42(9):2550–2555.
12. Bazan H, Pradhan S, Mojibian H, et al. Increased aortic arch calcification in patients older than 75 years: implications for carotid artery stenting in elderly patients. *J Vasc Surg.* 2007;46:841–845.
13. Li R, Duncan BB, Metcalf PA, et al. B-mode-detected carotid artery plaque in a general population. Atherosclerosis risk in communities (ARIC) study investigators. *Stroke.* 1994;25:2377–2383.
14. de Weerd M, Greving JP, Hedblad B, et al. Prevalence of asymptomatic carotid artery stenosis in the general population: an individual participant data meta-analysis. *Stroke.* 2010;41:1294–1297.

15. den Hartog AG, Algra A, Moll FL, de Borst GJ. Mechanisms of gender-related outcome differences after carotid endarterectomy. *J Vasc Surg*. 2010;52:1062–1071.
16. Walker MD, Marler JR, Goldstein M, et al. Endarterectomy for asymptomatic carotid artery stenosis. *JAMA*. 1995;273(18):1421–1424.
17. Halliday A, Mansfield A, Marro J, et al. Prevention of disabling and fatal strokes by successful carotid endarterectomy in patients without recent neurological symptoms: randomized controlled trial. *Lancet*. 2004;363:1491–1502.
18. Ballotta E, Renon L, Da Giau G, et al. Carotid endarterectomy in women: early and long-term results. *Surgery*. 2000;127(3):264–271.
19. Howard VJ, Voeks JH, Lutsep HL, et al. Does sex matter? Thirty-day stroke and death rates after carotid artery stenting in women versus men: results from the Carotid Revascularization Endarterectomy versus Stenting Trial (CREST) lead-in phase. *Stroke*. 2009;40:1140–1147.
20. Goldstein LJ, Kahn HU, Sambol EB, et al. Carotid stenting is safe and associated with comparable outcomes in men and women. *J Vasc Surg*. 2009;49(2):315–323.
21. Halliday A, Mansfield A, Marro J, et al. Prevention of disabling and fatal strokes by successful carotid endarterectomy in patients without recent neurological symptoms: randomized controlled trial. MRC Asymptomatic Carotid Surgery Trial (ACST) collaborative group. *Lancet*. 2004;363(9420):1491–502.

3

Restenosis Rates after CEA versus CAS: Analysis of the CREST Data

Brajesh K. Lal, MD

INTRODUCTION

Carotid endarterectomy (CEA) is the preferred treatment for symptomatic[1-3] and asymptomatic[4,5] patients with high-grade extracranial carotid stenosis compared to best medical therapy. The subsequent increase in the number of CEAs performed worldwide has resulted in a number of post-CEA carotid restenosis cases. Carotid artery stenting (CAS) has recently emerged as a less invasive alternative to CEA for cerebral revascularization. Our institution,[6-10] along with others,[11-14] has demonstrated that CAS is technically feasible and safe in high-risk patients. In the Carotid Revascularization Endarterectomy versus Stenting Trial (CREST), no difference was found between CAS and CEA for the composite endpoint of stroke, myocardial infarction, or death. A secondary analysis found that stroke occurred more frequently after CAS, while myocardial infarction was more common after CEA. That the frequency of the composite endpoint did not differ between the two procedures highlighted the need for a comparison of the anatomic durability of these revascularization procedures. Many participants in CREST were asymptomatic, so the long-term durability of revascularization becomes even more important. Finally, with the approval of CAS in the United States in high-risk patients with significant carotid stenosis ($\geq$70%) and neurological symptoms (ipsilateral stroke, transient ischemic attack, and amaurosis fugax), it is clear that the number of CAS procedures will continue to progressively increase. This will no doubt result in a number of post-CAS in-stent restenosis (ISR) cases.

Prior reports have indicated that the incidence of restenosis after CEA and CAS ranges from 1%–50% depending on its definition and the duration of follow-up. Considerable controversy still persists regarding the clinical significance, natural history, optimal diagnosis, threshold for management, and appropriate intervention for carotid restenosis. This review analyzes current information on this problem and presents recommendations for the diagnosis and management of recurrent carotid stenosis based on the results from CREST.

PATHOPHYSIOLOGY OF RESTENOSIS

Two mechanisms can account for the restenosis that occurs after carotid stenting. Restenosis early (<24 months) after the procedure is generally attributed to intimal hyperplasia. This is a universal response seen in any vascular bed subjected to vessel wall injury. The exact mechanisms of this response are not well known. The initial response to the stent is adherence of a fine film of protein on the metal surfaces and thrombus in the interstices.[15] This results in adherence of platelets and lymphocytes, and their activation leads to the release of cellular mediators. These mediators stimulate proliferation of smooth muscle cells and collagen matrix and result in neointimal hyperplasia. The injury from stenting is prolonged and robust compared to angioplasty alone and leads to a more vigorous reaction.[16,17]

Restenosis that occurs more than 24 months after carotid stenting is generally believed to be caused by progressive atherosclerosis.[18,19] The same mechanical, chemical, and physiologic processes that led to the primary carotid stenosis are presumably present and ongoing in the patient. These processes, over time, can lead to recurrent atherosclerotic lesions in the carotid artery.

Primary stenting prevents carotid artery recoil and constrictive remodeling. Therefore, the patterns of developing intimal hyerplasia (IH) lesions may reflect the aggressiveness of the intimal hyperplastic response and may also predict the future development of high-grade ISR (≥80%), necessitating reintervention. We have assessed the morphologic patterns of ISR using B-mode imaging[20] and identified patterns of post-CAS ISR that correlate with increasing severity (Fig. 3-1): type I (focal ≤10 mm end-stent lesions), type II (focal ≤10 mm, intrastent), type III (diffuse >10 mm, intrastent), IV (diffuse >10 mm proliferative, extending outside the stent), and V (total occlusion). Mapping these patterns during follow-up duplex ultrasonography (DU) after CAS may assist in determining the aggressiveness with which patients must be followed up for future high-grade restenosis.

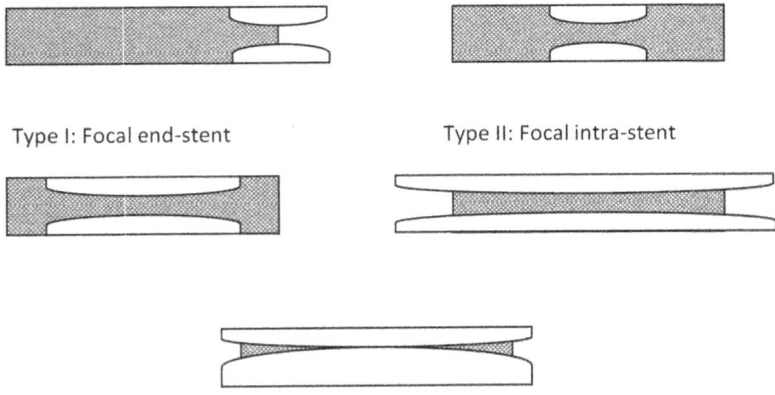

Type I: Focal end-stent   Type II: Focal intra-stent

Figure 3-1. Classification of post-CAS in-stent restenosis. Type I is a focal end stent lesion. Type II is a focal intrastent lesion. Type III is a diffuse intrastent lesion. Type IV is a diffuse proliferative lesion extending outside the stent. Type V is an occlusive lesion.

LONG-TERM DURABILITY OF CEA COMPARED TO CAS IN CREST

CREST enrolled symptomatic patients with more than or equal to 50% stenosis and asymptomatic patients with more than or equal to 70% stenosis at 117 clinical centers in the United States and Canada between December 21, 2000, and July 18, 2008. Patients were randomly assigned to either CEA or CAS. CEA was undertaken according to well-established techniques (standard or eversion endarterectomy) on the basis of the individual preferences of 477 surgeons. CAS was undertaken with a prespecified self-expanding nitinol stent and embolic protection device (RX Acculink and RX Accunet, Abbott Vascular, Santa Clara, CA, USA) by 224 participating interventionists. This randomized, well-characterized cohort of patients offered an optimal opportunity to measure and compare the long-term durability of the two revascularization procedures with respect to freedom from restenosis.

DIAGNOSIS OF IN-STENT RESTENOSIS

The standard diagnostic and screening tool used in the evaluation of primary carotid arterial stenosis and in the follow-up of patients who have undergone CEA is DU. DU correlates well with angiographic levels of stenosis in the native carotid artery. In addition, appropriate threshold velocity criteria for determination of various degrees of stenosis have been well established.[21–23]

In 2004, we reported that the placement of a stent altered the biomechanical properties of the carotid territory such that compliance was reduced[9] (Fig. 3-2). We proposed that the enhanced stiffness of the stent–arterial wall complex could render the flow–pressure relationship of the carotid artery closer to those observed in a rigid tube. The native artery allows some of the kinetic energy of blood to change to potential energy of the arterial wall. Since the compliance of the wall decreases with stenting, there is no transfer of this kinetic energy to the arterial wall. This could explain in part why the blood flow velocities would be increased in the presence of a stent. We compared post-CAS ultrasound velocities with angiographically measured residual in-stent stenosis after 90 CAS procedures. We concluded that revised velocity criteria would need to be developed to quantify ISR in stented carotid arteries.

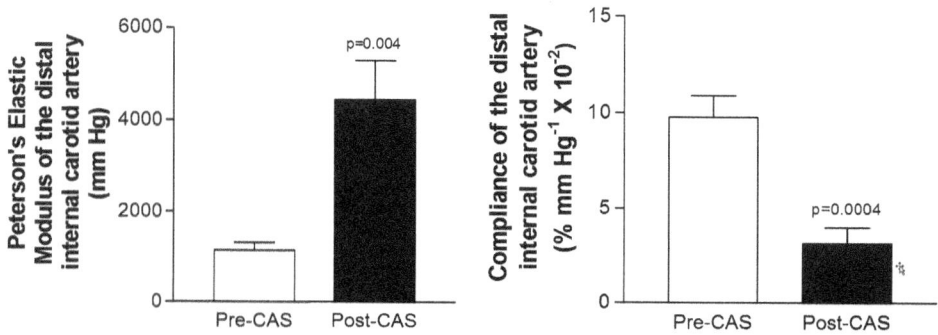

Figure 3-2. Carotid artery stenting alters the biomechanical properties of the stent–arterial complex. Measurement of elastic modulus (A) and compliance (B) of the native internal carotid artery versus stented internal carotid artery.

TABLE 3-1. REVISED VELOCITY CRITERIA FOR THE STENTED CAROTID ARTERY

	Stented Carotid Artery		Native Carotid Artery
0%–19%	PSV <150 cm/s and ICA/CCA ratio <2.15	0%–19%	PSV <130 cm/s
20%–49%	PSV 150–219 cm/s	20%–49%	PSV 130–189 cm/s
50%–79%	PSV 220–339 cm/s and ICA/CCA ratio ≥2.7	50%–79%	PSV 190–249 cm/s and EDV <120 cm/s
≥70%	PSV ≥300 cm/s	—	—
80%–99%	PSV ≥340 cm/s and ICA/CCA ratio ≥4.15	80%–99%	PSV ≥250 cm/s and EDV ≥120 cm/s, or ICA/CCA ratio ≥3.2

Abbreviations: CCA, common carotid artery; EDV, end-diastolic velocity; ICA, internal carotid artery; PSV, peak systolic velocity. PSV and EDV measurements for stented carotid arteries are performed within the stented segments.

In a subsequent report,[24] we compared DU velocity measurements with luminal stenosis measured by angiography or computed tomography angiography during follow-up of all our CAS patients (n = 310 observations). Receiver operating characteristic analysis demonstrated the following optimal threshold criteria: residual stenosis more than or equal to 20% (peak systolic velocity [PSV] ≥150 cm/s and internal carotid artery/common carotid artery (ICA/CCA) ratio ≥2.15), ISR more than or equal to 50% (PSV ≥220 cm/s and ICA/CCA ratio ≥2.7), and ISR more than or equal to 80% (PSV ≥340 cm/s and ICA/CCA ratio ≥4.15). Table 3-1 summarizes our recommended velocity criteria for the evaluation of stented carotid arteries.

DIAGNOSIS OF RESTENOSIS IN CREST

In CREST,[25] DU was performed at baseline and 1, 6, 12, 24, and 48 months after revascularization. DU was under taken at CREST-certified clinical center vascular laboratories with a standardized protocol that utilized the highest systolic velocity measurement from each treated carotid pathway to identify restenosis. Ultrasound images and Doppler waveforms were forwarded to a Core Laboratory for uniform assessment and coding. The main endpoint was a composite of restenosis, defined as more than or equal to 70% recurrent stenosis, or target-artery occlusion identified in ultrasound scans at 1, 6, 12, or 24 months. Based on our group's previous work, a diagnosis of restenosis was made when the PSV at any location within the treated internal or common carotid artery reached or exceeded 300 cm/s. Target-artery occlusion was diagnosed when no flow signal was detected at any location within the treated internal or common carotid artery.

SINGLE-INSTITUTION REPORTS OF ISR AFTER CAROTID ARTERY STENTING

DeGroote and associates[26] emphasized the importance of using life-table methods to determine the incidence of restenosis in the context of patients undergoing CEA. Calculation of an absolute restenosis rate (arteries with restenotic lesions/total carotid procedures) will generally underestimate the incidence of restenosis, because it is independent of the duration, frequency, and completeness of clinical follow-up. Using this principle, we had analyzed our own data and reported estimates of ISR after CAS.[10] Over a follow-up period of 1–74 months (mean 18.8 ± 10), the five-year rate of ISR more than or equal to 80% using

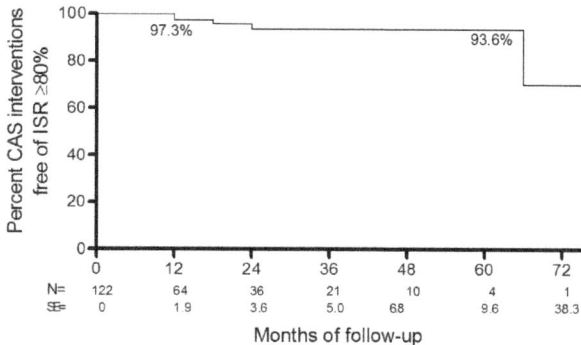

Figure 3-3. Incidence of in-stent restenosis after carotid artery stenting in a single-institution study. Kaplan–Meier cumulative event rates for clinically significant ISR more than or equal to 80% after carotid artery stenting. Number of patients at the beginning of each time interval and standard error are indicated below the X-axis of each graph. N, number at risk; SE, standard error.

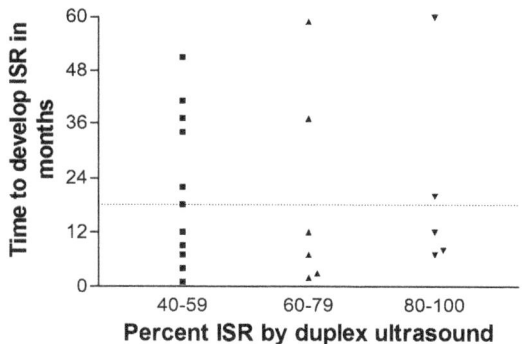

Figure 3-4. Distribution of in-stent restenosis cases based on time of diagnosis from initial carotid artery stenting procedure. Note that the majority of restenoses occurred within 18 months of the initial carotid artery stenting procedure. The dotted line identifies the 18 month postprocedure mark. ISR, in-stent restenosis.

life-table analysis was 6.4% (Fig. 3-3). These observations were subsequently confirmed by other authors.[27] The majority of restenoses in our series of CAS procedures occurred within 18 months of the procedure (Fig. 3-4). We concluded that ISR does not appear to occur at the high rates associated with coronary stenting. However, a substantial number of patients can be anticipated to progress to ISR. Therefore, surveillance is essential after CAS. We recommend that all patients undergoing CAS must be placed in a regular follow-up protocol with more frequent DU evaluations early after CAS. In our own practice, we evaluate patients every six months for the first two years and annually thereafter.

RESTENOSIS AFTER CEA VERSUS CAS IN CREST

In this study, 1086 patients undergoing CAS and 1105 patients undergoing CEA were compared with regards to durability of revascularization. The two cohorts were observed to be well matched with respect to demographics and patient characteristics (Table 3-2). Both groups were followed up for a median of 24 months. The composite outcome of restenosis

TABLE 3-2. CLINICAL CHARACTERISTICS OF THE CREST COHORT AND BY TREATMENT GROUP: CAROTID ARTERY STENTING AND CAROTID ENDARTERECTOMY

	CREST Cohort Analyzed (n = 2191)	CAS (n = 1086)	CEA (n = 1105)
Age	68.9 ± 8.8	68.6 ± 9.0	69.1 ± 8.7
Female sex (%)	33.9	35.2	32.6
White race	93.9	93.7	94.1
Symptomatic	52.9	52.6	53.2
Hypertension	85.3	84.7	86.0
Diabetes	30.5	30.0	31.0
Dyslipidemia	85.4	84.6	86.2
Current smoker	26.5	27.2	25.9
Previous cardiovascular disease or coronary artery bypass graft (CABG)	45.5	44.7	46.3
Pretreatment stenosis percent ≥70%	86.0	86.4	85.6
Blood pressure (mmHg), systolic	141.4 ± 20.0	141.4 ± 19.6	141.3 ± 20.5
Blood pressure (mmHg), diastolic	74.1 ± 11.5	74.0 ± 11.6	74.2 ± 11.4
Time from randomization to treatment (median number of days)	7	6	7
Lipid lowering treatment	92.0	92.7	91.4
Antiplatelet treatment	94.2	96.5	92.0
Antihypertensive treatment	96.1	95.2	97.0

Abbreviations: CREST, Carotid Revascularization Endarterectomy versus Stenting Trial; CAS, carotid artery stenting; CEA, carotid endarterectomy.

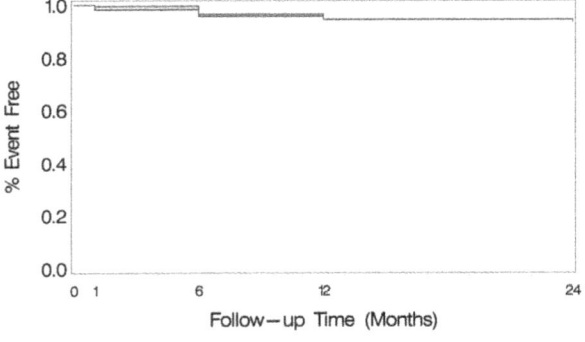

Figure 3-5. Kaplan–Meier graph showing proportion of patients free of restenosis after CEA versus CAS. Restenosis (≥70% diameter-reducing stenosis or occlusion) occurred in 120 patients (n = 58 after CAS; n = 62 after CEA).

or occlusion occurred in 120 patients, and there was no difference between the two types of revascularization procedures (58 CAS and 62 CEA). The Kaplan–Meier estimate for the frequency of the composite outcome at two years was 6.0% for CAS and 6.3% for CEA (hazard ratio [HR] 0.90, 95% confidence interval [CI] 0.63–1.29; $P = 0.58$) after adjustment for adjusted for age, sex, and symptomatic status (Fig. 3-5). Based on fewer patients, the Kaplan–Meier estimate for the frequency of the composite outcome at four years was 6.7% for CAS and 6.2% for CEA (HR 0.94, 95% CI 0.66–1.33; $P = 0.71$).

RISK FACTORS FOR THE DEVELOPMENT OF ISR

Predictors for neointimal hyperplasia are the subject of continued investigation, and there is limited information on which factors constitute risks for carotid ISR. Diabetes is a well-known predictor of early and aggressive IH and ISR after coronary artery stenting. One report has observed an increased incidence of ISR in patients with uncontrolled diabetes undergoing CAS.[28] Skelly et al.[29] analyzed 109 patients undergoing CAS for risk factors that may lead to restenosis. Asymptomatic restenosis occurred in 12 patients (11%); high-grade ISR necessitating reintervention occurred in 5 of those patients. Using Cox proportional hazards modeling, they identified prior neurological symptoms (stroke, transient ischemic attack, and amaurosis fugax) and prior cervical radiation as significant predictors of future ISR.

We have analyzed our own institutional data to identify risk factors for ISR.[20] We entered potential risk factors, including the pattern of ISR, age, gender, hypercholesterolemia, diabetes, hypertension, coronary artery disease, etiology of primary stenosis, prior symptomatic status, prior history of ISR, type of stent used, number of stents used, length of stent, and residual stenosis after CAS, into a multivariate regression model to determine independent predictors of future high-grade ISR. Eighty-five ISR lesions developed after 255 CAS procedures. Thirteen lesions were more than or equal to 80% diameter reducing and underwent endovascular reintervention. On univariate analysis, the need for reintervention was highest in type IV restenotic lesions ($P = 0.001$). A history of prior ISR ($P = 0.003$) and diabetes ($P = 0.02$) occurred more frequently with type IV ISR lesions. On multivariate analysis, only the type of ISR (odds ratio [OR] 5.1) and a history of diabetes (OR 9.7) were independent predictors of high-grade recurrent ISR and reintervention.

Therefore, follow-up duplex ultrasonography evaluations after CAS must include an assessment of the morphologic pattern of ISR so that patients with type IV lesions can be placed on a more intensive monitoring program (perhaps every six months for life). Similarly intensive monitoring is also warranted in patients with diabetes, in those with a history of cervical radiation, and in those who have been treated for ISR. We concluded that additional data were needed to validate these recommendations in prospectively implemented studies at multiple centers.

RISK FACTORS FOR RESTENOSIS AFTER CEA AND CAS IN CREST

Based on a univariate analysis of the CREST cohort, patients with the composite outcome of restenosis or occlusion (regardless of whether they underwent stenting or endarterectomy) were more likely to be younger, women, hypertensive, diabetic, and hyperlipidemic than were those who did not reach the outcome. Multivariate analysis identified female sex, diabetes, and hyperlipidemia to be independent predictors of restenosis after CEA or CAS. Interestingly enough, restenosis was more common in smokers than in nonsmokers who underwent CEA (10.6% vs. 4.7%, log rank $P = 0.0012$), but no difference was identified in those who underwent CAS.

MANAGEMENT OF CAROTID RESTENOSIS

The clinical significance of ISR is still debated. Due to the small number of patients who develop significant restenosis after CAS or CEA, and the lack of clinical trials following these patients for extended periods of time, it is a difficult issue to address. The incidence of symptomatic restenosis after CEA ranges from 0%–8.2%, while asymptomatic restenosis occurs in 1.3%–37%.[30] Consensus exists regarding the need for treatment for symptomatic restenosis. In asymptomatic patients, however, authors have acknowledged that the risk of stroke or progression to total occlusion is uncommon.[31] On the basis of low incidence of symptoms in this cohort of patients, these authors have proposed careful surveillance alone for asymptomatic patients. This recommendation was made in the absence of randomized trial data, with the belief that neointimal hyperplasia carries a low risk for embolization and that reoperation may carry an increased risk of perioperative neurological events and cranial nerve palsies.

Conversely, other surgeons have taken a more aggressive approach toward asymptomatic restenosis and elect to operate on high-grade (≥80%) asymptomatic lesions. O'Hara et al.[32] reported that of 206 redo-CEAs, only 43% had symptoms. Mansour et al.[33] operated on 82 restenoses, of which 66% were symptomatic and the remaining had high-grade asymptomatic stenoses more than or equal to 80%. The rationale for this approach is that it is extremely difficult to predict which high-grade lesions will progress to occlusion. Our group subscribes to this view, and we have reported our low complication rate with redo-CEAs for asymptomatic high-grade (>80%) and symptomatic (>50%) carotid restenosis.[6] Our recommendations for the management of ISR after CAS are based on the published experience with restenosis after CEA. Therefore, we recommend that symptomatic patients with ISR greater than 50% and asymptomatic patients with ISR greater than 80% should be considered for reintervention.

TREATMENT OF CAROTID RESTENOSIS IN CREST

There are several available techniques for reintervention. The fact that these multiple techniques have been used also implies that there is currently limited consensus regarding the most efficacious approach. Angioplasty alone is perhaps the simplest means of intervention; however, the hyperplastic lesions may recoil resulting in incomplete restoration of luminal diameters. In these situations, a cutting balloon may restore patency; however, on occasion, restenting may become necessary. Research continues in the fields of systemic or local pharmaceutical agents and local brachytherapy to prevent the neointimal hyperplasia. There is limited long-term follow-up on these patients, and further studies are needed to evaluate durability of the results. In our experience,[20] endovascular retreatment was required in 3 of 11 instances of type III ISR and 10 of 17 instances of type IV ISR (Table 3-3). The mean interval between CAS and reintervention was 18.2 months. We observed a significant increase in reintervention in association with increasing levels of ISR classification (0%, 0%, 27.3%, and 58.8% for types I–IV, respectively; χ^2 trend = 29.4, $P = 0.001$). Three of the patients have required repeat interventions. One patient has required two repeat interventions over a follow-up period of three years. We currently recommend angioplasty as the primary approach to these intimal hyperplastic lesions with restenting in those cases with suboptimal results.

In the CREST cohort, 43 patients had repeat revascularizations during two years of follow-up. Of those, 20 had previously undergone CAS and 23 had undergone endarterectomy ($P = 0.69$). Repeat angioplasty was the most frequently employed method of revascularization. However, repeat revascularization was not protocol driven; therefore reinterventions were performed at varied degrees of restenosis.

TABLE 3-3. DETAILS OF ENDOVASCULAR REINTERVENTIONS PERFORMED FOR IN-STENT RESTENOSIS AFTER CAROTID ARTERY STENTING

	Patterns of ISR			
	Focal End Stent I ($n = 34$)	Focal Intrastent II ($n = 22$)	Diffuse Intrastent III ($n = 11$)	Diffuse Proliferative IV ($n = 17$)
Incidence of TLR	0	0	27.3	58.8
Devices used for treatment of ISR (n)				
Balloon angioplasty	0	0	1	3
Stent	0	0	1	5
Cutting balloon	0	0	0	1
Cutting balloon + stent	0	0	1	1
Posttreatment result, % residual stenosis	N/A	N/A	10.4 ± 6.9	11.9 ± 6.1

Abbreviations: ISR, in-stent restenosis; TLR, target lesion revascularization.
Values are expressed as percentages.

CONCLUSIONS

CAS and CEA are associated with similar frequencies of restenosis over two and four years of follow-up in patients with symptomatic or asymptomatic carotid stenosis. Female sex, diabetes, and hyperlipidemia are independent predictors of restenosis after both CAS and CEA, while smoking is only associated with an increased likelihood of restenosis after endarterectomy. Morphologic classification of restenotic lesions after stenting may confer prognostic information that will assist in determining the frequency of follow-up evaluations. Restenosis after both endarterectomy and stenting can be successfully managed with endovascular techniques.

REFERENCES

1. North American Symptomatic Carotid Endarterectomy Trial Collaborators. Beneficial effect of carotid endarterectomy in symptomatic patients with high-grade carotid stenosis. *N Engl J Med.* 1991;325(7):445–453.
2. Randomised trial of endarterectomy for recently symptomatic carotid stenosis: final results of the MRC European Carotid Surgery Trial (ECST). *Lancet.* 1998;351(9113):1379–1387.
3. Barnett HJ, Taylor DW, Eliasziw M, et al. Benefit of carotid endarterectomy in patients with symptomatic moderate or severe stenosis. North American Symptomatic Carotid Endarterectomy Trial Collaborators. *N Engl J Med.* 1998;339(20):1415–1425.
4. Endarterectomy for asymptomatic carotid artery stenosis. Executive Committee for the Asymptomatic Carotid Atherosclerosis Study. *JAMA.* 1995;273(18):1421–1428.
5. Hobson RW II, Weiss DG, Fields WS, et al. Efficacy of carotid endarterectomy for asymptomatic carotid stenosis. The Veterans Affairs Cooperative Study Group. *N Engl J Med.* 1993;328(4):221–227.
6. Hobson RW II, Goldstein JE, Jamil Z, et al. Carotid restenosis: operative and endovascular management. *J Vasc Surg.* 1999;29(2):228–235; discussion 235–238.
7. Hobson RW II, Lal BK, Chakhtoura E, et al. Carotid artery stenting: analysis of data for 105 patients at high risk. *J Vasc Surg.* 2003;37(6):1234–1239.

8. Hobson RW II, Lal BK, Chakhtoura EY, et al. Carotid artery closure for endarterectomy does not influence results of angioplasty-stenting for restenosis. *J Vasc Surg.* 2002;35(3):435–438.

9. Lal BK, Hobson RW II, Goldstein J, et al. Carotid artery stenting: is there a need to revise ultrasound velocity criteria? *J Vasc Surg.* 2004;39(1):58–66.

10. Lal BK, Hobson RW II, Goldstein J, et al. In-stent recurrent stenosis after carotid artery stenting: life table analysis and clinical relevance. *J Vasc Surg.* 2003;38(6):1162–1168; discussion 1169.

11. Ohki T, Veith FJ. Carotid artery stenting: utility of cerebral protection devices. *J Invasive Cardiol.* 2001;13(1):47–55.

12. Roubin GS, New G, Iyer SS, et al. Immediate and late clinical outcomes of carotid artery stenting in patients with symptomatic and asymptomatic carotid artery stenosis: a 5-year prospective analysis. *Circulation.* 2001;103(4):532–537.

13. Vitek JJ, Roubin GS, New G, et al. Carotid angioplasty with stenting in post-carotid endarterectomy restenosis. *J Invasive Cardiol.* 2001;13(2):123–125; discussion 158–170.

14. Yadav JS, Wholey MH, Kuntz RE, et al. Protected carotid-artery stenting versus endarterectomy in high-risk patients. *N Engl J Med.* 2004;351(15):1493–1501.

15. Baier RE, Dutton RC. Initial events in interactions of blood with a foreign surface. *J Biomed Mater Res.* 1969;3(1):191–206.

16. Schwartz RS, Huber KC, Murphy JG, et al. Restenosis and the proportional neointimal response to coronary artery injury: results in a porcine model. *JACC.* 1992;19(2):267–274.

17. Kornowski R, Hong MK, Tio FO, et al. In-stent restenosis: contributions of inflammatory responses and arterial injury to neointimal hyperplasia. *JACC.* 1998;31(1):224–230.

18. Lattimer CR, Burnand KG. Recurrent carotid stenosis after carotid endarterectomy. *Br J Surg.* 1997;84(9):1206–1219.

19. Sterpetti AV, Schultz RD, Feldhaus RJ, et al. Natural history of recurrent carotid artery disease. *Surg Gynecol Obstet.* 1989;168(3):217–223.

20. Lal BK, Kaperonis EA, Cuadra S, et al. Patterns of in-stent restenosis after carotid artery stenting: classification and implications for long-term outcome. *J Vasc Surg.* 2007;46:833–840.

21. Faught WE, Mattos MA, van Bemmelen PS, et al. Color-flow duplex scanning of carotid arteries: new velocity criteria based on receiver operator characteristic analysis for threshold stenoses used in the symptomatic and asymptomatic carotid trials. *J Vasc Surg.* 1994;19(5):818–827; discussion 827–818.

22. Lal BK, Hobson IR. Carotid artery occlusive disease. *Curr Treat Options Cardiovasc Med.* 2000;2(3):243–254.

23. Mintz BL, Hobson RW II. Diagnosis and treatment of carotid artery stenosis. *J Am Osteopath Assoc.* 2000;100(suppl 11):S22–S26.

24. Lal BK, Hobson RW, Tofighi B, et al. Duplex ultrasound velocity criteria for the stented carotid artery. *J Vasc Surg.* 2008;47:63–73.

25. Lal BK, Beach KW, Roubin GS, et al.; for the CREST Investigators. Restenosis after carotid artery stenting and endarterectomy: a secondary analysis of CREST, a randomised controlled trial. *Lancet Neurol.* 2012;11(9):755–763.

26. DeGroote RD, Lynch TG, Jamil Z, Hobson RW II. Carotid restenosis: long-term noninvasive follow-up after carotid endarterectomy. *Stroke.* 1987;18(6):1031–1036.

27. Bosiers M, Peeters P, Deloose K, et al. Does carotid artery stenting work on the long run: 5-year results in high-volume centers (ELOCAS Registry). *J Cardiovasc Surg (Torino).* 2005;46(3):241–247.

28. Willfort-Ehringer A, Ahmadi R, Gessl A, et al. Neointimal proliferation within carotid stents is more pronounced in diabetic patients with initial poor glycaemic state. *Diabetologia.* 2004;47(3):400–406.

29. Skelly CL, Gallagher K, Fairman RM, et al. Risk factors for restenosis after carotid artery angioplasty and stenting. *J Vasc Surg.* 2006;44(5):1010–1015.

30. Beebe HG. Scientific evidence demonstrating the safety of carotid angioplasty and stenting: do we have enough to draw conclusions yet? *J Vasc Surg.* 1998;27(4):788–790.

31. Healy DA, Zierler RE, Nicholls SC, et al. Long-term follow-up and clinical outcome of carotid restenosis. *J Vasc Surg*. 1989;10(6):662–668; discussion 668–669.
32. O'Hara PJ, Hertzer NR, Karafa MT, et al. Reoperation for recurrent carotid stenosis: early results and late outcome in 199 patients. *J Vasc Surg*. 2001;34(1):5–12.
33. Mansour MA, Kang SS, Baker WH, et al. Carotid endarterectomy for recurrent stenosis. *J Vasc Surg*. 1997;25(5):877–883.

4

Revisiting Treatment Options for Asymptomatic Carotid Disease

Bruce A. Perler, MD, MBA

Cerebrovascular disease is the second leading cause of death worldwide and is responsible for approximately 9.5% of all mortalities. In the United States, stroke is responsible for approximately 137,000 deaths per year. According to the latest data from the American Heart Association, 795,000 strokes occur annually in the United States. Approximately 15% of strokes are fatal, 15%–20% are severely disabling, and at least 15%–20% of stroke survivors will experience a subsequent disabling stroke in the future. The financial cost of stroke to our healthcare system is now estimated to exceed $70 billion annually.

Approximately 80% of strokes are ischemic, and carotid artery disease is an important cause as a consequence of embolization from plaque at the carotid artery bifurcation, or in the common (CCA) or internal carotid (ICA) arteries, or due to low flow. Many of these strokes are therefore completely preventable by the timely performance of carotid endarterectomy (CEA) or carotid artery angioplasty and stent placement (CAS).

CEA was first performed in the 1950s, and the procedure experienced remarkable growth in performance during the next three decades after several natural history studies demonstrated that carotid stenosis was a risk factor for disabling stroke and death, and early clinical trials demonstrated that carotid surgery reduced the incidence of stroke associated with symptomatic carotid lesions. However, as the volume of procedures increased, subsequent reports documented high complication rates, which compromised the potential benefit of CEA, and the performance of CEA declined substantially in the 1980s. Subsequently, randomized controlled studies carried out in the 1990s established the safety and efficacy of CEA, and its superiority when compared to the best medical management of patients with symptomatic and asymptomatic carotid disease, and have provided Level I evidence to support the appropriate clinical indications for carotid intervention (Table 4-1).

TABLE 4-1. CEA VERSUS BEST MEDICAL THERAPY: RANDOMIZED TRIALS

Trial	Indication	Perioperative CVA/Death	Risk Reduction	P
NASCET	Sx: ≥70%	5.8%	16.5% / 2 years	<0.001
	Sx: 50%–69%	6.7%	10.1% / 5 years	<0.05
ECST	Sx: 70%–99%	7.5%	9.6% / 3 years	<0.01
ACAS	Asx: ≥60%	2.3%	5.9% / 5 years	0.004
ACST	Asx: >60%	3.1%	5.4% / 5 years	<0.0001

Abbreviations: ACAS, Asymptomatic Carotid Atherosclerosis Study; ACST, Asymptomatic Carotid Surgery Trial; Asx, Asymptomatic; ECST, European Carotid Surgery Trial; NASCET, North American Symptomatic Carotid Endarterectomy trial; Sx: Symptomatic.

INDICATIONS FOR CEA

The North American Symptomatic Carotid Endarterectomy Trial (NASCET) demonstrated a clear benefit of CEA and best medical management compared to best medical management alone for symptomatic patients with high-grade (70%–99%) ICA stenoses.[1] The same year the European Carotid Surgery Trial (ECST) demonstrated a similar but smaller benefit in symptomatic patients with 70%–99% ICA stenoses.[2] Analysis of a second cohort of symptomatic patients with moderate (50%–69%) stenoses in the NASCET trial demonstrated a smaller but statistically significant benefit as well.[3] Today, there continues to be a consensus that the patient with a ≥50% symptomatic ICA stenosis is optimally served by CEA.

Similarly, Level I evidence derived from randomized prospective clinical trials clearly established the indications for CEA among patients with asymptomatic ICA stenoses. The Asymptomatic Carotid Atherosclerosis Study (ACAS) demonstrated a significant benefit of CEA and best medical management compared to best medical management alone for patients with asymptomatic 60%–99% stenoses.[4] The inclusion criteria were similar, and the ACAS findings were confirmed, in the Asymptomatic Carotid Surgery Trial (ACST) in Europe.[5] In fact, based on this evidence, the recently published Society for Vascular Surgery (SVS) Clinical Practice Guidelines noted that CEA "should be considered" for asymptomatic patients with ≥60% stenoses if the patient can be assumed to have at least a 3- to 5-year life expectancy and if the perioperative stroke/death rate is ≤3%.

However, this recommendation has recently been challenged by respected leaders in the field. Specifically, it has been argued that in light of recent significant improvements in the medical management of cardiovascular disease in general and cerebrovascular disease in particular, most if not all patients with asymptomatic ICA stenoses should be treated medically without intervention.

SCOPE OF THE PROBLEM

In the current era of healthcare reform, shrinking resources, and increasing pressure for healthcare cost containment, the management of the patient with an asymptomatic carotid stenosis is emerging as an increasingly important issue. In fact, the SVS Research Council recently identified the nine most critical clinical research issues and the management of asymptomatic carotid disease was determined to be the most important. As noted earlier, cerebrovascular disease is a frequent cause of morbidity and mortality in the industrialized world, and asymptomatic carotid disease is a risk factor for ischemic stroke. In fact, it is estimated that asymptomatic carotid stenoses are responsible for 10%–21% of anterior circulation ischemic strokes.

Furthermore, asymptomatic carotid disease is very prevalent in western societies. Previous studies have demonstrated that the incidence increases among individuals over the age of 50 and may affect at least 10% of individuals aged 80 and older. For example, in one community-based study utilizing duplex ultrasound examination, a ≥50% asymptomatic ICA stenosis was identified in 6.4% of individuals between the ages of 50 and 79.[6] Another recent analysis documented a prevalence of significant asymptomatic carotid stenoses in 7% of women and more than 12% of men over the age of 70.[7] It is therefore not surprising that approximately 90% of CEA and CAS procedures in contemporary practice are being performed among patients with asymptomatic disease.[8] Currently, individuals over the age of 65, and especially those over the age of 75, represent the fastest growing segment of the population in the United States. Therefore, one can anticipate significant growth in the presentation of patients with asymptomatic carotid disease in the future so that determining the optimal treatment strategy is of paramount importance.

BEST MEDICAL THERAPY

Medical therapy for patients with cardiovascular disease has evolved over the past two decades and has clearly benefited patients with cerebrovascular disease in particular. Optimal medical therapy for patients with carotid artery disease includes both aggressive treatment of associated comorbid conditions and targeted pharmacologic management.

Hypertension is a well-known risk factor for stroke. For example, several studies have demonstrated that blood pressure elevation is a risk factor for carotid atherosclerosis. In fact, it has been demonstrated that there is a 30%–45% increase in the risk of stroke associated with each 10 mmHg elevation is systolic blood pressure, and conversely each 10 mmHg reduction in blood pressure among hypertensive patients reduces the risk of stroke by 33%. It is recommended that one should target a blood pressure of <140/90 in the patient with carotid artery disease.[9]

Although an elevated fasting glucose level is associated with an increased risk of stroke among patients with carotid artery disease, it is unclear whether strict reduction of A_{1c} levels is associated with a reduced stroke risk in this patient population. Likewise, although the association between elevated cholesterol levels and coronary artery disease is well established, the association between cholesterol levels and stroke is less clear. Nevertheless, while a recent meta-analysis demonstrated that the risk of stroke decreased by 15% for every 10% reduction in serum low density lipoprotein (LDL) level,[9] it is unclear whether the reduced risk of stroke is directly related to reduced cholesterol levels or the administration of statin medications to achieve that reduction.

The most important pharmacologic agent to treat cardiovascular disease in general and cerebrovascular disease in particular is a statin medication. There is a consensus that all patients with carotid artery disease should be treated with statin medications. Multiple clinical trials have demonstrated that statin therapy is associated with a 15%–30% reduction in stroke risk.[9] Although antiplatelet therapy and beta blocker administration have additional cardiovascular benefits, clearly statins are much more potent in terms of stroke-prevention.

In fact, it has been observed that these refinements in the medical management of patients with carotid artery disease, and their ubiquitous administration, have resulted in a reduced risk of stroke in this patient population. It has been argued that the incidence of stroke among patients optimally medically managed in contemporary practice has progressively declined in recent years and currently is lower than the rates of stroke observed in the medically treated patents in the randomized trials (Table 4-1). Specifically, it has been observed that the annual risk of any stroke has decreased approximately 60%, from 3.5% to 1.4% since the publication of ACAS, and the average annual risk of ipsilateral stroke has declined by 67% from 2.2% to 0.7% with best medical management.

Therefore, the performance of CEA and CAS among patients with asymptomatic carotid artery disease has been challenged on the basis of this circumstantial data, although there is to date no Level I evidence available to invalidate current treatment guidelines. In fact, those who advocate treating patients with asymptomatic carotid stenoses exclusively medically base that recommendation on relatively weak observational studies. For example, in the SMART study, 221 patients with asymptomatic carotid disease were followed prospectively, and the incidence of stroke was 2.7% at 6-year follow-up. However, individuals were included in the study with a peak systolic velocity of 150 cm/s, indicating relatively mild carotid disease. In addition, less than half of these patients had a >70% ICA stenosis, and 7% of the patients crossed over to CEA or CAS.[10] Likewise, in the Oxford Vascular Study, 101 patients with a >50% ICA stenosis were monitored, and the ipsilateral stroke rate was 0.34% annually. However, only 32 of these patients had a >70% stenosis, and the stroke rate among this cohort was 10%.[11] It seems clear that retrospective data analyses will not provide definitive evidence to challenge the role of carotid intervention for patients with asymptomatic carotid artery disease.

RATIONALE FOR INTERVENTION

Although it is clear that the prognosis of asymptomatic carotid disease has improved compared to historical controls, and it is not unreasonable to assume that at least some asymptomatic patients may be most appropriately treated today medically, there will nevertheless be others for whom carotid intervention is indicated. The rationale for a more aggressive approach to asymptomatic carotid disease is several-fold. This includes a risk of stroke in the asymptomatic patient without prior warning neurologic symptoms, the potential for silent long-term decline in cognitive function, and improved surgical outcomes of CEA when performed upon among asymptomatic patients in contemporary practice.

STROKE WITHOUT PRIOR TIAS IN ASYMPTOMATIC CAROTID DISEASE

Numerous studies have demonstrated that many patients with asymptomatic disease will experience a stroke without any warning transient ischemic attacks (TIAs). In fact, no more than 10%–30% of stroke patients report a history of a preceding TIA.[12,13] For example, in an early population-based study from Rochester, Minnesota, less than 10% of stroke patients reported a history of a TIA. Likewise, in the Oxfordshire Community Stroke Project, a history of prior TIAs was elicited from 15% of patients who experienced a stroke. In the Oxford Vascular Study, conducted 20 years later, the incidence of TIAs preceding a stroke was only 15%. Conversely, 35% of patients referred to the Mayo Clinic with a stroke diagnosis reported experiencing a history of TIAs. In the UK-TIA Aspirin Trial including 2435 patients, 23% of stroke patients reported experiencing a TIA before a stroke. Similarly, among 3018 patients in the ECST, TIAs were reported by 26% of patients who experienced a stroke. Furthermore, these investigations reveal that as many as 17% of the TIAs occurred on the day of stroke and 9% on the day before the stroke.[13] Although one may argue that recent advances in medical management may be contributing to a lower risk of stroke among patients with asymptomatic carotid disease, it is also possible that statins and other pharmacologic agents may be associated with a reduced incidence of warning TIAs in this patient population. For example, in a recent analysis of 16,409 stroke patients in 12 Ontario hospitals from 2003 to 2007, only 12.3% reported experiencing transient symptoms before the cerebral infarction, which is quite comparable to earlier reports.[14]

Furthermore, although contemporary medical therapy, and especially statin medications, appears to be associated with a reduced rate of ischemic strokes, many individuals still experience strokes while receiving optimal medical therapy. For example, in the REACH registry that followed 3164 patients with a ≥70% asymptomatic ICA stenosis, the stroke rate was 3.1% in one year. It is noteworthy that 70% of these patients were taking statins during this interval.

COGNITIVE DECLINE IN PATIENTS WITH ASYMPTOMATIC CAROTID DISEASE

Cognitive impairment is very common in the patient population with carotid atherosclerotic disease. The prevalence of cognitive impairment is 25% among individuals aged 65 and older and 65% among individuals aged 85 and older. Furthermore, there is growing evidence that so-called silent cerebral infarctions may contribute to long-term cognitive decline. A fundamental question is therefore whether asymptomatic carotid atherosclerotic lesions might predispose to long-term cognitive decline, and whether this risk might be ameliorated by timely carotid intervention. Preliminary evidence suggests that this might be the case.

In a study conducted at the West Haven Veterans Administration Hospital, for example, significant cognitive deficits in terms of immediate and delayed verbal memory, delayed visual recall, manual dexterity, visual scanning, and visual-spatial reasoning were identified among six patients with asymptomatic carotid stenoses but in none of six age-matched controls. In another larger study, 33 patients with significant carotid disease, including 28 symptomatic and 5 asymptomatic individuals, underwent neurocognitive testing. Deficits in mnemonic functions, attention under stress, and psychomotor function were identified in patients with stenoses or occlusions of the carotid arteries when compared to controls. The performance of the patients with asymptomatic disease was similar to that of patients with prior carotid symptoms. In a study from the Innsbruck Neurologic Clinic, 20 individuals with asymptomatic carotid disease underwent a battery of neurocognitive tests. Significant deficits in mental speed, learning, visuospatial abilities, verbal processing, and deductive reasoning were identified significantly more often in patients with asymptomatic carotid stenoses compared to controls. In a very recent study from the University of Pittsburgh, deficits in cognitive and physical functioning were identified among 79 patients with asymptomatic carotid stenoses, with the most widespread deficits in patients with severe stenoses as opposed to those with moderate stenoses. Of note, deficiencies in all cognitive domains were identified in patients with left-sided carotid or bilateral carotid disease, whereas deficiencies in visuospatial/constructional domain were found in patients with right-sided disease. This work was largely corroborated in the Cardiovascular Health Study. Among 4006 right-handed men and women aged 65 or older, there were 32 individuals with asymptomatic high grade (≥75%) left and 29 high grade (≥75%) right ICA stenoses who underwent the Modified Mini-Mental State Examination. After adjustment for right-sided stenosis, high-grade left ICA stenosis was associated with cognitive impairment (odds ratio 6.7 [95%CI, 2.4–18.1]) compared to individuals with no ICA stenosis. The persistence of this association after correction for right-sided disease suggests that it is not due to underlying risk factors for atherosclerotic disease in general.[15]

The impact of CEA on cognitive function is unclear. Although several studies have demonstrated an improvement in cognitive function after CEA, this has not been confirmed in other work. Nevertheless, the association of asymptomatic carotid disease and cognitive impairment does indicate that further study is necessary before concluding that medical therapy alone is the treatment of choice for patients with asymptomatic significant ICA stenoses.

IMPROVED SURGICAL OUTCOMES OF CEA FOR ASYMPTOMATIC DISEASE

The current role of CEA in the management of asymptomatic carotid atherosclerosis is largely based on Level I evidence derived from the ACAS and ACST investigations. However, it is argued that since medical therapy today is so much more effective than at the time of these trials, patients randomized to best medical therapy would have experienced much better neurologic outcomes had current therapy, and especially high-dose statin therapy, been utilized. Therefore, it is now argued by some that contemporary clinical guidelines should no longer be based on these results. It does seem clear that the stroke risk of the patient population with significant asymptomatic carotid disease is less than that observed in ACAS and ACST. However, it is also very clear that the surgical outcome of patients undergoing CEA in contemporary practice is superior to the outcomes noted in the 1990s, and including the ACAS and ACST studies. Therefore, it is not logical to assume a better outcome in the medical cohorts in these trials without also assuming a markedly improved outcome in the surgical cohorts as well. The improvement in surgical outcomes in contemporary clinical practice is related to better trained surgeons performing the operation and improved surgical technique but, perhaps most importantly, is related to the same improvements in medical therapy.

The perioperative stroke and death rates were 2.3% and 2.8% among patients undergoing CEA in ACAS and ACST, respectively. However, the rate of major complications associated with CEA has dramatically declined in recent years. For example, in the CREST investigation, the 30-day stroke and death rate after CEA for asymptomatic carotid stenoses was 1.4%, roughly half of what was observed in the asymptomatic randomized trials. Among CEA procedures performed for asymptomatic stenoses exclusively by vascular surgeons, the perioperative stroke and death rate was only 1.1%. Although it may be argued by some that these outstanding results reflect the strict credentialing criteria for operators in CREST, which limited participation to the most highly skilled practitioners, numerous reports have documented equally outstanding results of CEA in contemporary community practice. In the state of Maryland, for example, CEA was performed on 23,237 patients in 48 hospitals over a 10-year period. The indication for operation was asymptomatic disease in 85% of the patients. Stroke occurred in 169 (0.73%) and death in 125 (0.54%) of patients, yielding an in-hospital stroke and death rate of 1.3%. These results are consistent with a perioperative stroke and death rate of 1.4% after CEA among 1732 patients undergoing CEA for asymptomatic disease in a report from the Northern New England Vascular Study Group. Likewise, in a recent National Surgical Quality Improvement Program (NSQIP) report, the perioperative stroke and death rate was 1.7% among 5009 patients undergoing CEA for asymptomatic carotid stenoses.

Although better trained surgeons and improved surgical technique may be contributing to better outcomes among patients undergoing CEA, a major contributing factor appears to be improved perioperative medical management. The use of antiplatelet agents has been shown to be associated with a reduced rate of neurologic complications. Likewise, the use of beta blockers has been associated with a reduced rate of perioperative cardiac morbidity.

However, just as statins have been associated with effective primary stroke prevention among patients managed medically, there is also compelling evidence that statin medications are associated with a significantly improved outcome among patients undergoing CEA. In a report of 1566 CEAs performed at the Johns Hopkins Hospital, for example, the 30-day rates of stroke were 1.2% and 4.5% ($p = 0.002$) and death rates were 0.3% and 2.1% ($p = 0.002$) among statin users and nonusers, respectively. Multivariable analysis demonstrated that statin use was associated with a threefold reduction in stroke ($p = 0.019$) and fivefold reduction in death ($p = 0.049$) at 30-days following CEA. There was also a lower rate of 30-day myocardial infarction, 1.2% versus 2.1% ($p = 0.191$) among statin users and nonusers, respectively. The beneficial effects of statins among patients undergoing CEA have been corroborated in a population-based study from Canada among symptomatic patients undergoing CEA. One must conclude from these observations that although contemporary medical management has been associated with an improved outcome among patients with asymptomatic carotid stenoses managed medically, the outcome of CEA is also better than what was observed in historic randomized trials due to improved medical therapy as well. Therefore, one cannot simply dismiss the evidence with respect to the beneficial role of CEA among patients with asymptomatic carotid disease derived from these trials on the basis of improvement in the medical management of this patient population in contemporary practice.

SELECTION OF ASYMPTOMATIC PATIENTS FOR INTERVENTION

Severity of Stenosis

Historically, the decision to intervene on a patient with asymptomatic carotid disease was based on the severity of the stenosis, and this criterion remains relevant today. For example, in the Asymptomatic Carotid Stenosis and Risk of Stroke (ACSRS) trial, 1115 patients with an asymptomatic >50% ICA stenosis were followed for 6–84 (mean, 37.1) months. There were 108 hemispheric ischemic events ipsilateral to the significant stenosis, including amaurosis fugax (18), cortical TIAs (44), and ischemic strokes (46). The incidence of ischemic neurologic events increased progressively with increasing severity of the ICA stenosis. Using NASCET Duplex criteria, the incidence of ischemic neurologic events was 8.2% among those with a 50%–69%, 10.7% among those with a 70%–89%, and 19.3% among those with a 90%–99% ICA stenosis. The hemispheric stroke rate was 3.4% among those with a 50%–69% and 11.9% among those with a 90%–99% ICA stenosis.[16] These findings corroborate other studies that have demonstrated a relationship between the severity of the ICA stenosis and future ischemic neurologic events.

Progression in the Degree of Stenosis

In addition to the severity of the stenosis, there is evidence that progression in the degree of stenosis is also a risk factor for future ischemic neurologic events. In one recent study, for example, 1065 patients (63% male) with a median age of 69 underwent a baseline carotid duplex examination and then a follow-up examination from six to nine (median, 7.5) months later. Progression in the degree of stenosis was noted in 9% of the patients. During a median follow-up of 3.2 years, 56 (5%) strokes, including 53 ischemic and 3 hemorrhagic, occurred. There was a twofold increased risk of stroke among patients who experienced progression in the degree of stenosis.[17]

UNSTABLE PLAQUE

Morphologic Factors

Although the severity of the ICA stenosis correlates with the future risk of ischemic events, it has become well recognized that the character of the plaque may be a much more sensitive indicator of future ischemic events. Specifically, it is the unstable or vulnerable plaque that typically leads to acute ischemic events. Intraplaque hemorrhage, thinning of the fibrous capsule, and eventual plaque rupture not only lead to acute coronary events but also are likely responsible for carotid thromboembolism and the majority of TIAs and strokes. Our clinical challenge therefore is to identify the patient with an asymptomatic carotid stenosis who is most likely to experience plaque rupture and become symptomatic; that is, the patient with a vulnerable or potentially unstable plaque.

Over the past decade, numerous studies have identified morphologic factors that are suggestive of plaque instability. For example, MRI has been utilized to assess plaque morphology and correlate the findings to the risk of cerebral ischemic events. In one study a series of 154 patients ranging in age from 48 to 87 (mean, 71) years with a 50%–79% asymptomatic ICA stenosis underwent multicontrast-weighted MRI examinations and then were followed clinically. During a mean follow-up of 38 months, 14 patients experienced ischemic neurologic events, including six strokes, four TIAs, and four episodes of amaurosis fugax. Among a number of demographic and morphologic variables examined, plaques with intraplaque hemorrhage (HR, 5.2; 95% CI, 1.6–17.3; $p = 0.005$), larger mean intraplaque hemorrhage area (HR, for 10 mm^2 increase, 2.6; 95% CI, 1.4–4.6, $p = 0.006$), thin or ruptured fibrous cap (HR, 17.0; 95% CI, 2.2–132.0; $p < 0.001$), larger maximum percent of lipid-rich necrotic core (HR for 10% increase, 1.6; 95% CI, 1.2–2.0; $p = 0.004$), and maximum wall thickness (HR for 1 mm increase, 1.6; 95% CI 1.1–2.3; $p = 0.008$) were associated with the occurrence of subsequent ischemic neurologic events.[18] Kaplan–Meier analysis revealed that event-free survival was higher in patients with plaques without intraplaque hemorrhage ($p = 0.005$) and with thick fibrous capsules ($p < 0.01$).[18]

In the ACSRS study, 1121 patients with a 50%–99% asymptomatic ICA stenosis were followed for 6–96 (mean, 48) months. There were 130 ipsilateral cerebral or retinal ischemic events that occurred, including 59 strokes, 49 TIAs, and 22 episodes of amaurosis fugax. A number of clinical features were predictive of future cerebral ischemic events, including the severity of the stenosis, patient age, systolic blood pressure, serum creatinine level, smoking history, and a history of prior contralateral TIAs or stroke. However, a number of plaque morphologic characteristics were also highly predictive of future stroke. The most important plaque characteristics independently predictive of ipsilateral ischemic events included plaque area; a low gray scale median that is indicative of low echodensity; and a large discrete white area, indicative of hypoechoic areas that are associated with plaque vascularity and an increased concentration of macrophages.

Ultrasound studies have demonstrated that a juxtaluminal black (hypoechoic) area (JBA) in CEA specimens is associated with a large lipid core close to the lumen. The neurologic predictive value of the JBA was recently investigated in the ACSRS study among 1121 patients with a 50%–99% asymptomatic stenosis, and a linear relationship was identified. Specifically, the five-year stroke rate was 2% among 706 patients with a JBA < 4 mm^2, 7% among 46 patients with a JBA 8–10 mm^2, and 25% among 198 patients with a JBA > 10 mm^2. This analysis confirmed that the association between JBA and future risk of stroke persisted after controlling for other known risk factors. Although dedicated software that is not routinely available in clinical practice was utilized in this study to assess the JBA, the findings nevertheless help identify the plaque characteristics that may be indirectly detectable by more routine diagnostic methods.

In another recent study, the plaques were removed from 158 recently symptomatic patients at the time of CEA and were subjected to computerized ultrasound plaque analysis. Recurrent cerebral ischemic events occurred in 20 (12.7%) patients before undergoing CEA. Multivariate stepwise analysis revealed that a large lipid core (OR 4.00, 95% CI, 1.07–4.83, $p = 0.042$) and a low gray scale median (OR 6.21, 95% CI, 1.86–20.4, $p = 0.003$) were independently associated with recurrent cerebral events. Although these observations were obtained among symptomatic patients, it clearly identified anatomic plaque morphology that might identify the asymptomatic patient who is most prone to become symptomatic and therefore warrants intervention.[19]

Serologic Markers of Inflammation

Clinically useful measures of plaque instability to help identify patients with asymptomatic carotid stenoses at increased risk of future stroke are needed. For example, some work has focused on the potential benefit of serologic markers of an inflammatory state in identifying high-risk asymptomatic carotid stenoses. In one study of 62 both symptomatic and asymptomatic patients with a ≥70% carotid stenosis, high-sensitivity C-reactive protein (hs-CRP) levels were determined 48 hours before CEA, and levels >10 mg/L were considered abnormal. Histopathologic analysis was also carried out on the excised plaques. Unstable plaques were defined as those with endothelial ulceration or recent intraplaque hemorrhage. Patients with unstable plaques had significantly higher levels of hs-CRP when compared to patients with so-called stable plaques. In addition, there was a significant correlation between hs-CRP levels and the presence of macrophages in the plaques.

In another analysis of 40 patients with a ≥70% carotid stenosis who underwent CEA, including 13 who were asymptomatic, serum levels of metalloproteinase 2 (MMP-2) and metalloproteinase 9 (MMP-9) were measured, and the plaques underwent immunochemistry and histopathologic analysis. Elevated MMP-9 levels were associated with carotid plaque instability as well as the presence of macrophages within the plaques. Clearly, further study is necessary to identify potential serologic markers of patients with high-risk carotid plaques.

Clinical Indicators of Unstable Plaque: Silent Cerebral Infarcts

Although recent research studies have identified plaque morphologic features suggestive of vulnerable or unstable plaques and the potential for future cerebral ischemic events, other work has focused on identifying clinical factors suggestive of unstable plaque that might guide the practitioner evaluating the future stroke risk in the patient with asymptomatic carotid disease. One such clinical indicator to provide indirect evidence of unstable plaque is the presence of silent cerebral infarcts on brain imaging either utilizing CT or MRI. Previous work has associated silent infarcts with an increased risk of stroke in the general population, in the perioperative period among patients undergoing CEA, and during longitudinal follow-up after CEA. Recent evidence suggests that silent infarcts are an objective indicator of patients at risk of future stroke among the patient population with significant asymptomatic ICA stenoses.

For example, in the ASCRS study, 821 patients with a median age of 71 years and with asymptomatic ICA 50%–99% stenoses underwent CT scans and were monitored every six months for up to eight years. Excluding lacunar and watershed infarcts, clinically silent infarcts were identified in 146 (18%) patients. During a mean follow-up of 44.6 months, 102 ipsilateral cerebral hemispheric ischemic events occurred, including 47 strokes, 39 TIAs, and 39 episodes of amaurosis fugax. Among 462 patients with a 60%–99% stenosis, the cumulative stroke-free rate was 0.92 (1.0% annual stroke rate) when embolic infarcts were absent and 0.71 (3.6% annual stroke rate) when embolic infarcts were present ($p = 0.002$). The predictive value of silent infarcts was also observed among patients with moderate ICA stenoses. In the 216 patients with a 60%–79% stenosis, the cumulative stroke or TIA-free rate was 0.90 (1.3% annual rate) and 0.65 (4.4% annual rate) among patients without and with embolic infarcts, respectively.[20]

Clinical Indicators of Unstable Plaque: Cerebral Microemboli

Silent cerebral infarctions typically result from microemboli that can be detected in real time with transcranial Doppler (TCD) examination. In light of the relationship between silent cerebral infarction and future stroke among asymptomatic patients, it is not surprising that positive TCD studies are also predictive of future stroke risk in this patient population. For example, in the multicenter Asymptomatic Carotid Emboli Study (ACES) 467 patients with at least a 70% asymptomatic ICA stenosis in 26 centers underwent TCD studies at baseline and at 6, 12, and 18 months during follow-up. The absolute annual risk of stroke or TIA during two years of follow-up was 7.1% and 3.0% among those with positive and negative TCD studies, respectively. The hazard ratio for the risk of ipsilateral stroke and TIA during two years of follow-up was 2.54 (95% CI, 1.20–5.36, $p = 0.015$). The absolute annual risk of ipsilateral stroke was 3.6% and 0.7% for those with and without positive TCD studies, respectively. The hazard ratio for the risk of ipsilateral stroke during two years of follow-up was 5.6 (1.61–19.32, $p = 0.007$).[21]

In an earlier study, 319 patients with mean age of 70 years and a $\geq$60% asymptomatic ICA stenosis underwent TCD and positive studies were noted in 32 (10%) patients. The incidence of stroke during the first year of follow-up was 15.6% (95% CI, 4.1–79) versus 1% (95% CI, 1.01–1.36 (p < 0.0001) among individuals with positive and negative studies, respectively.[22] The prognostic significance of positive TCD studies among patients with asymptomatic carotid disease was further corroborated in a recent study. TCD was performed on 253 patients with a mean age of 70 years and a > 60% stenosis. Cerebral microemboli were detected in 11 (6%) patients. The three-year risk of stroke was 13.3% and 1.7% among those with positive and negative TCD studies, respectively (p = 0.04). The three-year risk of stroke and death was 20.0% and 1.7% among those with positive and negative TCD studies, respectively (p = 0.005).[23] These findings suggest that among asymptomatic carotid patients without TCD evidence of cerebral emboli, it is safe to consider continued medical management while positive studies might identify patients who would benefit from CEA.

Clinical Indicators of Unstable Plaque: Plaque Echolucency

TCD examination is difficult, requires a highly skilled sonographer, and in many older patients there is an inadequate temporal window to perform an adequate examination. On the contrary, cerebral CT and MRI studies are costly and not ideal as routine screening examinations among patients with asymptomatic carotid stenoses. In light of the morphologic plaque factors that have been found to be predictive of future stroke risk in research studies, increasing attention has focused on the utility of routine Duplex ultrasound to address this clinical challenge. Specifically, there is evidence that unstable or vulnerable plaque appears very echolucent on routine B-mode ultrasound imaging. For example, in an analysis of 435 patients with a mean age of 71.4 years and a $\geq$70% asymptomatic ICA stenosis in the ACES trial, the carotid plaques were graded as echolucent in 164 (38%) patients. Patients were followed for two years. The presence of echolucent plaque at the baseline examination was associated with a significantly increased risk of subsequent ipsilateral stroke. The hazards ratio was 6.43 (95% CI, 1.36–30.44, p = 0.019). Among patients with echolucent plaque at baseline and positive TCD studies, the hazards ration for ipsilateral stroke was 10.61 (95% CI, 2.98–37.82, p = 0.0003).[24] In the Cardiovascular Health Study, the largest investigation reported to date, 4886 patients $\geq$65 years of age with an asymptomatic carotid stenosis underwent carotid duplex examination. After controlling for risk factors, hypoechoic or echolucent plaque was associated with ipsilateral nonfatal stroke (RR, 2.78; CI, 1.36–5.69) with a mean follow-up of 3.3 years.[25]

ASYMPTOMATIC CAROTID DISEASE: CEA VERSUS CAS

A thorough analysis of the accumulated clinical experience with respect to the appropriate roles for CEA versus CAS is beyond the scope of this chapter. However, in a recent meta-analysis of 13 randomized clinical trials including nearly 7500 patients, CEA was found to be superior in terms of the endpoints of short-term stroke, long-term stroke, and long-term stroke and death, whereas CAS was found to be superior to CEA in terms of short-term myocardial infarction. This was clearly the observation in the recently completed CREST investigation, where the perioperative stroke and death rates were 1.4% and 2.5% among patients undergoing CEA and CAS, respectively, for asymptomatic disease. To date, reimbursement for CAS for asymptomatic disease is allowed only for patients enrolled in clinical trials. The recently published SVS Clinical Practice Guidelines stipulated that although CAS was appropriate for symptomatic patients considered high risk for CEA, asymptomatic patients who are considered high risk for CEA should be treated medically, rather than undergo CAS.

CONCLUSIONS

The evidence is compelling that the prognosis of patients with asymptomatic carotid disease is much better in contemporary practice than in previous years largely due to improvements in medical therapy. However, it is also very clear that the outcome of CEA in contemporary practice is better than at any time in the history of this operation due to better trained surgeons and also clearly due to these very same improvements in medical therapy in the perioperative period. Therefore, it does not seem reasonable to simply dismiss the conclusions of the ACAS and ACST investigations that CEA and best medical therapy is superior to best medical therapy along for patients with asymptomatic carotid disease. It is undeniable that asymptomatic carotid disease is a recognizable and therefore preventable cause of ischemic stroke. Although there may be many patients with asymptomatic carotid disease undergoing CEA or stent procedures unnecessarily, there are still many others who will benefit from these interventions to reduce their risk of developing an ischemic stroke. Our challenge is to accurately identify the patients at greatest risk and intervene safely. Although we have traditionally based the decision to intervene largely on the severity of an asymptomatic stenosis or progression in the degree of stenosis among patients managed medically, and although there is convincing evidence that the subsequent stroke risk correlates with stenosis severity and disease progression, it seems clear that the most important determinant of future stroke risk is the morphology of the plaque responsible for that stenosis. Currently we have relied on indirect indicators of unstable plaque such as the presence of silent cerebral infarctions on cerebral imaging studies or microemboli in real time using TCD, but ultimately we will have the necessary sophisticated duplex ultrasound technology to more precisely characterize plaque morphology and specifically to recognize those features most predictive of future cerebral ischemic events. Finally, based on the preponderance of evidence, CEA appears to be the treatment of choice for asymptomatic patients selected for intervention.

REFERENCES

1. North American Symptomatic Carotid Endarterectomy Trial Collaborators. Beneficial effect of carotid endarterectomy in symptomatic patients with high-grade stenosis. *N Engl J Med.* 1991;325:445–453.
2. European Carotid surgery Trialists' Collaborative Group. MRC European Carotid Surgery Trial: interim results for symptomatic patients with severe (70–99%) or with mild (0–29%) carotid stenosis. European Carotid Surgery Trial Collaborative Group. *Lancet.* 1991;337:1235–1243.
3. Barnett HJM, Taylor DW, Eliasziw M, et al. Benefit of carotid endarterectomy in patients with symptomatic moderate or severe stenosis. *N Engl J Med.* 1998;339:1415–1425.
4. Executive Committee for the Asymptomatic Carotid Atherosclerosis Study. Endarterectomy for asymptomatic carotid artery stenosis. Executive Committee for the Asymptomatic Carotid Atherosclerosis Study. *JAMA.* 1995;273:1421–1428.

5. Halliday A, Mansfield A, Marro J, et al. Prevention of disabling and fatal strokes by successful carotid endarterectomy in patients without recent neurological symptoms: randomised controlled trial. *Lancet.* 2004;363:1491–1502.

6. Mineva PP, Manchev IC, Hadjiev DI. Prevalence and outcome of asymptomatic carotid stenosis: a population-based ultrasound study. *Eur J Neurol.* 2002;9:383–388.

7. de Weerd M, Greving JP, de Jong AW, et al. Prevalence of asymptomatic carotid stenosis according to age and sex: systematic review and metaregression analysis. *Stroke.* 2009;40:1105–1113.

8. Schneider PA, Naylor AR. Asymptomatic carotid artery stenosis-Medical therapy alone versus medial therapy plus carotid endarterectomy or stenting. *J Vasc Surg.* 2010;52:499–507.

9. Ricotta JJ, AbuRahma A, Ascher E, et al. Updated Society for Vascular Surgery guidelines for management of extracranial carotid disease. *J Vasc Surg.* 2011;54:e1–e31.

10. Goessens BM, Visseren FL, Kappele LJ, et al. Asymptomatic carotid artery stenosis and the risk of new vascular events in patients with manifest arterial disease: the SMART study. *Stroke.* 2007;38:1470–1475.

11. Marquardt L, Geraghty OC, Mehta Z, Rothwell PM. Low risk of ipsilateral stroke in patients with asymptomatic carotid stenosis on the best medical treatment. A prospective, population-based study. *Stroke.* 2010;41:e11–e17.

12. Whisnanat JP. The decline of stroke. *Stroke.* 1984;15:160–168.

13. Rothwell PM, Warlow CP. Timing of TIAs preceding stroke: time window for prevention is very short. *Stroke.* 2005;64:817–820.

14. Hackam DG, Kapral MK, Wang JT, et al. Most stroke patients do not get a warning: a population-based cohort study. *Neurology.* 2009;73:1074–1076.

15. Johnston SC, O'Meara ES, Manolio T, et al. Cognitive impairment and decline are associated with carotid artery disease in patients without clinically evident cerebrovascular disease. *Ann Intern Med.* 2004;140:237–247.

16. Nicolaides AN, Kakkos SK, Griffin M, et al. Severity of asymptomatic carotid stenosis and risk of hemispheric ischaemic events: results from the ACSRS Study. *Stroke.* 2005;30:275–284.

17. Sabeti S, Schlager O, Exner M, et al. Progression of carotid stenosis detected by duplex ultrasonography predicts adverse outcomes in cardiovascular high risk patients. *Stroke.* 2007;38:2887–2894.

18. Takaya N, Yuan C, Chu B, et al. Association between carotid plaque characteristics and subsequent ischemic cerebrovascular events: a prospective assessment with MRI-Initial results. *Stroke.* 2006;37:818–823.

19. Salem MK, Sayers RD, Brown MJ, et al. Patients with recurrent ischemic events from carotid artery disease have a large lipid core and low GSM. *Eur J Vasc Endovasc Surg.* 2012;43:147–153.

20. Kakkos SK, Sabetai M, Tegos T, et al. Silent embolic infarcts on computed tomography brain scans and risk of ipsilateral hemispheric events in patients with asymptomatic internal carotid artery stenosis. *J Vasc Surg.* 2009;49:902–909.

21. Markus HS, King A, Shipley M, et al. Asymptomatic embolization for prediction of stroke in the Asymptomatic Carotid Emboli Study (ACES): a prospective observational study. *Lancet.* 2010;9:663–671.

22. Spence JD, Tamayo A, Lownie SP, et al. Absence of microemboli on transcranial Doppler identifies low-risk patients with asymptomatic carotid stenosis. *Stroke.* 2005;36:2373–2378.

23. Madani A, Beletsky V, Tamayo A, et al. High-risk asymptomatic carotid stenosis: ulceration on 3D ultrasound vs TCD microemboli. *Neurology.* 2011;77:744–750.

24. Topakian R, King A, Kwon SU, et al, for the ACES investigators. Ultrasonic plaque Echolucency and emboli signals predict stroke in asymptomatic carotid stenosis. *Neurology.* 2011;77:751–758.

25. Polak JF, Shemanski L, O'Leary DH, et al. Hypoechoic plaque at US of the carotid artery: an independent risk factor for incident stroke in adults aged 65 years or older. Cardiovascular Health Study. *Radiology.* 1998;208:649–654.

Complex Supra-Aortic Trunk Revascularization: Surgical Tips

Thomas C. Bower, MD

The supra-aortic trunks (SATs) are most often affected by occlusive disease and rarely by aneurysms. Savory and Broadbent first described occlusive disease of the SATs in the mid and late 1800s. Takayasu, Onishi, Martorell, and Fabre described the association between obliteration of the SATs, retinal changes in the eye, and absent radial artery pulses.[1] It wasn't until the 1950s and 1960s that great vessel reconstructions were undertaken. The use of homografts was reported by Bahnson.[2] Innominate endarterectomy through right thoracotomy and aortic-origin grafts were subsequently employed at several centers by Davis, DeBakey, Ehrenfeld, and associates.[3–5] Henceforth, both direct and extrathoracic reconstructions were utilized, including subclavian to carotid artery transposition and carotid to subclavian artery bypass.[6,7] Perioperative mortality and stroke rates are low with direct aortic-origin SAT reconstructions.[8–11]

Endovascular therapy has changed the approach to patients with isolated symptomatic lesions involving a single SAT. For this reason, complex open SAT reconstructions originating from ascending aorta include symptomatic patients who need multiple arteries reconstructed because of atherosclerosis or arteritis; those who need great vessel reconstruction as part of repair of ascending aortic and arch aneurysms or coarctation; patients with infections of previously placed prosthetic grafts; and the rare individual who needs resection of a great vessel for malignancy. The keys to successful outcome include patient selection, operative planning based on CT angiography, and adequate perfusion of the brain during the reconstruction.

ANATOMY

The SATs include the innominate, left common carotid, and left subclavian arteries. The innominate artery gives rise to the right common carotid and subclavian arteries. Anatomic variations are quite frequent and include a common brachiocephalic trunk in which the left common carotid artery arises in conjunction with the innominate artery; anomalous origin of the left vertebral artery between the left common carotid and the subclavian arteries; an aberrant right subclavian artery associated with a left-sided aortic arch; and a right-sided aortic arch.[1,12] Patients with a right-sided aortic arch often have an aberrant left subclavian artery that arises from the ascending aorta. In this situation, either the arch or the aberrant artery traverses behind the trachea and esophagus. Some patients with aberrant subclavian arteries have diverticula near the origins of them which may be aneurysmal. Hemodynamic forces, conformational changes, and the curve of the aortic arch are important considerations when hybrid reconstructions are done for arch aneurysms combined with SAT reconstruction.[12]

Atherosclerosis involves multiple SATs between 24% and 84% of the time and is the most common cause of occlusive disease of the great vessels.[1] Takayasu arteritis is predominantly seen in women, with occlusive lesions occurring more often than aneurysmal ones.[1,11] This inflammatory disease is the second leading cause of occlusive lesions of these arteries.[1] The subclavian artery is involved by arteritis in 93% of cases, followed by the common carotid artery in 58%, the vertebral in 35%, and the innominate artery in 27%.[1] Radiation-induced arteritis occurs, on average, 15 years following initial therapy and is most often found in patients who have had radiation treatment for head and neck malignancy, breast cancer, and lymphoma.[13] The specific vessels involved correlates to the mantle of the radiation field. Mediastinal radiation injury may also affect the ascending aorta and arch and lead to calcification of those vessels. Such wall changes have implications for inflow during open surgical reconstruction.

CLINICAL PRESENTATION AND DIAGNOSIS

Symptomatic patients with occlusive lesions present with thromboembolic events to the brain or upper extremity, or symptoms secondary to a low-flow state. The latter may cause upper extremity exertional fatigue, global ischemia, or vertebrobasilar symptoms.[1,8–11] Since most atherosclerotic lesions are irregular, and there is the potential for intimal disruption, patients with this pathology present more often with thromboembolic events compared to those with Takayasu arteritis, in which low-flow symptoms occur because the lesions are smooth and tapered.[1] Radiation-induced lesions cause either embolic or global ischemia problems.[1,13] In the Mayo Clinic report by Rhodes et al.[8] nearly two-thirds of patients treated with aortic-origin reconstructions secondary to atherosclerosis had embolic events, with 53% affecting the brain; 10%, the upper extremity; and 5%, both territories. Similar findings have been noted by others.[9,10]

The most common diagnostic methods include CT and MR angiography of the chest, neck, and head. These modalities allow for characterization of the type and extent of the occlusive lesion, the presence of soft tissue arterial inflammation and wall thickening, the severity of wall calcification, and the presence of intraluminal atheromatous debris.[1,12] Careful review of the imaging studies is necessary to plan the type of and approach to operation to minimize perioperative cardiac and neurologic morbidity. Advances in multidetector CT imaging should allow better anatomic definition when the aorta or SATs are calcified, which has been the bane of this modality. The need for iodinated contrast, radiation exposure, allergic reactions, and the potential for acute kidney injury are also drawbacks of CTA. MR provides assessment of the vessel wall and may have the potential to define plaque vulnerability in selected patients but has the drawback of gadolinium-associated nephrogenic systemic fibrosis in patients with chronic kidney disease.[1] Both CT and MR are useful for defining the extent of arch aneurysms and the presence of dissection, and newer dynamic imaging provides useful detail in this regard. Carotid duplex ultrasonography supplements CT or MR angiography for the evaluation of cervical carotid arteries.

AORTIC ARCH PATHOLOGY

Degenerative diseases from atherosclerosis or chronic inflammatory conditions are the most common etiologies that affect the aortic arch. Most of these patients are aged 60–70 years, have atherosclerosis in other vascular territories, and have the usual cardiovascular risk factors, including smoking, hypertension, and hyperlipidemia.[1,8–12,14] Three genetic disorders contribute to dissections and aneurysms in this location. These include Marfan syndrome, which is an autosomal dominant trait related to a defect in the *fibrillin 1* gene located on chromosome 15; type IV Ehlers–Danlos syndrome, caused by deficiency of the collagen type III, encoded by the *COL3A1* gene mutation; and Loeys–Dietz syndrome, caused by tumor growth factor beta receptor deficiency. Rarer conditions include individuals with familial thoracic aneurysmal disease, pseudoxanthoma elasticum, Erdheim's deformity, and inherited disorders, such as Turner syndrome.[12] Arteritides including Takayasu's disease, giant cell arteritis, temple arteritis, and polymyalgia rheumatica may lead to aneurysmal degeneration. Primary infected aneurysms are usually saccular, involve the inner curve of the aortic arch, and are caused by various bacterial species such as Staphylococcus, Streptococcus, Salmonella, and Pseudomonas. Syphilis and Mycobacteria should also be in the differential diagnosis.[12]

OPEN RECONSTRUCTION FOR OCCLUSIVE LESIONS

Direct transsternal aortic-based reconstructions are applicable to good-risk patients who are symptomatic.[1,8–12,14] These patients require a thorough evaluation for coexisting coronary artery disease, which occurs in nearly one-fourth of cases.[10,14] Cardiac stress testing and/or coronary arteriography is needed before operation. Pulmonary function tests and an arterial blood gas provide information about pulmonary risks. Echocardiography is important for individuals with Takayasu arteritis because of the propensity for valve disease, pulmonary hypertension, or left ventricular hypertrophy from longstanding hypertension. These particular individuals require assessment for stenotic lesions of the thoracic or abdominal aorta and the major branch arteries, including the renals. A few patients have conduction system abnormalities, and these can be screened for by electrocardiography.[1] It is paramount that the ascending aorta not be calcified, and this is best determined on the noncontrast CT images.

Exposure is done through a median or mini sternotomy, with the latter extended through the third intercostal space with transsection of the sternum at that level. The incision can be extended obliquely into either side of the neck as clinically necessary. Extension of the incision is more common when treating occlusive SAT lesions than when these arteries are reconstructed as part of an aortic arch repair. The left innominate vein is mobilized. Thymic and mediastinal fatty tissues can be resected to make room for the grafts. Our preference is to base the SAT reconstructions on an 8- or 10-mm single-limb polyester graft sewn to the lateral or anterolateral wall of the ascending aorta.[1,12] The patient's blood pressure is lowered to 90 mmHg before a partial occlusion clamp is applied to the aorta. An all-purpose aortic clamp works well, taking care to not increase cardiac afterload with application of the clamp. The graft is sewn to the ascending aorta with 4-0 polypropylene suture, buttressed by felt pledgets or strips as needed. Once the aortic anastomosis is completed, the patient's mean arterial blood pressure is maintained between 90 and 105 mmHg during reconstruction of the individual SATs. The graft can be tunneled beneath or on top of the left innominate vein. In rare circumstances, the vein is transected to make room for the graft.[1] Additional limbs are sewn end-to-side to this graft for reconstruction of the left common carotid and right subclavian arteries. The distal anastomoses are done end-to-end in most cases. In some cases, the right subclavian can be reimplanted onto the carotid graft limb and not separately bypassed. The left subclavian artery is rarely revascularized at the same time if the vertebral artery is patent, unless there is extensive disease involving that artery.[1] Should a graft limb be taken to the left subclavian artery in the supraclavicular fossa, the left common carotid artery either is separately reconstructed with a graft or reimplanted onto the subclavian limb (Fig. 5-1). Interrupted suture alone, or in combination with a running suture, is used to reimplant an artery if it is small. We prefer a single limb aortic origin graft over bifurcated grafts because of the bulk of the latter.[1,8] Should a bifurcated graft be used, it is best to keep the body long, to avoid the fibrosis from high flow and turbulence with a shorter length body, as we have experienced in some patients.[1] Additionally, there is more room in the mediastinum to allow closure with a single limb than with the bifurcated graft, which can buckle or kink. Some asthenic patients need resection of the soft tissues beneath the manubrium or even removal of part of the underside of the manubrium to make room for the bypass grafts.[1,12] Several adjuncts are used to perform the operation and keep it safe. These include continuous electroencephalographic monitoring and completion intraoperative duplex imaging to assess technical outcome. It is rare to have to shunt when the SATs are reconstructed by these methods. The sequence of reconstruction of multiple SATs is based on the preoperative anatomy, whether the arteries are stenotic or occluded, and the status of the intracranial circulation.

Although most patients with Takayasu arteritis have lesions isolated to the SATs, some individuals have long-segment occlusions or stenoses of the common carotid and subclavian arteries.[1,11] This may necessitate extension of the graft limbs to the carotid artery bifurcations, which usually are spared from inflammation in all but the most advanced cases of the disease. If the subclavian-axillary artery requires concomitant reconstruction to where the graft has to be passed between the clavicle and the first rib, it is important to ensure adequate space for that bypass graft. This may necessitate resection of a small segment of the first rib. The distal target arteries should be free of disease and inflammation. A specimen of the artery can be sent to the pathologist for frozen section to be certain that there are no giant cells or other inflammatory cells seen in the area. Our best graft patency occurs when reconstructions are performed to uninflamed arteries in patients with quiescent disease no longer requiring steroids. Our worst results have been in individuals with acute disease who either need steroids to control the inflammation or are unresponsive to steroids.[11]

Patients with radiation-induced SAT stenosis or occlusion pose special problems.[13] As mentioned previously, the surgeon needs to be certain that the ascending aorta is

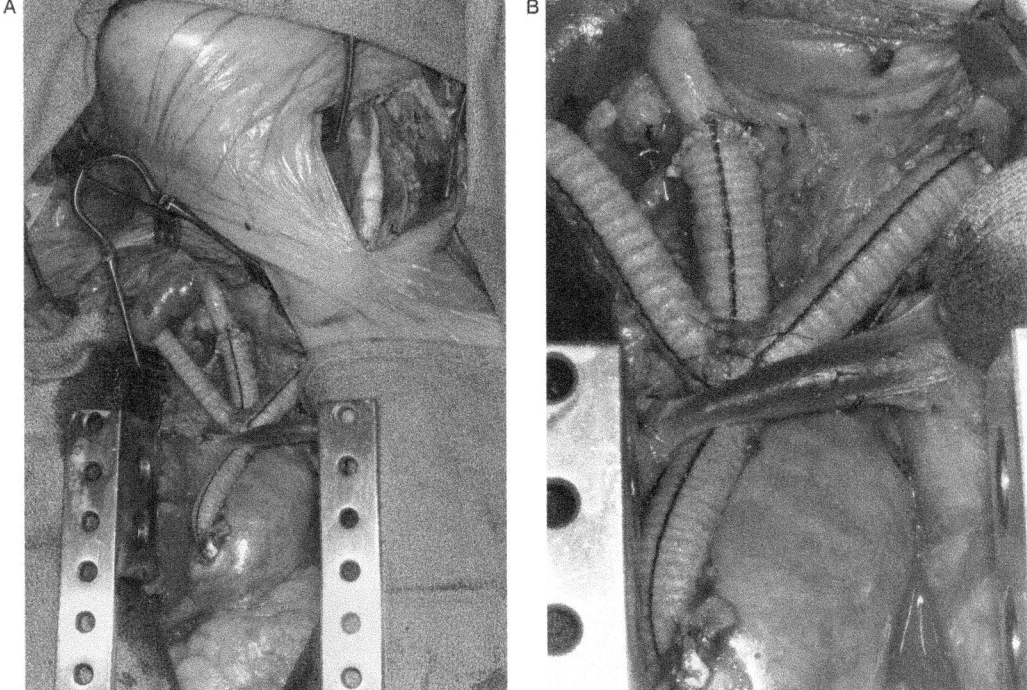

Figure 5-1. A patient with severely limiting and progressive bilateral upper extremity exertional fatigue secondary to atherosclerosis of multiple SATs. The left subclavian artery was chronically occluded, the aberrant right subclavian and right common carotid arteries were calcified and stenotic, and there was a pre-occlusive left carotid bifurcation stenosis. Reconstruction was done with an ascending aorto-right carotid bypass. Side arm grafts were taken to the left common carotid and right subclavian arteries. A left carotid endarterectomy and bovine pericardial patch angioplasty was also done. (A, B) After the reconstruction was completed, there was significant improvement in blood flow through the left subclavian through the vertebral artery, so that the subclavian was not bypassed.

free of calcification and that there is no coronary disease or significant valvular disease. The quality of the skin and subcutaneous tissues, the status of the internal mammary arteries, and the blood supply to the pectoralis major muscles have implications for wound healing. Some patients are best served by prophylactic rotation of a muscle flap into the neck to cover the prosthetic graft, should the incision extend that far. Since there is the potential for sternal wound healing problems, a more limited sternotomy is preferable if the operation can be safely performed through this exposure.

AORTIC ARCH REPAIR

Patients with extensive aneurysms involving the ascending aorta, arch, and thoracoabdominal aorta can be treated by open or hybrid techniques.[12,15–17] Reconstructions of the arch include reimplantation of the supraaortic trunks or separate bypass of them (Fig. 5-2). Cardiopulmonary bypass, deep hypothermic circulatory arrest, and antegrade or retrograde cerebral perfusion are utilized in these circumstances. Since mortality rates

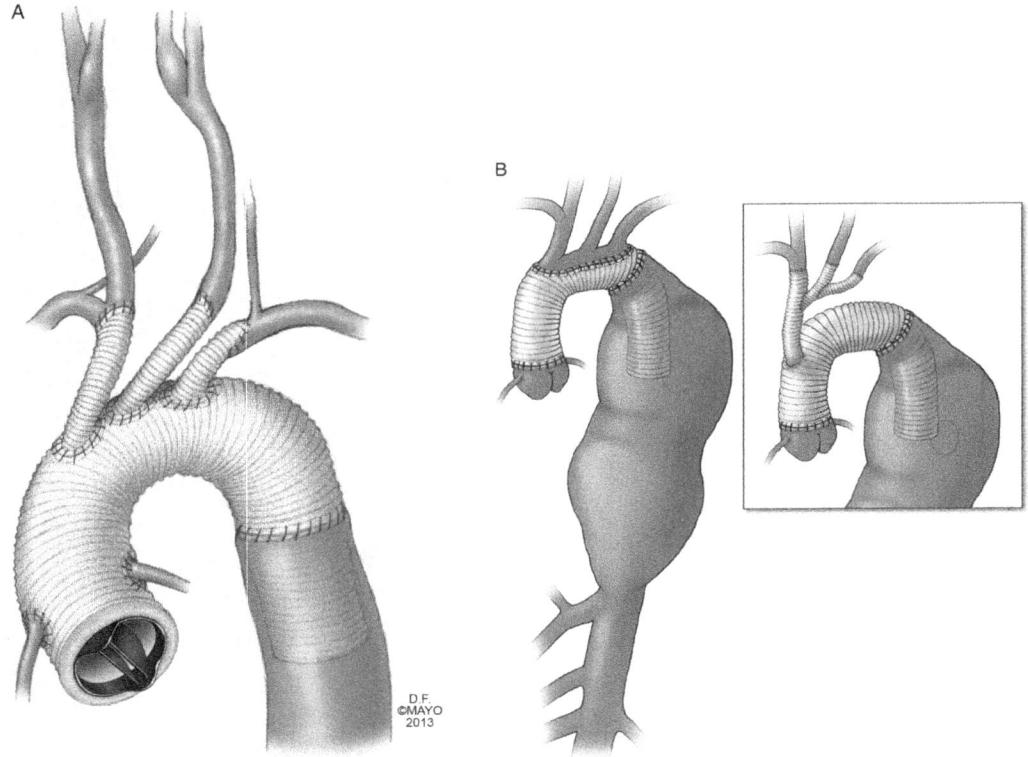

Figure 5-2. Schematic example of a patient who has an ascending aortic and total arch repair with an elephant trunk. The supra-aortic trunks are individually bypassed (A). Other methods to reconstruct these arteries are shown in B.

range between 6% and 20%, and stroke occurs in 4%–23% of patients, alternative surgical techniques have been trialed.[12] The elephant trunk operation was introduced by Borst et al. in 1983.[18] The procedure is two-staged, with the first stage involving open replacement of the ascending aorta and arch, leaving a distal segment of graft dangling freely into the descending thoracic aorta. The second stage is done through a left thoracotomy at a separate setting. The challenge with this technique is the mortality from each procedure alone, and the substantial number of patients who are unable to return for the second stage because of morbidity sustained during the first one. Safi and colleagues reported a 9% mortality rate for the first stage and 10% mortality rate in the second stage, with just over one-half of their 218 patients able to undergo both stages.[12,19] Similarly, the Cleveland Clinic group reported mortality rates of 2% for the first stage, 4% for the second stage, and a 12% interval mortality rate between the two stages. Over 40% of patients did not undergo the second operation.[12,20] These data have led vascular surgeons to utilize hybrid techniques for repair. The most common strategy is for patients to undergo ascending and arch repair with an elephant trunk procedure, followed by repair of the remaining aneurysmal aorta repair by endovascular means. The reverse and frozen elephant trunk techniques involve placement of an endovascular thoracic stent graft at, or proximal to, the left subclavian artery, with subsequent open repair of the ascending aorta and arch. The aortic graft is sewn to the stent graft and native aorta. These techniques are generally used when the quality of the aortic tissue is not deemed sufficient to support a standard elephant trunk procedure. The reverse elephant trunk technique implies a two-stage operation, whereas the frozen elephant trunk technique combines both the procedures in a single stage.[12] The SATs are reconstructed separately, or with an aortic conduit manufactured with a pre-sewn trifurcated graft on it.[16,17]

Another form of hybrid repair can be utilized for patients with arch aneurysms, with or without distal extension into the thoracic or thoracoabdominal aorta. In these cases, the SATs are reconstructed from the ascending aorta as described for patients undergoing multiple SAT construction for occlusive disease. A conduit is sewn onto the limb originating from the ascending aorta, through which a stent graft can be delivered antegrade.[12,15,17] More often, the conduit serves for through-and-through wire access so that the stent graft can be accurately positioned into the proximal arch or ascending aorta (zone 0,1) from the femoral artery. Placement of clips or a radiopaque ring at the ascending aorta anastomosis facilitates proper positioning of the stent graft.[12] Figure 5-3 highlights one of the challenges with this approach. During our treatment of a patient with a distal arch and descending thoracic aortic aneurysm associated with chronic dissection, placement of the device into the proximal ascending aorta created a bird's beak between the device and the inner curve of the aorta. Even after placement of a second device in the more proximal ascending aorta, the abnormality remained. There was no room for additional extension of the endograft as it was near the origin of the SAT graft. Rather than place the patient on hypothermic circulatory arrest to replace the remaining short segment of ascending aorta, the device was circumferentially secured around the ascending aorta with interrupted pledgeted sutures using fluoroscopic guidance.

The midterm results of a transcontinental registry targeting landing zone 0 for endovascular repair of arch aneurysms combine with total SAT reconstructions recently was reported by Czerny et al.[16] Sixty-six patients were treated at five centers in the United States and Europe between 2003 and 2011. Mean patient age was 70 years. Atherosclerotic aneurysm was the indication for repair in 48 patients, penetrating ulcer in 6, and 11 had prior type A or B dissection. In 33 patients (50%), the aneurysm began in the proximal arch, and in 32 the aneurysm began either in the ascending aorta or in the distal arch. The aneurysms extended into the distal arch in 28 patients, the descending thoracic aorta in 25, and below that level in the remaining 13. Three surgical strategies were used to reconstruct the SATs, with extra-corporeal circulation utilized in 39% of cases. The most common SAT reconstruction was a bifurcated graft to the innominate and left common carotid arteries (40%). A triple-branch graft was used in 39%, and a single innominate limb with a sidearm to the carotid or subclavian arteries was used in 21%. Retrograde placement of the aortic stent graft through the femoral artery was used in 33 patients (50%), antegrade placement through the arch was used in 27 (41%), and the others were done from the iliac artery or infrarenal aorta. Staged procedures were done in 28 patients (42%). The in-hospital mortality rate was 9%, major stroke rate 5%, and paraplegia rate 3%. Over a median follow-up of 25 months, six patients had late endoleaks. One- and five-year aorta-related survival rates were 96% each, and the overall one- and five-year survival rates were 81% and 72%, respectively.

Bavaria and colleagues at the University of Pennsylvania have described three methods to reconstruct SATs during hybrid aortic arch repair.[17] The first group

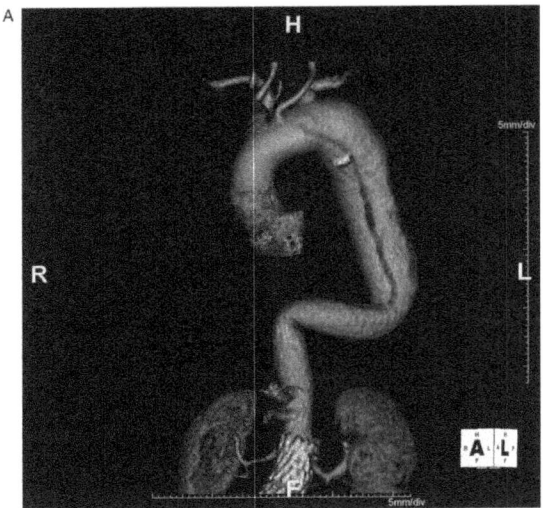

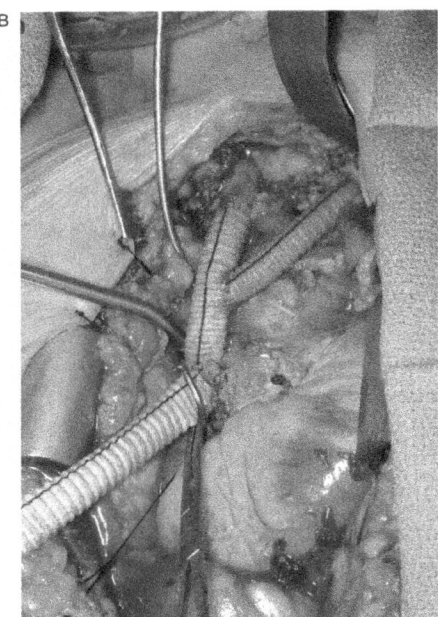

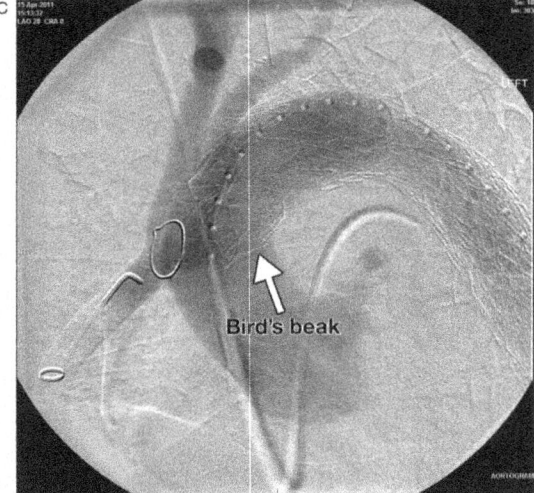

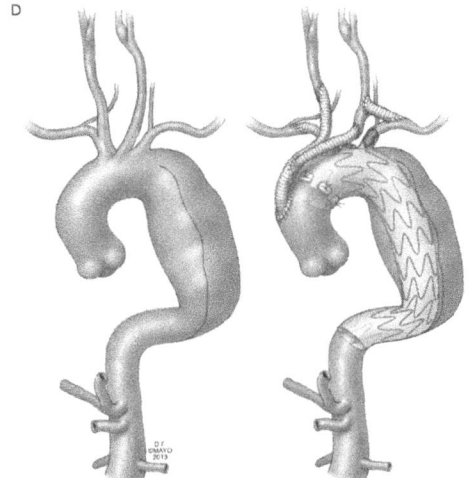

Figure 5-3. A patient with COPD and a 6 cm descending thoracic aortic aneurysm with chronic dissection (*A*). The upper extent of the aneurysm was just proximal to the left subclavian artery. He had a prior EVAR. He was not a candidate for an open repair, which would require cardiopulmonary bypass and a period of circulatory arrest to reconstruct the distal arch. He underwent staged reconstructions. The first operation was a left carotid to subclavian artery bypass. The second stage was a direct reconstruction of the carotid and right subclavian arteries from the ascending aorta, followed by endovascular repair of the aneurysm from the ascending to the lower descending thoracic aorta via a femoral approach utilizing a conduit on the aortic-origin graft (*B, C*). The proximal left subclavian artery was occluded with a plug. A bird's beak deformity occurred (*C*), so the endograft was circumferentially secured to the aortic wall with pledgeted sutures. Schematic representations are shown in *D*.

of patients have isolated arch aneurysms and good proximal landing zones in the ascending aorta and upper descending aorta. An innominate graft limb originates from the ascending aorta just above the sinotubular junction. Side arm grafts are used to reconstruct the other SATs. However, if the arch aneurysm extends into the ascending aorta so that an endograft cannot be safely placed without risking a retrograde type A dissection, the second method of reconstruction involves replacement of the ascending aorta, with the SAT graft originating from the aortic graft. These patients require cardiopulmonary bypass and may need a brief period of circulatory arrest. The authors recommend this type of repair if the ascending aorta exceeds 3.7 cm in diameter. The third type of reconstruction is for patients who require total open arch replacement with an elephant trunk. These individuals have SAT revascularization by separate grafts or with a trifurcated graft that has been pre-made onto an aortic graft.

Arch coarctation is rare, and the aortic and SAT reconstructions are done by pediatric cardiac surgeons. Recurrent coarctation in the adult is problematic and may require complex SAT revascularization, which involves the vascular surgeon. Figure 5-4 illustrates such a case in a young man who presented with a central retinal artery occlusion as a late complication from a prior arch coarctation repair at age 9 years. The original repair included an anterior routed ascending to descending aortic bypass through an anterior thoracotomy. Separate limbs had been used to reconstruct the right common carotid and left subclavian arteries, with those distal anastomoses done end-to-side. CT angiography at admission showed the old conduit to be calcified and stenotic, the carotid graft to have occluded, the left subclavian graft to be tightly stenotic, and the native innominate and left common carotid arteries to also be stenotic. The surgical challenge was to treat the coarctation and reconstruct the SATs while minimizing cerebral and cardiac malperfusion. We elected to do an ascending aorta to descending aortic bypass through the posterior pericardium to correct the coarctation and used the defect from the old proximal anastomotic site to originate the graft to reconstruct the great vessels. An 18- × 9-mm polyester graft was cut as a phlange so that the aortic defect was patched, and the 9-mm limb served as the right carotid bypass. A separate 8-mm limb was used to reconstruct the left subclavian in the supraclavicular fossa. The right subclavian and left common carotids were each reimplanted onto the graft limbs with a combination of running and interrupted suture. Cardiopulmonary bypass and a brief period of circulatory arrest were needed to perform the operation.

PROSTHETIC SUPRAAORTIC TRUNK GRAFT INFECTIONS OR TUMOR INVOLVEMENT

A dreaded complication of an aortic-origin SAT reconstruction is prosthetic graft infection. Treatment options in these cases are limited. Important decisions include in situ versus remote reconstruction and choice of conduit. Moreover, the presence of a pseudoaneurysm at the aortic anastomosis mandates redo sternotomy and possible cardiopulmonary bypass to avoid dehiscence and rupture as the sternum is reopened. The CT or MR scan defines the proximity of the aneurysm to the underside of the sternum. If the aneurysm is adherent to the sternum, cardiopulmonary bypass should be instituted through the femoral artery and vein before the sternum is opened. If a prosthetic graft infection involves a single limb to the innominate or left common carotid artery, remote reconstruction may be more

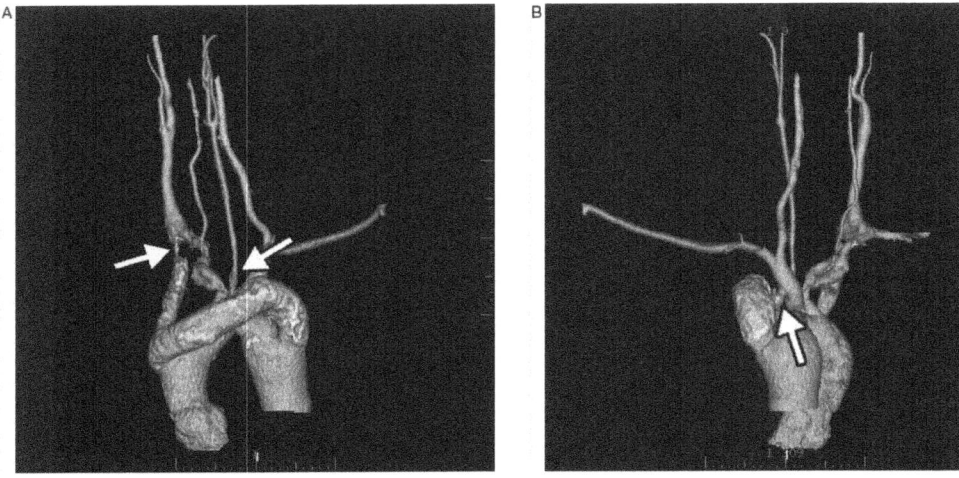

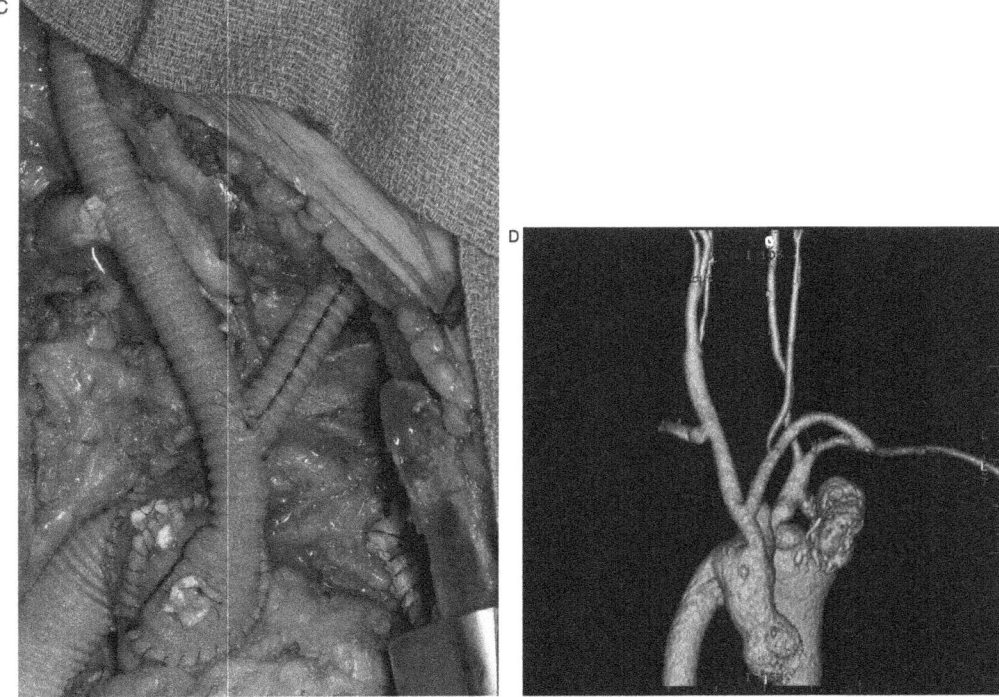

Figure 5-4. Patient with a central retinal artery occlusion as a late complication of prior aortic arch coarctation repair. The anterior and posterior CTA images (*A, B*) show the old conduit to be calcified and stenotic, the right common carotid graft to be occluded, and the left subclavian graft, native innominate and left common carotid arteries to be stenotic (arrows). Reconstruction was done with an ascending to descending aortic bypass. SAT reconstruction was done with grafts to the right common carotid and left subclavian arteries, with re-implantation of the right subclavian and left common carotid arteries onto the graft limbs (*C*). Postoperative CTA shows patent reconstructions (*D*).

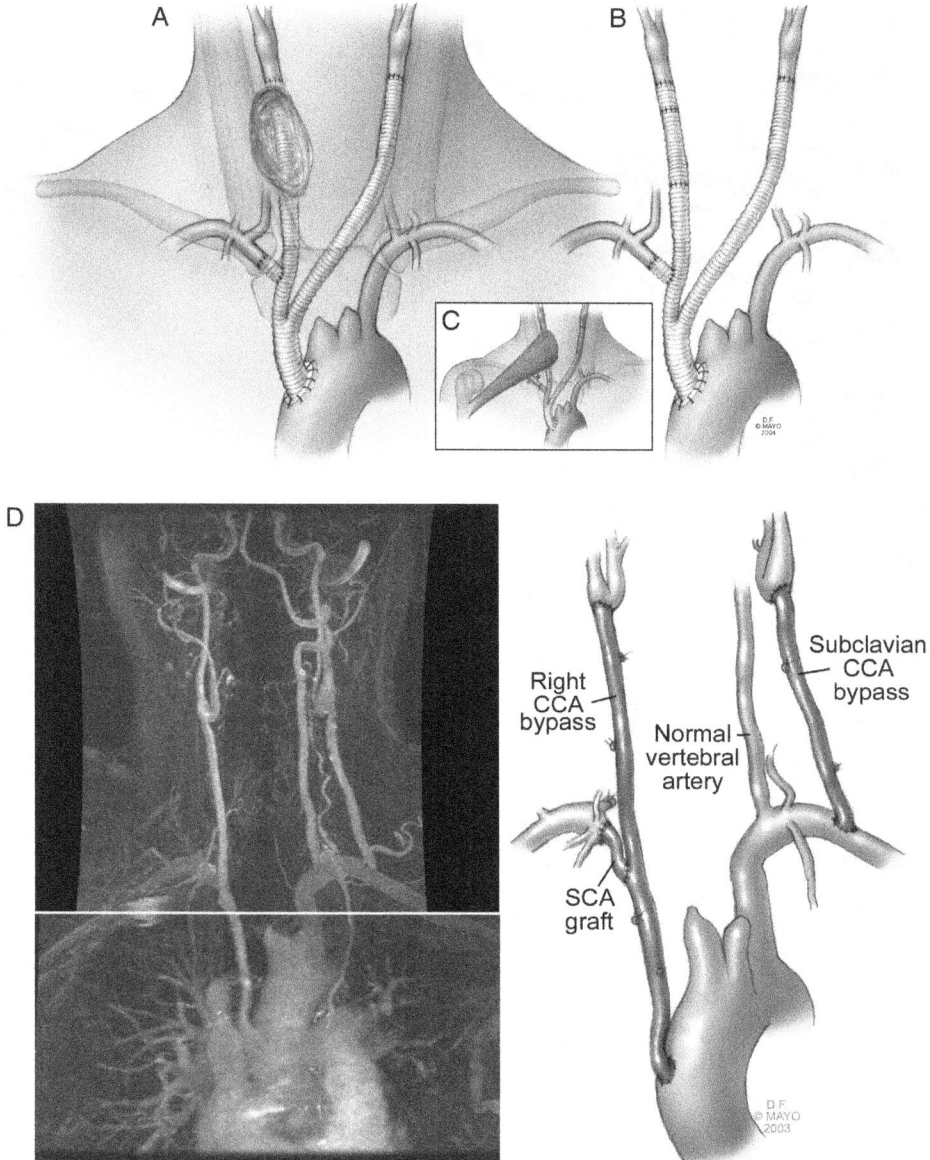

Figure 5-5. Patient with infection of an ascending aorto-bilateral distal carotid prosthetic bypass graft originally placed for Takayasu arteritis. Initially, the infection was isolated to the right neck. However, local reconstruction with an antibiotic-soaked interposition graft covered by a pectoralis major muscle flap failed (*A–C*). The patient returned with a mediastinal infection. The new arterial reconstruction was all done with superficial femoral artery. The left subclavian artery was free of disease. First, a left subclavian to carotid bifurcation bypass was done through a neck incision. There was no infection of the prosthetic here. The prosthetic graft was divided, oversewn, and pushed to the sternal notch. The neck incision and tunnel tract were closed. The sternum was re-opened. The infected prosthetic was resected, and the right carotid artery was reconstructed with an SFA graft from the ascending aorta. The right subclavian artery was re-implanted onto this graft. The pectoralis muscle was re-seated to cover the graft in the neck. A composite MRA picture at four-year follow-up and artistic rendition of the final reconstruction is shown in *D*.

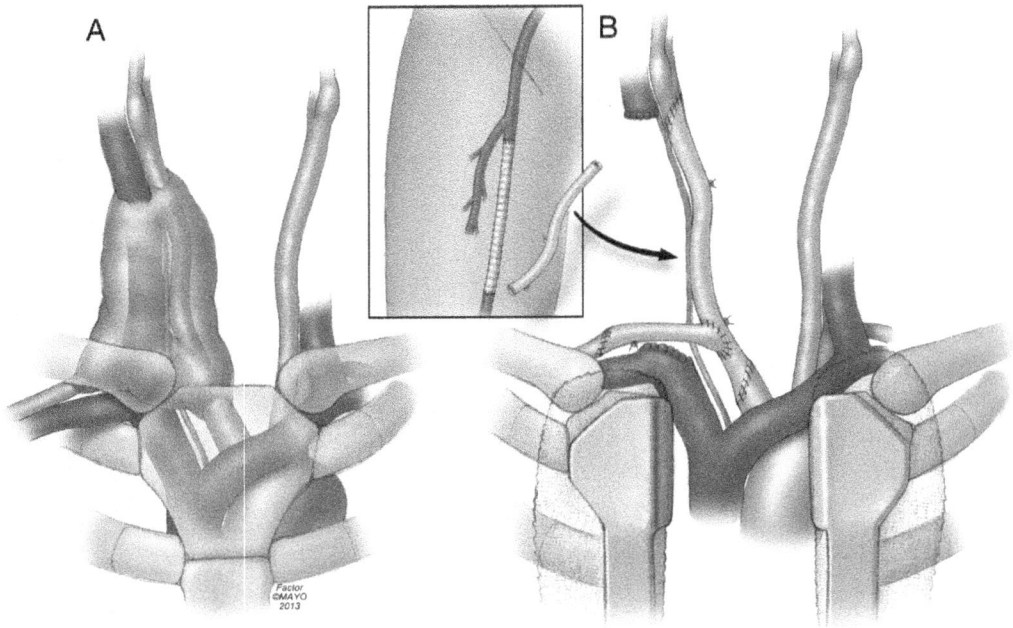

Figure 5-6. A young patient with an angiosarcoma that involved the innominate, right subclavian and cervical common carotid arteries, and the internal jugular vein (A). The tumor abutted the esophagus and trachea. The tumor was resected en bloc with the arteries, vein, and vagus nerve. The vertebral artery had been coil occluded before surgery. Arterial reconstruction was done with superficial femoral artery, and the SFA was replaced with an externally supported PTFE interposition graft (B).

applicable than a direct approach. Cervical debranching can be done before the infected conduit is removed. The ascending aorta requires a patch. Preparations should be made for cardiopulmonary bypass if there is extensive inflammation around the aortic graft anastomosis. In the case of infection of multiple SAT prosthetic graft limbs, in situ reconstruction is the only option.[21] Potential conduit includes superficial femoral artery, the native aortoiliac segment after it is replaced with prosthetic, homograft, or femoral or saphenous vein.[21–23] Antibiotic-impregnated polyester grafts have been used to treat low-grade bacterial abdominal aortic graft infections but have little utility in the mediastinum if there is an abscess or if the infection is secondary to methicillin-resistant *Staphylococcus aureus* or gram-negative species. Arterial conduits resist late aneurysmal degeneration better than vein grafts when they are sewn directly to the aorta.

We utilized superficial femoral artery to treat a patient with infection of an aortobilateral distal common carotid artery bypass graft originally placed for Takayasu arteritis (Fig. 5-5). Initially, the patient presented with a localized infection of the right limb of the graft in the neck. An attempt at local control of the infection failed, and the patient returned for more definitive treatment of a mediastinal abscess. We chose superficial femoral artery as the conduit because of the size match to the carotid arteries, the likelihood of better durability than a vein graft given the patient's young age, and because this conduit has successfully been used in contaminated fields for carotid artery replacement in patients with head and neck cancers treated by radiation therapy.[21]

It is rare that patients with malignancies in the mediastinum can be successfully treated with an R0 resection and great vessel reconstruction.[24] Reconstruction of the innominate veins or superior vena cava is more often possible than resection and replacement of the SATs. However, we have operated on a few patients with tumor involvement isolated to a single SAT or arteries on one side (Fig. 5-6). Reconstruction has been done with prosthetic or superficial femoral artery. Prosthetic works well when there is no violation of the aerodigestive tract and the risk of wound infection is low.[24] In irradiated fields, or those in which the tumor abuts or invades the esophagus or trachea, an arterial conduit is best.[23] In cases of malignancy involving the subclavian and vertebral arteries, a preoperative cerebral arteriogram with test balloon occlusion of the vertebral artery is done in advance of operation. If the intracranial circulation is intact, the contralateral vertebral artery is well developed, and there is no significant occlusive disease of the carotid arteries, the origin of the vertebral artery is occluded by coils within a day or two of surgery. This avoids the need for concomitant vertebral reconstruction, which would be done if a patient is intolerant of the test balloon occlusion or if the tumor involved the dominant vertebral artery.

SUMMARY

The most common indications for complex supraaortic trunk revascularization are symptomatic patients with multiple occlusive lesions, and those who require replacement of ascending aortic and arch aneurysms by open or hybrid techniques. Most patients have occlusive disease from atherosclerosis, Takayasu, or radiation arteritis. The most common presentations in these patients are thromboembolic complications or low flow states with global ischemia. Hybrid techniques to repair aneurysms of the aortic arch, with or without extent into the thoracic or thoracoabdominal aorta, seem to have improved outcomes compared to staged, open repairs. Aortic-based SAT reconstruction in any of these circumstances can be done safely with few graft-related complications. Rarely, patients require great vessel reconstruction for prosthetic graft infection or malignancy.

REFERENCES

1. Tracci MC, Cherry KJ. Surgical treatment of great vessel occlusive disease. *Surg Clin N Am.* 2009;89:821–836.
2. Bahnson HT. Consideration in the excision of aortic aneurysms. *Ann Surg.* 1953;138:377–386.
3. Davis JV, Grove WJ, Julian OC. Thrombic occlusion of branches of aortic arch. Martorell's syndrome: report of a case treated surgically. *Ann Surg.* 1956;144:124–126.
4. DeBakey, ME, Crawford ES, Cooley DA. Surgical considerations of occlusive disease of innominate, carotid, subclavian and vertebral arteries. *Ann Surg.* 1959;149:690–710.
5. Ehrenfeld WK, Chapman RD, Wylie EJ. Management of occlusive lesions of the branches of the aortic arch. *Am J Surg.* 1969;118:236–243.
6. Parrot JD. The subclavian steal syndrome. *Arch Surg.* 1969;88:661–665.
7. Diethrich EB, Garret H, Ameriso J, et al. Occlusive disease of the common carotid and subclavian arteries treated by carotid-subclavian bypass. Analysis of 125 cases. *Am J Surg.* 1967;114(5):800–808.

8. Rhodes JM, Cherry KJ Jr, Clark R, et al. Aortic-origin reconstruction of the great vessels; risk factors of early and late complications. *J Vasc Surg*. 2000;31(2):260–269.

9. Berguer R, Morasch MD, Kline RA. Transthoracic repair of innominate and common carotid artery disease: immediate and long-term outcome for 100 consecutive surgical reconstructions. *J Vasc Surg*. 1998;27(1):34–42.

10. Takach TJ, Reul GJ, Cooley DA, et al. Brachiocephalic reconstruction I: operative and long-term results for complex disease. *J Vasc Surg*. 2005;42:47–54.

11. Fields CF, Bower TC, Cooper LT, et al. Takayasu's arteritis: operative results and influence of disease activity. *J Vasc Surg*. 2006;43:64–71.

12. Oderich GS, Power AH. Hybrid repair of aortic arch aneurysms. In: Ascher E, et al., eds. *Haimovici's Vascular Surgery*, 6th ed. Hoboken and Chichester: Wiley-Blackwell; 2012:486–503.

13. Hassen-Khodja R, Kieffer E. Radiotherapy-induced supra-aortic trunk disease: early and long-term results of surgical and endovascular reconstruction. *J Vasc Surg*. 2004;40(2):254–261.

14. Takach TJ, Reul GJ, Duncan MD, et al. Concomitant brachiocephalic and coronary artery disease: outcome and decision analysis. *Ann Thorac Surg*. 2005;80:564–569.

15. Zhou W, Reardon M, Peden EK, et al. Hybrid approach to complex thoracic aortic aneurysms in high-risk patients: surgical challenges and clinical outcomes. *J Vasc Surg*. 2006;44(4):688–693.

16. Czerny M, Weigang E, Sodeck G, et al. Targeting landing zone 0 by total arch rerouting and TEVAR: midterm results of a transcontinental registry. *Ann Thorac Surg*. 2012;94:84–89.

17. Bavaria J, Vallabhajosyula P, Moeller P, et al. Hybrid approaches in the treatment of aortic arch aneurysms: postoperative and midterm outcomes. *J Thorac and Cardiovasc Surg*. 2013;145(3S):S85–S90.

18. Borst HG, Walterbusch G, Schaps D. Extensive aortic replacement using "elephant trunk" prostheses. *Thorac Cardiovasc Surg*. 1983;31(1):37–40.

19. Safi HJ, Miller CC 3rd, Estrera AL, et al. Staged repair of extensive aortic aneurysms: long term experience with the elephant trunk technique. *Ann Surg*. 2004;240(4):677–684.

20. Svensson LG, Kim KH, Blackstone EH, et al. Elephant trunk procedure: newer indications and uses. *Ann Thorac Surg*. 2004;78(1):109–116.

21. Fields CE, Bower TC. Use of superficial femoral artery to treat an infected great vessel prosthetic graft. *J Vasc Surg*. 2004;40(3):559–563.

22. Modrall JG, Joiner DR, Seidel SA, et al. Superficial femoral-popliteal vein as a conduit for brachiocephalic arterial reconstructions. *Ann Vasc Surg*. 2002;16:17–23.

23. Sessa CN, Morasch MD, Berguer R, et al. Carotid resection and replacement with autogenous arterial graft during operation for neck malignancy. *Ann Vasc Surg*. 1998;12:229–235.

24. Lee YS, Chung WY, Chang HS, Park CS. Treatment of locally advanced thyroid cancer invading the great vessels using a Y-shaped graft bypass. *Interactive Cardiovasc and Thorac Surg*. 2010;10:1039–1041.

Current Issues in Vascular Surgery

6

The Future of Vascular Surgery

Natalia Glebova, MD, PhD and Julie Freischlag, MD

We envision the future of vascular surgery as one of vast advances in patient care tempered by constraints of finances and resources. We will witness the development of exciting new technology, progress in basic and clinical research, and improvements in and streamlining of training. These advances will happen at a time of increasing concerns regarding delivery of affordable quality care and escalating financial regulation. As vascular surgeons, our goal will be to provide the best patient care with the available resources.

THE FUTURE OF PATIENT CARE

The future of patient care is one of collaboration and accountability. Vascular surgeons have a unique opportunity to be leaders in multidisciplinary patient care. Our patients have many comorbidities that contribute to the development and progression of vascular disease. Treating vascular disease without addressing diabetes, hypertension, hyperlipidemia, coronary artery disease, and smoking will invariably result in the need for further treatment. Evidence exists that collaboration between specialists in the management of these conditions leads to better patient care. For example, in Australia an Enhanced Primary Care (EPC) package was introduced in 1999 to promote the development of multidisciplinary healthcare plans. Retrospective analysis of the impact of this approach on the care of patients with diabetes shows that multidisciplinary care results in improved patient outcomes as reflected by several measured variables, including hemoglobin A1C.[1] Collaboration between podiatrists and vascular surgeons has also been shown to lead to better outcomes in limb salvage in diabetic patients.[2] Multidisciplinary diabetes care clinics, cardiovascular institutes, and other similar combined programs hold the promise of improving the care of vascular patients.

Advancements in patient care also hinge on evidence-based innovations in medical treatment. As vascular surgeons, we have a strong history of high-quality clinical research performed to guide our practice. In addition to generating many prospective randomized clinical trials, we as a group have established an initiative to improve patient care. The Society of Vascular Surgery Vascular Quality Initiative (VQI) is organized around regional quality groups.[3] It aims to improve the quality, safety, effectiveness, and cost of vascular health care. On the basis of a regional program developed in New England, this is a database of patient information that can be used for retrospective analysis of patient data with the goal of improving vascular surgical practice.[4] One hopes that in addition to advancing patient care, these research efforts will lead to more cost-effective treatments and positively contribute to healthcare reform. Such clinical outcomes research will also help us make better decisions for our patients in terms of the risks and benefits of our interventions.

THE FUTURE OF TRAINING

As healthcare and patient population change and as information and technology progress rapidly, the training of future vascular surgeons must evolve. Recently introduced integrated vascular surgery training programs have risen to the challenge of declining recruitment by offering more intense and less protracted training. These programs have attracted excellent applicants[5] and at least in surveys of trainees appear to provide equivalent if not superior vascular education as compared to traditional vascular fellowships.[6] Future developments in vascular surgeon training may involve early specialization of general surgery trainees,[7] as well as more use of simulation to supplement training.[8] Better education of our trainees also needs to include noninterventional skills including medication and diet management, lifestyle modification, image requesting and interpretation, and coordination of care.

THE FUTURE OF RESEARCH

From clinical trials to bench science, the future of research in vascular medicine and surgery is limitless. For example, controversies in the management of asymptomatic carotid artery disease will be addressed by trials such as Carotid Revascularization Endarterectomy versus Stent (CREST)-2 trial, which compares best medical management with carotid revascularization in asymptomatic patients. Translational research in the stem cell field promises the potential of treatment of critical limb ischemia with bone marrow stem cell therapy,[9] as well as for development of bioengineered tissues and organs for use in surgical treatment of vascular disease.[10] Advances in genomic research will lead to better understanding of mechanisms of development of vascular disease[11] and result in advances in its treatment.[12] This progress is tempered but one hopes not impeded by financial constraints. And in this age of international collaborations, research made more efficient by combining resources promises to lead to more shared knowledge and discoveries.[13]

THE FUTURE OF TECHNOLOGY

Technology research is rapidly leading to new discoveries and innovations in device development. Some examples of recent innovations include new types of endograft devices and peripheral arterial stents. The emergence of fenestrated devices is expanding the use of endovascular technology for the treatment of aneurysms. These endografts are used more and more for repair of juxtarenal abdominal and thoracoabdominal aneurysms.[14] Investigation into the outcomes and durability of these devices as compared to traditional open repair will help determine their applications in patient care. In peripheral arterial disease, the introduction of drug-eluting stents in treatment of infrapopliteal arterial occlusive disease holds promise for less restenosis and better durability based on randomized clinical trials.[15] Carotid stenting is entering into wider use,[16] but remains somewhat controversial when compared to carotid endarterectomy.[17] As more devices and treatments are developed, effective comparison research will help determine whether these new approaches are superior to established therapies.

The future of communication technology is seemingly unlimited. Social media, defined as forms of electronic communication through which people interact to create online communities to share information, hold promise to improve patient–physician communication. One must be mindful of the limitations on the use of social media in light of patient privacy concerns. Nevertheless, advancements in social media hold excellent potential for use in educating patients, developing and recruiting participants in clinical trials, and collaborating across institutions and countries.[18]

CONCLUSION

The future of vascular surgery is one of innovation in technology, research, education, and patient care. With confidence, we will continue to develop and advocate for our field and to provide the best care for our patients through interventions, medical management, and coordination of care. In the face of healthcare reform, we must keep discovery and innovation as part of our core values to ensure better care for our patients in the future.

REFERENCES

1. Zwar NA, Hermiz O, Comino E, et al. Do multidisciplinary care plans result in better care for patients with type II diabetes? *Aust Fam Phys*. 2007; 36(1/2):85–89.
2. Armstrong DG, Bharara M, White M, et al. The impact and outcomes of establishing an integrated interdisciplinary surgical team to care for the diabetic foot. *Diabetes Metab Res Rev*. 2012; 28:514–518.
3. Woo K, Eldrup-Jorgensen J, Hallett JW, et al. Regional quality groups in the Society for Vascular Surgery Vascular Quality Initiative. *J Vasc Surg*. 2013; 57:884–890.
4. Cronenwett JL, Kraiss LW, Cambria RP. The Society for Vascular Surgery Vascular Quality Initiative. *J Vasc Surg*. 2012; 55:1529–1537.
5. Zayed MA, Dalman RL, Lee JT. A comparison of 0+5 versus 5+2 applicants to vascular surgery training programs. *J Vasc Surg*. 2012; 56(5):1448–1452.
6. Dalsing MC, Makaroun MS, Harris LM, et al. Association of Program Directors in Vascular Surgery (APDVS) survey of program selection, knowledge acquisition, and education provided as viewed by vascular trainees from two different training paradigms. *J Vasc Surg*. 2012; 55(2):589–597.
7. Bass BL. Early specialization in surgical training: an old concept whose time has come? *Sem Vasc Surg*. 2006; 19(4):214–217.
8. Duran C, Bismuth J, Mitchell E. A nationwide survey of vascular surgery trainees reveals trends in operative experience, confidence, and attitudes about simulation. *J Vasc Surg*. 2013; 58(2):524–528.

9. Raval Z, Losordo DW. Cell therapy of peripheral arterial disease: from experimental findings to clinical trials. *Circ Res.* 2013; 112(9):1288–1302.

10. Bajpai VK, Mistriotis P, Loh Y-H, et al. Functional smooth muscle cells derived from human induced pluripotent stem cells via mesenchymal stem cell intermediates. *Cardiovasc Res.* 2012; 96(3):391–400.

11. Goldschmidt-Clermont PJ, Dong C, Seo DM, Velazquez OC. Atherosclerosis, inflammation, genetics, and stem cells: 2012 update. *Curr Atheroscler Rep.* 2012; 14(3):201–210.

12. Johnson JA, Cavallari LH. Pharmacogenetics and cardiovascular disease – implications for personalized medicine. *Pharmacol Rev.* 2013; 65(3):987–1009.

13. Adams J. Collaborations: the fourth age of research. *Nature.* 2013;497; 557–560.

14. Quinones-Baldrich WJ, Holden A, Mertens R, et al. Prospective, multicenter experience with the Ventana Fenestrated System for juxtarenal and pararenal aortic aneurysm endovascular repair. *J Vasc Surg.* 2013; 58(1):1–9.

15. Bosiers, M., Scheinert D, Peeters P, et al. Randomized comparison of everolimus-eluting versus bare-metal stents in patients with critical limb ischemia and infrapopliteal arterial occlusive disease. *J Vasc Surg.* 2012; 55(2):390–398.

16. Brott TG, Hobson RW, Roubin GS, et al. Stenting versus endarterectomy for treatment of carotid artery stenosis. *N Engl J Med.* 2010; 3636:11–23.

17. Davis SM, Donnan GA. Carotid artery stenting in stroke prevention. *N Engl J Med.* 2010; 363:80–82.

18. Indes JE, Gates L, Mitchell EL, Mush BE. Social media in vascular surgery. *J Vasc Surg.* 2013; 57:1159–1162.

7

Emotional Intelligence: Can It Enhance Your Personal and Professional Life?

Bruce L. Gewertz, MD

Irrespective of our life paths, the ability to initiate and sustain effective interactions with others is a key determinant of personal and professional success. This is particularly true for physicians who often find themselves in a wide variety of informal and formal leadership roles—in medical systems, clinics, and operating theatres. Furthermore, the stress and long hours involved in medical practice frequently put an additional burden on our personal relationships with family and friends. Successfully navigating these challenges requires a level of insight into our behaviors and the behaviors of others.

THE SCOPE OF EMOTIONAL INTELLIGENCE

The term "emotional intelligence" (EI) has been advanced to describe the set of personal attributes that enhance social and professional relationships. As developed by Goleman and others, the elements of EI encompass the full range of interactions between individuals and society including self-awareness, social awareness, self-regulation, and relationship management.[1,2]

Of these, the key constituents of EI are self-assessment and empathy. Most workers in the field believe that EI is not static but a set of skills that can be learned with commitment and behavioral modeling.[3]

Some practical aspects of each category are listed in the following text.

Self-awareness
  accurate self-assessment
  self-confidence
Social awareness
  empathy
  service orientation
  organizational insight

Self-regulation
  emotional control
  trustworthiness
  adaptability
  initiative
Relationship management
  communication
  conflict management
  teamwork

The increased interest in EI is supported by a growing compilation of data that demonstrate that enhanced social interactions improve personal performance in a wide range of settings. Boyatzis studied 2000 supervisors and executives and found that 14 of 16 distinguishing traits for success were emotional not cognitive.[4] Spencer and Spencer defined job competencies in 286 organizations and noted that 18 of 21 competencies associated with high performance were emotionally based.[5] Comparing "star" performers to average performers in diverse industries, Goleman found that emotional advantages were noted twice as frequently in high performers and were a much better predictor of achievement than cognitive superiority.[6]

EMOTIONAL INTELLIGENCE IN MEDICAL PRACTICE AND LEADERSHIP ROLES

Although having greater insight into one's feelings could be expected to correlate with success in leading others, supportive data in the medical field are not robust. That said, one could easily argue that the need for such informed and consistent leadership has never been greater. There is recent information that would argue that physicians are experiencing considerable emotional stress due to a host of financial and other pressures that are dramatically changing both the practice of medicine and how doctors perceive their role in society. A survey of 1951 full-time physicians and scientists from four geographically separated medical schools noted that 20% had significant depressive symptoms.[7] Depression and anxiety scores were higher in young physicians (<35 years of age) than in their more senior colleagues. Relevant to this discussion, the very highest depression and anxiety levels were noted in surgeons; the lowest scores were recorded in emergency medicine physicians who had high acuity challenges but "controllable lifestyles." This suggests that the context in which the stress occurs (e.g., the degree of personalization, total work hours) has more to do with adverse emotional effects than the level of stress itself.

It would be comforting to think that physician leaders, who are generally selected for both academic achievement and positive personal characteristics, might have better coping mechanisms and thus be well acquitted to serve as role models for their younger colleagues. Gabbe et al. surveyed 131 chairs of obstetrics and gynecology, achieving a 91% response rate.[8] A surprising 88% of chairs experienced moderate to severe "burnout" as measured by a standard inventory (MBI-HSS), which quantitated emotional exhaustion, depersonalization, self-efficacy, and personal achievement. The principle drivers of burnout were global and local financial pressures, Medicare audits, and hospital down-sizing not the traditional intramural academic conflicts of past times. The incidence of burnout did not correlate with experience or length of tenure as a leader.

As a rule, these most troubling problems had a single unifying theme—they were not directly controllable by the chairs. Dealing with them without undue personal strain would require a level of detachment coupled with strategic planning. For whatever reason, many of these experienced leaders were unable to maintain personal equanimity under these circumstances. One could reasonably conclude that the chairs' efficacy as role models for their junior faculty likely suffered in parallel.

It is clear that in such times of transition and challenge, optimal leadership is needed. What is less well defined is the specific actions that can improve the skill sets of modern surgical leaders and enhance their abilities to counsel and motivate their colleagues.

Although it is obvious that developing an improved understanding of one's emotions is the ideal first step in this process, achieving personal insight is often difficult. In designing a recent study of 43 highly successful business leaders, Bennis and Thomas postulated that the "more modern" leader would have fundamentally different skills and tactics than CEOs of a more traditional era.[9] In fact, their subsequent research demonstrated that the views of both sets of leaders were remarkably similar. One common experience was particularly revealing. A majority of those interviewed described an unplanned and usually traumatic incident in mid-life that caused them to reformat their personal views of achievement and develop a higher level of empathy for others. In nearly every instance, they credited this specific response for their improved leadership performance.

Certainly today's surgical leaders do not lack for such "learning opportunities." The challenge is using the experiences to grow rather than becoming frustrated. Since it is difficult to dispassionately analyze personal reactions during trying times, useful information can often be gained from the reactions of others experiencing the same environment. The further benefit is utilizing the information to better understand and address the dissatisfactions of the larger group.

At the University of Chicago, we were fortunate to collaborate on these issues with Harry Davis, professor in the Graduate School of Business. Professor Davis interviewed a representative group of faculty with different professorial ranks and areas of interest. On the basis of their detailed comments, he detected two distinctly different views of their professional situations that were, paradoxically, often expressed concurrently.

The first viewpoint could be characterized as the "half-full" glass. Physicians expressed pride in the mission of the department and university and general satisfaction in the degree of autonomy they enjoyed. They took pleasure in their achievements in the full range of academic activities including teaching, clinical care, and research. That said, the same individuals expressed considerable frustration in other elements of their job (the "half-empty" glass). They spoke of unity gained only through identification of "common enemies" such as hospital and university administrative restrictions. They bemoaned what they perceived as a "culture of expendability." They felt their value to the enterprise was real but transient and often felt that their contributions would soon be forgotten when they left. Finally, many described negative and unsettled feelings best described as "shattered dreams." Their expectations of a career in surgery were falling short due to the changes in reimbursement rates, malpractice expenses, and the unrelenting demand for clinical productivity. It was repeatedly stated that this emphasis on clinical volume made academic work only a secondary product. It was particularly revealing that despite their candor in all areas, dissatisfaction with compensation *per se* was not a prevalent complaint.

Our department leadership was impressed with the dichotomy of views. Most importantly, for perhaps the first time, we acknowledged the same feelings within ourselves. We discussed the findings with the entire faculty (and later the house staff) and focused on what specific steps we all could take to address the issues. Although our progress in these efforts has been, at times, tempered by reality, there has been considerable value to the open communication and frankness.

The information gained from the process continues to be relevant to my work with physicians. For the first few years, I kept a list of their underlying concerns on my desk. I am continually reminded of the legitimacy of the observations by how frequently specific complaints and behaviors by individual faculty can be directly traced back to the underlying "emotional" issues that were identified by Professor Davis. Addressing these deeper and highly personal concerns, not just the operational manifestations of those issues, often leads to more lasting solutions.

As just one example, these insights have been useful in assisting the "difficult" physician who disparages and turns over associates repeatedly. These poor working relationships were rarely the result of the skill level of the new colleague. Far more often they reflected some other issue entirely, such as the senior surgeon's discontent over perceived status in the organization. Although it was rarely easy to initiate, a frank discussion that identified the key driver and addressed it has been a far more efficient tact than recycling yet another young physician into an adverse environment. In addition to exploring the obvious (i.e., what the senior physicians could do to improve the comfort and performance level of their juniors), on a number of occasions deeper personal insight was gained. Quiet often, this self-knowledge translated to more collegial behavior in other areas.

Such successful "teaching" of EI requires an immediate and real-life context to both stimulate and reward skill acquisition. Personal insight is an important element, but it is useful to remember that efforts are most effective when directed toward modification of *behavior* not *personality*. The goal is a practical one—minimization of poor personal interactions by recognition and self-correction of nonproductive behavior. Although motivated learners can occasionally gain these skills by self-study, the presence of role models and mentors can greatly facilitate the process. As a consequence, surgical leaders must always be aware that their personal conduct and equanimity sends a strong signal to the entire group.

OPTIMISM

One of the key messages successful physician leaders must embody is optimism. For most surgeons in a clinical role, this should come easily. We all have had experience with patients who "feed off" our confidence, often demonstrating accelerated recoveries when they believe an operation has been successful. As well, a surgeon who does not demonstrate confidence is unlikely to garner much of a referral base and for good reason. Analogous to the aviation industry, no one wants to hear their airline pilot saying "I really hope I will be able to land this plane in Chicago."

There is some evidence that optimism has measurable physiologic consequences. In a now famous study of 941 people aged 65–85 years, Giltay and colleagues assessed cardiovascular and other risk factors and used a detailed questionnaire to separate the subjects into quartiles based on their disposition (optimistic vs pessimistic).[10]

Even after appropriate stratification for health measures, mortality over 9 years of observation was highly correlated with the degree of optimism. For example, 70% of the most optimistic men lived 9 years, whereas only 40% of the least optimistic survived the same interval.

Further support for this effect is provided by data from the so-called Nun study, most recently analyzed by Dunner et al.[11] Investigators had access to handwritten autobiographies of 180 nuns prepared when they entered their convents beginning in 1930. Entries were blindly coded for emotional content (i.e., positive, neutral, or negative in tone). All cause mortality was tracked late in their lives over a 10-year period. A positive attitude, expressed early in life, was a clear marker for greater longevity. Taken together, these studies strongly suggest that optimism and positivity have measurable physiologic benefits and likely reflect "hard wired" personal characteristics evident early in life.

THE CONCEPT OF "FLOW"

In addition to maintaining an optimistic attitude, enhanced EI necessarily includes the self-regulation of constructing a work and life environment that allows us to focus on the things that we consider important and fulfilling while limiting, as much as feasible, those tasks that are less rewarding. One of the most obvious issues to address might be the hectic pace of life in general and especially that associated with the delivery of health care.

In most surveys of full-time workers in the western world, those in the United Kingdom and United States work the longest hours by far. In 2002, one study documented that the US workers exceeded the hours worked by those in Europe by 25% with mean hours of 2000 per year (about 40 hours per week) in comparison with 1700 per year (about 30 hours per week).[12] I think we might agree that we know few surgeons—residents or attendings—who wouldn't exceed those numbers substantially. The Pew studies show conclusively that a hectic pace, associated with long hours and overlapping activities, clearly and adversely impacts personal satisfaction. In their most recent survey, only 27% of people who felt they were always rushed in daily life described themselves as "very happy" as compared to 42% who almost never felt rushed.[13]

In one sense, this feeling of "rushing around," which could be defined as urgency without importance, is unfortunately the single defining characteristic of many of our lives. Whether we are frantically thumbing our digital devices or mesmerized by CNN, I would argue that we too often spend our time on details and urgencies that lack much meaning.

To address this trap, my former University of Chicago colleague and prominent psychologist, Mihaly Csikszentmihalyi described a more purposeful ideal for our lifestyle, which he calls "flow."[14] Flow is characterized by complete immersion in a complex activity that is intrinsically motivated by our own talents and interests. The initial observations of this phenomenon were made in surgeons, athletes, and musicians who train for years to reach the high level of skill necessary for superior performance. In detailed interviews, all described a similar sense of clarity, serenity, and even ecstasy when purposefully engaged in the most challenging and difficult activities. Although flow shares some surface characteristics with other urgent tasks, it is elevated by the matching of hard-won skills and innate talents with a meaningful and noble purpose.

Csikszentmihalyi argues that true happiness is found in those who can find a way to maximize the time they are "in flow" in their personal and professional lives.

CONCLUSION

In the highly demanding environment of modern medical practice, positive interpersonal interactions are necessary to optimize clinical and academic productivity. Searching for a better understanding of others has the additional value of enhancing insights into our own actions and reactions, improving personal satisfaction. As the value of EI becomes even more evident, it is quite likely that more formal assessments of these skills will be used in selecting and training the surgical leaders of tomorrow.

REFERENCES

1. Goleman D. *Emotional Intelligence*. New York, NY: Bantam Books; 1995.
2. Mayer JD, Caruso D, Salovey P. Emotional intelligence meets traditional standards for an intelligence. *Intelligence*. 2000;27:267–298.
3. Taylor GJ, Parker JD, Bagby RM. Emotional intelligence and the emotional brain: points of convergence and implications for psychoanalysis. *J Am Acad Psychoanal*. 1999;27:339–354.
4. Boyatzis R. *The Competent Manager: A Model for Effective Performance*. New York, NY: John Wiley and Sons; 1982.
5. Spencer L, Spencer S. *Competence at Work*. New York, NY: John Wiley and Sons; 1993.
6. Goleman D. What makes a leader? *Harv Bus Rev*. 1998;76:62–93.
7. Schindler BA, Novack DH, Cohen DG, et al. The impact of the changing health care environment on the health and well-being of faculty at four medical schools. *Acad Med*. 2006;81:27–34.
8. Gabbe SG, Melville J, Mandel L, Walker E. Burnout in chairs of obstetrics and gynecology: diagnosis, treatment, and prevention. *Am J Obstet Gynecol*. 2002;186:601–612.
9. Bennis WG, Thomas RJ. Crucibles of leadership. *Harv Bus Rev*. 2002;80:39–45.
10. Giltay EJ, Geleijnse JM, Zitman FG, et al. Dispositional optimism and all-cause and cardiovascular mortality in a prospective cohort of elderly Dutch men and women. *Arch Gen Psychiatry*. 2004;61(11):1126–1135.
11. Dunner DD, Snowdon DA, Friesen WV. Positive emotions and longevity. *J Pers Soc Psych*. 2001;80:804–813.
12. Organisation for Economic Co-Operation and Development. *OECD Employment Outlook*. Paris: OECD; 2003:322.
13. Taylor P, Funk C, Craighill P. *Are We Happy Yet?* Washington, DC: Pew Research Center; 2006.
14. Csikszentmihalyi M. *Flow: The Psychology of Optimal Experience*. New York, NY: Harper & Row; 1990.

8

Top 10 Coding Tips

Sean P. Roddy, MD and Elizabeth L. Detschelt, MD

INTRODUCTION

Though patient care and quality outcomes are of highest importance, the process by which care is rendered must continuously be evaluated to optimize billing, coding, and, ultimately, reimbursement. A claim is generated when a diagnosis code is paired to a procedure code, and up to three modifiers are added. That claim is then submitted to an insurance carrier for payment, usually electronically. This chapter will describe coding tips identified through the Society for Vascular Surgery's coding course, discussion with other specialty societies on coding issues, and interaction with both governmental and private insurance carriers with regard to coverage determinations. They are presented in no particular order of importance. As always, please consult your local carriers for specific details on claim submission.

INVEST IN "SCRUBBING" SOFTWARE

Every physician office generates claims that will be submitted to the insurance carrier. The diagnosis code comes from the ninth edition of the *International Classification of Diseases Manual* (ICD-9) and the procedure codes come from the fourth edition of the *Current Procedural Terminology Manual* (CPT-4). When a claim is sent off to the insurance carrier, the insurance carrier will evaluate it for appropriateness. This is called "scrubbing" a claim. If the claim passes the insurance carrier's evaluation, payment is remitted. If there is something abnormal about the claim, it is rejected, and this requires further evaluation and possibly appeal by the provider. When the claims are entered in a physician office, this is termed "charge entry." Charge entry has potential for typographical errors as support staff enters data into the computer system or diagnoses for procedures may be chosen that are not appropriate from a medical necessity standpoint. Each of these inaccuracies can cause the claim to be rejected. If a physician practice has scrubbing software, the claims will be held if an error is detected. The first time a claim is submitted is the highest chance that it will ever be paid. With subsequent appeals, the chance of the physician practice ever seeing reimbursement goes down precipitously. In addition, appeals require the physician practice to pay for the staff's time and efforts to achieve remuneration. The billing software can be customized to ensure errors are identified before submissions. This includes both governmental and private carrier policies. Medicare has several levels of software scrubbing. There are national correct coding initiative edits, medical unlikely edits, local coverage determination medical necessity edits, and so forth. These as well as individual private carrier policies can be programmed to ensure that typographical errors are corrected to maximize reimbursement efforts; investment in scrubbing software more than pays for itself in the long term.

DO NOT IGNORE CLAIM REJECTIONS

Claims may be rejected for several reasons. The billing office in each physician practice should not ignore these claim rejections. Unfortunately, many believe that the emphasis should be placed on entering new claims and paying little to no attention to rejections. Claim denials should be analyzed for patterns. Such an analysis may reveal helpful information for future claim submission.

In some instances, the timeliness of the filing of the claim can be the culprit. Each insurance carrier requires that claims be submitted within a certain amount of time from the date of service. This can range from three months all the way to one year. In addition, when claims are rejected, there is a limited time period in which to appeal (e.g., with supporting documentation such as medical records). Either of these scenarios can result in denial for "timely filing." Once denied on these grounds, a claim will never receive reimbursement. Identifying this as the reason for claim denial can easily prevent future denials of the same kind.

Alternatively, analysis of rejected claims may reveal specific diagnoses that are not deemed medically appropriate for reimbursement. This is common at the local or regional level with vascular lab medical necessity policies.

Rarely, claim denial may reflect a larger issue. A recent national issue was identified whereby all bilateral diagnostic catheter-based selective carotid angiography claims were rejected. In the 2013 Medicare Physician Fee Schedule, an indicator is required after each CPT code to allow use of the -50 (bilateral) modifier. That indicator was incorrect for the selective carotid angiography claims (CPT codes 36222 through 36228), thus resulting in the rejections. The Society for Vascular Surgery and the American College of Radiology identified this issue. A letter was sent to the medical directors at the Centers for Medicare and Medicaid Services (CMS). They evaluated the issue and agreed. On April 1, 2013, the update sent to the local carriers for Medicare changed that indicator. This was retroactive through January 1, 2013 and was released as a CMS transmittal (http://cms.hhs.gov/Regulations-and-Guidance/Guidance/Transmittals/Downloads/R2677CP.pdf).

UNDERSTAND THE NUANCES OF IMAGING DONE BEFORE, DURING, AND AFTER OPEN REVASCULARIZATION

Completion angiography after open surgical revascularization is a bundled service. The introductory wording at the beginning of the "Arteries and Veins" section of the CPT manual states *"also included is that portion of the operative arteriogram performed by the surgeon, as indicated."* However, diagnostic angiography performed in the operating room or the angiography suite prior to open surgical revascularization is appropriate to bill if it fulfills specific criteria. To meet criteria for reimbursement, the operative report must state (1) that no prior catheter-based angiographic study is available, (2) that a full diagnostic study is performed, and (3) that the decision to intervene is based on the present diagnostic study. The CPT codes associated with catheterization and/or diagnostic imaging would require the 59 modifier, which certifies this as preoperative as opposed to postoperative and assumes that the dictation clearly outlines the three aforementioned criteria.

Intraoperative completion Duplex ultrasound evaluation of an arterial reconstruction after bypass grafting may be separately reportable. This is based on the current wording in the CPT manual and current National Correct Coding Initiative edits. For example, a lower extremity bypass is performed from the femoral artery to the popliteal artery. The completion Duplex scan is performed, and an ultrasound interpretation is placed in the patient's medical record. CPT code 93926 describes a lower extremity arterial unilateral or limited study. Provided all requirements for the code were fulfilled, this would be submitted with a -26 modifier (the professional fee and NOT the technical fee) since the hospital owns the equipment. A permanent copy of the ultrasound images would be required in the patient's medical record.

UNDERSTAND CPT CODE DEFINITIONS

There are multiple procedures in the CPT manual where two different CPT codes describe the same service. In that setting, it is important to understand the definition of each CPT code and what the options are for appropriate billing and reimbursement. For example, elective open surgical repair of a popliteal artery aneurysm is described by CPT code 35151. This has been assigned 38.22 total relative value units (RVUs) in the 2013 Medicare Physician Fee Schedule, which is substantially less than most limb salvage open surgical arterial reconstruction procedures. An alternative situation would be where a patient presents with a popliteal artery aneurysm that has thrombosed resulting in a limb-threatening acute arterial occlusion. To treat this latter situation, a patient may require a femoral to peroneal artery in situ bypass graft. This would be described by CPT code 35585 that has been assigned 51.61 total RVUs in the 2013 Medicare Physician Fee Schedule. When a popliteal artery aneurysm undergoes open reconstruction, CPT code 35151 is most appropriate and CPT code 35585 is not correct. When the aneurysm is occluded and the bypass is done for limb salvage, CPT code 35585 is appropriate and CPT code 35151 is not correct. This makes sense because there is a huge difference in the planning, the operation time and intensity, and the postoperative care between an elective popliteal artery aneurysm repair and the urgent in situ bypass for critical limb ischemia. The additional 13.39 RVUs compensate the physician. A lack of knowledge of these code definitions could result in significant financial loss to the provider if they were unaware of such a difference.

Not all aortic surgery is the same. Some abdominal aortic aneurysms are repaired with a tube graft, while others necessitate a bifurcated repair. Sometimes the aneurysm encroaches upon the renal arteries requiring a suprarenal clamp. Finally, patients may have occlusive disease that requires an aortobifemoral bypass. All these procedures have different CPT codes. A patient's surgical reconstruction may be performed for aneurysm, in which case the appropriate aortic aneurysm repair code should be

TABLE 8-1. COMPARISON OF ELECTIVE AND EMERGENT CPT CODES AND RVUS FOR AAA REPAIR

Procedure	CPT Code	Total RVUs
Open elective/emergent AAA tube repair	35081/35082	53.75/66.95
Open elective/emergent AAA bifurcated repair	35102/35103	58.06/68.71
Open elective/emergent juxtarenal AAA repair	35091/35092	54.84/79.64
Aorto-bifemoral bypass for occlusive disease	35646	52.73

*Using 2013 Medicare Physician Fee Schedule values without geographic adjustment.

chosen. If the patient's revascularization is for occlusive disease (with a diagnosis of claudication or critical limb ischemia), the aortobifemoral bypass with "other than vein" CPT code 35646 should be submitted to the insurance carrier. The elective and emergent interventions are listed in Table 8-1 with their associated total RVU content. Knowledge of the differences allows one to choose the appropriate CPT code for what was actually accomplished and thereby achieving appropriate reimbursement.

USE ADD-ON CODES

Add-on CPT codes describe services that cannot be reimbursed by themselves. They define more difficult situations and attempt to compensate the physician for added complexity and time. Submission of an add-on code to an insurance carrier requires clear documentation in the operative note. For example, the difference in the time and intensity of work when performing a first time leg bypass compared to a redo leg bypass is significant. No matter how fast a surgeon can dissect out the femoral artery, a reoperative groin with its scar tissue will be a longer and more arduous procedure with higher risk of vascular injury. CPT code 35700 is an add-on code that describes reoperative surgery and is submitted in addition to the leg bypass base code. The physician would be reimbursed for the base code and the add-on CPT code. In the 2013 Medicare Physician Fee Schedule, CPT code 35700 provides an additional 4.68 total RVUs. Another example includes splicing several pieces of vein together to create a conduit long enough to traverse the occlusive disease. Splicing three pieces of vein together from two or more locations to create an infrainguinal bypass conduit in the 2013 Medicare Physician Fee Schedule offers an additional 12.53 total RVUs. Table 8-2 describes some common add-on codes and their total RVU assignment.

CODE AND BILL FOR DIAGNOSTIC ANGIOGRAPHY COMPONENT OF ENDOVASCULAR PROCEDURES

There has been a significant increase in the treatment of arterial occlusive disease by endovascular methods. Diagnostic angiography performed at the time of an interventional endovascular procedure is separately reportable only if certain circumstances exist

TABLE 8-2. COMMON ADD-ON CPT CODES AND RVU VALUES

Procedure	CPT Code	Total RVUs
Redo carotid thromboendarterectomy	35390	4.86
Angioscopy during therapeutic intervention	35400	4.54
Redo infrainguinal leg bypass	35700	4.68
Single piece arm vein harvest for leg bypass	35500	9.78
Spliced vein conduit (2 pieces/3+ pieces)	35682/35683	10.78/12.53
Harvest of femoropopliteal vein	35572	10.52
Visceral artery reimplant during aortic surgery	35697	4.52
Distal anastomosis vein cuff w/ prosthetic graft	35685	6.10

*Using 2013 Medicare Physician Fee Schedule values without geographic adjustment.

as defined in the introductory wording for the "Vascular Procedures" section of the CPT manual. The requirements specifically state:

1. No prior catheter-based angiographic study is available.
2. A full diagnostic study is performed.
3. The decision to intervene is based on this study.

For example, a patient with critical limb ischemia may undergo an aortogram and a right lower extremity arteriogram. Based on this evaluation, a right superficial femoral artery stent is placed to improve extremity perfusion. If the patient had prior catheter-based angiography, only the stent CPT code 37226 would be reported. However, if the three aforementioned criteria are fulfilled, both the aortogram (75625) and the lower extremity arteriogram (75710) would be submitted in addition to 37226. A -59 modifier would be appended to the two imaging studies to certify that the three conditions were fulfilled.

CMS has a different definition for prior angiography. The CPT manual defines prior angiography as a catheter-based angiogram. CMS in the *National Correct Coding Initiative Policy Manual for Medicare Services* states that "*if a diagnostic angiogram (fluoroscopic or computed tomographic) was performed prior to the date of the percutaneous intravascular interventional procedure, a second diagnostic angiogram cannot be reported on the date of the percutaneous intravascular interventional procedure unless it is medically reasonable and necessary to repeat the study to further define the anatomy and pathology.*" This means that CMS defines a prior angiogram as either a catheter-based angiogram or a computed tomographic angiogram (CTA). There is no specific time limit; rather, "prior" relates to the clinical condition of the patient. For example, a CTA two months prior to an elective intervention with no change in symptoms between studies would qualify. Alternatively, an individual who develops rest pain ipsilateral to an iliac artery stent placed two days ago would have a change in clinical status necessitating a new diagnostic angiogram. Therefore, it is important to know whether a patient had diagnostic imaging before (either CTA or catheter-based contrast angiogram) and if the patient has Medicare as their insurance carrier when deciding what to bill.

DOCUMENT COMPLETELY

Many physicians wait until the end of their day before completing all surgery and angiography documentation. Prior to going home, they will dictate three or four procedure notes and try to do this quickly to get home to their family. The downside of dictating quickly at the end of the day is that information such as indications may be abbreviated or left out altogether. Also, certain portions of the procedure that are required for reimbursement may be omitted. In the billing and coding world, if something is not included in the procedure note, it did not happen and is therefore not reimbursable. Endovascular treatments, for which vascular surgeons do a large amount, require specifics for many of the CPT codes.

One complex example is as follows: a physician performs an endovascular infrarenal aortic aneurysm repair using a modular endoprosthesis with one contralateral docking limb followed by right external iliac and left common iliac artery stent graft extensions. The right hypogastric artery is coil embolized with selective catheterization of that vessel and then follow-up angiography confirms the embolization is appropriate. Bilateral femoral artery exposure is performed for vascular access with primary repair of the right common femoral artery and an endarterectomy of the left common femoral artery. A left renal stent is placed after selective catheterization of the artery. The contralateral femoral catheterization is nonselective in the aorta. In the process, a left external iliac artery stent is also placed. The complex procedure above may allow for submission of 16 CPT codes based on what is actually done and what is in the operative report. Every 1 of these 16 CPT codes would require adequate documentation for reimbursement and to defend the billing if audited by the carrier. Therefore, taking several extra minutes to place the indication and to dictate what truly happened in the operating room will be rewarding both from a legal and from a financial standpoint.

BE AWARE OF CARRIER-SPECIFIC BILLING RULES

Outpatient treatments for many private carriers require preauthorizations that are either date-specific or provider-specific. With these rules, physician groups need to decide exactly which provider is going to do the procedure on what date. In a large group where certain individuals will do the venous work, some carriers will approve a patient to only have one specific individual within that group do the procedure. If for some reason that provider changes, the carrier will need to reissue a new authorization or the claim may be denied. Also, if the patient's date of service for the procedure changes even by one day for any reason, the claim may be denied if a new preauthorization is not obtained.

Carriers may have modifier requirements. In Upstate New York, all vein ablation therapy submitted to Medicare is rejected if the -LT or the -RT modifier is not appended to the claim CPT codes. Finally, some private carriers will require a -50 modifier and others will require the CPT code with an -RT modifier on one line, and on a subsequent line, the CPT code is repeated with an -LT and a -59 modifier to indicated bilateral therapy. Knowledge of these rules will help facilitate reimbursement and lower denials/appeals.

KNOW YOUR LCDS

Medicare does not require authorizations for its procedures at this point in time. However, there are multiple local coverage determinations (LCDs) that govern care. In different regions of the country, the LCDs are the same. In other areas, they may differ. National Government Services in Upstate New York has a varicose vein treatment policy that considers varicose vein intervention medically necessary if the patient remains symptomatic after a six-week trial period of conservative therapy. There are private carriers that require three or six months of conservative treatment. Knowledge of what carrier a patient has and what their conservative therapy time requirements are helps facilitate follow-up visits and the timing of the intervention. The conservative therapy for the Medicare LCD requires weight reduction, a daily exercise plan, periodic leg elevation, and the use of graduated compression stockings. These four items should all be documented in the medical record. The policy also reads "radiofrequency/laser ablation is covered only for treatment of the lesser or greater saphenous vein to improve symptoms attributable to saphenofemoral or saphenopopliteal reflux. Coverage is only for FDA devices specifically approved for these procedures." Therefore, use of the device for alternate locations is not a covered service.

INCLUDE ALL APPROPRIATE CODES

Each procedure may be described by one or multiple CPT codes. When the latter is true, it is important for the provider to understand what each of those CPT codes describe so their operative report appropriately details all components of the service. For example, percutaneous embolization at this point in time is reported by CPT codes 37204 and 75894. CPT code 75898 that describes follow-up angiography after embolization is often ignored when billing these procedures. In the 2013 Medicare Physician Fee Schedule, this CPT code is valued at 2.44 total RVUs of additional revenue. CPT code 75898 is reportable if contrast is injected and filmed after placement of the occlusive material to ensure adequacy of the endovascular therapy. Most providers do this evaluation but don't realize that the additional CPT code is appropriate to submit. "CPT Assistant," a publication from the American Medical Association, which helps to clarify coding conundrums, in December 2007 confirms the use of all three codes as listed earlier.

SUMMARY

Vascular surgery coding is a complex process. Physicians must be involved to maximize their understanding of each service defined by one or several CPT codes. Operative notes and angiography reports are also "billing receipts." Treat them as such and include an appropriate diagnosis for medical necessity, a list of all imaging, catheterizations, and interventions for endovascular work, and individual procedures for open surgery. The physician must have a general understanding of what is billed in a given procedure so he or she can dictate a description that is clear and not disputable for each CPT code involved.

REFERENCES

1. *2013 Physicians' Professional ICD-9-CM International; Classification of Diseases*. Vol 1 & 2. Salt Lake City, UT: The Medical Management Institute; 2012.
2. *Current Procedural Terminology CPT 2013 Professional Edition*. Chicago, IL: American Medical Association; 2012.
3. *2013 Medicare Physician Fee Schedule Final Rule. Federal Register*. Vol. 77. No. 222. Friday, November 16, 2012.
4. *SVS 2013 Coding Guide*. 2nd ed. Version 2013.0.1. Chicago, IL.
5. *Bonus Feature: Surgery: Cardiovascular System. CPT Assistant*. December, 2007: 11.
6. *National Correct Coding Initiative Policy Manual for Medicare Services*. Chapter 9, page 8; 2013. http://www.cms.gov/Medicare/Coding/NationalCorrectCodInitEd/index.html?redirect=/nationalcorrectcodinited/.
7. National Government Services Local Coverage Determination L25519. *Treatment of Varicose Veins of the Lower Extremity*. 2013. http://www.ngsmedicare.com.

9

Legal Implications of Off-Label Device Use

O. William Brown, MD, JD

Rapid advancements in endovascular technology have resulted in vascular specialists being called upon to perform more complex procedures less invasively. In response to this request, vascular specialists have chosen to "push the endovascular envelope" by expanding the indications for endovascular techniques and modifying existing devices to meet the needs of individual patients. Thus, there has been a marked increase in the off-label use of vascular devices. Off-label use of medical devices has been defined as the use of a medical device for a purpose other than that approved by the FDA. Specifically, the intended use is not found in the cleared "indications for use." An example would be the use of an aortic stent graft for arterial occlusive disease of the aortoiliac segment. In addition, the use of a device for the purpose for which it was designed, but not in the manner for which it was approved, may also constitute off-label use of a medical device. An example of this type of use would be the placement of an aortic stent graft in a patient with an abdominal aortic aneurysm and a 1-cm aortic neck. These examples of off-label use should be differentiated from the use of an approved medical device that has been modified.

Technological advances in medical devices have revolutionized the treatment of patients with arterial and venous disease. Under the Federal Food, Drug and Cosmetic Act, before a medical device can be distributed into interstate commerce, it must be approved or cleared by the FDA for specific uses. Once a device is approved, the FDA rarely regulates how physicians use legally marketed devices. Historically, the Courts have recognized the importance of off-label use (Buckman, 531 U.S. at 350, 121S. CT.1012) and have gone so far as to note that such off-label use may in some instances constitute the standard of care. In 1997, an amendment to the Food, Drug, and Cosmetic Act stated, in part, that:

> Nothing in this Act shall be construed to limit or interfere with the authority of a health care professional to prescribe or administer any legally marketed device to a patient for any condition or disease within a legitimate health practitioner-patient relationship.

Today the off-label use of medical devices is quite common. Sutherell et al. found in their (noninvestigational) practice of pediatric interventional cardiology that 63%

of patients underwent procedures utilizing medical devices for off-label indications.[1] In Femrite v. Abbot Northwestern Hospital (568 N.W. 2d 535), the court concluded that a physician could use a legally marketed product for any reasonable clinical indication. As a result of the interpretation of the provisions on misbranding in the Federal Drug and Cosmetic's Act, this doctrine did not apply if the off-label use was in an effort to obtain data to gain FDA approval. Further, in the past, off-label use was not permitted to be actively promoted by the physician. Promotion, either by a company or a physician, has been defined as advertising the off-label use, dissemination of articles promoting the off-label use, physician training that includes training in off-label use, and reimbursement advice concerning off-label use. Reports concerning off-label use may be published, but must clearly state that the report constitutes an off-label use of the device. Finally, in the past, manufacturers could not use publications of off-label use to promote further off-label use of the device. However, in a recent court decision (United States of America v. Alfred Caronia (2012 WL5992141(C.A.(N.Y.))), the Federal court of appeals found that such promotion was protected by the Free Speech Clause of the First Amendment to the United States Constitution. In the Caronia case, Mr. Caronia, a manufactures representative, was recorded on two occasions promoting the off-label use of a drug. Mr. Caronia was also recorded suggesting the use of specific diagnosis codes for insurance purposes. At the initial trial, Mr. Caronia was found guilty. However, on appeal, Mr. Caronia argued that "the misbranding provisions of the FDCA prohibit off-label promotion, and therefore, unconstitutionally restrict speech. He further claimed that the First Amendment does not permit the government to prohibit and criminalize a pharmaceutical manufacturer's truthful and non-misleading promotion of an FDA-approved drug to physicians for off-label use where such use is not itself illegal and others are permitted to engage in such speech" (US v. Caronia). The government alleged that it did not prosecute Mr. Caronia for his speech, but rather, his promotion was "evidence of intent" that the off-label uses were the intended uses, and therefore, the present labeling failed to provide any directions. The Appellate Court disagreed with the government noting that the trial court record clearly established that Mr. Caronia was prosecuted for his speech. In Sorrell v. IMS Health, Inc. (131S.Ct 2653, 265), the court stated, "Speech in aid of pharmaceutical marketing…is a form of expression protected by the Free Speech Clause of the First Amendment." Further, the United States Supreme Court held that "creation and dissemination of information are speech within the meaning of the [Constitution]." The Court also raised concerns about restricting speech regarding off-label use when off-label use itself is not prohibited. Ironically, the FDA, in granting safe harbor to manufacturers by permitting the dissemination of off-label information through scientific journals, "recognizes public health can be served when health care professionals receive truthful and non-misleading scientific and medical information on unapproved uses" (US v. Caronia). At this time, it is uncertain when, or if, the government will appeal this ruling to the United States Supreme Court. However, as it stands now, it would seem that the promotion of off-label use, the presentation of off-label use at scientific meetings, and the publication of off-label use in scientific journals is, in fact, protected by the Free Speech Clause of the First Amendment. It should be stressed that there is a difference between the off-label use of a medical device, the modification of a medical device, and the clinical study of an off-label use of a medical device. Creating additional limbs on a graft that has been approved for implantation by the FDA may well be considered by the courts to constitute device modification. Under such circumstances, the courts might reach a very different conclusion concerning promotion, presentations, and publications. Therefore, caution must be taken in communicating data that was not captured within the applicable regulations.

With the current emphasis on minimally invasive treatment for all diseases, many vascular specialists have expanded the uses of endovascular medical devices to include off-label use. However, off-label use of medical devices is potentially associated with both civil and criminal liability. Should a medical malpractice suit arise out of the off-label use of a medical device, there is the potential for significant liability. This is especially true if the physician using the device in an off-label manner is not well versed in the use of the device for the approved indications. The legal system does not recognize a "learning curve" as a viable defense for complications associated with the off-label use of a medical device. Some courts have suggested that the off-label use of a medical device constitutes negligence per se, defined as "...negligence without any argument or proof as to the particular surrounding circumstances."[2] No expert witness is required in cases of negligence per se to establish negligence. Instead, the jury is permitted to assume that negligence has occurred.

Another potential cause of action is failure to obtain informed consent. Informed consent requires that five basic issues be discussed with the patient. These issues include (1) the diagnosis, (2) the treatment planned, (3) the risks and benefits of the proposed treatment plan, (4) other possible treatment options and their risks and benefits, and finally, (5) the natural history of the disease process without treatment. In Estrada v. Jaques (321 S.E.2d 240), a patient developed a false aneurysm of the superficial femoral artery as a result of a gunshot wound to the leg. The physicians involved chose to treat the aneurysm with coils. The patient went on to require an amputation. The patient filed suit alleging that he was not told that the procedure was "experimental". The court in this case stated that "...the rewards, financial and professional, attendant upon recognition of experiment success, increase the potential for abuse and strengthen the rationale for uniform disclosure." The court ruled that a physician must exercise reasonable care and inform a patient of the experimental nature of a procedure. The physician must also inform the patient not only of the risks associated with standard treatment but also of risks specifically associated with the new procedure. In this case, the specific risks of the new procedure were not addressed. In addition, courts have required that a physician provide the patient with the physician's individual experience and results with the planned procedure. In Johnson v. Kokemoor (545 N.W.2d 495), the court found that Kokemoor had not provided informed consent to his patient since Dr. Kokemoor misrepresented his experience.

Another component of informed consent involves the presence of a manufacturer's representative in the operating room during the use of a medical device. Most vascular specialists do permit, and in many cases require, the presence of a manufacturer's representative in the operating room during the implantation of aortic stent grafts. In fact, except in rare circumstances, device companies will not permit the implantation of a fenestrated aortic graft unless a representative is present in the operating room. The American College of Surgeons has addressed this issue requiring that "the patient should be informed of the presence and purpose of the [health care industry representative] in the [operating room] and give written, informed consent. This should be documented within the medical records."[3] Failure to obtain this consent could result in liability for the company and potentially for the physician under a theory of invasion of privacy. In fact, there is case law that supports such a claim. In De May v. Roberts (9N.W.146 (Mich.1881), the court found that a man, who accompanied a physician to a delivery, allegedly to help carry the physician's belongings, was guilty of invasion of privacy and responsible for damages. Although in the case of an aortic stent graft placement, it is the manufacturer's representative who is invading the patient's privacy, there is a strong legal argument that the responsibility for obtaining informed consent rests with the physician, and therefore, the financial liability will rest primarily with the physician.

Physicians should also realize that they are liable for all judgments made in the operating room regardless of whether the course of action taken was suggested by the representative. Not uncommonly, representatives, who often have much more experience with devices than individual physicians, will suggest a specific course of action in the operating room. They may attempt to bolster their recommendation by stating that they have used a particular technique on many occasions without any complications. Should complications occur as a result of the physician using the technique suggested by the representative, the courts have found, that under the learned intermediary doctrine, the physician will be held solely liable.

However, the requirement of informed consent does not require that the physician inform the patient of the FDA status of the device to be utilized. Specifically, the law does not require a vascular surgeon to inform his patient that an arterial stent that is to be used in the superficial femoral artery is FDA approved only for the biliary system. In Alvarez v. Smith (714 So.2d 652), the court did state that a physician was free to use medical judgment, but warned that a physician may be held liable for medical malpractice if that judgment violates the standard of care. The definition of standard of care is what the ordinary physician would do in like or similar circumstances. Currently, the use of a biliary stent in the superficial femoral artery is clearly within the standard of care for the endovascular treatment of a stenosis of the superficial femoral artery. Accordingly, this type of off-label use would not be subject to a claim of negligence per se.

Off-label use of a medical device could potentially result in criminal liability. Criminal liability may attach as a result of upgrading of services when submitting claims for payment. Under these circumstances, claims are most often brought under the False Claims Act. In order to apply the False Claims Act, the government must show the existence of three components: (1) a claim was submitted for payment, (2) a false statement was made, and (3) the individual knew that it was false. "Knowing" that a claim is false involves either actual knowledge or complete disregard as to whether the claim is true or false. Penalties for violating the False Claims Act can be very severe, ranging from three times the amount of the claim, plus fines of $5,500–$11,000 per claim. In addition, the government can file a regulatory action against a physician who knowingly causes a device to be shipped via interstate commerce for a purpose other than its approved use.

Finally, in considering the legal ramifications of off-label use of a medical device, one must consider the impact of the Medical Device Amendments (MDA) of 1976. "The federal government initially acquired oversight of medical devices through the Federal Food, Drug, and Cosmetic Act of 1938. However, the FDA lacked the authority to screen medical devices before they entered into the market until Congress passed the Medical Device Amendments of 1976."[4] Previously, the evaluation of new medical devices had been left to the individual states.

In Reigel v. Medtronic, Inc. (128 S Ct.999 (2008)), the court held that the MDA preempted certain tort law claims against manufacturers of medical devices that received premarket approval from the FDA. In contrast, in Medtronic, Inc., v. Lohr

(Medtronic v. Lohr, 518 U.S. 470 (1996)), the court determined that claims against manufacturers concerning substantially equivalent devices were not preempted.[4] The apparent conflict in these two rulings underscores the controversy surrounding the application of medical malpractice law to the off-label use of new medical devices. New Class III devices can only be marketed to the general public if they pass one of two FDA-mandated review processes: (1) substantial equivalence (501(k) review) or (2) premarket approval (PMA)[4]. Obtaining PMA involves a more rigorous evaluation than obtaining a substantially equivalent determination, and it is perhaps this distinction that led to the Court to distinguish between the Reigel and Lohr cases. Another possible reason for the conflicting opinions regarding the use of medical devices is that Congress was attempting to satisfy two competing aims. Congress was attempting to encourage the rapid development of new and beneficial medical devices, while at the same time attempting to assure public protection. This conflict continues to exist and has become accentuated by the public's thirst for minimally invasive techniques to treat all types of disease, especially vascular disease.

This conflict, and the resulting difficulty in filing a successful negligence claim against a manufacturer for a product that has been placed on the market as a result of a PMA, has placed physicians in a very precarious position. By essentially eliminating the manufacturer as a source of recovery, the patient is now forced to turn to the physician for compensation. Curfman et al. noted that "[if] injured patients are unable to seek legal redress from manufacturers of defective products, they may instead turn elsewhere."[5]

The legal implications of off-label use of a medical device are far-reaching, complex, and at this time, poorly delineated by the legal system. However, there are some basic principles that should be adhered to when using a device off-label. First and foremost, the physician should obtain full and complete informed consent. Second, if a physician is contemplating off-label use of a device, he or she should be well versed in the FDA-approved use of the device. Finally, care should be taken in billing for the services rendered. Off-label use of medical devices is an integral part of the development of new treatment paradigms. With proper preoperative planning and consent, the risks of criminal and civil liability can be significantly reduced.

Our legal system has had difficulty in finding an appropriate method to address the complex issue of off-label use of medical devices. Unfortunately, as in the case of medical malpractice law, physicians have chosen to complain about the failures of the legal system rather than assume the responsibility of monitoring, and in some manner regulating, the off-label use of medical devices. As discussed, off-label use is most often case specific. However, it is imperative that vascular societies, such as the Society for Vascular Surgery, establish some fundamental guidelines for the off-label use of medical devices. Such guidelines could include suggestions as to a minimum number of cases that should be performed "on-label" before off-label use is attempted. There is clearly precedent for these types of minimum requirements. Similar types of requirements have already been suggested for procedures such as carotid artery angioplasty and stenting. In addition, the vascular societies should take a strong stance against the publication and advertising of off-label use of medical devices by physicians or institutions solely for financial gain. In the past, physicians have chosen to take a passive role in stemming medical malpractice litigation by failing to aggressively pursue those physicians who provide inaccurate or false medical expert testimony. Physicians have relied upon the legal system to address the inequities associated with medical malpractice litigation. Clearly, physicians have been less than satisfied with the results of this approach. If the medical community chooses not to become actively engaged in the debate over off-label use of medical devices, it is doomed to the same outcome.

REFERENCES

1. Sutherell JS, Hirsch R, Beekman RH. Pediatric interventional cardiology in the United States is dependent on the off-label use of medical devices. *Congenit Heart Dis.* 2010;5(1):2–7.
2. Henry Campbell Black, M.A., *Black's Law Dictionary*, 6th edition, 1990, West Publishing Company, St. Paul, MN.
3. American College of Surgeons. Statement on Healthcare Industry Representatives in the Operating Room (revised 2005). http://www.facs.org/fellows_info/statements/st-33.html
4. 64 U. Miami L. Rev. 305
5. Curfman GD, Morrissey S, Drazen JM. Why doctors should worry about preemption. *N Engl J Med.* 2008;1(3):359.

10

Multiple Roles of the Surgeon: Informed Consent, Advance Directives, and Withdrawal of Support

Peter Angelos, MD, PhD

INTRODUCTION

Central to the contemporary practice of surgery is the surgeon's ability to confidently address a number of ethical issues that arise in the care of surgical patients. Obtaining informed consent from patients before proceeding with an operation, understanding how advance directives should be used to guide health care decision making, and understanding when it is appropriate to withdraw support from a patient are all important components of ethical issues in the care of surgical patients. Although none of these topics is unique to a vascular surgery practice, they are all clinically relevant and critically important to the ethical practice of vascular surgery.

Vascular surgery patients have higher rates of many medical comorbidities such as coronary artery disease, hypertension, and diabetes. As a result, these patients are often at higher risk for complications when entering the operating room. In this patient population, informed consent, advance directives, and withdrawal of support all require particular attention. Although these topics certainly do not exhaust the important ethical topics that arise in the care of surgical patients, these are three central topics in the area of surgical ethics.

INFORMED CONSENT

The necessity to obtain informed consent from the patient before surgery is well established in contemporary surgical practice. Yet the concept of informed consent is a recent one. For hundreds of years, doctors made decisions for their patients in a paternalistic fashion. The doctor–patient relationship was seen as one in which the doctor was like a parent making decisions for a child. According to this view, "the doctor knows best" because it is the doctor who has the medical knowledge. The patient is seen as the passive participant in the relationship who should accept the doctor's recommendation without question.

In recent decades, for many reasons, this paternalistic conception of the relationship between doctors and patients has changed.[1] The autonomous choices of patients are now considered important and necessary to respect. As a result, the context of contemporary decision making in surgery is one of "shared decision making" in which the values of the patient are critical and the patient participates in the decisions that are made about his or her health care.

In the current setting, once a surgeon has evaluated a patient and has determined that an operation is indicated, the surgeon must obtain the patient's informed consent before proceeding with the operation. Two important components of the informed consent process must be fulfilled. First, the patient (or surrogate decision maker) must have the capacity to give consent. In other words, the patient must have at the very least a level of consciousness to allow participation in the decision-making process. Second, the patient must be informed of the indications (benefits), risks, and alternatives to the surgery so that he or she can decide whether to proceed with the operation.

Although the informed consent process is ubiquitous in the clinical practice of surgery, a number of important ethical issues require specific attention. In emergency situations, when a patient is not able to give consent for surgery and there is no time to find a surrogate, how is the ethical requirement for informed consent met? Consider a patient with a known abdominal aortic aneurysm who is brought to the emergency room after fainting at work. The patient is unconscious and requires intubation for airway protection. A computed tomography scan reveals significant blood in the peritoneum consistent with ruptured aneurysm. In this emergency situation with an unconscious patient, the patient lacks the capacity to make decisions. If a surrogate decision maker is readily available, the surgeon should discuss the situation with that person to obtain informed consent before attempting life-saving surgical interventions. If there is no surrogate readily available from whom consent could be obtained, a judgment is made by the surgeon whether to go to the operating room. In this context, no informed consent is possible. Rather than simply ignoring the importance of informed consent, the surgeon must make a decision on the basis of "presumed consent." We presume that a patient would want us to make decisions that would lead to the overall medical benefit of the patient.

This notion of presumed consent is similarly the basis for any attempted cardiopulmonary resuscitation when a patient suffers a cardiac arrest. There is never time in that circumstance to seek a surrogate from whom informed consent can be obtained. Instead the assumption is made that patients would want us to try to save their lives. This is the basis for presumed consent.

CHALLENGES TO INFORMED CONSENT

Even though most surgeons are well versed in the importance of informed consent and have obtained consent from hundreds of patients, ethical challenges, nevertheless, remain. An important consideration in the context of informed consent for surgery centers on the question of whether the ethical requirement is for the patient to actually be knowledgeable about the recommended surgical procedure or only that the patient has had the opportunity to have questions about the procedure answered. In other words, if a patient needs a carotid endarterectomy for critical carotid stenosis and the surgeon has recommended the operation, can the patient decline the opportunity to be informed? Can the patient simply state, "I have been told you are a good surgeon and I trust you. I am willing to sign anything that you want, but I don't want to hear the risks"? This scenario raises the question of whether the requirement for informed consent is that the patient is actually informed of the indications, risks, and alternatives of the surgery or simply that they have the *opportunity* to be informed.

Although most surgeons would not feel comfortable without attempting to discuss risks of an operation with a patient, the evidence suggests that even when an attempt has been made to inform patients of the risks of an operation, few patients actually remember the risks.[2-5] How, then, should a surgeon respond to a patient's stated desire not to be told the risks? Most surgeons would appropriately emphasize that it is important to know that there are risks and push the patient to at least hear in general terms about the risks. Few patients when told by their surgeon that the information is critically important for them to hear will persist in declining to hear about the risks of an operation. Ultimately, patients can decline to be informed much as they can decline recommended surgical procedures, but surgeons should be very careful to document the attempts made to inform the patients as well as the patient's wishes not to be informed.

Another challenge to the contemporary practice of informed consent for surgery is when the operation recommended for the patient is an innovative procedure. According to the Society for University Surgeons Taskforce on Surgical Innovation, an innovative operation is one that has not been described in a North American surgical textbook.[6] Although many surgeons would argue that at any time a large number of well-accepted surgical procedures may not yet have been described in a North American surgical text, there are certainly situations in which surgeons are recommending procedures that are novel. In such circumstances, the surgeon recommending the innovative procedure may strongly believe that it is better than the conventional procedure. However, when discussing the benefits and risks of an innovative operation with a patient, the surgeon must clearly describe the uncertainties associated with the new procedure. In such cases, as long as the lack of information about the risks and benefits is clearly explained to the patient, informed consent for the innovative procedure can be obtained. The challenge in such cases is to fully acknowledge the uncertainties in assessing the risks and benefits for novel operations.

ADVANCE DIRECTIVES

Advance directives are methods designed to respect a patient's wishes at a point when the patient can no longer make autonomous choices. Advance directives are most commonly informal and take the form of verbal statements about what the patients might or might not want done for them if they were in specific health conditions. Informal advance directives often take the form of, "If I were in serious condition X, I would never want to have treatment Y done to me." Although discussing one's feelings about different classes of interventions can be very helpful for family members or close friends that might someday be called upon to make decisions on behalf of a patient, such informal advance directives are often less helpful than we might think. Since such statements are usually not documented anywhere, they are commonly ignored at the time when they might be most helpful. In addition, the exact condition that the patient might have discussed is often not exactly the situation in which he or she is now present. This often creates doubt as to whether the patient's informal advance directive is really applicable.

In an attempt to avoid some of the problems with informal advance directives, in recent decades, there has been an emphasis on encouraging patients to have formal advance directives. Formal advance directives may take the form of a living will that is designed to specify the decisions that I would want made if I were no longer able to make them myself. Living wills are better than informal advance directives in that everyone involved in the health care decision making for a patient can read the document to see what the patient's wishes are with respect to a particular health condition. Thus, in comparison to informal advance directives, living wills allow the patient to more specifically direct the decision making on their own behalf when they can no longer participate. However, it may sometimes be difficult to ensure that the patient's condition matches the condition in the living will adequately enough to specifically direct the decision making.

An alternative approach to the living will is the durable power of attorney for health care (DPAHC) that designates a specific person to make choices for the patient if the patient is no longer able to make such choices. If I have signed a DPAHC that, for example, names my adult daughter to make choices for me if I cannot do so myself, then at the point when I lack the capacity to participate in the decision making, my daughter will make decisions for me. In some circumstances, the choices that my DPAHC makes for me may not be the same decisions that I would have made, but the fact that I chose the person to make those choices validates the choices that are made on my behalf.

PRACTICAL ISSUES FOR SURGEONS

Although there is nothing inherently more difficult for surgeons or surgical patients when it comes to advance directives, there are several ethical issues that seem to arise with regularity. It is clear that a patient might be fully participating in decision making prior to surgery, but unable to participate in any decision making right after surgery. Consider a 78-year-old man who consented to an endovascular repair of a complex thoracic aortic aneurysm. Such a patient might have been very willing to accept the risks of the operation and might also have requested that the surgeon be aggressive in doing everything possible to help the patient to return to his preoperative state. If this patient has a DPAHC that specifies his wife to make decisions, then if the patient has a myocardial infarction intraoperatively and requires postoperative ventilation and sedation, the wife would be designated as the appropriate surrogate. However, if the wife wants to immediately minimize interventions to "keep the patient from suffering," the surgeon might object based on his or her prior conversations with the patient.

In such a circumstance, it might not be in the patient's best interest to abide by the decision of the DPAHC rather than the stated wishes of the patient. In an effort to avoid conflicts such as this, many surgeons have adopted the strategy of including the surrogate decision makers in the preoperative discussions so that all parties have the benefit of hearing the patient's wishes first hand.

Even though formal advance directives are designed to allow the patient's choices to be expressed and respected even at the point when the patient lacks capacity to participate in the decision making, they do not eliminate all of the ethical issues in the perioperative period. Knowing what a patient might want done in certain circumstances is helpful, as is knowing who the patient wants to be making the decisions if he or she is unable to do so. However, also critical is that the patient and potential surrogates have the appropriate expectations for recovery. In other words, if it is expected that the patient may be intubated and sedated for some period of time after the surgery, then the surgeon should make clear that the consent for surgery extends into that immediate postoperative situation. Although advance directives can be valuable aids to surgeons and families facing difficult decisions for patients that cannot participate in the decision making, they should not be used prematurely to detour the patient's wishes as expressed at the time of surgical consent.

WITHDRAWAL OF SUPPORT

It is widely accepted that patients can decline medical and surgical therapies even if doing so will jeopardize their medical condition. Since respect for the autonomous choices of patients is given tremendous weight in contemporary health care, it is no longer the case that patients must go along with their surgeon's recommendations. Just as we have come to accept a patient's prerogative to decline any therapy, so too, have we come to accept a patient's right to discontinue any unwanted medical or surgical therapy even against the doctor's recommendations.

Today, it is widely accepted that there is no ethical difference between not starting a therapy (withholding) and stopping a therapy (withdrawal).[7] However, even as recently as the 1970s, the suggestion was often made that it is ethically acceptable not to start a therapy that might be effective, but unethical to stop that same therapy that has been proven to be ineffective once it has been started. In the landmark case of Karen Ann Quinlan in 1975, one of the central issues was whether the hospital should abide by the family's request to withdraw ventilator support. The hospital had refused to withdraw the ventilator claiming that to do so would be euthanasia and therefore unethical.[8] After a number of landmark court cases as well as a shift in the opinion of the public and the medical profession, we now no longer believe that it is any more ethically problematic to, for example, stop dialyzing a patient whose renal failure is not improving, than to never start dialysis.

An important concept when caring for critically ill patients is the "time-limited therapeutic trial." If a patient is in the surgical intensive care unit postoperatively and he or she develops acute renal failure, it may be optimal to begin dialysis in the hopes that the renal function will improve over time. Even though there is no fundamental ethical difference between stopping the dialysis if the renal function does not improve as opposed to never starting it, from the standpoint of the patient's surrogate decision makers, there often feels like a difference. In this context, starting a therapy with the idea that it will be only continued if it is effective at reversing the patient's overall condition often makes the later discussions about withdrawing treatment easier to undertake.

In the context of patients who are near the end of life, the term "futility" is often raised. Often the concept of futility is raised when a patient is critically ill and his or her doctors no longer believe that a particular therapy will result in benefit. As the general argument goes, "since doctors need not provide futile treatments, if a treatment is defined by the doctors as futile, it need no longer be provided to the patient." This line of argument suggests that futility is an objective fact that can be assessed by the physician. Despite early attempts at defining futility as a medical fact,[9,10] most physicians now acknowledge that a treatment can only be determined to be futile relative to a specific goal or objective.[11] What is now clear is that since futility is a value-laden term (i.e., something can only be determined as futile relative to an individual's goals and objectives), it is best to avoid use of the term and instead explain why a specific treatment is or is not likely to help the patient meet a specific goal or objective.

CONCLUSIONS

Although the aforementioned short discussion of specific topics in the ethical care of surgical patients is in no way comprehensive, it nevertheless addresses several of the central ethical issues that arise in the contemporary care of surgical patients. Vascular surgeons, in particular, should be well versed in the ethical issues involved in informed consent, advance directives, withdrawal of care because of the high acuity of the patients, and the high risks associated with many of the operations.

Even a few short decades ago, many in medicine considered the concept of "surgical ethics" to be an oxymoron. However, it is now increasingly well accepted that surgical ethics relates to an important set of ethical issues that are particularly relevant to the care of surgical patients. Although surgical ethics is not completely different from medical ethics, the nature of surgical practice raises several important differences as compared to nonsurgical practices. First, the relationship between the surgeon and the patient is particularly uneven with the patient being forced to accept a very high level of trust in the surgeon who performs potentially highly morbid and life-threatening procedures when the patient is most vulnerable (in the operating room under a general anesthetic). Second, by virtue of the physical nature of surgery and what surgeons do in the operating room, surgeons feel a higher level of responsibility for the outcomes of their patients compared to any other doctor. As medical sociologist Charles Bosk has written, the action of the surgeon is more closely linked to the outcome of the patient than it is for any other doctor.[12] Third, because innovation is expected in surgery and there is no oversight of how surgeons do specific operations, the manner in which innovation should be managed in surgery is critical and unlike other areas of medical care. In the years to come, even as the technological advances provide even more options for surgeons to take care of critically ill patients, there will be increasingly a need for surgeons to be comfortable with the ethical issues central to the care of surgical patients.

REFERENCES

1. Angelos P. Orlo Clark and the rise of surgical ethics. *World J Surg.* 2009;33:372–374.
2. Godwin Y. Do they listen? A review of information retained by patients following consent for reduction mammoplasty. *Br J Plast Surg.* 2000;53(2):121–125.

3. Sahin N, Ozturk A, Ozkan Y, Demirhan EA. What do patients recall from informed consent givenbefore orthopedic surgery? *Acta Orthop Traumatol Turc.* 2012;44(6):469–475.

4. Krupp W, Spanehl O, Laubach W, Seifert V. Informed consent in neurosurgery: patients' recall of preoperative discussion. *Acta Neurochir (Wein).* 2000;142(3):233–238; discussion: 238–239.

5. Fagerlin A, Lakhani I, Lantz PM, et al. An informed decision? Breast cancer patients and their knowledge about treatment. *Patient Educ Couns.* 2006;64(1–3):303–312.

6. Biffl WL, Spain DA, Reitsma AM, et al. Responsible development and application of surgical innovations: A position statement of the Society of University Surgeons. *J Amer Coll Surg.* 2006;202:990.

7. Pawlik TW. Withholding and withdrawing life-sustaining treatment: A surgeon's perspective. *J Amer Coll Surg.* 2006;202:990.

8. In re Quinlan. 355 A2d 647 (NJ). Vol. 429 US 9221976.

9. Blackhall LJ. Must we always use CPR? *N Engl J Med.* 1987;317:1281–1285.

10. Schneiderman LJ, Jecker NS, Jonsen AR. Medical futility: its meaning and ethical implications. *Ann Int Med.* 1990;112:949–954.

11. Grossman E, Angelos P. Futility: what Cool Hand Luke can teach the surgical community. *World J Surg.* 2009;33:1338–1340.

12. Bosk CL. *Forgive and Remember: Managing Medical Failure.* 2nd ed. Chicago, IL: University of Chicago Press; 2003.

Vascular Access

11

Is Preemptive Vascular Access Warranted?

Mark R. Nehler, MD

KIDNEY DISEASE OUTCOMES QUALITY INITIATIVE

The National Kidney Foundation's Kidney Disease Outcomes Quality Initiative (KDOQI) for vascular access states that patients in need of long-term, permanent access for hemodialysis (HD) should undergo native arteriovenous fistulas (AVFs) creation over other access types (e.g., grafts or central catheters, central venous catheterization [CVC]).[1] This should be done preferably at least six months before the anticipated start of HD—generally, chronic kidney disease (CKD) stages 4 and 5.[2] Once patients are identified, three action items include the following: avoid CVC, protect potential access sites and conduit, and maximize the creation of "useable" fistulas as the best long-term access choice. The guidelines emphasize targets for permanent HD access placement to include a rate of functional AVFs greater than 50% in incident HD patients and at least 67% in prevalent cases, with long-term CVC use in less than 10%.[2,3] The Centers for Medicare and Medicaid Services embraced this idea with the development of the National Vascular Access Improvement Initiative (NVAII) and the Fistula First Breakthrough Initiative (FFBI) to usher in these guidelines with the medical community. In January 2013, performance goals limiting the number of patients in HD centers using a CVC for access without financial penalty began. It is important to remember that large portions of the access practice guidelines for KDOQI are not significantly based on level-one data.

Once the AVF is in place, it should be monitored by either nephrology or surgery and if it does not mature satisfactorily within four to six weeks a fistulogram and intervention is recommended. Central to these initiatives is the presumption that preemptive HD access planning will increase the likelihood of fistula construction and successful maturation prior to initiating HD treatments. The actual results nationwide are more sobering. In 2010 FFBI data, only 15% of incident patients were using an AVF, with 82% starting dialysis with a CVC—78% as their only access option and the remainder with a potentially maturing AVF. A recent study demonstrated only 52% of end stage renal disease (ESRD) patients saw a nephrologist prior to the onset of HD, and only 17% of incident patients had a functioning AVF at onset. Given the obvious disparity between FFBI goals and actual achievements in incident patients, it is useful to examine the factors involved to see if they are modifiable.

PATIENT POPULATION

CKD afflicts 14%–16% of the general population of the United States.[4] Patients with CKD are classified into one of five stages according to the presence of kidney damage or the glomerular filtration rate. The prevalence of stages 3–5 CKD has grown by 40% in the last decade.[5] There is significant racial disparity in the rate of ESRD incidence—Hispanics have 1.5 times the rate as non-Hispanics and African Americans 3.5 times the rate of whites. The incidence of patients with ESRD who are over 65 years has risen over 30% in the last decade. As seen from the risk factors affecting successful placement of an AVF, these racial and age disparities have impact on the success of FFBI.

Mortality is another issue that clearly impacts the efficacy of preemptive HD access. Table 11-1 demonstrates the expected survival in years for patients with ESRD compared to age-matched controls. The population over age 65 on HD has an abbreviated life expectancy that is similar to that of advanced stages of malignancy. The top causes of death in ESRD patients (Table 11-2) include cardiac causes as the top two, followed by sepsis and withdrawal of dialysis. The latter two can clearly be influenced by type of access or complications of the same. The large contribution to mortality of withdrawal of dialysis in the older ESRD cohort also has implications on quality of life. In summary, it is clear that in many older patients with ESRD HD is palliative in nature with modest results of the same, which calls into question the efficacy of preemptive access in this subgroup.

TABLE 11-1. MEAN LIFE EXPECTANCY IN YEARS FOR PREVALENT USRDS DIALYSIS POPULATION 2006

Age Group	All	Male	Female
0–14	19.8	19.1	20.5
15–19	17.6	18.5	16.6
20–24	14.9	15.8	13.9
25–29	13.2	13.9	12.3
30–34	11.4	11.8	10.8
35–39	9.9	10.3	9.5
40–44	8.6	8.8	8.4
45–49	7.4	7.5	7.3
50–54	6.5	6.6	6.4
55–59	5.6	5.7	5.6
60–64	4.8	4.8	4.9
65–69	4.1	4.0	4.1
70–74	3.4	3.4	3.5
75–79	2.9	2.8	2.9
80–84	2.4	2.3	2.5
85+	1.9	1.9	2.0

Source: U.S. Renal Data System.[4]

TABLE 11-2. UNADJUSTED ANNUAL MORTALITY RATES PER 1000 BY CAUSE OF DEATH IN PREVALENT USRDS DIALYSIS PATIENTS 2005–2007

Cause	0–19	20–44	45–64	65–74	75+
Myocardial infarction	0.4	2.2	7.3	13.7	19.1
Hyperkalemia	0.1	0.5	0.6	0.9	2.2
Pericarditis	—	0.1	0.1	0.2	0.2
Atherosclerotic cardiac	—	0.4	1.6	4.4	8.6
Cardiomyopathy	0.4	0.7	2.0	5.3	10.3
Cardiac arrhythmia	0.4	1.5	3.8	7.3	12.1
Cardiac arrest	3.0	11.6	26.5	48.5	82.8
Valvular cardiac	—	0.2	0.4	0.9	1.7
Pulmonary edema	0.3	0.3	0.5	0.8	1.6
Congestive heart failure	0.2	0.6	2.0	5.8	13.1
AIDS	—	—	<0.05	<0.05	—
Cachexia	0.1	0.3	1.3	3.7	10.8
Cerebrovascular	0.7	2.4	5.1	8.6	13.5
Gastrointestinal hemorrhage	0.1	0.2	0.7	1.3	2.7
Other hemorrhage	0.2	0.7	1.2	2.1	3.3
Sepsis	1.4	4.5	11.5	20.7	29.9
Pulmonary infection	0.4	0.8	1.8	4.5	10.5
Viral infection	<0.05	<0.05	0.2	0.1	0.1
Other infection	0.4	1.0	1.9	3.2	4.5
Malignancy	0.7	1.1	4.7	10.5	14.1
Withdrawal of dialysis	0.5	1.5	5.3	16.4	44.9
Other	16.1	18.4	37.1	65.4	105
Unknown	—	—	<0.05	<0.05	<0.05

Source: U.S. Renal Data System.[4]

SUCCESS OF AVF CREATION

Much of the literature on AVF placement demonstrates rather sobering results with most series demonstrating maturation failure rates of 40%–45%,[6-10] with a single recent report being slightly better at only 30%.[11] In addition, some patients undergoing AVF placement in the preemptive strategy may never require HD and are exposed to unnecessary morbidity. Risk factors for failure of AVF maturation are generally not modifiable. They include advanced age, female gender, diabetes, and non-white race. The size of the vein and the creation of upper versus forearm AVFs (likely interrelated) have some potential modification in planning with targeting a certain extremity/vein and so forth. Current recommendations for acceptable vein diameter range from 2.5 to 3 mm with veins 4 mm or greater having the best chance of AVF success. If, however, the plan was to only perform AVFs on younger nondiabetic white males with large veins, the fraction of patients undergoing AVF would be minimal and, although maturation success would be much higher, the overall percent of incident patients using an AVF at HD onset would remain very low.

These contributions can be seen in the regional variability of prevalent AVF usage in FFBI data. Regions such as Colorado, Oregon, New Hampshire, Rhode Island, and Washington are at or above the target of two-thirds prevalent AVF usage. Conversely, regions such as South Carolina, Virginia, District of Columbia, Alabama, and Arkansas are only slightly above 50% prevalent usage. It would seem safe to assume that much of these differences are due to nonmodifiable issues within the respective populations they are caring for rather than any inherent skill set differences between the providers.

The major morbidity of AVF creation is lack of maturation and failure to mature for use, necessitating additional procedures as stated earlier. Other issues include steal in 1%–8% of patients, arm edema due to unmasked central venous stenosis, and rarely ischemic monomelic neuropathy. All of these require secondary procedures up to and including abandoning the access. The incidence of these complications increases with age and diabetes.

THE MORBIDITY OF CENTRAL CATHETERS

Published reports about late referral for vascular access evaluation demonstrate poor global outcomes such as increased CVC use; increased morbidity, such as line sepsis and central venous stenosis; and ultimately increased mortality.[12,13] Recent United States Renal Data System (USRDS) data demonstrated markedly increased rates of admissions for infection in patients with CVCs compared to either arteriovenous graft (AVG) or AVF (Table 11-3). Although the rate of infection in AVG patients was larger than that in AVF patients, it is markedly less than that in patients using a CVC.

A large review of access and mortality in the Fresenius dialysis database[14] demonstrated that the mortality rates of patients with CVC access was markedly greater than those of AVG or AVF patients adjusted for other risk factors. Patients who were female, African American, and also had onset of HD for less than one year were much more likely to be using CVC access. There is no argument regarding the morbidity and mortality of CVC. What is not proven is whether preemptive AVFs would reduce this

TABLE 11-3. ADJUSTED RATES OF ADMISSION FOR VASCULAR ACCESS INFECTION IN PREVALENT PATIENTS BY ACCESS TYPE, RACE, AND VINTAGE, 2008

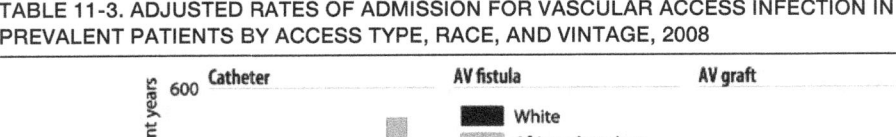
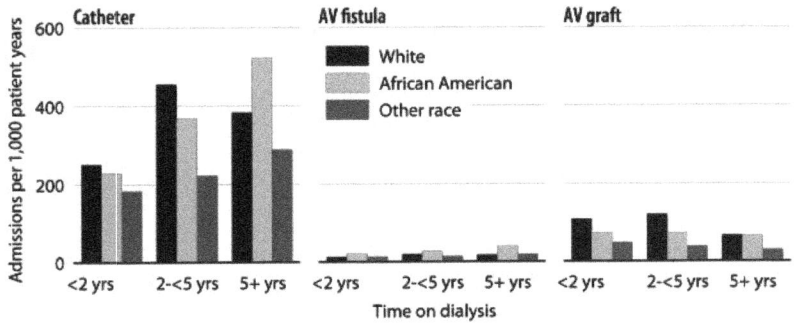

Prevalent HD patients, aged 20 and older, reaching day 90 of ESRD on or before October 1, 2007, and followed for admissions in 2008; ESRD CPM & Medicare claims data. Adj: age/gender/ primary diagnosis.
Source: USRDS 2010.

and also whether an increased placement of AVGs would be beneficial given the poor results with AVFs in certain patient and anatomic scenarios.

RESULTS OF PREEMPTIVE DIALYSIS ACCESS

Study Design

The study[15] was a retrospective review from the vascular surgery practices at the University of Colorado at Denver (Denver Veterans Affairs Medical Center and University of Colorado Hospital) and the Portland Veterans Affairs Medical Center. Consecutive patients with late-stage CKD who underwent preemptive AVF creation (AVF prior to the onset of HD per NVAII and FFBI and in accordance with KDOQI principles)[2,3,5] between January 2003 and December 2007 were entered into a registry database. Patients were excluded if they had a previous vascular access procedure (e.g., fistula, graft, or catheter), were receiving HD treatments, or initiated the same within one week of the vascular access consultation.

Baseline demographics and comorbidities were collected. Technical operative data included preoperative vein mapping and type of AVF created. Preoperative vein mapping data included the cephalic and basilic veins above and below the elbow. Adequate vein size for AVF creation was qualified as ≥2.5 mm per the guidelines recommended by Silva et al.[16] Radiocephalic AVF was considered as the first-line option if the cephalic vein size was adequate.

The primary objectives were to determine the efficiency of a preemptive AVF strategy by examining over time success of predicting the need for HD and success of AVF maturation/use. To accomplish this, patients were stratified into one of four subgroups (groups A–D) over the follow-up period: those on HD using their fistulas (group A—ideal result); those not on HD with patent fistulas (group B—near ideal); those on HD with a secondary access type (failed fistulas; group C—succeeded in predicting HD but failed in AVF maturation and function); and those not on HD with an abandoned AVF due to death, refusal of HD, kidney transplant, or fistula failure (group D—failed on both goals).

Patient-related outcomes determined over the follow-up included incidence of HD initiation and all-cause mortality. The fistula-specific outcomes assessed were mean maturation time (i.e., time interval from creation to first cannulation), cumulative functional patency at 6 and 12 months, mean number of interventions per fistula, most frequent complications, and total AVF abandonment over time.

Results

Demographics

The study cohort included 150 late-stage CKD patients (85% male; median age 63 years) referred for first-time AVF creation over a four-year period at the combined sites (Portland Veterans Affairs Medical Center, Denver Veterans Affairs Medical Center, and University of Colorado Hospital). Table 11-4 lists baseline demographics and clinical characteristics of the study group. Most patients were Caucasian (66%), with African American (15%) and Hispanic (11%) comprising the largest two minority groups.

The majority of patients referred were CKD stage 4. Over two-thirds of the patients were diabetic, and the majority smoked. Consistent with the high incidence

TABLE 11-4. DEMOGRAPHICS OF 150 CKD PATIENTS UNDERGOING
PREEMPTIVE AVF CONSTRUCTION

Variable	N	Percentage
Smoking		
Current	36	23
Former	75	48
Never	45	29
Diabetes	104	69
Hypertension	100	67
Median BMI	30	—
CKD		
Stage 3	7	5
Stage 4	108	73
Stage 5	34	23

Source: Reproduced with permission from Kimball et al. *J Vasc Surg.* 2011;54:760–766.[15]

TABLE 11-5. TYPES OF PREEMPTIVE AVF CONSTRUCTED

AVF type	N	Percentage
Forearm	72	48
Upper arm	78	52
Brachial cephalic	58	74
Basilic vein transposition	20	26

Source: Reproduced with permission from Kimball et al. *J Vasc Surg.* 2011;54:760–766.

of diabetes in this population, patients were frequently obese with a median body mass index (BMI) of 30. A total of 142 patients (92%) underwent preoperative vein mapping. One hundred and fifty AVFs were created (54% in upper arm and 46% in the forearm). The majority of forearm AVFs were constructed at the Portland Veterans Affairs Medical Center, and most of the basilic vein transpositions were constructed in Denver (Table 11-5).

Patient-Related Outcomes

At a median follow-up of 10 months (Fig. 11-1), 74 (49%) patients were receiving HD and 48 of the 74 (65%) were using their AVF (group A), while 26 of the 74 (35%) were not due to AVF failure (group C). Thirty-four (23%) patients never initiated HD treatments but had a patent AVF (group B), and 42 patients (28%) never initiated HD and abandoned their AVF (group D). Thirty-four (23%) of all patients had died.

Fistula-Specific Outcomes

Mean maturation time of all AVFs that were cannulated was 285 days (median 185 days, range 30–1265 days). Cumulative functional patency values for all AVFs were 19% and

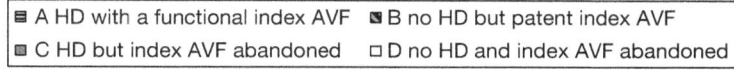

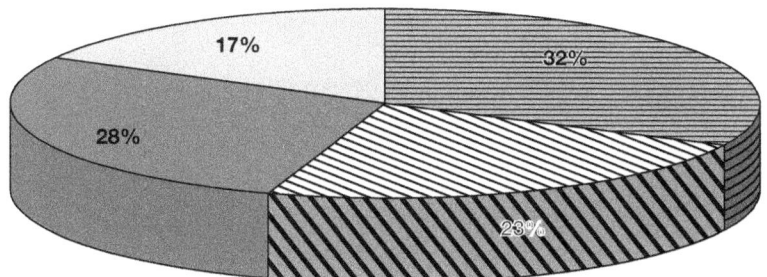

Figure 11-1. Clinical fate at a mean of 10 months of 150 Chronic Kidney Disease Patients undergoing preemptive arteriovenous fistula construction. (Reproduced with Permission from Kimball et al. *J Vasc Surg* 2011;54:760–6.[15])

TABLE 11-6. PATIENT AND OPERATIVE PREDICTOR VARIABLES ON TIME TO AVF ABANDONMENT

Strata	Test	Chi-Square	DF	Pvalve
Gender	Log-rank	0.5065	1	0.4767
Race	Log-rank	0.3751	1	0.5402
Smoking	Log-rank	0.5717	1	0.4496
Institution	Log-rank	3.9371	2	0.1397
Age 75	Log-rank	0.0163	1	0.8984
BMI 30	Log-rank	0.1938	1	0.6598
Procedure	Log-rank	2.5937	5	0.7623

Source: Reproduced with permission from Kimball et al. *J Vasc Surg.* 2011;54:760–766.
Note: DF = Degrees of freedom

27% at 6 and 12 months, respectively, with a mean number of two interventions per AVF (range 1–10). The top five complications encountered were maturation failure for cannulation (15%), focal stenosis requiring intervention (13%), inadequate flows on HD (9%), steal syndrome (9%), and thrombosis (8%). A time-dependent Cox proportional-hazard model found no influence from patient and operative predictor variables on time to AVF abandonment (Table 11-6). Upper extremity fistulas were abandoned less often than forearm fistulas during the short term (<2 years), although this comparison was not statistically significant over the entire time interval (Fig. 11-2; $p > 0.872$). The overall AVF abandonment incidence was 51%.

DISCUSSION

Preemptive AVF placement in the present series demonstrated that predicting HD needs at 10 months was only 50%. Mortality was quite high, which calls into question a preemptive strategy. Of the patients on HD, two-thirds were using their index AVF for access. However, in terms of functional patency for all 150 AVFs, the results were quite poor at 6 and 12 months. Reasons for these results include size criteria for vein and the usual factors that make AVF maturation difficult.

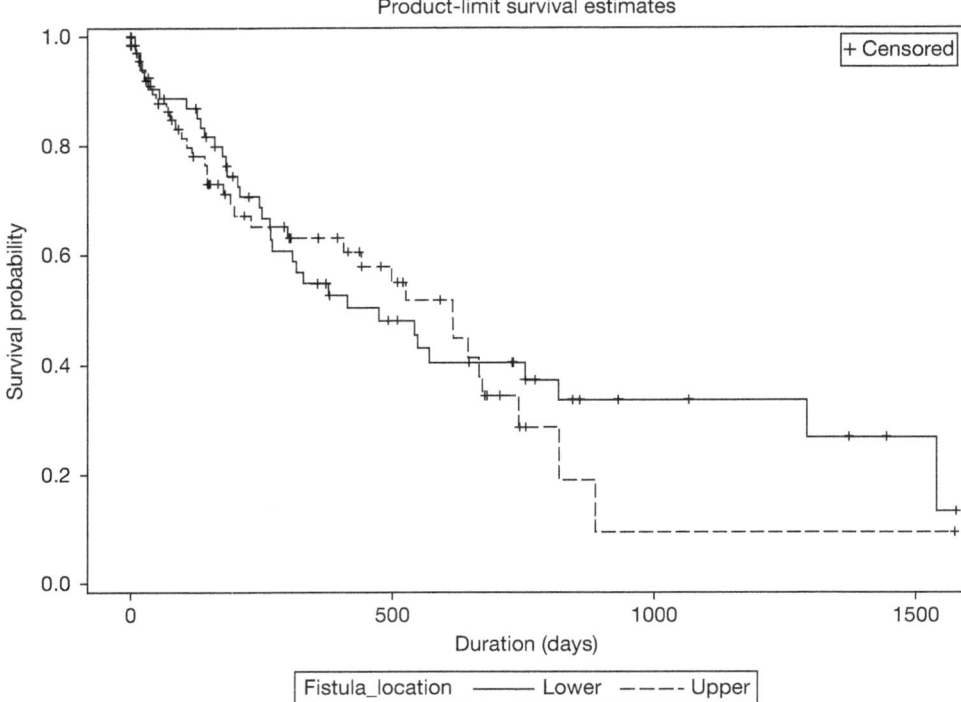

Figure 11-2. Freedom from abandonment of 150 pre-emptive arteriovenous fistulas comparing upper arm and forearm. (Reproduced with Permission from Kimball et al. *J Vasc Surg* 2011;54:760–6.[15])

Do these results justify a preemptive AVF access strategy? In comparison to other prophylactic treatment strategies in vascular surgery—abdominal aortic aneurysm (AAA) repair[17,18] and asymptomatic carotid revascularization[17]—the strategy's success in the current series is lower. Even taking into account that the natural history of many patients with asymptomatic AAA and carotid stenosis is to remain so, the long-term success of the revascularizations is markedly better than the success rate of AVFs. Only half of the preemptive AVF population benefit from the procedure with intermediate term patency, and the other half actually progress to HD during near-term follow-up. However, the argument can be made that the perioperative risk of the AVF is less than AAA repair or carotid revascularization.

Comparing the hypothetical benefits of preemptive AVF construction with operative management of small AAAs prior to the major randomized trials[18,19] is instructive. The assumption for small AAAs was that all patients became worse operative risks over time. Furthermore, it was established that small AAAs would grow over time and that rupture risk was related to increased size. Therefore, it made intuitive sense to operate on good-risk patients with small AAAs provided the repair could be done with a small perioperative mortality risk. These assumptions, however, were not confirmed when tested in randomized trials using open[18,19] or endovascular[20] techniques despite having excellent technical success.

Preemptive AVF construction is similar in many ways. The assumption is that patients become worse access candidates over time as potential vein sites are exhausted with intravenous lines, and so forth. It is established that CVCs have significant septic and thrombotic morbidity[21] and once patients initiate HD with a CVC their mortality rates increase[14] and are often reluctant to agree to surgery for a better access option. Patients with CKD stages 4 and 5 have a high rate of requiring near-term HD[22] and the maturation time for AVFs is often measured in months not weeks. Therefore, it makes intuitive sense to construct AVFs preemptively on patients with late-stage CKD.

However, there are some major issues with this argument. As stated earlier, the global success of AVF construction in the vast majority of recent reported series[6–10,23,24] is modest—50% despite preoperative assessment per KDOQI—including one randomized trial. One major principle of prophylactic vascular care is to focus on good-risk patients with a life expectancy that justifies the up-front morbidity and potential mortality of the procedure. However, KDOQI does not focus on good-risk patients. Unfortunately, the mortality rate of a modern renal failure population is substantial—especially older patients.[4,25] The quality of life of many older patients on HD is questionable—withdrawal of HD is a major cause of death in a USRDS report.[4] Just as patients are reluctant to undergo surgery for an AVF once they have CVC access on HD, they are also often reluctant to undergo surgery for an AVF when their CKD does not yet require HD.

The argument for preemptive AVF construction would be much stronger if the success rate of the procedure was improved. Although there is no general agreement, perhaps our criteria for acceptable venous conduit are not stringent enough. In this study, veins 2.5 mm or greater were considered usable for AVF construction, as recommended by Silva et al.[15] However, this differs from the best report on lower extremity venous bypass, the Prevent III trial.[26] In that study, a venous conduit <3.5 mm was considered high risk[27] and those grafts had worse patency rates and greater number of interventions compared to grafts constructed with venous conduits ≥3.5 mm. A recent report on AVF construction demonstrated that veins ≥4 mm had much better maturation rates.[11] Unfortunately, in our practice very few patients would qualify for an attempt at preemptive AVF construction if those criteria were used; but the 3.5 mm vein requirement could be a compromise. One of the authors in the present report uses ≥3 mm rather than 2.5 mm as the size for acceptable venous conduits for AVFs.

Regardless of changes in strategy, the plan for preemptive AVF placement for all patients is not realistic. Many patients would likely be better served with an AVG and a focus on reducing the need for CVC rather than increasing the percentage of AVFs. Certain patient populations (obese, female, and African American) have poor AVF maturation rates. It would seem a reasonable compromise to focus preemptive AVF placement in the population most likely to have successful maturation to make the risk–benefit ratio justifiable.

REFERENCES

1. KDOQI Clinical Practice Guideline for Diabetes and CKD: 2012 Update. *Am J Kidney Dis.* 2012;60(5):850–886.
2. Fistula First Breakthrough. End-Stage Renal Disease Quality Initiative. The Centers of Medicare and Medicaid Services. www.cms.hhs.gov/ESRDQualityImproveInit/04_ FistulaFirstBreakthrough.asp. Accessed March 2008.
3. Clinical practice guidelines for vascular access. *Am J Kidney Dis.* 2006;48(suppl 1):S248–S273.
4. U.S. Renal Data System, USRDS 2008 Annual Data Report: Atlas of Chronic Kidney Disease and End-Stage Renal Disease in the United States. Bethesda, MD: National Institutes of Health, National Institute of Diabetes and Digestive and Kidney Diseases; 2008.

5. Clinical practice guidelines for vascular access. *Am J Kidney Dis*. 2006;48(supp l):S176–S247.
6. Feldman HI, Joffe M, Rosas SE, et al. Predictors of successful arteriovenous fistula maturation. *Am J Kidney Dis*. 2003;42(5):1000–1012.
7. Lok CE, Allon M, Moist L, et al. Risk equation determining unsuccessful cannulation events and failure to maturation in arteriovenous fistulas (REDUCE FTM I). *J Am Soc Nephrol*. 2006;17(11):3204–3212.
8. Lee T, Barker J, Allon M. Comparison of survival of upper arm arteriovenous fistulas and grafts after failed forearm fistula. *J Am Soc Nephrol*. 2007;18(6):1936–1941.
9. Dember LM, Beck GJ, Allon M, et al. Effect of clopidogrel on early failure of arteriovenous fistulas for hemodialysis: a randomized controlled trial. *JAMA*. 2008;299(18):2164–2171.
10. Biuckians A, Scott EC, Meier GH, et al. The natural history of autologous fistulas as first-time dialysis access in the KDOQI era. *J Vasc Surg*. 2008;47(2):415–421; discussion 420–421.
11. Lauvao LS, Ihnat DM, Goshima KR, et al. Vein diameter is the major predictor of fistula maturation. *J Vasc Surg*. 2009;49(6):1499–1504.
12. Goransson LG, Bergrem H. Consequences of late referral of patients with end-stage renal disease. *J Intern Med*. 2001;250(2):154–159.
13. Lhotta K, Zoebl M, Mayer G, Kronenberg F. Late referral defined by renal function: association with morbidity and mortality. *J Nephrol*. 2003;16(6):855–861.
14. LacsonE, Jr, Wang W, Lazarus JM, Hakim RM. Change in vascular access and mortality in maintenance hemodialysis patients. *Am J Kidney Dis*. 2009;54(5):912–921.
15. Kimball, T.A. et al., *Efficiency of the kidney disease outcomes quality initiative guidelines for preemptive vascular access in an academic setting*. J Vasc Surg, 2011. 54(3): p. 760–765; discussion 765–766.
16. Silva MB, Jr, Hobson RW, 2nd, Pappas PJ, et al. A strategy for increasing use of autogenous hemodialysis access procedures: impact of preoperative noninvasive evaluation. *J Vasc Surg*. 1998;27(2):302–307; discussion 307–308.
17. Halliday A, Harrison M, Hayter E, et al. Prevention of disabling and fatal strokes by successful carotid endarterectomy in patients without recent neurological symptoms: randomised controlled trial. *Lancet*. 2004;363(9420):1491–1502.
18. Lederle FA, Wilson SE, Johnson GR, et al. Immediate repair compared with surveillance of small abdominal aortic aneurysms. *N Engl J Med*. 2002;346(19):1437–1444.
19. Mortality results for randomised controlled trial of early elective surgery or ultrasonographic surveillance for small abdominal aortic aneurysms. The UK Small Aneurysm Trial Participants. *Lancet*. 1998;352(9141):1649–1655.
20. Lederle FA, Wilson SE, Johnson GR, et al. Outcomes following endovascular vs. open repair of abdominal aortic aneurysm: a randomized trial. *JAMA*. 2009;302(14):1535–1542.
21. Lorente L, Henry C, Martiín MM, et al. Central venous catheter-related infection in a prospective and observational study of 2,595 catheters. *Crit Care*. 2005;9(6):R631–R635.
22. Johnson ES, Thorp ML, Platt RW, Smith DH. Predicting the risk of dialysis and transplant among patients with CKD: a retrospective cohort study. *Am J Kidney Dis*. 2008;52(4):653–660.
23. Patel ST, Hughes J, Mills JL, Sr. Failure of arteriovenous fistula maturation: an unintended consequence of exceeding dialysis outcome quality initiative guidelines for hemodialysis access. *J Vasc Surg*. 2003;38(3):439–445; discussion 445.
24. Weale AR, Bevis P, Neary WD, et al. Radiocephalic and brachiocephalic arteriovenous fistula outcomes in the elderly. *J Vasc Surg*. 2008;47(1):144–150.
25. Biesenbach G, Hubmann R, Grafinger P, et al. 5-year overall survival rates of uremic type 1 and type 2 diabetic patients in comparison with age-matched nondiabetic patients with end-stage renal disease from a single dialysis center from 1991 to 1997. *Diabetes Care*. 2000;23(12):1860–1862.
26. Conte MS, Bandyk DF, Clowes AW, et al. Results of PREVENT III: a multicenter, randomized trial of edifoligide for the prevention of vein graft failure in lower extremity bypass surgery. *J Vasc Surg*. 2006;43(4):742–751; discussion 751.
27. Schanzer A, Hevelone N, Owens CD, et al. Technical factors affecting autogenous vein graft failure: observations from a large multicenter trial. *J Vasc Surg*. 2007;46(6):1180–1190; discussion 1190.

12

Nuts and Bolts of Basilic Vein Transposition

Sunny Fink, MD and Anton Skaro, MD, PhD

INTRODUCTION

There are more than five hundred thousand individuals suffering from end-stage renal disease (ESRD) in the United States.[1] Additionally, nearly 20% of the US population has chronic kidney disease (CKD), many of whom will develop ESRD in their life-time.[1] While a consensus statement from the National Kidney Foundation (NKF) suggests that preemptive kidney transplantation is the optimal treatment for patients with ESRD,[2] an imbalance in the supply of and demand for donor kidneys limits transplantation.[3]

Hemodialysis, which was developed in 1944, serves as a life-sustaining renal replacement therapy (RRT) for patients with ESRD.[4] However, hemodialysis depends on suitable vascular access sites that can be exhausted due to a life-long need for RRT. Alternatives to central venous catheter (CVC)-based hemodialysis, which is associated with a greater hazard of mortality due to infection, include arteriovenous grafts (AVG) also prone to infection or the creation of autologous arteriovenous fistulae (AVF).[5]

Since the release of the NKF-sponsored Kidney Disease Outcomes Quality Initiative (KDOQI) guidelines in 1997,[6] and subsequent revisions,[7] increasing attention has been paid to the impact of vascular access on outcomes of hemodialysis patients. These guidelines promote a peripheral-to-central sequence and favor the creation of autogenous AVF over CVC and synthetic grafts to improve patency and contain costs, providing adequate flow rates, low rates of complications and fistula longevity. Recognizing the disadvantages (see Table 12-1) associated with CVC[5] the Centers for Medicare and Medicaid Services (CMS) have intensified efforts to promote AVF utilization by introducing the Fistula First Initiative that reduces reimbursement for hemodialysis using a CVC.[8] While this program has not reached its goal of 65% AVF compliance, many centers now achieve rates of 90% or more.

TABLE 12-1. DISADVANTAGES OF CENTRAL VENOUS CATHETER (CVC)-BASED HEMODIALYSIS

Morbidity and mortality secondary to thrombosis/infection

Central venous stenosis

Cosmetically unpleasing and uncomfortable

Low flow rates and longer hemodialysis duration

The most commonly performed primary and secondary AVF are the radial-cephalic and brachiocephalic fistulae first introduced by Brescia in 1966[9] and Cascardo in 1970,[10] respectively. However, in the setting of failure or nonviable primary or secondary options basilic vein transposition (BVT) has emerged as a legitimate secondary/tertiary access site for chronic hemodialysis after its initial description in 24 patients by Dagher et al. in 1976.[11] BVT has reduced the need for AVG fashioned from synthetic or homografts that are associated with higher complication and poorer patency rates compared to autologous AVF.[12]

PREOPERATIVE EVALUATION FOR BASILIC VEIN TRANSPOSITION

Patients with ESRD and associated comorbid conditions pose a substantial challenge in the perioperative period that necessitates careful preoperative evaluation, risk stratification, and optimization to facilitate the safe conduct of the surgical procedure. As with any AVF creation, there must be suitable venous and arterial vasculature available, which is typically the rate-limiting step (see Fig. 12-1). Consequently, a clinical assessment of the arterial and venous anatomy of the upper extremities is essential.

On the venous side, the basilic vein often exceeds 4 mm in the upper arm[13] and 2.5 mm in the forearm[14] as assessed by either duplex ultrasound mapping or venography (see Fig. 12-2) in order to create a successful AVF for BVT. A sufficient length of basilic vein before confluence with the brachial/axillary venous system is necessary to provide adequate distance to allow for migration of cannulation sites (see Fig. 12-3). In addition to a basilic vein of suitable caliber and quality, adequate venous outflow for the remainder of the arm is necessary to avoid arm edema. In the event of concerns of or risk factors for central vein stenosis (see Table 12-2) central venography should be performed (see Fig. 12-4).

From an arterial perspective either the radial or brachial artery can be used for AVF creation with subsequent BVT. According to the Society of Vascular Surgery (SVS) vascular access guidelines a proximal radial artery that exceeds 1.5 mm is appropriate for AVF creation preserving the brachial for future use.[13] Moreover, the radial artery that is less than 1.5 mm based on duplex ultrasound measurement is associated with poor fistula maturation.[13]

The basilic vein is deep and protected from injury caused by venipuncture making it an ideal hemodialysis conduit but requiring elevation. The BVT produces a straight, lengthy, and superficial fistula that is easily amenable to cannulation. Moreover, BVT maintains anatomic continuity with the axillary vein for optimal fistula outflow creating hemodynamic parameters compatible with high flow rates. In addition, BVT obviates the need for grafts when other primary and secondary sites have been exhausted.

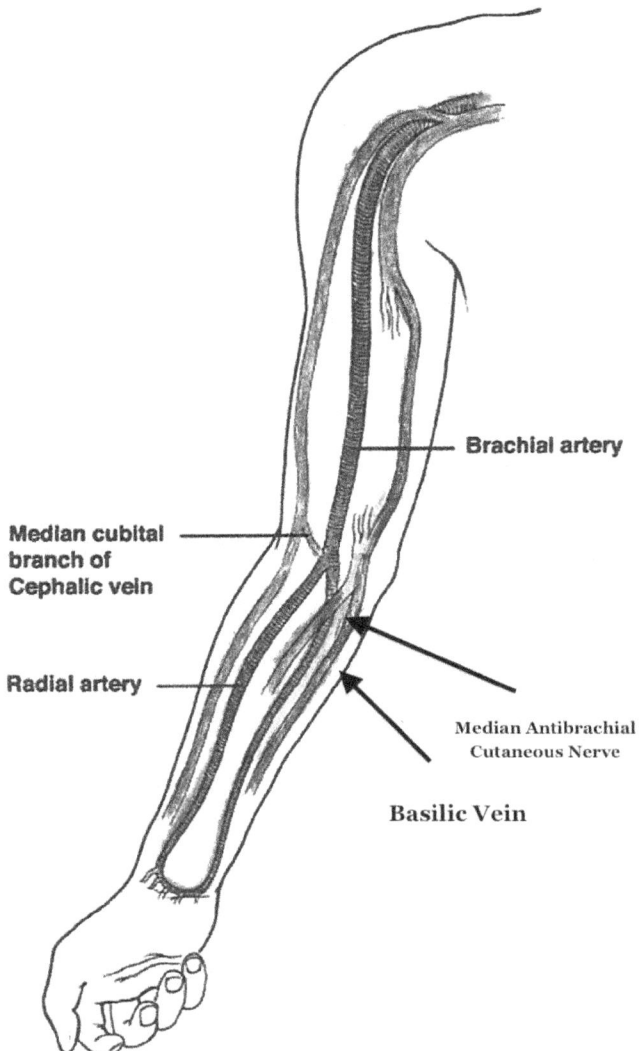

Figure 12-1. Venous and arterial vasculature of the arm.

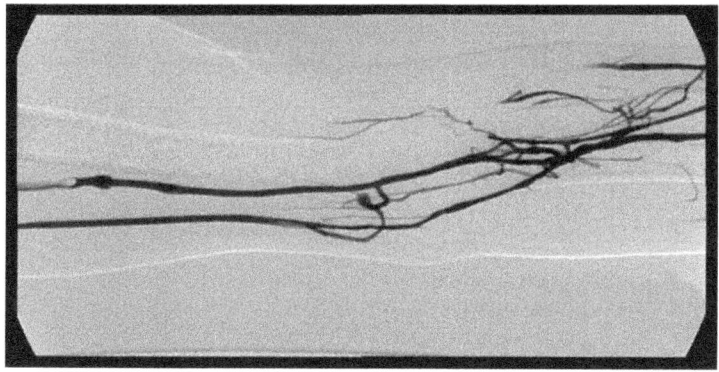

Figure 12-2. Imaging of basilic vein.

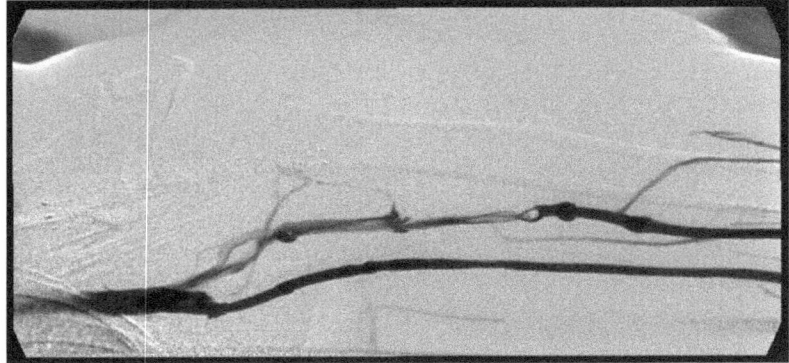

Figure 12-3. Site of confluence of basilic vein with the brachial/axillary venous system.

TABLE 12-2. INDICATIONS FOR CENTRAL VENOGRAPHY

Extremity edema

Venous collaterals

Ipsilateral subclavian catheter placement

Ipsilateral transvenous pacemaker

Neck, arm, or chest trauma

Previous vascular access surgery

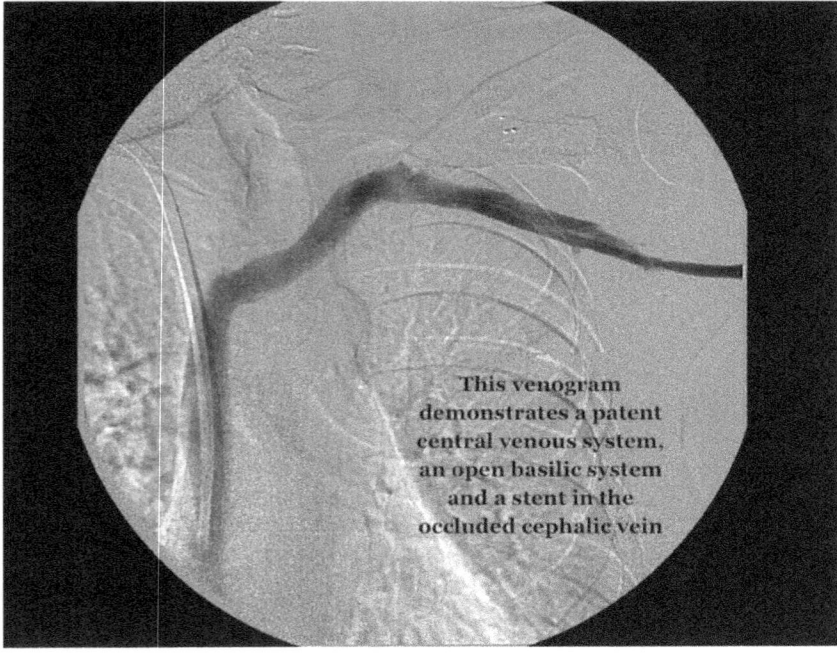

This venogram demonstrates a patent central venous system, an open basilic system and a stent in the occluded cephalic vein

Figure 12-4. Example of central venography.

SURGICAL TECHNIQUE OF BASILIC VEIN TRANSPOSITION

The procedure can be performed under local or regional and less commonly general anesthesia in an ambulatory surgery setting. Mobilization of the basilic vein has been described using a single large incisionb[15] or two[51,16] or more smaller incisions.[11] After mobilization and ligation of collaterals, an end-to-side anastomosis of the basilic vein with the brachial artery is fashioned using polypropylene sutures. In addition, either transposition through a subcutaneous tunnel or simply elevation such that the deep fascia is closed beneath the fistula, which rests immediately under the incision, can be undertaken. More recently, video-assisted elevation and transpositions using minimally invasive techniques have been described but are not in widespread use.[17] Hemodialysis using the BVT is initiated after fistula maturation and wound healing usually 4–6 weeks after the procedure.

LOCATION—FOREARM VERSUS UPPER ARM

BVT can be performed in either the upper arm or the forearm. Consistent with KDOQI guidelines a proximal-to-central sequence of forearm followed by upper arm BVT is favored. Such an approach preserves the more proximal vessels for future access sites given the life-long need for RRT among ESRD patients. However, success rates greatly depend on inflow and outflow vessel size and quality, and other patient-related factors including but not limited to presence of thrombophilia, poor hemodynamics, and cardiac function.

Forearm Basilic Vein Transposition

The radial/ulnar-to-basilic forearm transposition is a valid secondary/tertiary AVF option that should be considered when radial- and/or brachial-to-cephalic options have been exhausted. This procedure was first described by Silva et al.[14] First, duplex ultrasonography was used to demonstrate appropriate vein size and compressibility along the entire basilic distribution of the forearm. An incision is then made along the length of the vein from distal to proximal for venous mobilization. The artery is then identified and mobilized. Caution is taken to preserve nerve branches, such as the superficial branch of the radial nerve. Next, a superficial tunnel is created and transposition of the basilic vein and end-to-side radial/ulnar-to-basilic anastomosis is accomplished. According to Weiswasser et al., 91% of forearm BVT achieved maturation with 84% and 69% patency at 12 and 30 months, respectively.[18] However, forearm BVT, particularly those using ulnar artery inflow, are prone to steal syndrome especially among patients with previous failed radial procedures.

Forearm Loop Basilic Vein Transposition

The forearm loop BVT is another technique in which the mobilized distal basilic vein is tunneled as a loop for anastomosis to the brachial artery in the antecubital fossa.[19] Owing to anastomosis of the distal basilic vein of the forearm with the larger caliber brachial artery, more favorable results among diabetics has been observed.[19] Hence, this type of BVT is indicated for patients with a satisfactory basilic vein in the forearm but an inadequate radial or ulnar artery for anastomosis.

Upper Arm Basilic Vein Transposition

The most proximal of the BVT is the upper arm brachial artery-to-basilic vein AVF. This AVF represents the original description of BVT by Dagher et al.[11] The procedure involves distal division of the basilic vein, mobilization, elevation, and transposition with end-to-side anastomosis of the basilic vein to the brachial artery. The upper arm BVT procedure includes modification from a single-stage to a two-stage procedure.

One-Stage Versus Two-Stage Upper Arm Basilic Vein Transposition

The two-stage technique entails anastomosis of the basilic vein to the brachial artery in the antecubital fossa (see Fig. 12-5) and later, after maturation (see Fig. 12-6) has occurred and during a subsequent surgical procedure, elevation and transposition (see Fig. 12-7) to facilitate cannulation. During the second stage of BVT a longitudinal incision is made over the basilic vein, and care is taken to preserve the adjacent median

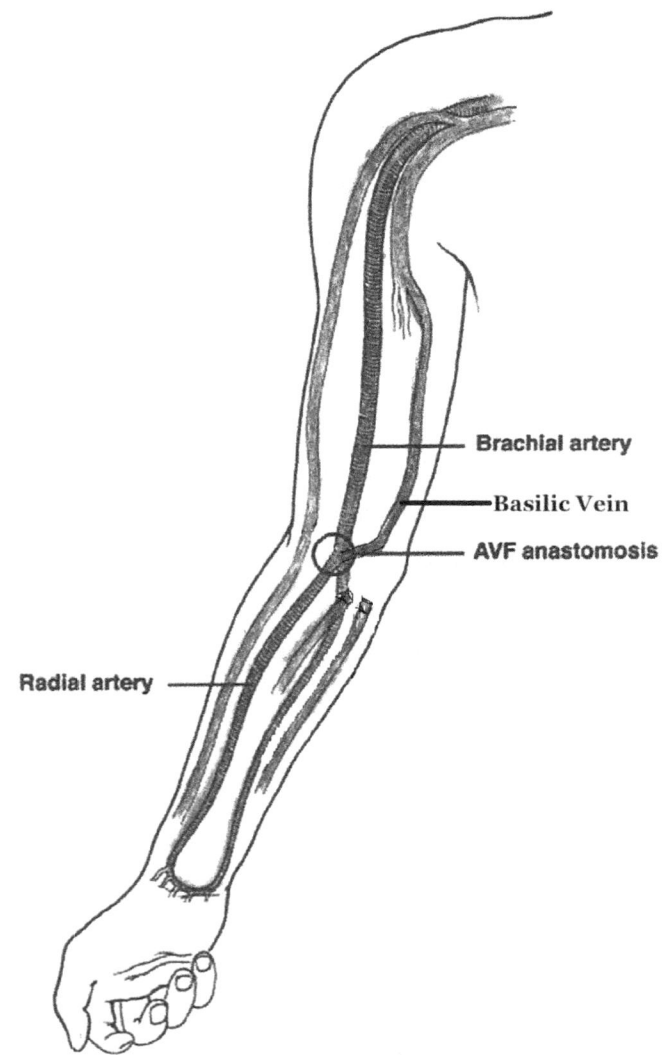

Figure 12-5. Anastomosis of the basilic vein.

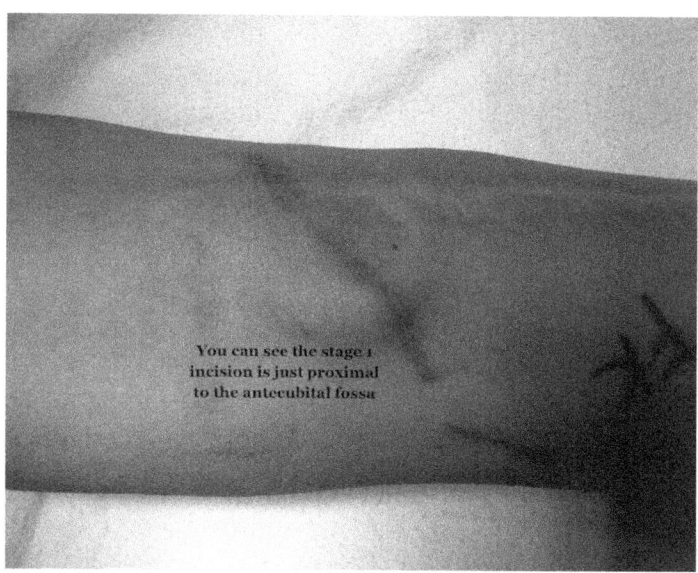

You can see the stage 1 incision is just proximal to the antecubital fossa

Figure 12-6. Location of stage 1 incision.

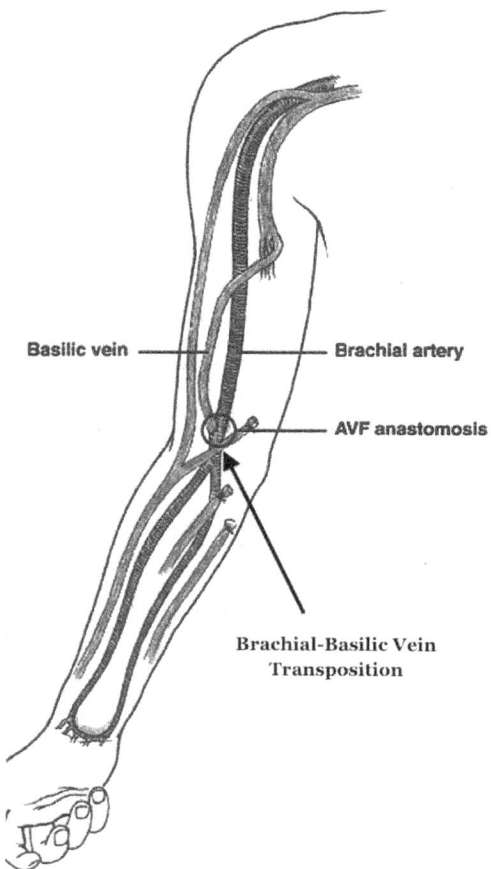

Basilic vein ———————— Brachial artery

———— AVF anastomosis

Brachial-Basilic Vein Transposition

Figure 12-7. Brachial-basilic vein transposition.

antebrachial cutaneous nerve (see Fig. 12-8). The basilic vein is identified and traced proximally. Its branches are ligated and the dissection continues proximally up toward axilla. Once the vein has been completely mobilized, it is marked for orientation, and a subcutaneous tunnel is created laterally (see Fig. 12-9). Proximal and distal control of the vein is established using vascular clamps, the vein transected and care is taken to ensure that the vein maintains proper orientation as it traverses the tunnel to avoid obstruction that could leave the fistula prone to thrombosis (see Fig. 12-10). After transposing the vein it is flushed with heparinized saline to remove any blood and confirm orientation. The vein is then re-anastomosed end-to-end using polypropylene sutures. Flow is again

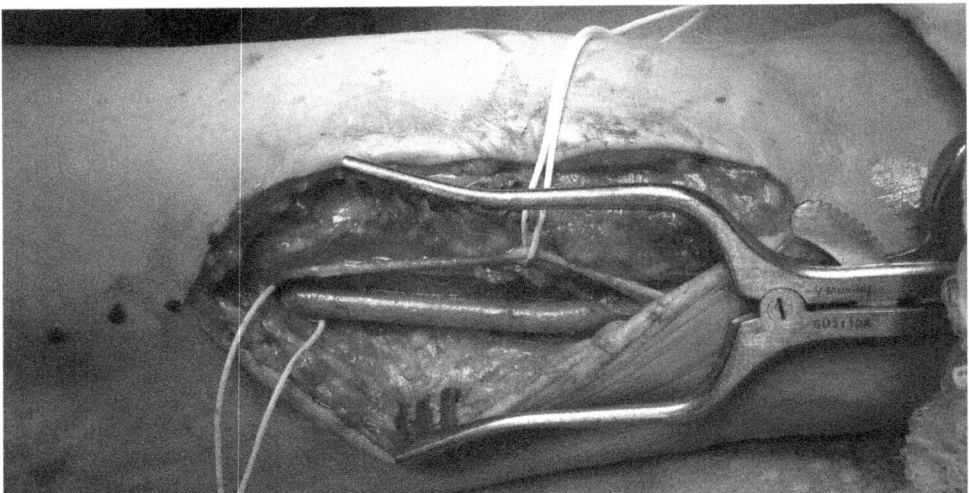

Figure 12-8. Stage 2 BVT incision.

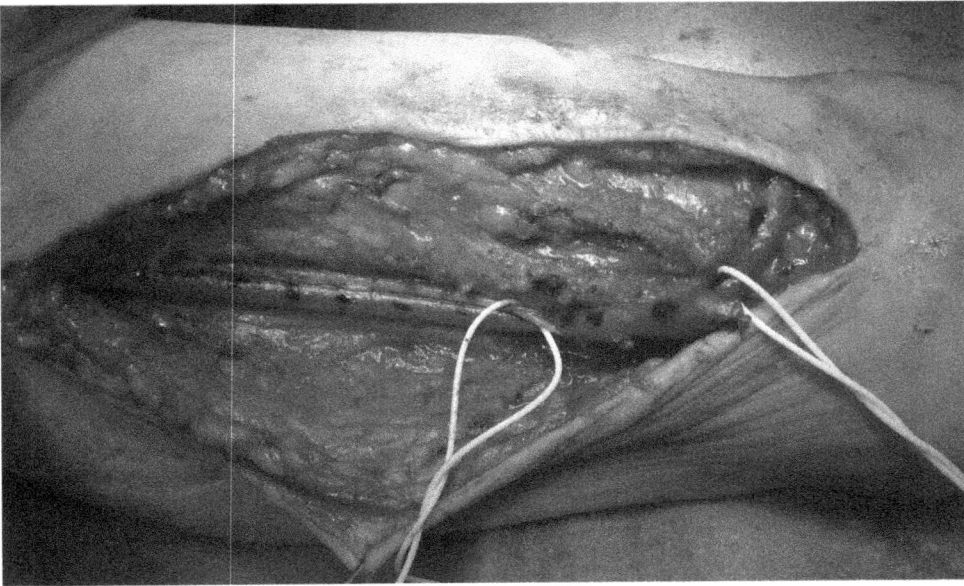

Figure 12-9. Vein is fully mobilized, marked for orientation, and subcutaneous tunnel created.

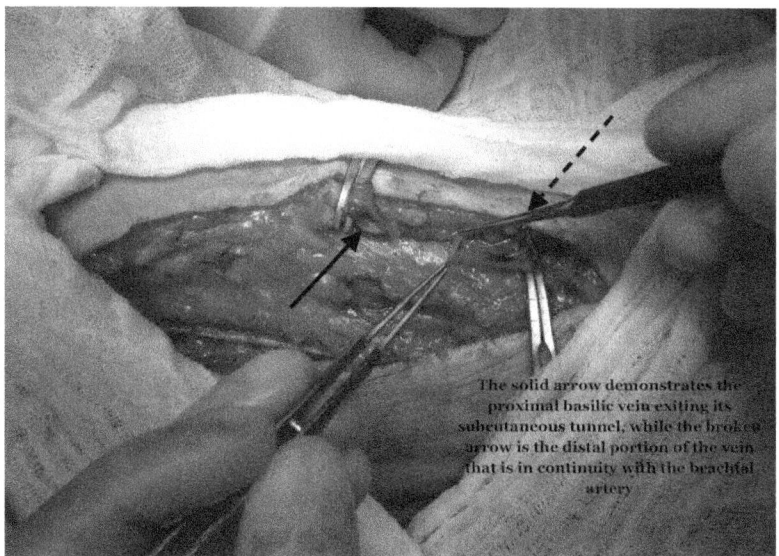

Figure 12-10. Transection of vein.

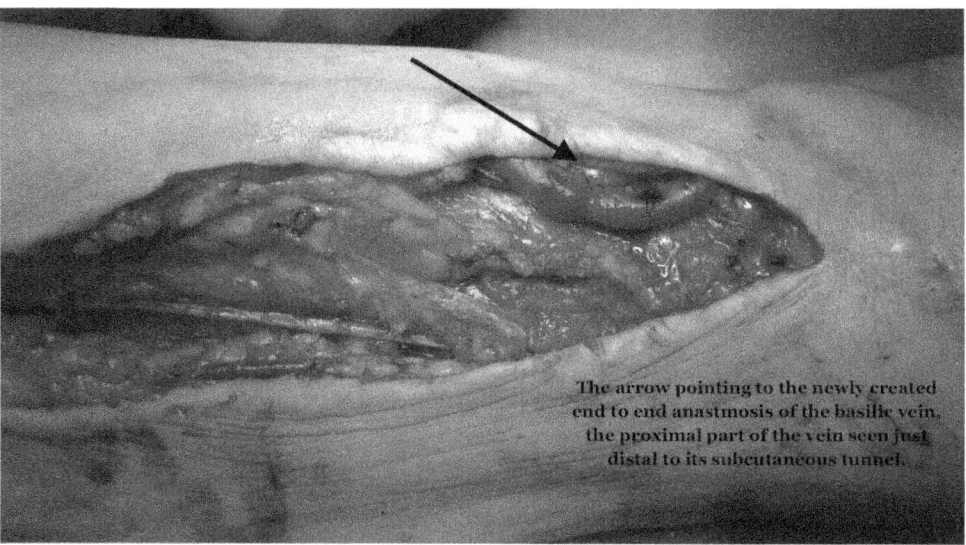

Figure 12-11. Flow re-established in preparation for closing wound in layers.

established, and once hemostasis has been assured, the wound is then closed in layers (see Fig. 12-11).

BVT is increasingly being performed as a two-stage procedure. In a randomized control trial, El Mallah compared 40 patients undergoing the one-stage or two-stage BVT and observed primary patency rates of 50% and 80%, respectively, at a median follow-up of 15 months.[20] However, in a smaller retrospective study, Hossny demonstrated similar patency rates (90% and 84%) for one- and two-stage procedures.[21]

The advantage of the two-stage approach is the avoidance of a long, potentially nonhealing, incision among patients who do not experience fistula maturation. Moreover, the two-stage BVT also allows time for the hypertrophy of venous outflow or the development of venous collaterals that promote venous drainage limiting the formation of arm edema. Also, the staged procedure may give the vein time to arterialize and strengthen such that it is less prone to thrombosis during elevation and transposition. The higher failure rates observed after the one-stage procedure may reflect damage during extensive dissection of the basilic vein. In contrast, as is implied a one-stage BVT involves arteriovenous anastomosis after elevation and transposition during the same surgical procedure. The advantages of a single-stage BVT include the formation of only a single vascular anastomosis, and the ligation of collaterals theoretically might augment flow through the fistula and enhance the likelihood of maturation.

TRANSPOSITION VERSUS ELEVATION

As mentioned earlier in text, the brachial-to-basilic AVF can be either elevated such that the fistula rests beneath the incision or transposed through a subcutaneous tunnel to the more lateral aspect of the arm. It has been suggested that the incisional morbidity of BVT is prohibitive in certain populations at risk for wound complications including patients with diabetes and morbid obesity. This has led to the application of endoscopic vein harvest for BVT.[17] The same endoscopic techniques used for saphenous vein harvesting during cardiac surgery have been applied to BVT. The first endoscopic-assisted BVT was reported by Martinez et al. in 2001.[22] Preoperative ultrasonography is used to mark the vein and location of large branches that will require ligation. One downside to this technique is that the vein harvesting apparatus is disposable, and this coupled with longer procedure time can add significantly to the cost. Irrespective of the technique used for transposition, it achieves several important objectives including (1) excluding the fistula from the incision and any issues related to wound healing; (2) re-location of the fistula laterally to improve the ease of cannulation; and (3) movement away from the adjacent median antebrachial cutaneous nerve protects the nerve from injury and improves patient comfort during cannulation. Despite the theoretical advantages associated with transposition, the change in location and trajectory might negatively impact fistula patency. Hossny studied the impact of different techniques including a comparison between transposition and elevation.[21] Seventy brachial-to-basilic AVF were constructed, transposed in 30 patients and elevated in 40 patients (20 in one stage and 20 in two stages). Patency rates at one year were 87%, 90%, and 84% in the transposed, elevated in one-stage, and elevated in two-stage groups, respectively. The rate of complications was substantially higher in the elevation group (71.4% versus 28.6%). In addition, transposition was favored among dialysis staff due ease of access, patient comfort, and the lower rate of complications.

ARTERIOVENOUS FISTULA PATENCY RATES

The 12-month primary patency rates of radial-cephalic (62%–91%),[23,24] brachial-cephalic (70%–84%),[25,26] and prosthetic grafts (62%–87%)[27,28] are favorable making them suitable primary, secondary, and tertiary options, respectively, for hemodialysis as outlined in the KDOQI guidelines.[7] While a meta-analysis has suggested that radial-cephalic patency rates can be as low as 62%,[23] their distal nature and favorable complication profile make it the ideal primary AVF option. Historically, on the basis of a data-driven selection process, the KDOQI investigators have favored the brachial-cephalic AVF with its favorable (70%–84%) patency rates[24,25] as the secondary option of choice.[7] However lower longer term patency rates have been observed. For instance, Dunlop et al., observed an overall patency rate of 57% at 2 years, and 50% at 3 years among 81 fistulas performed in 77 patients.[26] Subsequently, controversy has emerged regarding the favored tertiary option since the development of synthetic grafts and BVT as viable procedures.

ARTERIOVENOUS GRAFTS USING POLYTETRAFLUOROETHYLENE COMPARED TO BASILIC VEIN TRANSPOSITION

A common alternative to autogenous AVF creation when sites are either exhausted or not viable is the insertion of an AVG using synthetic material such as polytetrafluoroethylene (PTFE). AVG using PTFE have demonstrated one-year primary patency rates ranging between 62% and 87%.[27,28] When BVT was directly compared to AVG using PTFE, patency of BVT was higher (90% versus 70% at 12 months; and 86% versus 49% at 24 months).[29] Keuter et al., in a multicenter randomized study also demonstrated superior patency for BVT compared to PTFE grafts.[30] In a high-risk population including patients of advanced age, diabetics, peripheral vascular disease, previous access failure, Gonzalez et al., found superior patency of the two-stage BVT compared to PTFE AVG.[31] Furthermore, fewer interventions are necessary to maintain patency with fewer complications among BVT compared to PTFE grafts.[30]

Perhaps more striking is the inferiority of PTFE grafts (43%) compared to BVT (17%) regarding all complications. Similarly, Matsuura et al. observed higher thrombosis (51% versus 30%) and infection (10% versus 0%) rates of AVG using PTFE compared to BVT.[32] However, complications related to cannulation including bleeding and hematoma formation were worse for the BVT group (20% versus 5%).[32] Nonetheless, Coburn and Carney suggested that AVG using PTFE was technically easier to perform, could be cannulated sooner, and produced higher flow rates.[29]

BASILIC VEIN TRANSPOSITION PATENCY RATES

In a recent study, Glowinski et al, reviewed patients who underwent forearm BVT after failing a radial-cephalic fistula.[33] They observed 100% maturation with 93% patency at 1 year, 78% at 2 years, and 55% after 3 years.[33] Gormus et al. studied the outcomes of forearm and upper arm BVT.[33] They reported slightly better short-term (10 month) primary patency rates in radial-to-basilic fistulas created in the forearm compared with brachial-basilic fistulas created at the elbow (90% versus 80%), but with more complications.[34] Despite being the earliest experience of BVT, Dagher et al. reported an 8-year patency rate of 70% for the two-stage procedure.[11] These favorable outcomes have generated great interest to supplant brachiocephalic AVF and PTFE grafts as secondary and tertiary options. Consequently, many recent studies have reported outcomes of BVT. A systematic review of BVT was performed by Dix et al. in 2006, and we have expanded this search to include publications as of June 2013. Briefly, the MEDLINE, EMBASE, and Cochrane Library databases were searched and supplemented by review of conference proceedings and publication bibliographies. All original studies of basilic arteriovenous fistula reporting patency outcomes at 1 year, 2 years, and 3 years were included and are presented in (Table 12-3). These data establish BVT as a legitimate tertiary if not secondary option.

TABLE 12-3. PATENCY RATES OF BASILIC VEIN TRANSPOSITION ARTERIOVENOUS FISTULA

Author	Year	N	Primary Patency (months)		
			12	24	36
Jennings et al.	2013	30	57%	N/A	N/A
Ayez et al.	2012	151	40.80%	30.20%	N/A
Matsumoto et al.	2012	41	68.10%	55.00%	N/A
Morosetti et al.	2011	30	61%	60%	N/A
Smith et al.	2011	34	41%	20%	N/A
Paulson et al.	2011	49	72%	54%	54%
Korkut et al.	2010	350	92%	78%	64%
Paul et al.	2010	98	58.4%	31.8%	N/A
Paul et al.	2010	78	45.7%	27.6%	N/A
Son et al.	2010	461	67.6%	53.9%	N/A
Glass et al.	2010	215	63%	40%	26%
Veeramani et al.	2010	14	78.6%	N/A	N/A
Kim et al.	2010	31	91%	N/A	N/A
Koksoy et al.	2009	100	86%	N/A	73%
Hashemi et al	2009	293	95%	N/A	N/A
Chemla et al.	2008	34	73%	69%	N/A
Casey et al.	2008	59	50%	N/A	N/A
Haricharan et al.	2008	18	74%	N/A	N/A
Keuter et al.	2008	52	46%	N/A	N/A
Moosavi et al.	2008	58	56.5%	N/A	N/A
Pflederer et al.	2008	161	58%	44%	N/A
Bronder et al.	2008	295	60%	46%	N/A
Torina et al.	2008	141	45%	N/A	N/A
Beaulieu et al.	2007	543	42%	N/A	N/A
Weale et al.	2007	71	45.3%	40%	N/A
Woo et al.	2007	120	71%	N/A	N/A
Yilmaz et al.	2007	42	71.4%	54.7%	N/A
Wolford et al.	2005	87	23%	11%	N/A
El Sayed et al.	2005	162	52.2%	41.6%	30.3%
Keuter et al.	2005	31	58%	47%	N/A
Hill et al.	2005	32	66%	N/A	N/A
Rao et al.	2004	56	35%	N/A	N/A
Taghizadeh et al.	2003	75	92%	N/A	N/A

Author	Year	N	Primary Patency (months)		
			12	24	36
Segal et al.	2003	99	47%	41%	N/A
Tsai et al.	2002	54	90%	73%	65%
Murphy et al.	2002	74	68%	54%	44%
Gibson et al.	2001	181	44%	28%	N/A
Humphries et al.	1999	67	84%	N/A	73%
Matsuura et al.	1998	30	70%	70%	N/A
Stonebridge et al.	1994	19	79%	N/A	N/A
Coburn et al.	1994	59	90%	86%	N/A
Elcheroth et al.	1994	80	76.7%	N/A	N/A
Hatjibaloglou et al.	1992	25	81%	N/A	N/A
Hibberd et al.	1991	15	70%	50%	N/A
Davis et al.	1986	66	83.3%	N/A	N/A
Dagher et al.	1986	96	70%	N/A	N/A
Koontz et al.	1983	12	75%	N/A	N/A
Cantelmo et al.	1982	68	70%	66%	57.2%
Dagher et al.	1980	90	78%	N/A	N/A
Barnett et al.	1979	16	94%	N/A	N/A
LoGerfo et al.	1978	25	85%	N/A	N/A

COMPLICATIONS OF BASILIC VEIN TRANSPOSITION

Surgical procedures to create an AVF are complex in nature, and the ESRD patient population is equally complex with multiple comorbidities including peripheral vascular disease, hypertension, and diabetes. Moreover, ESRD and associated comorbid conditions are often predictors of complications after AVF creation in general and BVT in particular.

A failure to create the fistula (up to 7%)[29] or failure of maturation (up to 38%)[35] due to either an inadequate basilic vein or arterial inflow are reported complications of BVT. These events are often associated with advanced patient age. Interestingly, maturation rates among diabetics were more favorable for BVT (100%) compared to radial-cephalic fistulas (30%) supporting BVT as a primary option in these patients.[36]

While pain is often not a reported outcome after vascular access procedures, BVT performed using a single lengthy incision might be expected to generate substantial pain. A lengthy incision and extensive vascular dissection renders BVT prone to the complications of bleeding and hematoma formation. Of the studies included in the systematic review performed by Dix et al., hematomas developed in 3.8% and fistula rupture occurred in 0.25% of cases.[12] While fistula rupture can be life threatening, hematoma formation can lead to compression of the fistula and subsequent failure necessitating early evacuation if compromise is suspected. Indeed, Hossny identified hematoma formation as an important predictor of BVT failure.[21] Hematoma formation commonly occurs after early attempts at cannulation before healing and obliteration of the tunnel surrounding the BVT. Consequently, a period of at least 6 weeks following BVT to allow for maturation and healing is advisable.

Infections are also a consideration after fistula surgery, particularly after BVT due to the lengthy incision used for the procedure. While infections are more frequent after PTFE grafts, infections of the wound or fistula are reported in up to 3.6% of BVT cases based on the systematic review by Dix and colleagues.[12]

Steal syndrome is a well-recognized complication of fistula formation. If blood preferentially flows from the brachial artery into the fistula without providing sufficient flow to the hand symptoms of pain, cold temperature, nerve injury, and hand necrosis may develop. The size of the arteriovenous anastomosis often determines whether steal syndrome develop. For instance, an anastomosis that is too small can lead to stenosis and ultimately thrombosis and fistula failure. Too large an anastomosis will lead to excess flow through the low resistance fistula and insufficient flow to the hand generating symptoms of steal syndrome. After BVT, steal syndrome has been reported in up to 5.4% of cases.[35] Many authors have suggested the use of digital-brachial index as an intraoperative predictor of the development of symptomatic steal syndrome.

In contrast, stenosis, which can lead to thrombosis and failure, increasingly can be treated using endovascular techniques.[37] The causes of stenosis can be multiple including poor anastomotic surgical technique, poor fistula orientation, and injury to the fistula due to cannulation. The two-stage BVT that necessitates two anastomoses might be particularly prone to stenosis. However, a favorable stenosis rate of only 2.3% and thrombosis rate of 9.7% has been observed after BVT.[12]

Pseudoaneurysm formation can develop after repeated venipuncture of the AVF at the same site. Consequently, KDOQI guidelines suggest that cannulation sites be migrated regularly to obviate the development of pseudoaneurysms. Aneurysm formation can develop at the site of anastomosis and might result as a consequence of cannulation at this site or due to infection with the suture material acting as a nidus. Pseudoaneurysm formation complicates BVT in approximately 2% of cases.[12] In addition, the flow through the fistula is most profoundly impacted by the luminal diameter so that pseudoaneurysm formation might profoundly increase flow to the detriment of the dialysis patient. Indeed, high-output cardiac failure can be precipitated due to high fistula flow rates among aneurysmal fistulae, or alternatively, normal flow rates can be problematic for ESRD patients with numerous cardiovascular risk factors that are prone to heart failure. The incidence of high output cardiac after BVT is reported to be less than 0.2%.[28]

Finally, arm edema is an important complication following AVF creation. Given that BVT is often regarded as a tertiary option, the rate of arm edema, which is greatly impacted by previous failed vascular access procedures, might inflate the risk of arm edema. The rate of arm edema after BVT ranges between 3.7% and 21%.[12,21]

CONCLUSION

BVT represents a safe and efficacious tertiary if not secondary option for hemodialysis access. BVT demonstrates a favorable patency to complication ratio and hence should be considered before AVG insertion. Furthermore, randomized studies with sufficient sample size are necessary to address whether outcomes after BVT are not inferior to those obtained for brachial-cephalic AVF creation.

REFERENCES

1. Collins AJ, Foley RN, Herzog C, et al. US renal data system 2010 annual data report. *Am J Kidney Dis.* 2011;57:A8, e1–526.
2. Abecassis M, Bartlett ST, Collins AJ, et al. Kidney transplantation as primary therapy for end-stage renal disease: a national kidney foundation/kidney disease outcomes quality initiative (nkf/kdoqitm) conference. *Clin J Am Soc Nephrol: CJASN.* 2008;3:471–480.
3. Matas AJ, Smith JM, Skeans MA, et al. Optn/srtr 2011 annual data report: kidney. *Am J Transplant.* 2013;13(Suppl 1):11–46.
4. Kolff WJ, Berk HT, ter Welle M, et al. The artificial kidney: a dialyser with a great area. 1944. *J Am Soc Nephrol:JASN.* 1997;8:1959–1965.
5. Moist LM, Trpeski L, Na Y, Lok CE. Increased hemodialysis catheter use in Canada and associated mortality risk: data from the canadian organ replacement registry 2001–2004. *Clin J Am Soc Nephrol:CJASN.* 2008;3:1726–1732.
6. NKF-DOQI clinical practice guidelines for vascular access. National kidney foundation-dialysis outcomes quality initiative. *Am J Kidney Dis.* 1997;30:S150–191.
7. Ascher E, Hingorani A. The dialysis outcome and quality initiative (doqi) recommendations. *Semin Vasc Surg.* 2004;17:3–9.
8. Lok CE. Fistula first initiative: advantages and pitfalls. *Clin J Am Soc Nephrol:CJASN.* 2007;2:1043–1053.
9. Brescia MJ, Cimino JE, Appel K, Hurwich BJ. Chronic hemodialysis using venipuncture and a surgically created arteriovenous fistula. *N Engl J Med.* 1966;275:1089–1092.
10. Cascardo S, Acchiardo S, Beven EG, et al. Proximal arteriovenous fistulae for haemodialysis when radial arteries are unavailable. *Proc Europ Dial Transplant Assoc.* 1970;7:42–46.
11. Dagher F, Gelber R, Ramos E, Sadler J. The use of basilic vein and brachial artery as an a-v fistula for long term hemodialysis. *J Surg Res.* 1976;20:373–376.
12. Dix FP, Khan Y, Al-Khaffaf H. The brachial artery-basilic vein arterio-venous fistula in vascular access for haemodialysis—a review paper. *Eur J Vasc Endovasc Surg.* 2006;31:70–79.
13. Glass C, Porter J, Singh M, et al. A large-scale study of the upper arm basilic transposition for hemodialysis. *Ann Vasc Surg.* 2010;24:85–91.
14. Silva MB, Jr, Hobson RW 2nd, Pappas PJ, et al. Vein transposition in the forearm for autogenous hemodialysis access. *J Vasc Surg.* 1997;26:981–986; discussion 987–988.
15. Davis JB Jr, Howell CG, Humphries AL Jr. Hemodialysis access: Elevated basilic vein arteriovenous fistula. *J Ped Surg.* 1986;21:1182–1183.
16. LoGerfo FW, Menzoian JO, Kumaki DJ, Idelson BA. Transposed basilic vein-brachial arteriovenous fistula. A reliable secondary-access procedure. *Arch Surg.* 1978;113:1008–1010.
17. Tordoir JH, Dammers R, de Brauw M. Video-assisted basilic vein transposition for haemo-dialysis vascular access: preliminary experience with a new technique. *Nephrol Dial Transpl.* 2001;16:391–394.
18. Weiswasser JM, Kellicut D, Arora S, Sidawy AN. Strategies of arteriovenous dialysis access. *Semin. Vasc Surg.* 2004;17:10–18.
19. Gefen JY, Fox D, Giangola G, et al. The transposed forearm loop arteriovenous fistula: A valuable option for primary hemodialysis access in diabetic patients. *Ann. Vasc Surg.* 2002;16:89–94.
20. El Mallah S. Staged basilic vein transposition for dialysis angioaccess. *Int Angiol.* 1998;17:65–68.
21. Hossny A. Brachiobasilic arteriovenous fistula: different surgical techniques and their effects on fistula patency and dialysis-related complications. *J Vasc Surg.* 2003;37:821–826.
22. Martinez BD, LeSar CJ, Fogarty TJ, et al. Transposition of the basilic vein for arteriovenous fistula: an endoscopic approach. *J Am Coll Surg.* 2001;192:233–236.
23. Foran RF, Shore EH, Levin PM, Treiman RL. Bovine heterografts for hemodialysis. *West J Med.* 1975;123:269–274.

24. Rooijens PP, Tordoir JH, Stijnen T, et al. Radiocephalic wrist arteriovenous fistula for hemodialysis: meta-analysis indicates a high primary failure rate. *Eur J Vasc Endovasc Surg.* 2004;28:583–589.

25. Dunlop MG, Mackinlay JY, Jenkins AM. Vascular access: experience with the brachiocephalic fistula. *Ann R Coll Surg Engl.* 1986;68:203–206.

26. Bender MH, Bruyninckx CM, Gerlag PG. The gracz arteriovenous fistula evaluated. Results of the brachiocephalic elbow fistula in haemodialysis angio-access. *Eur J Vasc Endovasc Surg.* 1995;10:294–297.

27. Tellis VA, Kohlberg WI, Bhat DJ, et al. Expanded polytetrafluoroethylene graft fistula for chronic hemodialysis. *Ann Surg.* 1979;189:101–105.

28. Anderson CB, Sicard GA, Etheredge EE. Bovine carotid artery and expanded polytetrafluroethylene grafts for hemodialysis vascular access. *J Surg Res.* 1980;29:184–188.

29. Coburn MC, Carney WI Jr. Comparison of basilic vein and polytetrafluoroethylene for brachial arteriovenous fistula. *J Vasc Surg.* 1994;20:896–902; discussion 903–894.

30. Keuter XH, De Smet AA, Kessels AG, et al. A randomized multicenter study of the outcome of brachial-basilic arteriovenous fistula and prosthetic brachial-antecubital forearm loop as vascular access for hemodialysis. *J Vasc Surg.* 2008;47:395–401.

31. Gonzalez E, Kashuk JL, Moore EE, et al. Two-stage brachial-basilic transposition fistula provides superior patency rates for dialysis access in a safety-net population. *Surgery.* 2010;148:687–693; discussion 693–684.

32. Matsuura JH, Rosenthal D, Clark M, et al. Transposed basilic vein versus polytetrafluoroethylene for brachial-axillary arteriovenous fistulas. *Am J Surg.* 1998;176:219–221.

33. Glowinski J, Glowinska I, Malyszko J, Gacko M. Basilic vein transposition in the forearm for secondary arteriovenous fistula. *Angiology.* 2013.

34. Gormus N, Ozergin U, Durgut K, et al. Comparison of autologous basilic vein transpositions between forearm and upper arm regions. *Ann Vasc Surg.* 2003;17:522–525.

35. Rao RK, Azin GD, Hood DB, et al. Basilic vein transposition fistula: a good option for maintaining hemodialysis access site options? *J Vasc Surg.* 2004;39:1043–1047.

36. Hakaim AG, Nalbandian M, Scott T. Superior maturation and patency of primary brachiocephalic and transposed basilic vein arteriovenous fistulae in patients with diabetes. *J Vasc Surg.* 1998;27:154–157.

37. Rivers SP, Scher LA, Sheehan E, et al. Basilic vein transposition: An underused autologous alternative to prosthetic dialysis angioaccess. *J Vasc Surg.* 1993;18:391–396; discussion 396–397.

13

Alternative Conduits for Hemodialysis Access

Vivian Marie Torres, MD, Ravi Kapadia, MD, and William Frank Oppat, MD

ALTERNATIVE CONDUITS FOR HEMODIALYSIS ACCESS

End-stage renal disease (ESRD) and the population of patients treated for ESRD in the United States are rising at an alarming rate. The cost of caring for patients with need for renal replacement therapy has soared. It is currently estimated that the cost to Medicare for providing one year of hemodialysis is over $43 thousand, a staggering figure when the average yearly healthcare cost of a retired Medicare recipient is $7654.[1] Surprisingly, the care and maintenance of access for hemodialysis is one of the biggest drivers of healthcare expense in patients afflicted with ESRD.

The adjusted prevalence rate of ESRD rose 1.7% in 2010 to 1763 per million in the American population. When compared to the prevalence rate in the year 2000, the current rate is 21% higher. The annual rate of increase in the number of Americans who develop ESRD has remained between 1.7% and 2.3% since 2004. Clearly, the population of patients who will require dialysis access continues to grow. As of December 31, 2010, the total treated ESRD population in the United States was 593,086; of these, 383,992 where on hemodialysis[2] Figures 13-1 and 13-2). Hemodialysis is the most common and effective means of therapy for ESRD. Ninety-one percent of patients starting dialysis therapy will start on hemodialysis.[2] Furthermore, the mortality for patients with ESRD on dialysis has decreased over the years.

Among the patients who require renal replacement therapy, hemodialysis access failure and the complications associated with dialysis access are the commonest causes of hospitalization and are responsible for the greatest number of hospitalized days.[3] As patients receiving hemodialysis live longer, the need for effective, durable access becomes more obvious, especially in an era of increasingly limited funds for chronic care of Medicare recipients.

Longitudinal population studies convincingly demonstrate dialysis access by means of an autologous AV fistula provides the best, most durable option for patients with ESRD who require hemodialysis. In 1993, the year for which peak data are

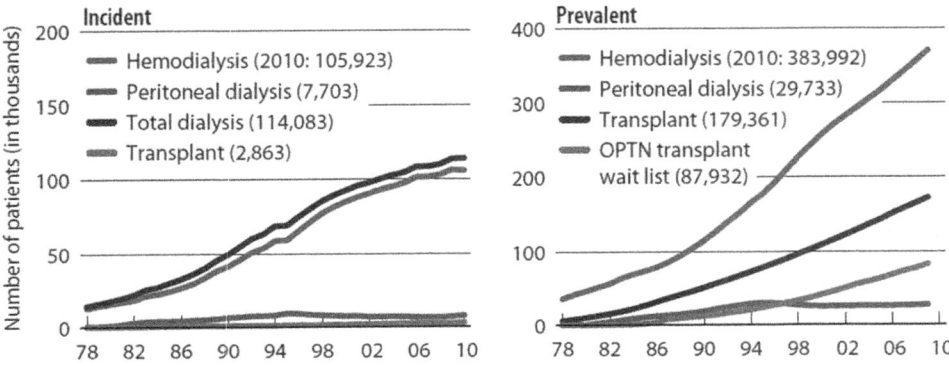

Figure 13-1. Incident and prevalent patient counts (USRDS) by modality.

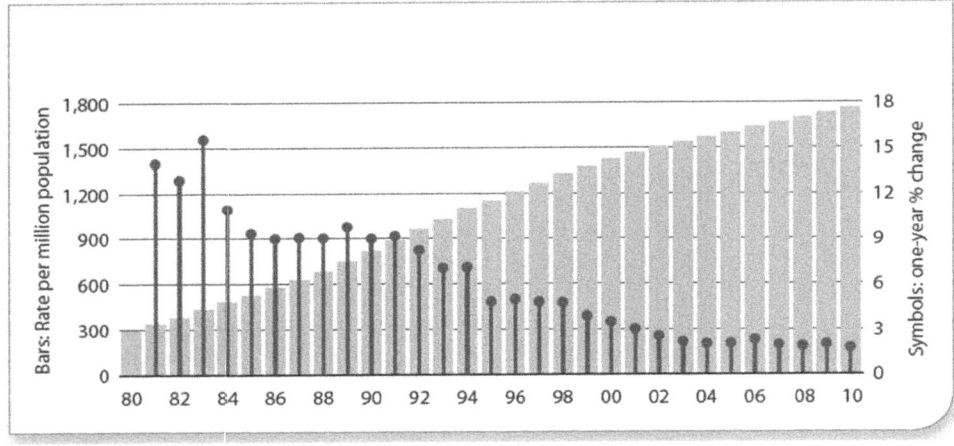

Figure 13-2. Adjusted prevalent rates of ESRD and annual percent change.

currently available, 73% of incident patients had a hemodialysis access bridge graft constructed from polytetrafluoroethylene (PTFE).[4] In 1997, the National Kidney Foundation (NKF)-Kidney Disease Outcomes Quality Initiative (KDOQI) Clinical Practice Guidelines were published in an effort to increase autogenous access placement as a means to control runaway cost and improve quality. The NKF-KDOQI data-driven initiative has been hugely successful. Nationally, arteriovenous fistula (AVF) prevalence rates have increased to nearly reach the goals of 65%.[3]

However, despite their purported advantages, autologous AVF ultimately have a finite life expectancy and will eventually require revision or replacement. Furthermore, the increase in the ESRD patient population aged 65–74 (baby boomers), many of whom are diabetic seem to lack adequate native vessels suitable for creation of a functional, durable arteriorvenous fistula (AVF). Therefore, it is imperative that access surgeons are familiar with readily available alternative conduits for hemodialysis, including their advantages and limitations. This requires a familiarity with alternative techniques and new technology coupled with a certain level of creativity to provide new options for hemodialysis access once the standard access sites and conduit has reached its useful life expectancy.

Objectively analyzed, the ideal nonautogenous hemodialysis access system must be durable, must enjoy prolonged patency, must provide adequate flow rates for effective dialysis, and must display resistance to infection and degeneration with low complication rates and pseudoaneurysm formation. The ideal conduit has to be accessible and easy to cannulate for the technician.

We expect to review some of the current alternative conduits that exist for hemodialysis when autogenous vessels are inadequate or have failed. We will review strategies that we have utilized to overcome inflow or outflow issues.

SYNTHETIC AV GRAFTS

Despite the heightened awareness of the effectiveness of autologous AVF are directly attributable to success of the well-publicized and data-driven NKF-DOKI guidelines, nearly half of the ESRD patient population currently receive HD through a synthetic AV graft.[3] Reasons for alternative conduits are utilized to provide access for hemodialysis have been analyzed and fall into three major categories.

Even though the attempt to create a primary AVF has dramatically increased, as many as 30% of AVF fail to mature.[5] Once a fistula is created, it must develop to the point that it is usable. Basically, maturation requires two things—adequate arterial inflow and physical characteristics of the vein that allow for repetitive cannulation. Without adequate inflow, the fistula will simply not develop. The suitability of the fistula to tolerate repetitive cannulation is somewhat harder to judge. Maturation in essence relates to the diameter of the AVF and how the flow feels (the thrill). There are other characteristics of the AVF that are also important for cannulation and successful hemodialysis, such as its position on the arm, its configuration, and its depth. The increasing drive to comply with the national KDOQI guidelines may lead access surgeons to create AVF in patients with unsuitable or less than ideal anatomy in an effort to meet the KDOQI guidelines. In the United States, an increase in the elderly population who develop ESRD and initiate HD tend to be diabetic, and the diabetic subset of patients has a higher fistula failure rate with higher likelihood of steal development. The subset of women initiating hemodialysis is also at increased risk of autogenous access failure, presumably due to smaller arteries and veins in the upper extremity. Synthetic bridge grafts are a sensible initial conduit for the creation of dialysis access in many elderly, diabetic patients who do not have suitable anatomy for the creation of autologous access or the life expectancy needed to reach maturation of an autologous fistula.

Furthermore, in many regions of the United States, a delay between the initiation of hemodialysis and the referral to an access surgeon still exists. Temporary centrally placed venous catheters provide urgent access for the initiation of HD. The KDOQI data clearly demonstrate that patients with ESRD who initiate hemodialysis through catheters suffer more complications primarily as a result of infections and the development of central venous stenosis. In patients with shortened life expectancy, it might be more appropriate to create the prosthetic bridge shunt that is more likely to be successful, at least in the short term, to limit the time with an indwelling catheter and its associated complications.

Prosthetic bridge shunts have several advantages. Recognizing that a successful fistula or shunt must have good inflow, unobstructed outflow, and a healthy conduit, the questionable autologous vein seen in many of the elderly is eliminated from the list of reasons that AFV fail to provide durable access. Assuming that the inflow and outflow are adequate, the creation of a bridge shunt is straightforward, and it can be performed quickly under minimal anesthesia. Most patients will have vessels adequate for placement of AV graft, even if the bridge shunt must be based on more proximal axillary inflow and outflow vessels. Other advantages of bridge shunts include increased early tolerance to access when compared to AVF and increased ease of cannulation for the dialysis technician. Despite the recognized advantages of bridge shunts, an AVF continues to be the ideal conduit as prosthetic grafts are associated with higher morbidity, primarily due to infection. Other major drawbacks associated with synthetic grafts are stenosis secondary to intimal hyperplasia with or without graft thrombosis, and vascular steal syndrome. Unlike autologous conduits that have a propensity to heal post cannulation, bridge shunts do eventually wear out. A 2008 single center, single surgeon experience of 1700 procedures showed no significant difference in patency between prosthetic AV graft and AV fistula, with a median patency time of 10 months for both groups. However, the infection rate was significantly higher for AV grafts (9.5%) than the fistulas (0.9%). Thrombosis occurred in 24.7% of grafts and 9.0% of fistulas.[6]

Several modifications have been made to grafts in an attempt to reduce infection and thrombosis. Despite these modifications, thrombosis and infection continue to be significant source of morbidity for this population.

PTFE GRAFTS

PTFE is the most commonly used material for prosthetic AV access construction because it most closely satisfies the criteria for an ideal conduit. PTFE handles well and is readily available in a variety of sizes at most institutions. Also, the material is partially anti-thrombogenic and non-antigenic. Although there is a higher incidence of infection, the material is more resistant to disintegration under these circumstances. The use of PTFE synthetic grafts has been associated with higher incidence of arterial steal. Tapered grafts are used in an effort to reduce this complication. The most commonly used diameter of PTFE is 6mm and 40–45 cm length; up to 8mm diameter grafts are used for hemodialysis access. The larger diameter graft may prolong the patency of the venous anastomosis, which is susceptible to intimal hyperplasia albeit at a higher risk for the development of steal. The thicker wall of the 8mm grafts may provide a longer duty cycle for repeated cannuulations.

Despite the recommendations in the KDOQI and their justifications based on retrospective reports in multiple subsets of the population, no randomized controlled trials or meta-analyses comparing AVF to prosthetic access exists. However, Hubert et al.[7] conducted a formal systematic review of the literature comparing the patency rates of upper extremity PTFE and autogenous accesses in adults. There were 34 studies included in the review, with the majority composed of case series or nonrandomized controlled studies with the data collected in a retrospective fashion. The primary annual patency rates for the autogenous and PTFE accesses were approximately 60% and 40%, respectively, whereas the corresponding secondary patency rates were 80% and 60% (Figure 13-3).

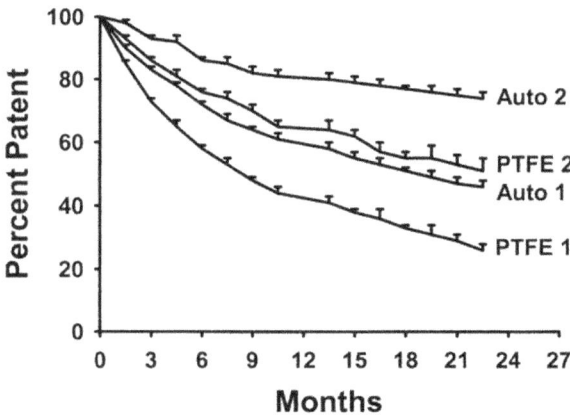

Figure 13-3. Primary annual patency rates for the autogenous and PTFE accesses.

The KDOQI guidelines recommend PTFE over other prosthetic or biologic conduits for patients who are not candidates for autogenous AVF access. The guidelines state that the access may be configured straight, looped, or curved, with the ultimate objective of optimizing the surface area available for cannulation. A review of evidence-based medicine for the hemodialysis surgeon was published by Huber et al. in 2004.[8] In this review, the authors were unable to identify any randomized controlled trials examining the various locations or configurations for the prosthetic grafts. The DOQI recommends that the configuration should be optimized surface area and the location should be dictated by individual patient's anatomy, the surgeon's skill and preference as well as the anticipated period of time the access will be required; all these recommendations seem reasonable, although largely opinion.

In addition to being used as a primary hemodialysis conduit in patients with no available vessels for the creation of an AV fistula, PTFE grafts can provide an option for the salvage for fistulas that are failing while preserving proximal vein for future conduit creation. PTFE grafts may be used as an interposition graft as a means to surgically revise failing fistulas with lesions such as stenosis, pseudoaneurysm, or sclerosed cannulation segments. A prospective review published by Georgiadis et al.[9] addressed the use of a PTFE interposition graft as a means to surgically revise failing or failed autogenous AV fistulas. A total of 59 pts were followed for a mean 16.7 months; roughly half (30) were revised surgically with a short segment (<6 cm) 6 mm PTGE graft for venous stenosis. The rest of the patients were surgically revised with a new autologous fistula or with resection and primary anastomosis of the affected venous segment. Postintervention primary cumulative patency in PTFE group was 100% at 6 months, 88% at 12 months, and 82% at 18 months, whereas the corresponding patency for autologous group was 90% at 6 months, 82% at 12 months, and 71% at 18 months. No statistical differences in postintervention patency rates were observed between the two groups (Figures 13-4 and 13-5).

In a retrospective analysis to be presented at the Midwestern Vascular Society meeting in September 2013, we review our experience with 19 patients who received 8-mm PTFE graft as a means of surgically revising a failing autologuous AV fistula. From 2000 to 2011, 19 patients who presented with failing AVF but preserved arterial

Access characteristics	Group I (PTFE) (%)	Group II (autologous) (%)	P
Type of autogenous AVF before revision			.275*
Lower arm accesses	20 (67)	23 (79)	
Upper arm accesses	10 (33)	6 (21)	
Brachiocephalic access	6 (20.0)	3 (10)	
Brachiobasilic access	4 (13)	3 (10)	
AVF condition before revision			.953*
Failing	25 (83)	24 (83)	
Failed	5 (17)	5 (17)	
Previous accesses on ipsilateral arm			1.00†
0-2	26 (87)	25 (86)	
>2	4 (13)	4 (14)	
Lesions detected			.691*
Type I stenosis	15 (50)	16 (55)	
Type II stenosis	15 (50)	5 (17)	
Steal syndrome	—	2 (7)	
Difficult vein cannulation segment	—	2 (7)	
Low inflow state	—	2 (7)	
Anastomotic aneurysm	—	1 (3)	
Vein aneurysm rupture	—	1 (3)	

PTFE, Polytetrafluoroethylene; AVF, arteriovenous fistula.
*χ^2 test.
†Fisher-exact test, two-tailed P values.

Figure 13-4. Post-intervention primary cumulative patency in PTFE and autogenous groups.

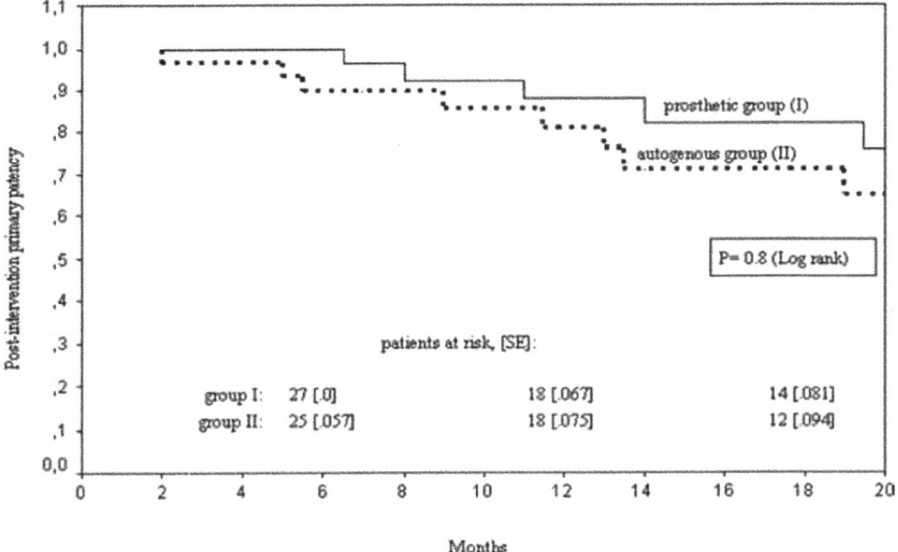

Figure 13-5. Kaplan-Maier postintervention primary patency curves. SE = standard error.

inflow and venous outflow and no steal symptoms were converted to 8-mm PTFE interposition shunt. Maximum length of interposition graft used was 40 cm. Assisted primary patency exceeded two years in 8/17 patients. Of these, only one patient developed steal symptoms requiring ligation four months after placement. We believe that a greater diameter PTFE with a thicker wall provides a more durable alternative to more proximal AVF formation, thereby preserving options for future conduits without significant development of steal.

CUFFED PTFE GRAFTS

A major cause of failure of prosthetic grafts is outflow stenosis believed secondary to intimal hyperplasia of the venous anastomosis. In fact, the most common cause of graft dysfunction is the development of a stenosis. It occurs most commonly in AVF at the graft vein and juxta-anastomotic vein segment and is primarily due to venous intimal hyperplasia.[10] Many factors are thought to contribute to the development of intimal hyperplasia at the venous anastomosis in prosthetic bridge shunts; the most significant is the presence of flow disturbances at this site. The surgical trauma at the time of AV surgery, hemodynamic shear stress at the vein graft outflow anastomosis, graft bio-incompatibility, vessel injury due to repeated cannulations, uremia resulting in endothelial dysfunction, and repeated angioplasties that result in further endothelial injury are all factors that contribute to the development of intimal hyperplasia.[11] In an attempt to reduce the flow disturbances leading to intimal hyperplasia and stenosis at the venous outflow anastomosis, the geometry of the outflow anastomosis has been modified and assessed for extension of graft patency. The use of cuffed PTFE has resulted in improved patency rates in various studies. Sorom et al.[12] reported in a prospective evaluation that PTFE grafts configured with a PTFE cuff (Venaflo, Impra) had superior one-year patency rates than noncuffed stretch PTFE grafts (Gore). They reported a one-year secondary patency of 64% for cuffed grafts versus 32% for noncuffed. None of the grafts failed as a result of venous outflow stenosis. Tsoulfas et al.[13] retrospectively reviewed a total of 67 patients who underwent placement of either cuffed or standard PTFE grafts and analyzed primary and secondary patency rates at one to three years. They found a trend toward better primary graft patency rates in the cuffed versus the standard PTFE and a significant difference in secondary one-year patency rates between the two (81.8% for cuffed PTFE vs 56.1% for noncuffed PTFE). This increased secondary patency was sustained at two- and three-year analysis. Neither of these studies' author formulated an explanation of why the advantage of the cuffed is only observed in secondary patency rates and not in primary patency rates.

Interestingly, the use of a vein cuff at the venous anastomosis has not translated into improved patency rates of PTFE AV grafts. Lemson et al.[14] reported that the use of a venous anastomotic cuff did not improve patency when used with a thin wall PTFE (Gore) graft. Furthermore, Gagne et al.[15] reported a decrease in patency rate with the use of a vein cuff resulting in premature end to his study. It is not clear why the use of vein cuff not only did not improve patency rates of PTFE grafts but resulted in decreased patency grafts when compared to standard noncuffed grafts. As of now, there is no compelling evidence to use any type of cuffed PTFE graft for AV anastomosis, although some dialysis access surgeons might still see and advantage to using nonvein cuffed PTFE grafts.

EARLY ACCESS GRAFTS

Typically, graft longevity is extended if two to four weeks before a prosthetic graft is accessed for hemodialysis. It appears that the delay from placement to access permits tissue incorporation (scarring around the prosthetic graft) and allows for repeated puncture without perigraft hematoma formation or intimal hyperplasia within the body of the graft. Therefore, many patients require central venous hemodialysis catheters as a bridge during this period of time of healing to receive therapy. Central venous catheters place patients at higher risk of infectious complications, central venous stenosis/thrombosis, and overall delay in patients from seeking more permanent access and repetitive needle punctures. The catheters do not provide optimal flow rates for hemodialysis and result in increased healthcare costs per patient. Ultimately, central venous stenoses from dialysis catheters complicate the placement and/or lifespan of AVF or grafts.

In an effort to reduce the use of central venous catheters as a bridge for hemodialysis access while the prosthetic bridge shunt incorporates, grafts that allow for early cannulation have been developed with acceptable patency rates and low complication rates when compared to PTFE grafts. The Flixene (Atrium, Hudson, NH) graft is a three-layer graft (Figure 13-6) that can be accessed within 24–48 hours in most patients. Owing to its tri-laminate composition and thickness, the graft is in theory more resistant to repeat puncture as well as external compression and kinking. Schild et al.[16] reported on a prospective two-center trial including 33 patients who had a Flixene AV early access graft place. Patients were followed for six months to evaluate early cannulation success, postoperative complications, primary patency, and primary assisted patency. Dialysis center complications related to early cannulation was also documented. Early cannulation was successful in all patients. Primary and secondary patency rates at six months were equivalent to other data reported on PTFE grafts. No seroma or pseudoaneurysm formation was documented at six months. Owing to its relatively thick wall, this graft is more difficult to handle during creation of the anastomosis, and it can be difficult to palpate at the time of cannulation.

Another available early access cannulation graft is the Vectra (Thoratec Laboratories, Pleasanton, PA). This graft is a polyetherurethaneurea (PVAG) graft that was designed to be cannulated within 24 hours after implantation. Glickman et al.[17] reported on a randomized, prospective, multicenter study comparing the PVAG with standard PTFE: specifically patency, complication rates, time to first dialysis access,

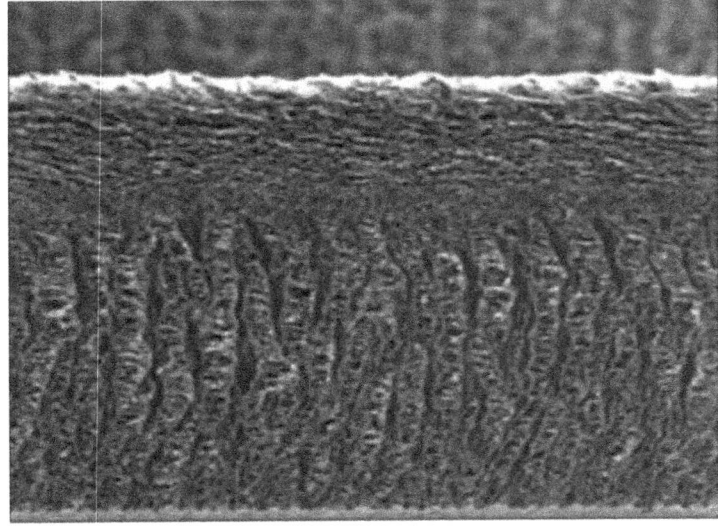

Figure 13-6. The Flixene (Atrium, Hudson, NH) graft.

and time to hemostasis after needle removal. He concluded that no significant difference in patency rates existed between the two grafts. All grafts were cannulated before nine days after implantation. PVAG grafts did achieve a shorter time to hemostasis after cannulation. The PVAG graft did have higher kinking rates when compared to PTFE. The authors concluded that the Vectra graft can be accessed early without having any detrimental effects in long-term patency or increased bleeding after cannulation.

CRYOPRESERVED ALLOGRAFT

Cryopreserved vein allografts represent an expensive but viable option for alternative nonautologous hemodialysis access when an autogenous AVF cannot be created. Most of the experience with cryopreserved allografts comes from its use as an alternative conduit for infected bypass grafts used for arterial reconstruction. Although cryopreserved allograft is less likely to become infected, the cryopreserved grafts appear to have a low resistance to infection and cases of graft rupture in the presence of infection have been reported. Mousavi et al.[18] conducted a prospective randomized study of 70 patients comparing PTFE and cryopreserved saphenous vein for hemodialysis access. They found no difference in flow rates or rate of thrombosis after a one-year follow-up. They did find an increased rate of infection in the PTFE group with none of the cryovein grafts infected at one-year follow-up. Cryopreserved femoral vein has also been used as an alternative conduit for hemodialysis with similar results as cryopreserved saphenous vein. Owing to the increased cost of cryopreserved allograft, these grafts are generally considered only for in situ replacement of arterioveous grafts when alternative sites are exhausted or infected.

BIOSYNTHETIC GRAFT

Biosynthetic grafts were more widely used in the past but have fallen from favor once PTFE grafts were successfully deployed. In theory, biosynthetic products should have similar compliance to autogenous veins and demonstrate increased resistance to intimal hyperplasia, infection, and degeneration. Bovine carotid artery, ureter, and mesenteric vein have been used as alternative conduits for hemodialysis. Kennealey et al.[19] recently reported their findings regarding the use of bovine carotid artery as an alternate hemodialyisis access. They conducted a prospective, randomized comparison of bovine carotid artery and PTFE graft. Fifty-seven patients were prospectively randomized to receive either the Artegraft bovine carotid graft (Artegraft, North Brunswick, NJ) or cuffed PTFE graft (Venaflo, Bard Peripheral Vascular, Tempe, AZ). Primary patency and primary assisted patency was significantly higher in the bovine artery group with rates of 60.5% for both. Patients with bovine artery graft also required fewer interventions to assist primary patency. The authors do note a decreased assisted primary patency rate of their cuffed PTFE group compared to previous reports with a primary assisted patency rate of 20.8% at one year. The small number of procedures might contribute to this discrepancy. Although more data are needed, bovine carotid artery seems to be a viable alternative to standard PTFE for secondary alternative nonautogenous dialysis access.

Bovine ureter has also been proposed as a biosynthetic alternative graft. Specifically, Das et al.[20] reported the results of a single center experience with this graft in the United Kingdom. Their results were not as favorable as those seen for the bovine carotid artery. They used a SynerGraft (S100; CryoLife Europa, Guildford UK) on 43 patients during a seven-year period. Their primary patency at one year was 13.9%, much lower than that reported for PTFE. Secondary patency improved to 70.1%, which is comparable to PTFE. These grafts responded well to percutaneous intervention after thrombosis, resulting in increased secondary patency. At this time this graft is not in the market. There is no clear advantage to using this graft over PTFE considering the lack of quality data and poor patency rates observed in the currently reported patency rates.

HYBRID DEVICES

In an attempt to reduce intimal hyperplasia and graft thrombosis, devices have been developed that eliminate the need for a sutured venous anastomosis. In theory, this strategy should reduce intimal hyperplasia by limiting the alteration in flow dynamics into the vein and the endothelial response to suture material used to create the venous anastomosis. An endoluminal anastomosis should also reduce venous manipulation and dissection. Recently, GORE® (Flagstaff, AZ) developed a hybrid "stent-graft" that can be applied not only in arterial bypasses for peripheral arterial obstructive disease but also as a hybrid vascular access graft. The GORE® hybrid graft is a PTFE graft that has a section reinforced with nitinol. The nitinol-reinforced section is partially constrained to allow for endoluminal insertion. There are no prospective trials to date reporting on patency or complication rates as compared to standard PTFE nonhybrid grafts. Therefore, it is premature to make any conclusions regarding the advantages of using this type of graft for dialysis access.

Another device designed to mitigate the effects of a venous anastomosis is the Atrium® (Hudson, NH) intraluminal flow guard (IFG) device. Similar to the hybrid graft, the IFG has a nitinol stent that deploys at the venous anastomosis. The IFG is a Flixene® graft ending in a T shape that is fitted into the vein through a small venotomy. The T-shape portion contains the nitinol reinforcement, thereby eliminating the need for a sutured anastomosis (Figure 13-7).

Mistry et al.[21] reported their prospective experience with the IFG device in a series of 12 patients who were then followed for a mean of 393 days. Primary patency,

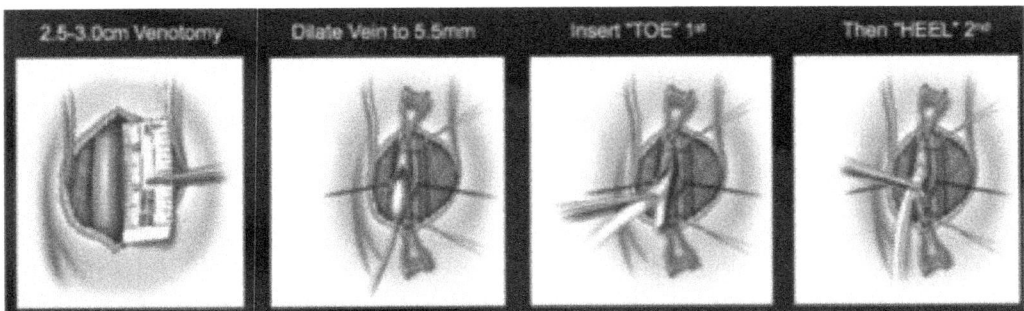

Figure 13-7. Intraluminal Flow Guard (IFG) device.

assisted primary patency, and secondary patency were 38.9%, 56.3%, and 64%, respectively. They did observe that three patients developed venous stenosis, two immediately adjacent to the venous stent and one proximal to it. The authors noted that these responded well to angioplasty. Even though the IFG device is a safe and effective method of establishing venous access for hemodialysis, further studies are needed in order to determine if it effectively reduces or eliminates intimal hyperplasia resulting from flow disturbances and ultimately avoids premature graft thrombosis.

A hybrid catheter commercially available for patients with limited and complex access options is the Hemodialysis Reliable Outflow catheter (HeRO®, Hemosphere, Eden Prairie, MN). The HeRO device is a clever alternative used to reestablish central venous access in dialysis patients with either central venous stenosis or occlusion. The main goal of the HeRO is to render patients free of tunneled central venous catheters while avoiding lower extremity access. In patients with central venous limitations, the HeRO has been successfully utilized to create a new access, "rescue" a failing access, and has also been used to address symptoms associated with severe upper extremity venous hypertension.

Tunneled central venous catheters and lower extremity catheters are linked to a higher rate of systemic infection. Tunneled central venous catheters place this patient group at risk for bacteremia and blood-related infections. Unfortunately, close to 80% of patients who initiate hemodyalisis will initiate with a catheter.[2] Among hemodialysis patients, admissions for vascular access infection rose steadily until 2005, but since have fallen 24% in 2010. Despite the improvement in dialysis access, admissions for bacteremia/sepsis remain highest for hemodialysis patients, at 116 per 1000 patient years in 2010.[2] The majority of infections are attributed to the presence of tunneled central venous catheters.

The study with the largest amount of patients was a multicenter, retrospective evaluating the use, longevity, and complications of the HeRO catheter conducted by Gage et al.[22] and sponsored by the manufacturer, Hemosphere Corp. The study included a total of 164 patients who underwent successful HeRO implantation across four medical centers, resulting in an accumulation of 2092.1 HeRO months. Follow up ranged from 0.07 to 32.9 months with a mean of 12.8. The access-related infection rate was 4.3% or 0.14 per 1000 catheter days. Primary and secondary patency at 12 months was 48.8% and 90.8%, respectively. At 24 months primary patency was 42.9% and secondary patency was 86.7%. There was no significant difference in terms of patency across the four centers. The authors concluded that the HeRO device is superior to tunneled dialysis catheters in terms of patency, intervention, and infection rates when compared to the available literature. They also found no difference in patency rates when compared to the available data for prosthetic grafts (Figure 13-8).

In contrast to this study, a single-institution, retrospective review by Wallace et al.[23] reported high complication rates and low secondary patency rates associated with the HeRO device. This study included 19 patients who underwent 21 consecutive attempts at HeRO implantation between June 2010 and January 2012. They report a 6- and 12-month primary patency rates of 6% and 11%, respectively. The 6- and 12-month secondary patency rates were 60% and 32%, respectively. They had an infection rate of 0.5 per 1000 catheter days, much higher than the 0.14 per 1000 catheter days reported by Gage et al.[22] but still lower than the rates reported for tunneled dialysis catheters. In addition, four patients (22%) developed steal, which required removal of the graft in the immediate postoperative period. Despite the study's small sample size and retrospective nature, it is the largest non-industry-sponsored study to date reporting the experience with HeRO device for patients with central venous stenosis or occlusion.

Variable	% [95% CI]
HeRO Patency[a]	
Primary at 6 months	60.0% [51.7, 67.3]
Secondary at 6 months	90.8% [84.9, 94.4]
Primary at 12 months	48.8% [39.9, 57.0]
Secondary at 12 months	90.8% [84.9, 94.4]
Primary at 24 months	42.9% [33.3,52.0]
Secondary at 24 months	86.7% [78.9,91.8]
HeRO intervention rate[b]	1.5/year [1.30, 1.67]
Access-related infections[c,d]	4.3% (6/140)

[a] Kaplan-Meier estimates with corresponding 95% CI.
[b] Rate per patient-year of follow-up; 257 events in 174.4 total patient years.
[c] % (n/N).
[d] Data only available from 3 sites.

Figure 13-8. HeRO patency, intervention, and infection data.

Use of the HeRO device appears beneficial for avoidance of long-term tunneled dialysis catheters and as a sensible option before moving to the lower extremity for graft placement secondary to central venous stenosis. With the purpose of comparing infection rates between lower extremity AVG and the HeRO graft, Steerman et al.[24] published a retrospective review of LE-AVG and HeRO implants from 2004 to 2010 performed at a single institution. During this time, 60 HeROs were placed in 59 patients and 22 lower extremity AV grafts were placed in 21 patients. When accessing infection rates, lower extremity AV grafts became infected at a rate of 0.71 per 1000 days, whereas HeROs became infected at a rate of 0.61 per 1000 days, with P value being nonsignificant. Overall, 13 of 59 HeROs (22.0%) and 6 of 20 lower extremity AV grafts (30%) became infected over the study period. Overall, they found no significant difference in rates of secondary patency, infection, and all-cause mortality between the implanted HeRO grafts and lower extremity AV grafts. Sample size was too small to evaluate primary patency rates due to statistically unreliable data. The advantage of the HeRO is that it maintains an upper extremity in the presence of central venous stenosis or obstruction. HeRO is useful particularly in patients with peripheral arterial disease and in the obese population, because it preserves the lower extremities for future access options as a last resort in a patient population that is at increased risk of complications from a lower extremity AV graft. The HeRO device has shown promise as an alternative to catheter dependence as means for permanent hemodialysis access and hopefully could reduce the morbidity, the mortality, and healthcare costs associated with tunneled dialysis catheters. Data from additional prospective, randomized trials could add further clarity on the Hero's performance and its use as an alternative to tunneled dialysis catheters and lower extremity catheters.

CONCLUSION

The population of ESRD patients requiring hemodialysis in the United States continues to grow. As medical advances permit improved care of this patient population, patients receiving renal replacement through dialysis live longer. This means that many patients outlive their autogenous AV fistula by years. This requires the access surgeon to keep up with the new technology available as well as be creative in order to continue to provide new options for the patient once their conduit has reached its life expectancy. The ideal alternative conduit needs to be tailored to the patient's anatomy and co-morbid conditions contributing to their morbidity and mortality as well as previous access history. High-quality data are lacking addressing the available alternative access for dialysis in patients that have exhausted their autogenous access conduits. As the newest devices and grafts in the market are used more frequently and in patients with variable characteristics, more information will be available to guide the surgeon in the choice of the best access option that will be tailored to a specific patient characteristics and needs.

REFERENCES

1. Medicare Payment Advisory Commission (MEDPAC); *A Data Book: Healthcare spending and the Medicare program*, June 2009. http://www.medpac.gov/chapters/jun09databooksec12.pdf
2. US Renal Data System, USRDS. *2012 Annual Data Report: Atlas of Chronic Kidney Disease and End-Stage Renal Disease in the United States.* Bethesda, MD: National Institutes of Health, National Institute of Diabetes and Digestive and Kidney Diseases; 2012.
3. Sidawy AN, Spergel LM, Besarab A, et al. The society for vascular surgery: clinical practice guidelines for the surgical placement and maintenance of arteriovenous hemodialysis access. *J Vasc Surg.* 2008;48(5):2S–25S.
4. U.S. Renal Data System. *U.S. Renal Data System 1997 Annual Report.* Chap. X. Washington, DC: 1997:143–161. http://www.usrds.org/chapters/ch10.pdf
5. Schild F. Maintaining vascular access: the management of hemodialysis arteriovenous grafts. *J Vasc Access.* 2010;11(2):92–99.
6. Schild AF, Perez E, Gillaspie E, et al. Arteriovenous fistulae vs. arteriovenous grafts: a restrospective review of 1,700 consecutive vascular access cases. *J Vasc Access.* 2008;9:231–235.
7. Huber TS, Carter JW, Carter RL, Seeger JM. Patency of autogenous and polytetrafluoroethylene upper extremity arteriovenous hemodialysis access: a systematic review. *J Vasc Surg.* 2003;39:491–496.
8. Huber TS, Buhler AG, Seeger JM. Evidence-based data for the hemodialysis access surgeon. *Semin Dial.* 2004;17(3):217–223.
9. Georgiadis GS, Lazarides MK, Lambidis CD, et al. Use of short PTFE segments (6 cm) compares favorably with pure autologous repair in failing or thrombosed native arteriovenous fistulas. *J Vasc Surg.* 2005;41:76–81.
10. Basile C, Konner K, Lomonte C. The haemodialysis arteriovenous graft: is a new era coming? *Nephrol Dial Transplant.* 2012;27:876–878.
11. Lee T. Hemodialysis vascular access dysfunction In: Carpi A, Donadio C, Tramonti G eds. *Progress in Hemodialysis from Emergent Biotechnology to Clinical Practice.* 2011. www.intechopen.com
12. Sorom AJ, Hughes CB, McCarthy JT, et al. Prospective, randomized evaluation of a cuffed expanded polytetrafluoroethylene graft for hemodialysis vascular access. *Surgery.* 2002;132:135–140.
13. Tsoulfas G, Hertl M, Dicken SCK, et al. Long-term outcome of a cuffed expanded PTFE graft for hemodialysis vascular access. *World J Surg.* 2008;32:1827–1831.
14. Lemson MS, Tordoir JHM, Van Det RJ, et al. Effects of a venous cuff at the venous anastomosis of polytetrafluoroethylene grafts for hemodialysis vascular access. *J Vasc Surg.* 2000;32:1155–1163.

15. Gagne PJ, Martinez J, DeMassi R, et al. The effect of a venous anastomosis tyrell vein collar on the primary patency of arteriovenous grafts in patients undergoing hemodialysis. *J Vasc Surg.* 2000;32:1149–1154.

16. Schild AF, Schuman ES, Noicely K, et al. Early cannulation prosthetic graft (FlixeneTM) for arteriovenous access. *J Vasc Access.* 2011;12(3):248–252.

17. Glickman MH, Stokes GK, Ross JR, et al. Multicenter evaluation of a polyurethaneurea vascular access graft as compared with the expanded polytetrafluoroethylene vascular access graft in hemodialysis applications. *J Vasc Surg.* 2001;34:465–473.

18. Mousavi SR, Moatamedi MRK, Akbari MM. Comparing frozen saphenous vein with goretex in vascular access for chronic hemodialysis. *Hemodial Int* 2011;15:559–562.

19. Kennealey PT, Elias N, Hertl M, et al. A prospective, randomized comparison of bovine carotid artery and expanded polytetrafluoroethylene for permanent hemodialysis vascular access. *J Vasc Surg.* 2011;53:1640–1648.

20. Das N, Bratby MJ, Shrivastava V, et al. Results of a seven-year, single-centre experience of the long-term outcomes of bovine ureter grafts used as novel conduits for haemodialysis fistulas. *Cardiovasc Intervent Radiol.* 2011;34:958–963.

21. Mistry H, Stephenson MA, Valenti D. Early outcomes of the intraluminal flow guard device for secondary renal access. *J Vasc Access.* 2012;14(2):131–134.

22. Gage SM, Katzman HE, Ross JR, et al. A multi-center experience of 164 consecutive hemodialysis reliable outflow [HeRO] graft implants for hemodialysis treatment. *Eur J Vasc Endovasc Surg.* 2012;44:93–99.

23. Wallace JR, Chaer RA, Dillavou ED. Report on the Hemodialysis Reliable Outflow (HeRO) experience in dialysis patients with central venous occlusions. *J Vasc Surg.* 2013; Published online April 15, 2013.

24. Steerman SN, Wagner J, Higgins JA, et al. Outcomes comparison of HeRO and lower extremity arteriovenous grafts in patients with long-standing renal failure. *J Vasc Surg.* 2013;57:776–783.

14

Contemporary Management of Access-Related Aneurysms

George H. Meier III, MD

INTRODUCTION

For many patients, achieving successful dialysis access is only the first step in a long line of interventions necessary to maintain continuous hemodialysis. Although access thrombosis is an obvious concern leading to premature loss of access, the problems generated from access-related aneurysms are nearly as critical. Although the short-term aneurysms of the access may not lead to thrombosis, decreased access function and deterioration of the access are clearly long-term problems. Functional access patency depends on the continued ability to use the patient's access for successful hemodialysis. Without question, access-related aneurysms shorten the useful lifespan of the access and lead to limitations in the quality of hemodialysis in other cases.

WHY DO ACCESS-RELATED ANEURYSMS OCCUR?

Intrinsically, maturation of in arteriovenous fistula is associated with an increase in flow-mediated venous remodeling.[1] The hope is that the access conduit will enlarge sufficiently to allow for easy cannulation and provide adequate flow for high-flux dialysis. In the simplest explanation for access aneurysms, this process continues unchecked allowing continued enlargement of the access conduit until it becomes an aneurysm. Generally, a new arteriovenous access enlarges to a fixed limit beyond which further dilatation will not occur under normal circumstances. Additional factors may impact this to extend the limits of enlargement further but in general this is a biologic limit related to the tissue response to elevated arteriovenous flows. Although diffuse enlargement of access can occur (Fig. 14-1), it is probably a less common cause than some of the explanations that follow.

One of the common issues with any dialysis access is the development of venous outflow stenosis. Venous outflow stenosis is the most common mechanism for dialysis

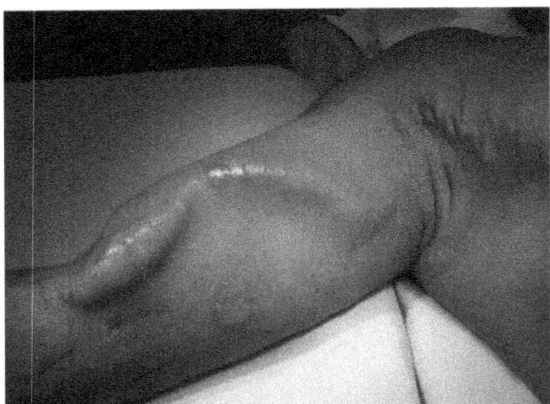

Figure 14-1. Diffuse enlargement of the upper extremity autogenous access associated with routine hemodialysis.

access failure or dysfunction. Once a stenosis develops, then turbulence occurs at that point and poststenotic dilatation may result downstream with aneurysmal enlargement of the conduit itself. Characteristically, this is a low shear stress segment of the access outflow with diminished pulsatility distally while at the same time having increased pulsatility proximal to the stenosis. In this situation the aneurysm is developing downstream from the stenosis; in other circumstances the outflow stenosis helps to generate the aneurysmal enlargement.

The development of access-related pseudoaneurysms often begins with the cannulation of the access for its initial use for hemodialysis.[2] As needles are passed through the skin and into the access, the sharpened edges of the needle lead to laceration of the underlying tissues and skin that weakens the wall of the access (Fig. 14-2). This weakening may lead to gradual enlargement of the access or alternatively may lead to the development of a pseudoaneurysm due to extravasation of blood from the needle hole. Once the extravasation occurs, persistent flow through the needle hole may result in excavation of the clot within the pseudoaneurysm allowing the enlargement to occur. As discussed later in this chapter, retrograde needle access appears to increase this risk.

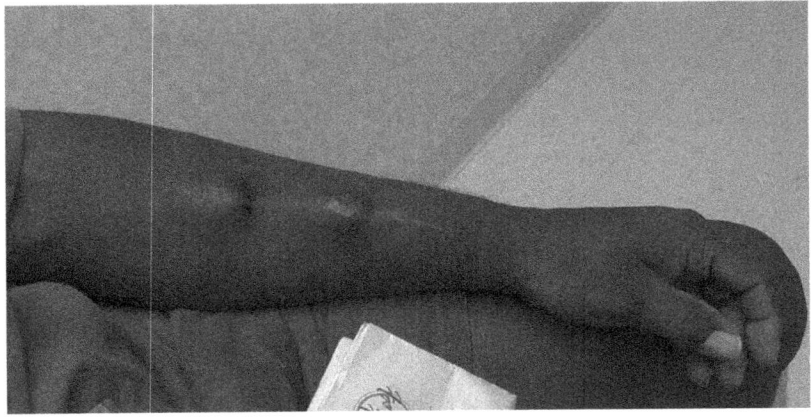

Figure 14-2. Access-related aneurysms associated with the "area" technique of cannulation.

Intrinsic to this process of aneurysm formation is the patient's ability to heal at the site of access cannulation. If the patient has poor wound healing overall, then repair of the access puncture may take longer than the interval between accesses at that site. Gradually this can lead to weakening of the wall in areas of repeated access. Over the span of months or years the access will degenerate, forming aneurysms along its course.

WHAT EFFECT DOES AN ACCESS ANEURYSM HAVE ON ACCESS FUNCTION?

The function of a dialysis access is dependent on the flow present at the site of needle cannulation. As the aneurysm develops, laminar thrombus is deposited along the wall in an attempt to remodel flow within the access. This remodeling increases the flow velocity above the thrombotic threshold but the presence of thrombus in the aneurysm may make cannulation more difficult and more unpredictable. Accessing the flow lumen through this thrombus can be difficult since much of the aneurysm is filled by laminar thrombus. In some cases the needle may push the thrombus away from the wall toward the flow lumen. If the needle is inserted into the thrombus itself, this can limit the ability to cannulate the access reliably, leading to a need for access revision.

If the access aneurysm is sufficiently large so that both needles are placed within the aneurysm, then recirculation can become a significant issue. Recirculation occurs when freshly dialyzed blood is sucked back in to the arterial intake needle. If a pool

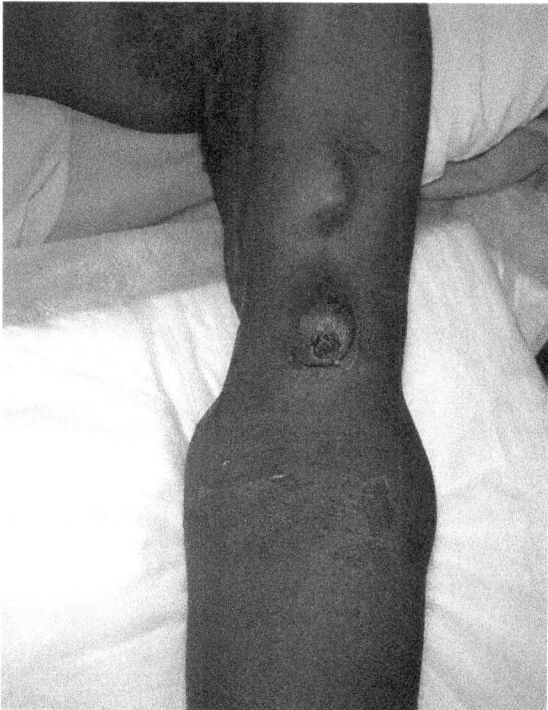

Figure 14-3. Area of skin necrosis associated with acute hematoma in the area of an access-related aneurysm. This area will need replacement, avoiding the area of necrosis and infection.

of partially cleansed blood is then used for dialysis inflow, less effective dialysis will result. Again, recirculation is an issue only when the needles are close enough so that the same pool of arterial inflow and returned blood are in immediate contact. Nonetheless, as diffuse enlargement of an access occurs, the risk of significant recirculation increases. If significant recirculation is present, further needle separation may allow continued use of the access.

More importantly, access aneurysms results in deterioration of the access conduit hastening the abandonment of the access.[3] As the aneurysms enlarge, limitations in the ability to access the conduit occur and complications increase. As the puncture sites encroach on aneurysmal segments where the wall tension is increased, the risk of hematoma, pseudoaneurysm, and further aneurysmal degeneration continue. Skin necrosis may ensue (Fig. 14-3). Ultimately, as conduit degeneration becomes confluent, abandonment of the access becomes an issue.

AVOIDING ACCESS-RELATED ANEURYSMS

Access-related aneurysms are most commonly associated with needle access into the conduit to attach the patient to the dialysis machine. There are several components that deserve further discussion relative to avoiding the formation of these aneurysms. Nonetheless, the underlying patient physiology and biology have a profound influence on the development of aneurysms, and these predispositions may overwhelm any other factors related to aneurysm formation.

The first issue concerning access-related aneurysms is the direction of needle puncture. In many dialysis centers the arterial needle is placed facing the flow of blood, retrograde into the access. The venous needle is placed along the axis of flow and antegrade into the access. When the access is cannulated retrograde into the flow stream, the hole in the wall of the access is held open by the flow stream once the needle is removed. This results in more hematoma formation from the cannulation puncture. The first and simplest thing to do to decrease hematomas and pseudoaneurysms is to cannulate both the arterial and the venous needles anterograde along the access flow (Fig. 14-4). As a result of the simple maneuver, the hole in the wall of the access will tend to seal itself once the needle is removed. Although a misdirected puncture can still result in access complications and pseudoaneurysm formation, needle hole hematomas can be diminished.

In the United States the most popular approach for needle access of dialysis conduits is referred to as the "rope ladder" or area technique. These two techniques are actually slightly different in that the area technique tends to perform access cannulation in the same areas repetitively. In the "rope ladder" technique the cannulation sites are progressively moved along the access so that recurrent punctures in the same general vicinity are less likely. In this method of access the needle sites are rotated from site to site with each dialysis session. The theory is that this will minimize injury in any one area and prevent aneurysmal degeneration. Nonetheless, this results in a more diffuse injury pattern to the access.

In the "area" access technique cannulation of the access is generally performed in the same locations repetitively. Although this results in small aneurysmal degeneration of the access, the focus is to limit the size of the aneurysmal segments to prevent larger aneurysms or diffuse conduit enlargement. Additionally, the larger size of

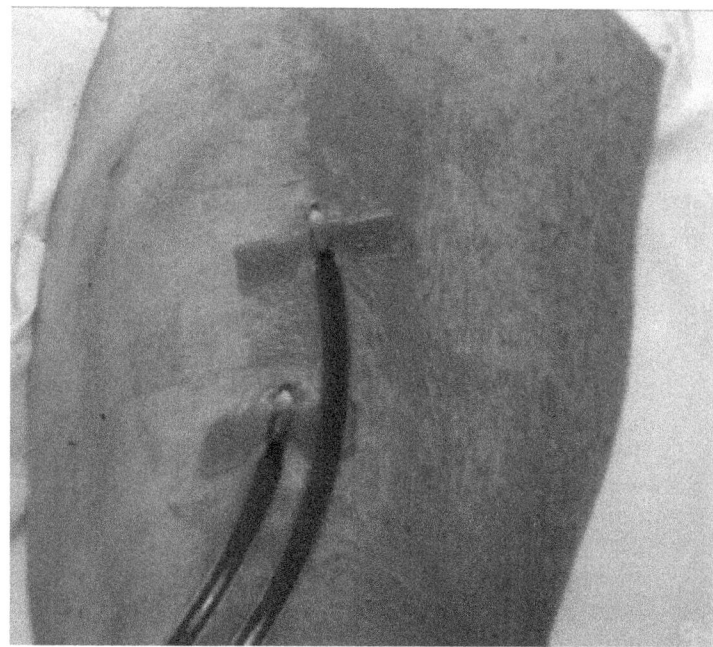

Figure 14-4. Antegrade access with both needles to avoid creating a flap that would predispose to hematoma formation.

the conduit in the area of repetitive access makes for easier puncture for the dialysis nurse.

In Europe and the Far East a different technique is more common. The "buttonhole" technique repetitively accesses the same point on the dialysis conduit, emphasizing the same angle, location, and depth for needle insertion during each dialysis session.[4] This technique results in a chronic scar at the point of access, often resulting in dimpling of the skin over the access in the area where the needles are routinely placed (Fig. 14-5). The scab from the previous access session is teased away before inserting a tapered, blunt tipped needle (Fig. 14-6) into this chronic tract for each dialysis session. Comparative trials of these two distinct techniques show that pseudoaneurysms are much less common with the buttonhole technique at the expense of some increase in the risk of local infectious complications.[5–7] The main limitation to broader

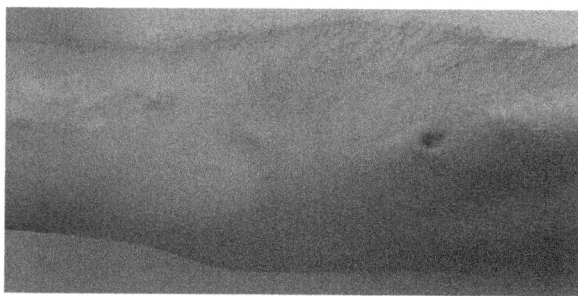

Figure 14-5. Skin dimple associated with the use of the "buttonhole" technique of needle cannulation.

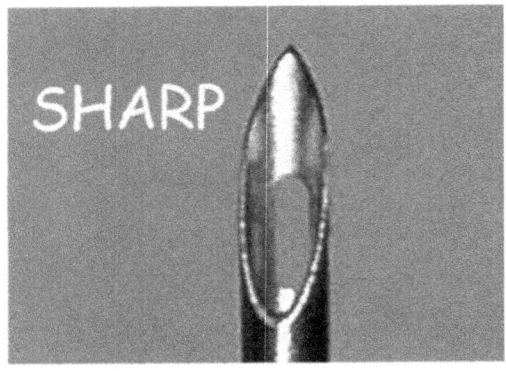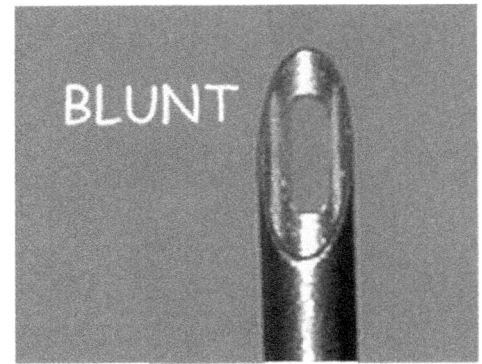

Figure 14-6. Traditional dialysis needle compared to the "blunt" needle used for the buttonhole technique.

implementation of the buttonhole technique in the United States is the limited experience of the dialysis unit staffs in this country.

Finally, the issue of venous outflow stenosis raises concerns that high outflow resistance may contribute to the development of access related aneurysms. Under this scenario, high outflow resistance as is commonly seen in failing dialysis access results in hemodynamic effects on the dialysis access conduit. As a result, enlargement of the access can occur even to the extent of frank aneurysmal degeneration. Recent studies looking at outflow stenosis and aneurysm formation confirm this association, particularly as it relates to brachiocephalic fistulas.[8]

OPEN MANAGEMENT OF ACCESS-RELATED ANEURYSMS

In its simplest form, surgical management of access-related aneurysms is relatively simple, requiring only replacement of that segment of conduit where the aneurysm has formed. This is relatively minimal in the setting of a dialysis access prosthetic graft where the aneurysmal portion of the graft can be easily replaced with prosthetic material available off the shelf. With autogenous access however this can be quite a bit more complicated since equivalent conduit may not be readily available.[9]

First and foremost in the management of access-related aneurysms is an attempt to maintain continuous dialysis access, avoiding catheter placement. This requires that an adequate segment of conduit is available that can be accessed for the continuing dialysis. In a forearm loop graft, it is rare that the entire graft degenerates concurrently. In this setting, a segmental replacement can be undertaken to replace the involved segments without complete graft replacement. Alternatively, an early access prosthetic graft can be inserted into the old dialysis graft, allowing dialysis to be continued even in the newly inserted graft segment.

With autogenous access, the challenge is increased since additional conduit is not often available to replace the degenerate, aneurysmal segment. Direct treatment of the aneurysmal segment by surgical reduction has been used and remains favored by some.[10] Despite some success, the risk of recurrent aneurysmal degeneration remains. This technique of endoaneurysmorrhaphy has been used since the initial descriptions of autogenous access with varying degrees of success.

In some cases aneurysmal enlargement may result in lengthening of the conduit as well as increasing diameter, allowing resection of aneurysmal segments to be performed with direct reanastomosis. Generally, insertion of prosthetic graft into an autogenous fistula that has become aneurysmal is a last resort maneuver since the patency of the autogenous conduit will be adversely affected by the prosthetic segment. Harvesting a vein segment to replace an aneurysmal segment can be difficult since most veins available for ready harvest will be too small in diameter to complement the mature fistula that is being inserted into. Occasionally, harvest of femoral or basilic vein may allow replacement of an aneurysmal segment with conduit of similar diameter. Nonetheless, the segment that is replaced will need to mature before allowing needle puncture within the new vein segment.

ENDOVASCULAR MANAGEMENT OF ACCESS-RELATED ANEURYSMS

An appealing alternative to open revision for access-related aneurysms is the use of endovascular covered stents to remodel areas of enlargement. With a conceptually simple percutaneous procedure, the aneurysmal segment can be relined with a graft covered stent, allowing continued use of the access[11,12] (Fig. 14-7). Despite the appeal of this approach, there are many limitations associated with endovascular treatment for access-related aneurysms.[13] The natural history of covered stents within aneurysmal accesses is still awaiting further study.

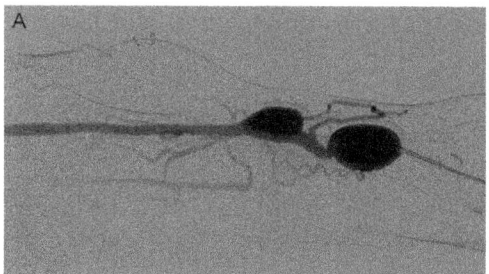
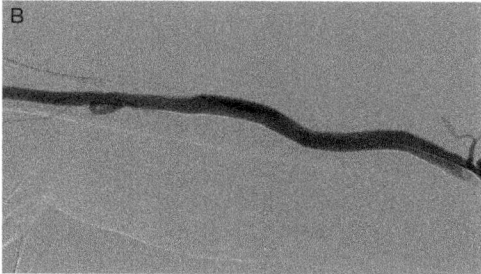

Figure 14-7. *A,* Two pseudoaneurysms associated with repetitive puncture for dialysis. *B,* Coverage of the aneurysmal segment using a Viabahn stent graft (Gore). Reproduced with permission from the *Journal of Vascular Surgery.*[15]

First, these covered stent grafts have not been designed to stand up to repetitive needle sticks in areas of high use, such as seen with dialysis access. The fabric on the stent grafts is typically thinner and more fragile than that more commonly used for dialysis access grafts. As a result, recurrent pseudoaneurysms may occur due to the difficulty in sealing needle holes in these stent grafts. Additionally, the stent itself limits the introduction of the dialysis needle and may lead to collapse of the stent graft with repetitive access. Many of these stent grafts are self-expanding, and needle access force may ultimately collapse the graft leading to stenosis or thrombosis.

Second, stent grafts are often placed in areas of pseudoaneurysm and hematoma and may be somewhat free-floating within the areas of aneurysmal degeneration. This results in a large area of hematoma around the stent graft with a risk of secondary infection or re-bleeding into the pseudoaneurysm. Infection particularly appears to be associated with use of stent grafts within the pseudoaneurysms and may ultimately lead to loss of access.[14]

ABANDONMENT OF ACCESS DUE TO ACCESS-RELATED ANEURYSMS

As multiple open or endovascular procedures accrue, the challenges of maintaining the access increase. If the access cannot be used reliably, then abandonment may ultimately be necessary. The challenge in abandonment is anticipating when this may occur; ideally, a new access should be in place once abandonment is anticipated. If it is apparent that the access is threatened by the presence of aneurysmal degeneration, an alternative autogenous access should be placed as soon as feasible. In this manner, hopefully catheter-dependent dialysis can be avoided.

The decision to abandon an access is not a simple one. The emotional investment of the patient and the physicians in the access may limit the ability to anticipate abandonment. In many cases excessive optimism relative to the long-term prognosis for the access may lead to a delay in placement of an alternative access. Nonetheless, once complications occur, the risk of abandonment of the access increases dramatically.[15]

CONCLUSIONS

Access-related aneurysms remain a substantial limitation in our utilization of dialysis conduits for hemodialysis. Although the aneurysms are rarely directly threatening to the dialysis conduit, as the complications accumulate the risk of abandonment increases. Preventing access-related aneurysms is the key to avoiding access abandonment due to aneurysmal degeneration. Nonetheless, there is no sure way to avoid access-related aneurysms, and for this reason their management is often more art than science. Until a less traumatic, more consistent method for accessing the dialysis conduit is available, access-related aneurysms will continue to occur and continue to limit dialysis access in patients with end-stage renal disease.

REFERENCES

1. Achneck HE, Sileshi B, Li M, et al. Surgical aspects and biological considerations of arteriovenous fistula placement. *Semin Dial*. 2010;23(1):25–33.
2. Wang A, Silberzweig JE. Brachial artery pseudoaneurysms caused by inadvertent hemodialysis access needle punctures. *Am J Kidney Dis*. 2009;53(2):351–354.
3. Siedlecki A, Barker J, Allon M. Aneurysm formation in arteriovenous grafts: associations and clinical significance. *Semin Dial*. 2007;20(1):73–77.
4. van Loon MM, Goovaerts T, Kessels AG, et al. Buttonhole needling of haemodialysis arteriovenous fistulae results in less complications and interventions compared to the rope-ladder technique. *Nephrol Dial Transplant*. 2010;25(1):225–230.
5. Smyth W, Hartig V, Manickam V. Outcomes of buttonhole and rope-ladder cannulation techniques in a tropical renal service. *J Ren Care*. 2013;39(3):157–165.

6. Grudzinski A, Mendelssohn D, Pierratos A, Nesrallah G. A systematic review of buttonhole cannulation practices and outcomes. *Semin Dial.* 2013;26(4):465–475.

7. Verhallen AM, Kooistra MP, van Jaarsveld BC. Cannulating in haemodialysis: rope-ladder or buttonhole technique? *Nephrol Dial Transplant.* 2007;22(9):2601–2604.

8. Rajput A, Rajan DK, Simons ME, et al. Venous aneurysms in autogenous hemodialysis fistulas: is there an association with venous outflow stenosis. *J Vasc Access.* 2013;14(2):126–130.

9. Georgiadis GS, Lazarides MK, Panagoutsos SA, et al. Surgical revision of complicated false and true vascular access-related aneurysms. *J Vasc Surg.* 2008;47(6):1284–1291.

10. Pierce GE, Thomas JH, Fenton JR. Novel repair of venous aneurysms secondary to arteriovenous dialysis fistulae. *J Vasc Endovasc Surg.* 2007;41(1):55–60.

11. Barshes NR, Annambhotla S, Bechara C, et al. Endovascular repair of hemodialysis graft-related pseudoaneurysm: an alternative treatment strategy in salvaging failing dialysis access. *J Vasc Endovasc Surg.* 2008;42(3):228–234.

12. Najibi S, Bush RL, Terramani TT, et al. Covered stent exclusion of dialysis access pseudoaneurysms. *J Surg Res.* 2002;106(1):15–19.

13. Niyyar VD, Moossavi S,. Vachharajani TJ. Cannulating the hemodialysis access through a stent graft—is it advisable? *Clin Nephrol.* 2012;77(5):409–412.

14. Kim CY, Guevara CJ, Engstrom BI, et al. Analysis of infection risk following covered stent exclusion of pseudoaneurysms in prosthetic arteriovenous hemodialysis access grafts. *J Vasc Interv Radiol.* 2012;23(1):69–74.

15. Zink JN, Netzley R, Erzurum V, Wright D. Complications of endovascular grafts in the treatment of pseudoaneurysms and stenoses in arteriovenous access. *J Vasc Surg.* 2013;57(1):144–148.

15

Management of Infected Arteriovenous Grafts

Audra A. Duncan, MD

The Society for Vascular Surgery clinical practice guidelines and the KDOQI fistula first initiatives recommend the preferential use of autologous arteriovenous fistulae in most cases before resorting to the use of prosthetic material.[1,2] Regardless of attempts to place a fistula first, approximately 20% of the 400,000 US hemodialysis patients dialyze with prosthetic grafts.[3] A meta-analysis by Murad et al. did not demonstrate significant differences in infection between autologous and prosthetic access conduit.[4] However, when graft infections occur, the downstream complications can be significant. Graft infections occur in 8%–40% of patients and result in prolonged hospitalizations, systemic complications, longer catheter dependence, and death.[5] Approximately 20%–36% of deaths in dialysis patients are caused from complications of infection, and renal failure patients have 100- to 300-fold higher risk of death caused by sepsis compared to a matched patient in the general population.[5,6] A series from UAB identified 90 graft infections over 4.5 years with 1104 graft-years of follow-up resulting in a rate of 8.2 infections/100 graft-years.[7] Repeated needle cannulation, chronic illness in renal failure patients, the presence of tunneled catheters, and the need for lower extremity access are risk factors for arteriovenous (AV) dialysis graft infections. Several authors have noted that many graft infections occur in the first year after graft placement, but the incidence decreases in subsequent years.[8]

RISK FACTORS

Uremia can interfere with T-cell and B-cell dysfunction, macrophage phagocytosis, and antigen presentation, thus increasing the overall risk of infections in patients with renal failure.[9] Dialysis patients are often hospitalized more frequently for chronic and acute illnesses, which correlates with high infection rates.[10] In addition, personal hygiene was found to be a significant independent risk factor for infectious complications, as patients with poor hygiene had significantly higher concentrations of *Staphylococcus aureus* on the skin at the access site after application of antiseptic than patients with good hygiene.[10] In Minga et al. series, patients with graft infections had a lower serum albumin

157

level (<3.5 g/dL) in the month preceding infection compared to a noninfected hemodialysis cohort (73% vs. 18%, P < .001).[7] Multiple interventions (thrombectomies, thrombolysis, and fistulograms) may predispose patients to infection by introducing bacteria. In cases when AV graft pseudoaneurysms are treated percutaneously with covered stent grafts, there is a higher risk of graft infections than when covered stents are used for other reasons, or bare metal stents are used.[11] Therefore, one must be cautious in using percutaneous covered stents to treat graft pseudoaneurysm and consider using open techniques.

As patients with renal failure live longer on hemodialysis, the need for multiple access sites increases. Many patients require lower extremity AV grafts after upper extremity options have been exhausted. Geenan et al. reported 153 femoral AV grafts placed in 127 patients with primary and secondary patency rates of 54% and 75%, respectively. Infection occurred in 41 (27%) of grafts, which is comparable to upper extremity AV graft infection incidence.[12] Therefore, if needed, one can offer a lower extremity AV graft without a prohibitive infection risk.

DIAGNOSIS

History and Clinical Exam

Graft infections are often identified early after they appear due to the superficial nature of the grafts and the frequency with which renal failure patients are seen by physicians or other health-care providers. Patients may present with erythema, tenderness, and swelling over the graft with concomitant fever or chills. Severe infections may present with hypotension from sepsis or anastomotic hemorrhage. Clinical exam may reveal an exposed graft, draining sinus tract, or a fluctuant or painful mass over the graft. Laboratory studies may reveal leukocytosis; however, the lack of leukocytosis in chronically immunosuppressed renal failure patients does not eliminate the possibility of significant infection.

Imaging

Diagnosis is typically made with physical exam, but ultrasound can also be used to distinguish between a seroma, hematoma, or abscess (Fig. 15-1). In patients with fever of

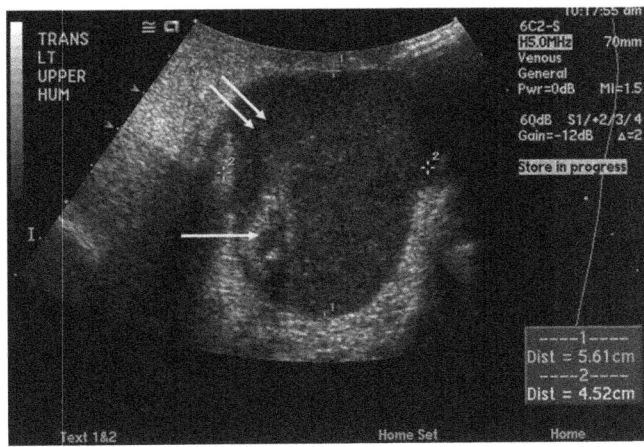

Figure 15-1. Ultrasound of infected brachial artery to axillary vein PTFE graft (single arrow) with a large debris-filled surrounding abscess (double arrows).

unknown origin, radiolabeled white blood cell scans can be sensitive (95%–100%) and specific (90%–93%) for confirming a graft infection. In a series of 30 scans in 26 patients, 16 patients with normal physical exams had a positive scan result, and infection was confirmed at the time of graft removal.[13] These white blood cell scans may be particularly important to eliminate the AV graft as an infectious source in a patient with an unknown infectious etiology, to be able to keep the graft intact if it is not clinical infected. In cases of complex graft anatomy, several sinus tracts, or to determine extent of the infection, computed tomography may be of use (Fig. 15-2).

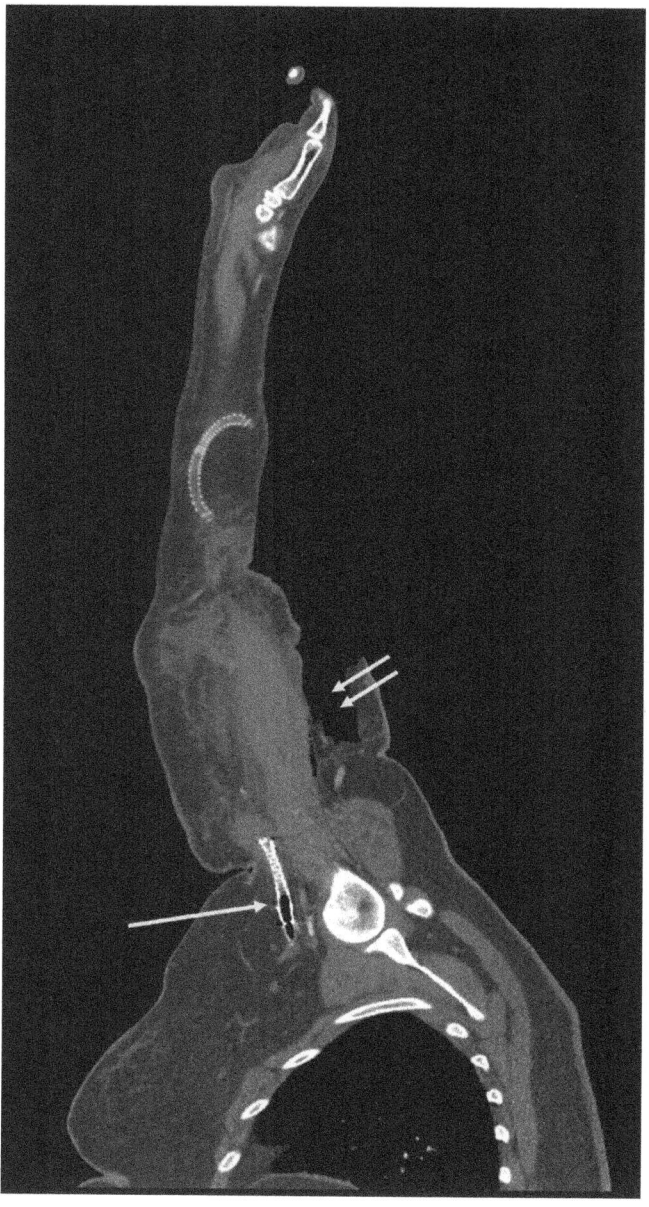

Figure 15-2. Computed tomography of a 27-year-old with multiple previous access attempts with an infected AV graft with air-filled vein thrombus (single arrow) and an open draining wound (double arrows).

TREATMENT

Most authors agree that the standard of care for graft infections include prompt hospital-ization and systemic antibiotics followed by surgical excision of the graft and open wound packing. To maintain arterial continuity, the arterial defect is patched with autogenous vein or primarily repaired. Veins are ligated or primarily repaired. Risks of graft removal include bleeding, ischemia, nerve injury, and loss of the site for future access.

The surgical wound is treated with delayed primary or secondary closure.[7] If a graft can be removed without a large incision, drains are left in the graft bed in the subcutaneous tunnel. If needed, a tunneled central venous catheter is placed for dialysis, preferably after the graft is removed and bacteremia resolved if possible. After removal of the infected graft, patients are often dependent on catheter-based dialysis for a median of 4 months with a risk of bacteremia.[7] Once the surgical wound is healed, a new permanent dialysis access is placed. Consideration should be given to identify an autologous conduit, even in the dominant arm, and also to discuss the option of peritoneal dialysis.

In rare cases, brachial artery ligation (BAL) may be considered. Schanzer et al. reported a series of 45 infected AV grafts in 43 patients, with demonstrated arterial anastomotic involvement requiring BAL in 21 patients.[14] Most (95%) of these patients had an upper extremity graft, 90% of which were polytetrafluoroethylene (PTFE). All patients were followed at least one month, and 67% followed up to six months, with no patients having ischemic or septic complications after BAL. The authors concluded that BAL was an effective yet safe way to manage infected AV grafts.[14]

Although complete resection of prosthetic graft is the gold standard for manage-ment of any infected graft, the morbidity of resection and the loss of a permanent access site have prompted several authors to create a strategy for partial resection. Ryan et al. reported a graft preservation technique in patients without sepsis (i.e., normal hemodynamics, mildly elevated or normal white blood cell count, and absent or low-grade fever).[15] In these patients, a 2-3mm cuff of well-incorporated prosthetic adjacent to the underlying artery can be left in place while the remainder of the graft is excised. This technique reduces the risk of hemorrhage or nerve injury. If the infec-tion is isolated to one portion, a new graft is tunneled through sterile tissue planes, followed by resection of the infected graft. This technique allows the incorporated por-tions of the graft to be used immediately for dialysis, thereby eliminating the need for a temporary tunneled access catheter. Ryan et al. reported their experience treating 51 infected PTFE AV grafts in 45 patients employing 13 successful total graft excisions, 15 subtotal graft excisions with graft cuffs left, and 23 partial graft excisions leaving a por-tion of usable graft. Of these 23, six patients ultimately required total graft excision due to nonhealing wounds with an overall success rate of 74%.[15] Similar attempts at partial excision was reported by Walz et al.[16] In their series, 84 excisions of an infected AV graft were done in 77 patients, with 26 (31%) being treated with complete excision with no further infection noted; 28 (33%) with partial resection and no new graft placed had four (14%) episodes of future infection; 30 (36%) had partial excision with a new inter-position graft resulting in 14 (47%) cases of reinfection at the incision site. The authors conclude that although partial excision with graft restoration is possible in an attempt to avoid catheter placement for dialysis, the resulting incidence of reinfection is high.[16]

Based on the use of cryopreserved allograft for treatment of aortic and peripheral graft infections, cryopreserved human vein allografts have been reported as an acceptable option in difficult AV graft situations. Lin et al. reported 45 cryopreserved femoral vein allografts that were used as AV graft conduits in 38 patients for indications of infected AV graft (22), remote bacteremia or sepsis (14), or compromised central vein outflow (2).[17] One year cumulative patency rate was 68% and no evidence of reinfection. Aneurysmal degeneration, however, was seen in two patients near the puncture site access at 12 and 14 months. Based on this small series, cryopreserved femoral vein allografts may be a reasonable alternative for conduit in complex patients with infected AV graft. Reinfection is infrequent and patency is comparable to prosthetic AV grafts, although high cost must be considered.[17]

In many patients with complex AV graft histories, multiple previous grafts may have thromboses and left in place. Many renal failure patients are immunocompromised based on chronic illness or after renal transplant. In this patient group, old nonfunctioning AV grafts can become infected and cause life-threatening sepsis. In a series of five patients, Nassar et al. noted that the patients presented with highly variable symptoms.[18] Only two patients had clinical signs of infection in the thrombosed grafts. Of the other three, one had a diagnosis of graft infection made by radiolabeled indium white blood cell scan, the second had bacterial endocarditis and a positive indium scan, and the third had failure to thrive with positive indium scan.[18] Although there is little literature on this topic, the tendency to leave nonfunctioning AV grafts in place without standardized screening may need to be reconsidered. Since many of these infections are occult, but can develop quickly into life-threatening sepsis, one must have a low threshold to image the grafts with indium scans and remove if indicated.

Antibiotics

When organisms are identified, the pathogens are frequently gram-positive, including *S. aureus*, *Staphylococcus epidermidis*, other *Staphylococcus* species, *Streptococcus* species, and enterococci.[7] This trend is greatly different than the organisms encountered in infections from tunneled catheters that are more frequently (24%–45%) gram-negative.[19] However, because of the risks of untreated infections, early empiric antimicrobial coverage often includes gram-negative coverage until culture results are known. In addition, Harish and Allon reported a comparison of infections in upper and lower extremity grafts, which confirmed that thigh graft infections are more likely to be caused by gram-negative bacteria and are more likely to have systemic complications.[20] Therefore, those with lower extremity AV graft infections should receive gram-negative coverage until organisms are identified.

SUMMARY

Infections in hemodialysis AV grafts can be life-threatening, but often are identified early and treated with excision and antibiotics. The extent of excision, management of the brachial artery anastomosis, and the timing and conduit used for future access should be managed on a case-by-case basis, since data is limited. If temporary access is required, the patients are at further infection risk from the tunneled catheters and should be converted to permanent access as soon as it is feasible. The best management for AV graft infection is prevention with good hygiene, fewer hospitalizations, good nutrition, and minimizing interventions.

REFERENCES

1. Sidawy AN, Spergel LM, Besarab A, et al. The Society for vascular surgery: clinical practice guidelines for the surgical placement and maintenance of arteriovenous hemodialysis access. *J Vasc Surg*. 2008;48:2S–25S.
2. National Kidney Foundation. KDOQI guidelines. http://www.kidney.org/professionals/ KDOQI/guideline_upHD_PD_VA/index.htm. Accessed December 9, 2007.
3. Lynch JR, Wass H, Armistead NC, McClellan W. Achieving the goal of fistula first breakthrough initiative for prevalent maintenance hemodialysis patients. *Am J Kidney Dis*. 2011;57:78–89.
4. Murad MH, Elamin MB, Sidawy AN, et al. Autogenous vs prosthetic vascular access for hemodialysis: a systematic review and meta-analysis. *J Vasc Surg*. 2008;48(suppl S):34S–47S.
5. Mailloux LU, Bellucci AG, Wilkes BM, et al. Mortality in dialysis patients: analysis of the causes of death. *Am J Kidney Dis*. 1991;18:326–335.
6. Sarnak MJ, Jaber BL. Mortality caused by sepsis in patients with end-stage renal disease compared with the general population. *Kidney Int*. 2000;58:1758–1764.
7. Minga TE, Flanagan KH, Allon M. Clinical consequences of infected arteriovenous grafts in hemodialysis patients. *Am J Kidney Dis*. 2001;38:975–978.
8. Miller PE, Carlton D, Deierhoi MH, et al. Natural history of arteriovenous grafts in hemodialysis patients. *Am J Kidney Dis*. 2000;36:68–74.
9. Pesanti EL. Immunologic defects and vaccination in patients with chronic renal failure. *Infect Dis Clin North Am*. 2001;15:813–832.
10. Kaplowitz LG, Comstock JA, Landwehr DM, et al. A prospective study of infections in hemodialysis patients: patient hygiene and other risk factors for infection. *Infect Control Hosp Epidemiol*. 1988;9:534–541.
11. Kim CY, Guevara CJ, Engstrom BI, et al. Analysis of infection risk following covered stent exclusion of pseudoaneurysms in prosthetic arteriovenous hemodialysis access grafts. *J Vasc Interv Radiol*. 2012;23:69–74.
12. Geenan IL, Nyilas L, Stephen MS, et al. Prosthetic lower extremity hemodialysis access grafts have satisfactory patency despite a high incidence of infection. *J Vasc Surg*. 2010;52:1546–1550.
13. Palestro CJ, Vega A, Kim CK, et al. Indium-111-labeled leukocyte scintigraphy in hemodialysis access-site infection. *J Nucl Med*. 1990;31:319–324.
14. Schanzer A, Ciaranello AL, Schanzer H. Brachial artery ligation with total graft excision is a safe and effective approach to prosthetic arteriovenous graft infections. *J Vasc Surg*. 2008;48:655–658.
15. Ryan SV, Calligaro KD, Scharff J, Dougherty MJ. Management of infected prosthetic dialysis arteriovenous grafts. *J Vasc Surg*. 2004;39:73–78.
16. Walz P, Ladowski JS. Partial excision of infected fistula results in increased patency at the cost of increased risk of recurrent infection. *Ann Vasc Surg*. 2005;19:84–89.
17. Lin PH, Brinkman WT, Terramani TT, et al. Management of infected hemodialysis access grafts using cryopreserved human vein allografts. *Am J Surg*. 2002;184:31–36.
18. Nassar GM, Ayus JC. Infectious complications of old nonfunctioning arteriovenous grafts in renal transplant recipients: a case series. *Am J Kidney Dis*. 2002;40:832–836.
19. Tanriover B, Carlton D, Saddekni S, et al. Bacteremia associated with tunneled dialysis catheters: comparison of two treatment strategies. *Kidney Int*. 2000;57:2151–2155.
20. Harish A, Allon M. Arteriovenous graft infection: a comparison of thigh and upper extremity grafts. *Clin J Am Soc Nephrol*. 2011;6:1739–1743.

Lower Extremity Venous Disease

16

Early Thrombus Removal for Acute Iliofemoral Deep Vein Thrombosis

Mark H. Meissner, MD

Venous thromboembolism (VTE) is the third most common cardiovascular disorder in Western populations, following myocardial infarction and stroke. The management of acute deep venous thrombosis (DVT) is accordingly guided by high-quality evidence from randomized clinical trials that have been incorporated into widely disseminated practice guidelines.[1] Such trials have generally considered DVT to be confined to the calf veins ("distal DVT") or to involve the popliteal or more proximal veins ("proximal DVT"). However, it is becoming increasingly clear that not all "proximal" venous thrombi are equivalent—those involving the iliac and common femoral veins (iliofemoral DVT) have a distinctly different natural history and prognosis than those confined to the femoropopliteal veins.

Furthermore, clinical trials regarding the management of proximal DVT have often been industry driven and have focused on the short-term outcomes of recurrent VTE and bleeding. Unfortunately, such a limited view ignores differences related to the anatomic location of an acute proximal DVT as well as important late consequences such as the post-thrombotic syndrome (PTS). Although anticoagulant strategies have been well validated for the treatment of "proximal DVT," it is likely that adjunctive strategies employing early thrombus removal may have a role in reducing post-thrombotic morbidity in those with iliofemoral DVT. From a theoretical perspective, early thrombus removal strategies including venous thrombectomy, catheter-directed thrombolysis (CDT), and pharmacomechancial thrombolysis (PMT), may reduce post-thrombotic morbidity by restoring venous patency and preserving venous valvular function. Although the outcomes of randomized clinical trials are pending, the early evidence does suggest that these strategies have a role in the management of patients with iliofemoral DVT.

ANTICOAGULANT TREATMENT OF ACUTE DEEP VENOUS THROMBOSIS

The treatment of acute DVT is directed toward preventing its two primary complications, recurrent VTE and PTS, and anticoagulation is well recognized as standard therapy. Current guidelines recommend initial treatment with a parenteral anticoagulant (low-molecular-weight heparin, fondaparinux, or unfractionated heparin) for at least five days and until the INR is ≥2 for at least 24 hours. A vitamin K antagonist should be started on the first treatment day with a target INR of 2.0–3.0 and compression therapy and early ambulation instituted as soon as feasible.[1]

Adequate anticoagulation reduces the risk of clinically significant recurrent VTE from 20% to 50% to less than 5% during treatment with unfractionated or low-molecular-weight heparin followed by warfarin for at least three to six months. Standard anticoagulation is also safe; initial treatment with unfractionated or low-molecular-weight heparin being associated with only a 2% risk of major hemorrhage.

Unfortunately, most clinical trials have failed to address long-term outcome after DVT and it is clear that standard anticoagulation provides imperfect protection against manifestations of PTS, including pain, edema, hyperpigmentation, and ulceration. The development of PTS is highly associated with an inferior quality of life[2] and the associated medical costs have been estimated to account for 40% of the total cost of episode of acute DVT.[3] Although a higher incidence was suggested by historical series with many methodological flaws, contemporary series suggest that 20%–50% of patients will develop objectively documented PTS, although symptoms are mild in the majority of patients. Among 355 patients with a first episode of DVT, the cumulative incidence of any and severe PTS at five years was 28% and 9.3%, respectively.[4]

IS ILIOFEMORAL THROMBOSIS DIFFERENT FROM "PROXIMAL" DVT?

Thrombus involves the common femoral and iliac veins in up to 24.3% of patients with acute unilateral DVT,[5] and it is clear that these thrombi differ in a number of respects from those confined to the femoropopliteal segment. Chronic iliac vein lesions, frequently arising from arterial compression of the left common iliac vein (May–Thurner syndrome), underly many of these events[6] (Fig. 16-1). Furthermore, the hemodynamic effects of proximal venous obstruction are substantially more severe than in femoropopliteal DVT. Acute iliofemoral thrombosis is often accompanied by more severe pain and swelling and rarely phlegmasia cerulea dolens (PCD), a clinical presentation that may be complicated by venous gangrene, amputation, and death.

In the long term, iliofemoral DVT is associated with higher rates of recurrent VTE and PTS. Despite the initial efficacy of anticoagulation, the late natural history of DVT is dominated by recurrent thrombotic events. Among 1626 consecutive patients followed after a first symptomatic DVT or pulmonary embolism (PE), the overall incidence of recurrent VTE was 22.9% after a median follow-up of 50 months.[7] Many factors, including an idiopathic etiology, underlying thrombophilia, a shorter duration of anticoagulation, and advanced age contribute to the risk of recurrent DVT. However, perhaps most importantly, iliofemoral DVT is associated with at 2.4-fold higher risk of recurrent DVT than is femoropopliteal DVT.

Patients with iliofemoral DVT are also more likely to develop PTS. Important predictors of this syndrome include age, obesity, female gender, previous ipsilateral DVT, and quite importantly, iliofemoral DVT.[8] Venous claudication develops in as many as 43.6% of these patients[9] and objective post-thrombotic scores are significantly higher than in patients with femoropopliteal DVT.[8]

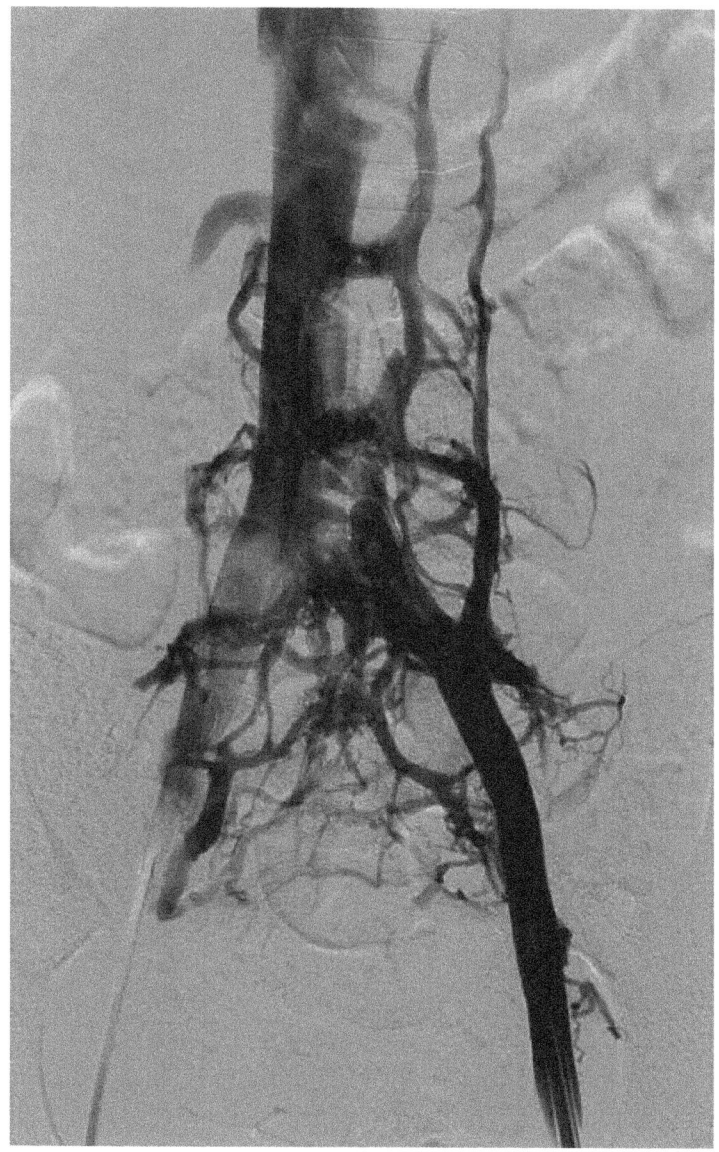

Figure 16-1. Chronic obstructive lesion of the left common iliac vein, most likely due to arterial compression, uncovered after thrombolytic treatment for acute iliofemoral DVT. Note the prominent transpelvic, paravertebral, and ascending lumbar venous collaterals.

THE THEORETICAL BENEFITS OF EARLY THROMBUS REMOVAL

Despite the epidemiologic importance of these predictors, such observations provide little insight into how PTS might be prevented. Rather, prevention requires some understanding of the natural history of DVT and the pathophysiology of PTS. Several factors related to the natural history of acute DVT are important determinants of PTS. These include the rate and degree of recanalization, the development of valvular incompetence, and the occurrence of recurrent venous thrombosis.

The more severe manifestations of the PTS result from ambulatory venous hypertension or a failure to lower venous pressures with exercise in the upright position. The highest ambulatory venous pressures occur in limbs with both reflux and obstruction. Not surprisingly, limbs with advanced PTS, that is those with skin changes and ulceration, are more likely to have a combination of reflux and obstruction than either abnormality alone. Persistent proximal venous obstruction not only increases venous pressure but may also contribute to distal valvular incompetence. Although the majority of incompetent venous segments are rendered so by the presence of thrombus, valves in uninvolved segments may also become incompetent in the presence of a proximal venous obstruction.[10] Among 113 patients treated with conventional anticoagulation and followed with venous ultrasound, complete recanalization required 2.3 to 7.3 times longer in segments developing reflux than in segments in which valve function was preserved.[11] Rapid recanalization thus appears to preserve valve function. Finally, recurrent thrombotic events are very deleterious to valve function, the incidence of reflux being significantly higher in venous segments sustaining more than one thrombotic event. Clinically, ipsilateral recurrence is associated with a 2.4-fold higher risk of PTS.[4]

Appropriate anticoagulation does address some of these factors. Insuring an appropriate intensity and duration of anticoagulation is likely very important in reducing the risk of PTS. The amount of time that the INR is in the therapeutic range has been shown to independently predict the development of PTS. It is also likely that newer anticoagulants may reduce anticoagulant variability and correspondingly the risk of PTS. In comparison to treatment with vitamin K antagonists, three months of anticoagulation with enoxaparin was associated with significantly higher rates of recanalization (49.1% vs. 24.0%) and lower five-year recurrence rates (19.3% vs. 36.3%).[12,13] Although not statistically significant, the incidence of severe PTS was also lower after three months of enoxaparin treatment (19.6% vs. 29.5%).

However, despite careful attention to anticoagulation, these drugs do little to promote active recanalization and early thrombus removal strategies have far greater potential to address the factors underlying the development of PTS. Only 24% of iliofemoral thrombi treated with anticoagulation will be patent at one year.[14] In contrast, early thrombus removal strategies have the potential to both relieve proximal venous obstruction and preserve valvular function. Although definitive evidence is lacking, it is also likely that relief of underlying anatomic abnormalities reduces the risk of recurrent thrombosis and its deleterious effects on valve function.

THROMBOLYTIC THERAPY FOR ACUTE DEEP VENOUS THROMBOSIS

A variety of strategies for early thrombus removal have been developed including open surgical thrombectomy, systemic thrombolytic therapy, CDT, and pharmacomechanical thrombolysis (PMT). Although surgical thrombectomy may reduce the risk of PTS, meta-analysis has demonstrated a trend toward better outcomes with the percutaneous thrombolytic techniques.[15] Although there may still be a role for surgical thrombectomy in highly selected patients, thrombolytic approaches are less invasive and have replaced surgical thrombectomy in many parts of the world.

The earliest clinical trials utilized systemically administered thrombolytic agents and not surprisingly demonstrated these agents to be more effective than unfractionated heparin in producing at least some degree of thrombolysis. However, widespread adoption was limited by long infusion times, low rates of complete thrombolysis, significant bleeding risks, and failure of trials to demonstrate a clear clinical benefit. Major bleeding events occurred in 13.2% of patients treated with systemic streptokinase or tissue plasminogen activator (t-PA) in comparison to only 3.5% of patients treated with heparin.[16] Approximately four patients needed to be treated with systemic recombinant tissue plasminogen activator (rt-PA) to achieve >50% lysis in one patient at the expense of one major hemorrhage for every 15 patients treated.[17]

CDT, with direct infusion of thrombolytic agents into the thrombus, theoretically allows a high concentration of the lytic agent to be delivered locally, promoting more efficient lysis, reducing infusion times, and reducing bleeding complications. Among 303 limbs treated with CDT in a national venous registry, complete lysis was achieved in 31%; 50%–99% lysis in 52%; and <50% lysis in 17% of infusions. Several comparative studies,[14,18–20] including two randomized trials, have subsequently suggested a clinical benefit of CDT over standard anticoagulation. A small randomized trial including 35 patients found more patients treated with catheter-directed streptokinase to be without reflux or obstruction (72%) than those treated with anticoagulation (12%).[19] In the largest clinical trial to date, the CaVenT investigators randomized 209 patients to either standard anticoagulation or CDT in addition to standard anticoagulation.[20] At 24 months, there was a modest 14.4% reduction in the incidence of PTS. There were 20 overall bleeding complications, five of which were clinically relevant giving a number needed to treat of seven and number needed to harm of 17. A recent systematic review evaluating comparative trials of CDT found the overall quality of the data to be poor and complications to be poorly reported. However, in comparison to standard anticoagulant therapy, catheter-directed thrombolytic therapy was associated with significant reductions in the risks of PTS (RR 0.19; 95% CI 0.07–0.48) and venous obstruction (0.38; 0.18–0.37), with a trend toward less venous reflux (0.39; 0.16–1.00)[15] (Fig. 16-2).

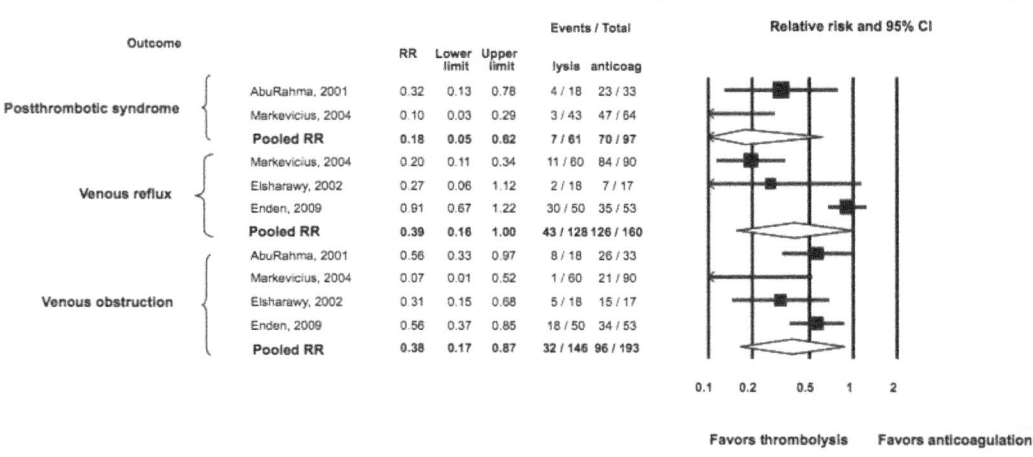

Figure 16-2. Meta-analysis of four studies comparing catheter-directed thrombolysis with standard anticoagulation. Catheter-directed thrombolytic therapy was associated with significant reductions in the risks of PTS and venous obstruction, with a trend toward a lower risk of reflux. Reprinted with permission from Casey et al.[15]

The limitations of both systemic and catheter-directed lysis have led to a variety of pharmacomechanical strategies directed toward increasing lytic efficiency while reducing procedural times. This theoretically would translate into fewer bleeding complications, decreased hospital and intensive care unit stays, and reduced cost. Amongst several mechanical thrombolytic devices, three have been widely utilized in the venous system—the Angiojet power pulse system (MEDRAD Interventional, Minneapolis, MN), the Trellis infusion catheter (Covidien, Mansfield, MA), and the EKOS ultrasound accelerated thrombolysis catheter (EKOS Corporation, Bothell, WA). The isolated use of mechanical devices is rarely successful and their use in combination with thrombolytic drugs is usually required.[21]

Two small cohort studies have directly compared PMT with CDT. Lin found rates of complete thrombolysis to be similar for PMT and CDT (75% vs. 70%), although infusion times (76 ± 34 minutes vs. 18 ± 8 hours) and costs (mean difference $37, 609) were significantly less with PMT.[22] A second small study (N = 45) also demonstrated shorter treatment times (30.3 ± 17.8 vs. 56.5 ± 27.4 hours) and lower urokinase doses (2.95 ± 1.8 million U vs. 6.70 ± 5.90 million U) for PMT in comparison to CDT alone.[23] There was no difference in major bleeding complications between the two approaches in either study. Although randomized trials are currently lacking, the early data does support a role for these pharmacomechanical approaches and their use is recommended over CDT alone if expertise and resources are available.[24]

INDICATIONS FOR EARLY THROMBUS REMOVAL

Although more efficacious than anticoagulation alone in the treatment of iliofemoral DVT, the associated cost, resource utilization, and potential for bleeding complications mandate careful consideration of the potential benefits and risks in the individual patient. Ambulatory patients with good functional capacity and a reasonable life expectancy are most likely to benefit from these procedures. Given the poor outcome associated with standard anticoagulation, patients with phlegmasia cerulea dolens and limb threatening thrombosis should also be considered for such treatment. Several case reports have established the efficacy of CDT in restoring venous outflow and arresting tissue ischemia. Contraindications to thrombolytic treatment are shown in Table 16-1.[21]

The benefits of early thrombus removal are likely to be far greater for iliofemoral venous thrombosis that for femoropopliteal thrombosis. Persistent femoral venous obstruction appears to be better tolerated, likely due to the development of robust collaterals between the popliteal and profunda femoris veins. Femoropopliteal thrombosis is accordingly associated with a lower risk of both PTS[8] and recurrent DVT[25] and the one-year patency after thrombolysis is considerably lower (47% vs. 64%) than for iliofemoral DVT.[6] The role of thrombolytic treatment in femoropopliteal thrombosis is currently being evaluated in randomized clinical trials, but for the present, a higher threshold should probably be utilized in evaluating such patients for these procedures.[21]

Duration of symptoms of less than 14–21 days has variously been recommended for consideration of early thrombus removal. Although a benefit in patients with a longer duration of symptoms cannot be excluded, chronic thrombosis is clearly associated with inferior results.[6]

TABLE 16-1. CONTRAINDICATIONS TO THROMBOLYTIC THERAPY

Active Internal Bleeding
Recent cerebrovascular accident or intracranial bleeding, trauma, or tumor
Major trauma or surgery within 10 days
Recent serious gastrointestinal bleeding
Severe uncontrolled hypertension
Pregnancy
Endocarditis or intracardiac thrombus
Known right to left shunt
Coagulopathy, thrombocytopenia, or absolute contraindications to anticoagulation
Suspected septic thrombus
Allergy to thrombolytic agents

Source: Adapted from Vedantham et al.[21]

THROMBOLYTIC TREATMENT: TECHNICAL DETAILS

Although some details are specific to the patient, the resources available, and the skills of the interventionalist, many technical aspects of the procedure are similar. Evaluation of the most proximal extent of thrombus with computed tomography (CT) is often suggested before intervention. If inflow to the popliteal vein is patent, ultrasound guided puncture of the popliteal vein using a micropuncture set is preferred by many interventionalists, with more distal access through the posterior tibial vein, small saphenous vein, or great saphenous vein (with deep system access through a perforator) being alternatives. Initial venography is performed to document the extent of thrombus and a wire is advanced across the thrombus. CDT, using a multiside hole infusion catheter, or PMT is then instituted (Fig. 16-3). The Angiojet and Trellis devices theoretically allow treatment in a single setting, although placement of an infusion catheter for completion of thrombolysis is not infrequently required. Although the EKOS catheter may speed the lytic process, it does not have the potential for single setting treatment. If follow-up CDT is required, current guidelines suggest t-PA infusion at a rate of 0.5–1 mg/h. High-volume infusions are generally preferred in the venous system and follow-up venography is indicated at 12–24 hours.[21] Systemic anticoagulation, usually with unfractionated heparin, is utilized during the procedure, usually at a reduced dose to avoid bleeding complications.

Adjunctive procedures are a critical component of the thrombolytic strategies. The Venous Registry reported a low incidence (1%) of symptomatic pulmonary embolism with CDT[6] and it is generally accepted that routine placement of an IVC filter is unnecessary in this setting. However, there is not yet consensus regarding the use of retrievable inferior vena caval (IVC) filters in high-risk situations, such as in those with thrombus extending into the inferior vena cava or undergoing PMT. Current guidelines suggest a careful consideration of risk versus benefit and cost in such situations.[24]

Thrombolysis will uncover an underlying iliac vein lesion in 45%–60% of patients presenting with a left-sided iliofemoral DVT. Such lesions most commonly occur at the crossing of the left common iliac vein by the right common iliac artery (May–Thurner syndrome), but may occur on the right side as well. Failure to treat such lesions with self-expanding stents is associated with a high rate of recurrent thrombosis and

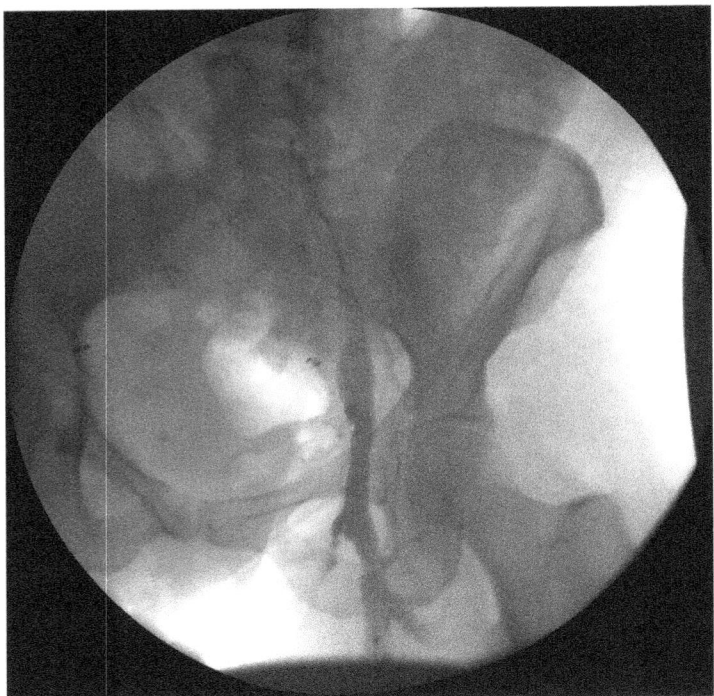

Figure 16-3. Multiside hole infusion catheter in place across an acutely thrombosed left common iliac vein (patient is prone).

thrombolytic failure.[6] Current studies suggest that when an iliac vein stenosis is present, self-expanding metallic stents improve one-year venous patency rates from 53% to 74%. Although the data regarding infrainguinal stents is limited, it is likely a stented, refluxing femoropopliteal venous segment is more deleterious than a chronically obstructed segment. Stenting of the femoropopliteal venous segment is not currently recommended.[24]

Conventional anticoagulation, based on current guidelines,[1] is necessary after the procedure. As prevention of the PTS is the primary goal of early thrombus removal, all patients should be discharged with knee-high 30–40–mm Hg compression stockings that should be continued for at least two years.

SUMMARY

The safety and efficacy of anticoagulation with intravenous unfractionated heparin or subcutaneous low-molecular-weight heparin followed by warfarin for the treatment of acute DVT has been well validated by randomized clinical trials. Less than 5% of patients treated with appropriate anticoagulation will sustain a recurrent thromboembolic event. However, anticoagulation is substantially less efficacious in the treatment of PCD and in preventing the PTS.

Early thrombus removal strategies have the potential to relieve venous obstruction and preserve valvular function and are an attractive adjunct to anticoagulation in selected patients. Initial experience with systemic and CDT was characterized by prolonged infusion times, significant rates of partial lysis, and high rates of bleeding complications. Pharmacomechanical approaches are attractive in that they have the potential to minimize treatment times, with corresponding decreases in cost and bleeding complications. Unfortunately, such approaches are only beginning to be evaluated in rigorous randomized trials. However, the current evidence does suggest that early thrombus removal strategies reduce the incidence of the PTS in appropriately selected patients. Pending the results of randomized clinical trials, these include ambulatory patients with a first episode of iliofemoral thrombosis of less than 14–21 days duration and lacking contraindications to thrombolytic drugs. Guidelines for early thrombus removal have been summarized in a recent document from the Society for Vascular Surgery and the American Venous Forum.[24]

REFERENCES

1. Kearon C, Akl EA, Comerota AJ, et al. Antithrombotic therapy for VTE disease: antithrombotic therapy and prevention of thrombosis, 9th ed: American College of Chest Physicians Evidence-Based Clinical Practice Guidelines. *Chest*. 2012; 141:e419S–e494S.
2. Kahn SR, Shbaklo H, Lamping DL, et al. Determinants of health-related quality of life during the 2 years following deep vein thrombosis. *J Thromb Haemost*. 2008; 6:1105–1112.
3. Bergqvist D, Jendteg S, Johansen L, et al. Cost of long-term complications of deep venous thrombosis of the lower extremities: an analysis of a defined patient population in Sweden. *Ann Intern Med*. 1997; 126:454–457.
4. Prandoni P, Villalta S, Bagatella P, et al. The clinical course of deep-vein thrombosis. prospective long-term follow-up of 528 symptomatic patients. *Haematologica*. 1997; 82:423–428.
5. Bochanen N, Van Schil P, De Maesaneer M, editors. *Characterization of Thrombus Extent in Pateints with Acute Lower Limb Deep Venous Thrombosis*. 14th Annual Meeting of the European Venous Forum; 2013; Belgrade, Serbia.
6. Mewissen MW, Seabrook GR, Meissner MH, et al. Catheter-directed thrombolysis of lower extremity deep venous thrombosis: report of a national multicenter registry. *Radiology*. 1999; 211:39–49.
7. Prandoni P, Noventa F, Ghirarduzzi A, et al. The risk of recurrent venous thromboembolism after discontinuing anticoagulation in patients with acute proximal deep vein thrombosis or pulmonary embolism. A prospective cohort study in 1,626 patients. *Haematologica*. 2007; 92:199–205.
8. Kahn SR, Shrier I, Julian JA, et al. Determinants and time course of the postthrombotic syndrome after acute deep venous thrombosis. *Ann Intern Med*. 2008;149:698–707.
9. Delis KT, Bountouroglou D, Mansfield AO. Venous claudication in iliofemoral thrombosis: long-term effects on venous hemodynamics, clinical status, and quality of life. *Ann Surg*. 2004; 239:118–126.
10. Caps MT, Manzo RA, Bergelin RO, et al. Venous valvular reflux in veins not involved at the time of acute deep vein thrombosis. *J Vasc Surg*. 1995; 22:524–531.
11. Meissner MH, Manzo RA, Bergelin RO, et al. Deep venous insufficiency: the relationship between lysis and subsequent reflux. *J Vasc Surg*. 1993; 18:596–608.
12. Gonzalez-Fajardo JA, Arreba E, Castrodeza J, et al. Venographic comparison of subcutaneous low-molecular weight heparin with oral anticoagulant therapy in the long-term treatment of deep venous thrombosis. *J Vasc Surg*. 1999; 30:283–292.
13. Gonzalez-Fajardo JA, Martin-Pedrosa M, Castrodeza J, et al. Effect of the anticoagulant therapy in the incidence of post-thrombotic syndrome and recurrent thromboembolism: comparative study of enoxaparin versus coumarin. *J Vasc Surg*. 2008; 48:953–959.

14. AbuRahma A, Perkins SE, Wulu JT, Ng HK. Ileofemoral deep vein thrombosis: conventional therapy versus lysis and percutaneous transluminal angioplasty and stenting. *Ann Surg.* 2001; 233:752–760.

15. Casey ET, Munrad MH, Zumeta Garcia M, et al. Treatment of acute iliofemoral deep vein thrombosis: a systematic review and meta-analysis. *J Vasc Surg.* 2012; 55:1463–1473.

16. Lensing AWA, Hirsh J. Rationale and results of thrombolytic therapy for deep vein thrombosis. In: Bernstein EF, editor. *Vascular Diagnosis.* 4th ed. St. Louis, MO: Mosby; 1993.

17. Forster A, Wells P. Tissue plasminogen activator for the treatment of deep venous thrombosis of the lower extremity. *Chest.* 2001; 119:572–579.

18. Comerota AJ, Throm RC, Mathias SD, et al. Catheter-directed thrombolysis for iliofemoral deep vein thrombosis improves health-related quality of life. *J Vasc Surg.* 2000; 32:130–137.

19. Elsharawy M, Elzayat E. Early results of thrombolysis vs anticoagulation in iliofemoral venous thrombosis. A randomised clinical trial. *Eur J Vasc Endovasc Surg.* 2002 24:209–214.

20. Enden T, Haig Y, Klow NE, et al. Long-term outcome after additional catheter-directed thrombolysis versus standard treatment for acute iliofemoral deep vein thrombosis (the CaVenT study): a randomised controlled trial. *Lancet.* 2012; 379:31–38.

21. Vedantham S, Thorpe PE, Cardella JF, et al. Quality improvement guidelines for the treatment of lower extremity deep vein thrombosis with use of endovascular thrombus removal. *J Vasc Interv Radiol.* 2006; 17:435–447.

22. Lin PH, Zhou W, Dardik A, et al. Catheter-direct thrombolysis versus pharmacomechanical thrombectomy for treatment of symptomatic lower extremity deep venous thrombosis. *Am J Surg.* 2006; 192:782–788.

23. Kim HS, Patra A, Paxton BE, et al. Adjunctive percutaneous mechanical thrombectomy for lower-extremity deep vein thrombosis: clinical and economic outcomes. *J Vasc Interv Radiol.* 2006; 17:1099–1104.

24. Meissner MH, Gloviczki P, Comerota AJ, et al. Early thrombus removal strategies for acute deep venous thrombosis: clinical practice guidelines of the Society for Vascular Surgery and the American Venous Forum. *J Vasc Surg.* 2012; 55:1449–1462.

25. Douketis JD, Crowther MA, Foster GA, Ginsberg JS. Does the location of thrombosis determine the risk of disease recurrence in patients with proximal deep vein thrombosis? *Am J Med.* 2001; 110:515–519.

17

Iliofemoral Thrombolysis without Inferior Vena Caval Interruption

Robert I. Hacker, MD; Efthimios Avgerinos, MD;
Rabih Chaer, MD; and Eric S. Hager, MD

INTRODUCTION

Deep vein thrombosis (DVT) is estimated to affect five per 10,000 people annually and remains a significant cause of post-thrombotic syndrome (PTS), pulmonary embolism, and death.[1] The burden of patient morbidity coupled with the staggering cost of treatment caused the surgeon general in 2008 to issue a Call to Action for the prevention and treatment of DVT. In response, the American College of Chest Physicians (ACCP) issued guidelines for the prophylaxis and treatment of DVT and for the first time made recommendations on invasive treatment therapies aimed at rapid dissolution of acute DVT.[2]

Invasive treatment modalities most commonly include catheter-directed thrombolysis (CDT) and pharmacomechanical thrombolysis (PMT). These minimally invasive endovascular techniques have been shown to rapidly reduce thrombus burden and provide immediate symptom relief. Many studies have suggested that early thrombus removal can lead to superior long-term symptom relief and improvement in the patient's quality of life by preventing PTS.[3] The major risks of these treatments are secondary to bleeding due to delivery of thrombolytics and potential for embolization during catheter manipulation.[4] To mitigate the risk of bleeding, most hospitals have protocols in place with strict guidelines for thrombolytic dose, patient monitoring and frequent laboratory surveillance of hemoglobin, coagulation panels, and fibrinogen levels. Iatrogenic pulmonary embolism remains a potentially serious but clinically rare event during CDT.[5-8] Despite this, some interventionalists routinely insert inferior vena cava (IVC) filters before CDT/PMT although there is no current literature to support this practice. The purpose of this chapter is to present the current guidelines on vena cava interruption during lytic therapy and to review the current literature and indication for the use of filters in that setting.

CURRENT GUIDELINES

Current guidelines for the treatment of DVT recommend anticoagulation as the primary modality to prevent thrombus propagation, recurrence, and embolization.[9] This, in conjunction with compression stockings, can help reduce the incidence of PTS. Despite these therapies, it is estimated that 20%–50% of patients with thrombus above the level of the popliteal vein will develop PTS.[10] The spectrum of PTS can range from mild symptoms to debilitating chronic limb swelling, pain, ulceration, and reduction of quality of life.[5] To help decrease the incidence of PTS, therapy has been directed to rapid removal of proximal iliofemoral thrombus. The efficacy and durability of CDT and PMT in removing thrombus has been evaluated in multiple studies,[11–13] but it was not until the Norwegian Catheter-directed Venous Thrombolysis study made the correlation between catheter-directed lysis of iliofemoral DVT and long-term reduction of PTS rates.[14] They reported an absolute risk reduction of 14.4% of PTS in patients treated with CDT versus anticoagulation alone. Despite the relative lack of robust randomized data showing a benefit to CDT, it has become common practice among interventionalists.

The updated 2012 ACCP guidelines have softened their verbiage on catheter-directed lysis stating that "Patients who are most likely to benefit from CDT have iliofemoral DVT, symptoms for less than 14 days, good functional status, life expectancy of greater than 1 year, and a low risk of bleeding (level 2C evidence)," although they go on to say that simple anticoagulation alone is acceptable in all patients that do not have impending venous gangrene as the absolute risks/benefits of CDT are uncertain.[9] In addition to this recommendation, they do not endorse the use of IVC filters during CDT, but again this is based on low level evidence. The current ACCP guidelines on treatment of iliofemoral DVT are in contradistinction to the other guidelines proposed by administrative and regulatory bodies.

American Heart Association (AHA) guidelines recommend CDT or PMT in patients with impending venous gangrene or limb threat secondary to venous obstruction, in patients with rapid thrombus extension despite anticoagulation and as a first-line therapy for treatment of iliofemoral DVT, and in patients with symptoms less than 21 days and who are at low risk of bleeding complications.[15] The AHA recommendations are similar to the Society of Interventional Radiologists (SIR) who published their position statement in 2009 recommending PMT or CDT supporting the use of CDT and PMT in patients with symptoms less than 14 days, with limb threatening phlegmasia.[16] The SIR statement essentially mirrors that of the current Society for Vascular Surgery consensus on treatment of iliofemoral DVT. They suggest that CDT or PMT be utilized for the first episode of acute iliofemoral deep venous thrombosis, symptoms ≤14 days, patients with low risk of bleeding, and in patients that are ambulatory with good functional capacity and an acceptable quality of life.[17]

TREATMENT STRATEGIES FOR PREVENTION OF POST-THROMBOTIC SYNDROME

PTS can be a devastating chronic complication of proximal DVT. Thus, invasive therapies have been designed to reduce the thrombus burden and therefore help prevent the long-term sequelae of PTS by maintaining vein patency and preserving valve function. The most commonly employed methods to treat proximal venous thrombosis are CDT with or without ultrasound-accelerated catheters (EKOS) and PMT (Trellis/Angiojet).

CATHETER-DIRECTED THROMBOLYSIS

CDT is performed by placing a specialized multihole catheter into the bulk of the thrombus. Once positioned, thrombolytic agents (i.e., tissue plasminogen activator) are infused through the catheters directly into the thrombus thereby reducing the overall amount of thrombolytic needed and decreasing the risk of serious bleeding complications that were seen in systemic lysis.[18]

The surgical approach to CDT is typically through the popliteal, small saphenous or femoral veins under ultrasound guidance. Placement of the catheter into the thrombus allows direct infusion to maximize the surface area exposed to the lytic agents. Early studies reported bleeding complications as high as 11% although this was hypothesized to be due to the high dose of lytic agents initially used. Contemporary studies have reported bleeding complication rates, which approach 1% primarily due to the shorter infusion times as well as lower does lytic agent used.[5]

EKOS Catheter

The EKOS catheter (EKOS Corp., Bothell, WA) is similar to standard CDT catheters except for a proprietary ultrasound core wire that generates ultrasound waves during lytic infusion. Utilizing ultrasound accelerates the contact of the lytic agent with the plasminogen receptor sites within the thrombus, thus augmenting the speed in which the lytic can penetrate and therefore reduce treatment times.[19]

PHARMACOMECHANICAL THROMBOLYSIS

Angiojet

The Angiojet (Bayer, Warrendale, PA) is a commonly used device that utilizes the Bernoulli effect to rapidly decrease thrombus burden. The catheter design allows high pressure saline to be directed through the distal tip of the catheter, thereby creating a vacuum with pressures less than –600 mm Hg. The vacuum exerts its effect by mechanically loosening the thrombus, fragmenting it, and extracting it through outflow holes in the body of the catheter. The device has two settings, power pulse mode and thrombectomy mode. Power pulse mode uses Tissue Plasminogen Activator instead of saline, which is infused through the catheter and allowed to dwell within the thrombus. This helps soften the thrombus and improve dissolution when the catheter is placed in thrombectomy mode. After a 10–15-minute dwell time, the device is switched to thrombectomy mode to aspirate the dissolved column of thrombus and residual TPA, therefore reducing the overall amount absorbed.

Trellis Device

The Trellis device (Covidien, Mansfield, MA) works through mechanical and pharmacologic mechanisms to dissolve thrombus. The catheter has two occlusive balloons that are placed proximally and distally to the treatment segment. TPA is infused through side holes located in the catheter between the balloons. A wire then rotates at 1500 revolutions per minute to fragment the thrombus and mix the TPA that is then aspirated before deflation of the balloons. This technique potentially isolates the TPA and fragmented thrombus from the systemic circulation and allows for rapid thrombus removal.

IVC FILTER USE

All of these treatment strategies have a theoretic risk of embolization during catheter placement and manipulation or during the treatment duration. The current 9th edition of the ACCP Evidence-Based Clinical Practice Guidelines does not endorse routine use of IVC filters in patients undergoing CDT. This recommendation is based on low level evidence as there has been no large randomized study to evaluate the need for routine placement of IVC filters before PMT or CDT.

The US National Venous Registry reported on 473 patients who underwent lysis without IVC filter placement and reported a clinical pulmonary embolism rate of just 1%.[20] This correlated with pooled data from 19 published studies of CDT or PMT, which reported a 0.9% rate of clinically significant pulmonary embolism.[21] These reports contradicted earlier series that reported high rates of IVC filter–captured emboli. These older studies reported on outdated technology and lacked control groups.[22] Thus, utilizing current thombolytic technology seems to carry a relatively low risk of pulmonary embolism. Identification of risk factors of those patients that did suffer clinically significant PE remains controversial.

The UPMC experience

A recent retrospective study[23] from our group sought to examine the outcomes of 80 patients that underwent CDT and/or PMT with and without filter placement. The patients were divided into two groups: those with IVC filters ($n = 41$) and those with no effective IVC interruption ($n = 39$). We found no clinically significant pulmonary embolism in either group although in group A there were nine patients (22%) with documented embolic clot within the filter nest. The entrapped clot was deemed to be of significant size (>1/3 filter volume) in two patients (4.9%) (Fig. 17-1). Multivariate analysis of patients with embolization found female gender (OR 5.833, CI 95% 1.038–32.797, $P = .032$) and preoperative clinical PE (OR 5.6, CI 95% 1.043–30.081, $P = .054$). In addition, there was a trend for increased embolization seen with a higher average number of DVT risk factors (1.44 vs. 1, $P = .065$) and when PMT was used as the single treatment modality (OR 4.32, CI 95% 0.851–21.929, $P = .087$). Our data suggested that IVC filter placement should be selectively performed in patients with preoperative clinical pulmonary embolism, in females, and potentially in patients who are to undergo a single PMT session or in patients with a large number of DVT risk factors.

In 2012, Sharifi and colleagues described their experience with 141 patients who underwent percutaneous endovenous intervention for deep venous thrombosis and randomized them to IVC filter placement ($n = 70$) or no filter ($n = 71$). They reported an eightfold increase in iatrogenic symptomatic PE in those patients not receiving a filter. Their multivariate analysis identified several risk factors for development of PE: (1) pulmonary embolism identified at admission, (2) involvement of two or more adjacent venous segments with acute thrombus, (3) inflammatory DVT (erythema, pain, and edema), and (4) vein diameter ≥7mm.[24]

In addition to these relative indications for IVC filter placement, it seems appropriate that patients with a poor cardiopulmonary reserve may benefit from caval interruption due to the potential for hemodynamic collapse with further insult. Despite lack of evidence, patients with free floating thrombus extending into the IVC who underwent PMT were traditionally considered high risk for PE and were selected for IVC filter replacement.[25] Table 17-1 summarizes the aggregated suggestions for placement of IVC filters when performing CDT or PMT in patients with iliofemoral DVT.

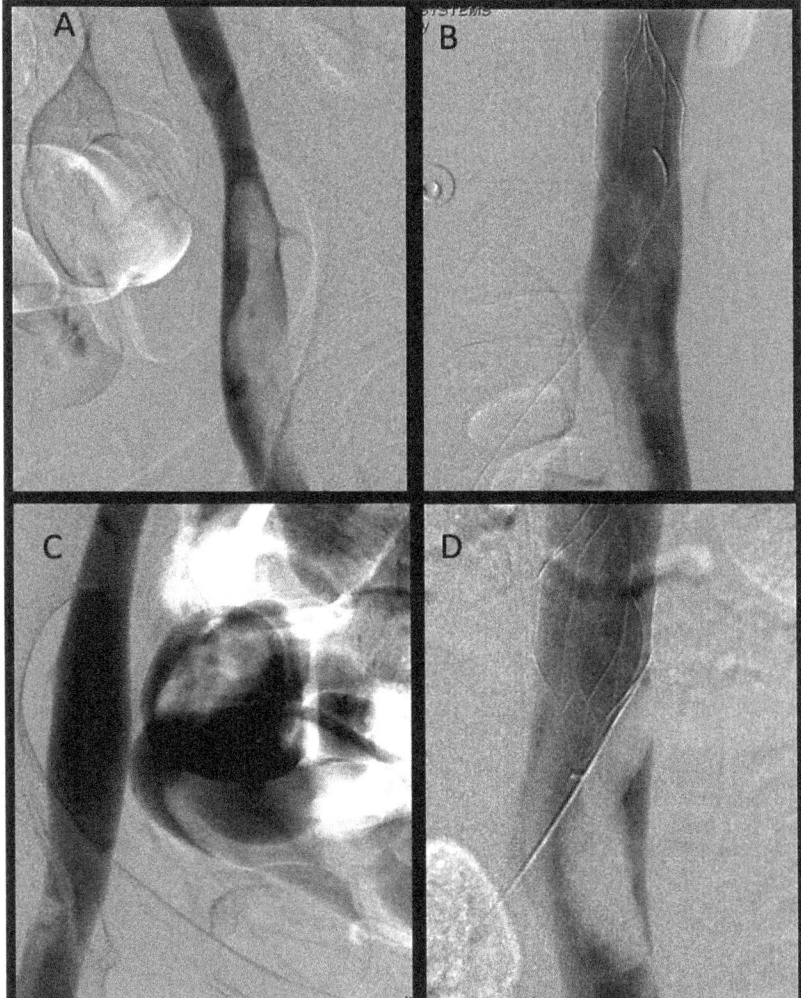

Figure 17-1. A patient with presenting with a pre-procedure PE and iliofemoral DVT. Venogram showing, *A*, preoperative left iliofemoral DVT, *B*, IVC filter free of thrombus, *C*, left iliac vein after treatment, and, *D*, IVC filter with trapped thrombus.

TABLE 17-1. AGGREGATE RECOMMENDATIONS FOR IVC FILTER PLACEMENT BASED ON SUBGROUP ANALYSIS (AVGERINOS, PROTACK, SHARIFI)

Patients in whom placement of IVC filters may be warranted

Pulmonary embolism diagnosed

Acute thrombus in two or more venous segments

Inflammatory DVT (edema, pain, erythema)

Vein diameter ≥7 mm

Single PMT session planned

Female gender

Patients with poor cardiopulmonary reserve

CONCLUSION

The associated morbidity with DVT, especially in the iliofemoral segment, has driven interventionists toward more invasive treatments strategies. PMT and CDT provide rapid dissolution of the thrombus burden with an acceptable complication profile and help prevent PTS. Overall, clinically significant pulmonary embolism rates are reported to be approximately 1% or less in the majority of the published literature. Therefore, routine placement of IVC filters during lysis does not seem to be justified, and the identification of select patient who might benefit from caval interruption is warranted. Current guidelines suggest that caval interruption not be undertaken routinely in patients undergoing iliofemoral lysis although this recommendation is based on weak evidence. Multiple retrospective reviews have attempted to identify high-risk patients in whom filter placement is beneficial. Our data and that of others suggest the selective use of IVC filters before the interventional treatment of DVT, particularly in patients with pre-procedural PE, females, and those in whom a single session of PMT is planned. Data from larger ongoing randomized trials may further clarify the role of IVC filters in patients undergoing lytic therapy for iliofemoral DVT.

REFERENCES

1. Fowkes FJ, Fowkes FG. Incidence of diagnosed deep vein thrombosis in the general population: systematic review. *Eur J Vasc Endovasc Surg.* 2003;25(1):1–5.
2. Kearon C, Agnelli G, Goldhaber S, et al. Antithrombotic therapy for venous thromboembolic disease: American College of Chest Physicians Evidence-Based Clinical Practice Guidelines (8th Edition). *Chest.* 2008;133:454S–545S.
3. Kahn SR, Shrier I, Julian JA, et al. Determinants and time course of the postthrombotic syndrome after acute deep venous thrombosis. *Ann Intern Med.* 2008;149(10):698–707.
4. Haig Y, Enden T, Slagsvold CE, et al. Determinants of early and long-term efficacy of catheter-directed thrombolysis in proximal deep vein thrombosis. *J Vasc Interv Radiol.* 2013; 24(1):17–24; quiz 26.
5. Casey ET, Murad MH, Zumaeta-Garcia M, et al. Treatment of acute iliofemoral deep vein thrombosis. *J Vasc Surg.* 2012;55(5):1463–1473.
6. Kolbel T, Alhadad A, Acosta S, et al. Thrombus embolization into IVC filters during catheter-directed thrombolysis for proximal deep venous thrombosis. *J Endovasc Ther.* 2008; 15(5):605–613.
7. Baekgaard N, Broholm R, Just S, et al. Long-term results using catheter-directed thrombolysis in 103 lower limbs with acute iliofemoral venous thrombosis. *Eur J Vasc Endovasc Surg.* 2010;39(1):112–117.
8. Enden T, Klow NE, Sandvik L, et al. Catheter-directed thrombolysis vs. anticoagulant therapy alone in deep vein thrombosis: results of an open randomized, controlled trial reporting on short-term patency. *J Thromb Haemost.* 2009;7(8):1268–1275.
9. Kearon C, Akl EA, Comerota AJ, et al. Antithrombotic therapy for VTE disease: antithrombotic therapy and prevention of thrombosis, 9th ed: American College of Chest Physicians Evidence-Based Clinical Practice Guidelines. *Chest.* 2012;141(2_suppl):e419S–e494S.
10. Kahn SR. The post-thrombotic syndrome. ASH Education Program Book, 2010. *Hematology Am Soc Hematol Educ Program.* 2010;2010(1):216–220.
11. Elsharawy M, Elzayat E. Early results of thrombolysis vs anticoagulation in iliofemoral venous thrombosis. a randomised clinical trial. *Eur J Vasc Endovasc Surg.* 2002;24(3):209–214.

12. AbuRahma AF, Perkins SE, Wulu JT, Ng HK. Iliofemoral deep vein thrombosis: conventional therapy versus lysis and percutaneous transluminal angioplasty and stenting. *Ann Surg.* 2001;233(6):752–760.

13. O'Connell JB, Russell MM, Davis G, et al. Thrombolysis for acute lower extremity deep venous thrombosis in a tertiary care setting. *Ann Vasc Surg.* 2010;24(4):511–517.

14. Enden T, Haig Y, Klow NE, et al. Long-term outcome after additional catheter-directed thrombolysis versus standard treatment for acute iliofemoral deep vein thrombosis (the CaVenT study): a randomised controlled trial. *Lancet.* 379(9810):31–38.

15. Jaff MR, McMurtry MS, Archer SL, et al. Management of massive and submassive pulmonary embolism, iliofemoral deep vein thrombosis, and chronic thromboembolic pulmonary hypertension: a scientific statement from the American Heart Association. *Circulation.* 2011; 123(16):1788–1830.

16. Vedantham S, Millward SF, Cardella JF, et al. Society of Interventional Radiology position statement: treatment of acute iliofemoral deep vein thrombosis with use of adjunctive catheter-directed intrathrombus thrombolysis. *J Vasc Interv Radiol.* 2009; 20(7 suppl):S332–S335.

17. Meissner MH, Gloviczki P, Comerota AJ, et al. Early thrombus removal strategies for acute deep venous thrombosis: Clinical Practice Guidelines of the Society for Vascular Surgery and the American Venous Forum. *J Vasc Surg.* 2012;55(5):1449–1462.

18. Broholm R, Jensen LP, Baekgaard N. Catheter-directed thrombolysis in the treatment of iliofemoral venous thrombosis. A review. *Int Angiol.* 2010; 29(4):292–302.

19. Grommes J, Strijkers R, Greiner A, et al. Safety and feasibility of ultrasound-accelerated catheter-directed thrombolysis in deep vein thrombosis. *Eur J Vasc Endovasc Surg.* 2011; 41(4):526–532.

20. Mewissen MW, Seabrook GR, Meissner MH, et al. Catheter-directed thrombolysis for lower extremity deep venous thrombosis: report of a national multicenter registry. *Radiology.* 1999; 211(1):39–49.

21. Vedantham S, Thorpe P, Cardella JF, et al. Quality improvement guidelines for the treatment of lower extremity deep vein thrombosis with use of endovascular thrombus removal. *J Vasc Interv Radiol.* 2009;20(7 suppl): S227–S239.

22. Lorch H, Welger D, Wagner V, et al. Current practice of temporary vena cava filter insertion: a multicenter registry. *J Vasc Interv Radiol.* 2000;11(1):83–88.

23. Avgerinos ED, Jyabalan G, Marone L, et al. Vena cava interruption during thrombolysis for acute iliofemoral deep vein thrombosis. *J Eur Vasc Surg.* 2013; publication pending.

24. Sharifi M, Bay C, Skrocki L, et al. Role of IVC filters in endovenous therapy for deep venous thrombosis: the FILTER-PEVI (filter implantation to lower thromboembolic risk in percutaneous endovenous intervention) trial. *Cardiovasc Intervent Radiol.* 2012;35(6):1408–1413.

25. Arko FR, Davis CM, 3rd, Murphy EH, et al. Aggressive percutaneous mechanical thrombectomy of deep venous thrombosis: early clinical results. *Arch Surg,* 2007;142(6):513–518; discussion 518–519.

18

Practice Guidelines for Varicose Veins

Robert B. McLafferty, MD

INTRODUCTION

Affecting upwards of one-quarter of the United States population, the spectrum of chronic venous disease (CVD) in the lower extremities ranges from subtle telangiectasias to severe skin changes with ulceration.[1] The majority of this group with CVD are made up of patients with "classic" varicose veins, and within this group, a wide variety of signs and symptoms can exist. Once thought to be a purely cosmetic problem, we now know that varicose veins can often be a cause of significant symptoms such as aching, pain, heaviness, throbbing, urticaria, and tenderness.[2] Furthermore, these symptoms can significantly hamper quality of life.[3]

Over the past 30 years there has been an explosion in information and innovation concerning the evaluation and treatment of CVD. This has been especially true in caring for patients with varicose veins—given the ubiquity of the clinical problem. Many areas of advancement have occurred in areas that include the development of classifications, duplex ultrasound, percutaneous ablation techniques, sclerotherapy, and outcome measurement. All have changed the way varicose veins are evaluated and treated.[4-8] What was once a clinical problem that required general anesthesia, an open surgical stripping procedure, and considerable recovery time, has evolved into treatments that are purely office-based needing only local anesthesia.

Now more than ever, given the commonality of varicose veins and the fact that technology has allowed for office-based less invasive procedures, is there a need for evidence-based guidelines to assist practitioners in optimizing choices for treatment. In 2011, the Society for Vascular Surgery and the American Venous Forum published clinical practice guidelines as a supplement in the Journal of Vascular Surgery entitled "The Care of Patients with Varicose Veins and Associated Chronic Venous Diseases."[9] This sentinel publication represented years of work by experts around the world using sound evidence-based methodology to create comprehensive recommendations surrounding the care of patients with varicose veins. The majority of what follows will summarize key salient points made in this important document. It should be emphasized that guideline recommendations do not necessarily translate into "standard of care." All patients differ in clinical presentation, comorbidities, and socioeconomically, thus allowing for variance in how these guidelines are applied. Nevertheless, they provide the framework for evaluation and treatment so as to drive continuity of the best possible care according to the best and most current medical evidence.

EVIDENCE-BASED METHODOLOGY

The clinical practice guidelines on the treatment of varicose veins put forth by the Society for Vascular Surgery and the American Venous Forum in 2011 use the Grading of Recommendations Assessment, Development and Evaluation (GRADE) system as described by Guyatt et al.[9,10] In the GRADE system, strength of recommendation and level of evidence are noted by 1 or 2 and A, B, or C, respectively. The number 1 represents a strong recommendation and 2 gives a weak recommendation. Likewise, the letter A represents high-quality evidence, B for moderate-quality evidence, and C for low-quality evidence. The term "we recommend" is used for strong GRADE 1 recommendations, whereas "we suggest" is used for weak GRADE 2 recommendations. Additionally for a GRADE 1 recommendation, benefits are clearly higher than risks and for a GRADE 2 recommendation, benefits cannot be clearly defined as outweighing risks.

Experts from the Society for Vascular Surgery and the American Venous Forum made up the Venous Guideline Committee. GRADE methodology was based on an extensive review of the scientific literature including, but not limited to, previously published consensus documents and guidelines, meta-analyses, reports from the 2006 and 2009 Venous Summits held at the Pacific Vascular Symposium and other recommendations within the third edition of the *Handbook of Venous Disorders, Guidelines of the American Venous Forum.*[11–13]

DEFINITIONS AND CLASSIFICATIONS

A varicose vein is defined as a subcutaneous dilated vein that is greater than or equal to 3 mm while in the standing position. Standardized nomenclature for veins in the lower extremity was updated in a consensus publication by Caggiati et al. in 2005 in the *Journal of Vascular Surgery.*[14] In this publication many of the veins with a person's name tagged to it were given more appropriate anatomic names. For example, the vein of Giacomini is now the intersaphenous vein. Cockett perforators in the medial calf that arise from the posterior accessory saphenous vein are now categorized as upper, middle, and lower posterior tibial perforating veins. Probably the most notable change was the "lesser" saphenous vein being renames as the small saphenous vein.

"CVD" involves the entire spectrum of venous abnormalities that occur over the long time. Although it excludes acute deep venous thrombosis and its immediate signs and symptoms, chronic symptoms that develop are secondary and part of CVD spectrum. Primary CVD develops when inherent abnormalities of the vein wall lead to dilatation, valve dysfunction, and reflux.

To better classify the continuum of CVD, the CEAP criteria were developed.[4] In this comprehensive classification system, C is for classification, E for etiology, A for anatomy, and P for pathophysiology. Within each category, there are further sub-categories under each main category that allow for a detailed description of the current status of CVD. Most commonly, classification is used to speak the "common" language of the current status of a patient and their lower extremity examination. Classification ranges from C_0 to C_6 with the following definitions:

C_0—No visible or palpable signs of venous disease
C_1—Telangiectasias or reticular veins
C_2—Varicose veins
C_3—Edema
C_{4a}—Pigmentation and/or eczema
C_{4b}—Lipodermatosclerosis and/or atrophie blanche
C_5—Healed venous ulcer
C_6—Active venous ulcer

Objectively defining how CVD changes over time also remains an important piece of reporting in CVD. One of the most common tools is the Venous Clinical Severity Score (VCSS).[15] By assigning an objective numeric scoring system of mild, moderate, and severe to such areas as pain, varicose vein burden, venous edema, skin pigmentation, inflammation, induration, and ulcer burden, a consistent method arises to assess the natural history of CVD. Additionally, the VCSS becomes a very important tool when objectively assessing the effectiveness of similar and different treatments for the same level of disease. This has become increasingly important in the treatment of varicose veins or C_2 disease as many new treatments have or are being developed. These include new types of surgery, new ablative technologies, and new drugs and formations of sclerosing agents.

GUIDELINES

The clinical practice guidelines of the Society for Vascular Surgery and the American Forum consist of 14 different guideline categories and a summation of 42 recommendations or suggestions according to evidence-based GRADE criteria.[9] What follows are selected verbatim guidelines from this publication. These selected guidelines are chosen as they are particularly important to understand for the busy venous practitioner. Following each selected guideline, comments follow to further clarify and discuss certain controversies that still may exist despite what the evidence puts forth.

Guideline 2.3—GRADE 1A
> We recommend that reflux to confirm valvular incompetence in the upright position of the patients be elicited in one of two ways: either with increased intra-abdominal pressure using a Valsalva maneuver to assess the common femoral vein and the saphenofemoral junction or for the more distal veins, use of manual or cuff compression and release of the limb distal to the point of examination.

This recommendation brings clarity to the role of the Valsalva maneuver in providing reliable value for the determination of reflux. Note that the popliteal vein or the small saphenous vein should be assessed with the use of cuff deflation and not Valsalva.

Guideline 2.4—GRADE 1B

We recommend a cutoff value of 1 s for abnormally reversed flow (reflux) in the femoral and popliteal veins and 500 ms for the great saphenous vein, the small saphenous vein, the tibial, deep femoral, and the perforating veins.

There has been continued debate as to what the cutoff value should be with regard to 1 s or 500 ms. Here this delineation is clearly made and relates to triaging what veins play the biggest role in the development of clinically relevant venous reflux. Interestingly, the classic definition of a perforator diameter of greater or equal to 3.5 mm is mentioned in a separate recommendation and must be under an open or healed ulcer.

Guideline 3.1—GRADE 2C

We suggest that venous plethysmography be used selectively for the noninvasive evaluation of the venous system in patients with simple varicose veins (CEAP class C_2).

Despite many venous specialists using venous air plethysmography to assess the physiologic function of the venous system, there is little evidence that these test changes add information that could change the course of treatment. Perhaps as more study is performed on calf muscle pump dysfunction, the measurement of calf vein ejection fraction will become more relevant to assess before and after a directed treatment.

Guideline 4.1—GRADE 1B

We recommend that in patients with varicose veins and more advanced CVD, computed tomography venography, magnetic resonance venography, ascending and descending contrast venography, and intravascular ultrasonography are used selective for indications, including but not limited to postthrombotic syndrome, thrombotic or nonthrombotic iliac vein obstruction (May–Thurner syndrome), pelvic congestion syndrome, nutcracker syndrome, vascular malformations, venous trauma, tumors, and planned open or endovascular venous interventions.

This may be one of the most important and overlooked areas of investigation for patients presenting with varicose veins and "more advanced" CVD. This recommendation begs close inspection of a patient's leg that has varicose veins. Additional evidence of nonpitting edema in addition to the presence of ipsilateral varicose veins constitutes more advanced disease. Therefore, in the large majority of patients, further imaging is necessary to assure no further presence of obstruction. Vascular specialists should have a low threshold to obtaining further imaging and be familiar as to what particular type of advanced imaging is best suited to use in their institution. If ultimately a therapeutic venogram is performed, intravascular ultrasound represents the criterion standard to further assure the presence of an obstruction or stenosis. Although this technical consideration does not constitute a recommendation within the current guidelines, it does represent more the norm among those venous endovascular specialists who commonly perform venous angioplasty and stenting.

Guideline 6.1—GRADE 1A

We recommend that the CEAP classification be used for patients with varicose veins. The basic CEAP classification is used for clinical practice, and the full CEAP classification system is used for clinical research.

CEAP classification, as developed by experts within the American Venous Forum, has become the standard for assuring a consistent communication system of CVD severity. Furthermore, the more detailed use of the "EAP" in research provides the opportunity to compare "apples to apples." Given the gamut of symptomatology associated with varicose veins as well as the spectrum of technology now being developed for treatment, use of the full CEAP classification system becomes vitally important as more research spawns.

Guideline 7.1—GRADE 1B

We recommend that the revised VCSS is used for assessment of clinical outcomes after therapy for varicose veins and more advanced CVD.

The revised VCSS has become a valuable tool in following outcome after treatment of varicose veins. Like CEAP, it not only allows a better assessment of outcome to observe to what degree clinical improvement occurred but also allows comparison of the effectiveness of two different modalities for treatment of varicose veins. For the busy vascular specialist who treats varicose veins, CEAP and VCSS are indispensable tools in correctly classifying severity of CVD from varicose veins and how effective outcomes are for certain treatments. Thus a common language of classification and outcome can be spoken among the clinical and the research teams.

Guideline 9.1—GRADE 2C

We suggest compression therapy using moderate pressure (20–30 mmHg) for patients with symptomatic varicose veins.

Guideline 9.2—GRADE 1B

We recommend against compression therapy as the primary treatment of symptomatic varicose veins in patients who are candidates for saphenous vein ablation.

Guidelines 9.1 and 9.2 are among the most powerful when considering how to primarily treat symptomatic varicose veins. In correct contradiction to the large majority of insurance carrier policies, Guidelines 9.1 and 9.2 give strong evidence that patients will get the most relief by undergoing ablation. The fact that most insurance companies require a mandatory waiting period to "fail" compression therapy for the treatment of varicose veins only further delays the proper treatment, when the evidence is closely examined. Interestingly, Guideline 9.2 does not add to its statement any mention of stab phlebectomy of branch varicosities or stripping of the saphenous vein.

Guideline 10.4—GRADE 1A

To decrease recurrence of venous ulcers, we recommend ablation of the incompetent superficial veins in addition to compression therapy.

Recurrence of venous ulcers continues to be a major problem for patients and the current guideline lends credence to assuring that all patients with leg ulcers that clinically appear to be of venous origin have reflux testing of the deep and superficial veins. The basis of this guideline comes from the results of the ESCHAR study, which randomly compared compression alone to compression in addition to open venous surgery.[16,17] Ablation was not used in the ESCHAR study, yet the GRADE in this guideline is 1A. Note also that ablation is recommended with no mention of the status of reflux in the deep venous system. Indeed, reflux in the deep system can often show evidence of improvement with ablation of the great saphenous vein.

Guideline 11.2—GRADE 1B

Because of reduced convalescence and less pain and morbidity, we recommend endovenous thermal ablation of the incompetent saphenous vein over open surgery.

Guideline 11.2 defines the standard of modern treatment of varicose veins stemming from an incompetent saphenous vein. Despite the evidence leading to this guideline, controversy and differing opinions exist as to its validity. Great Britain has struggled with the notion that thermal ablation shows superiority over open surgery. Neovascularization, a phenomena leading to recurrence following open stripping of the great saphenous vein is not mentioned as another detrimental outcome of open venous surgery in comparison with thermal ablation.

Guideline 12.1—GRADE 1B
    We recommend liquid or foam sclerotherapy for telangiectasia, reticular veins, and varicose veins.

Given the scope of use of sclerotherapy, Guideline 12.1 represents an interesting recommendation in that there is no comparison or recommendation in preference to stab phlebectomy. Moreover, stab phlebectomy for the treatment of varicose veins receives little if any attention throughout the entire guideline publication. Guideline 12.1 and the absence of any superiority over stab phlebectomy does not necessarily mean that liquid or foam schlerotherapy should be used in preference. Rather, sclerotherapy can certainly be used as a primary treatment of branch varicosities, despite its failure rate and clinical sequela (such as hyperpigmentation).

Guideline 13.1—GRADE 1B
    We recommend against selective treatment of incompetent perforating veins in patients with simple varicose veins (CEAP class C_2).

Although incompetent perforation veins may play a role in ulcer healing and recurrence, they do not warrant treatment if identified with CEAP class C_2 disease. Alternatively stated, treatment of an incompetent saphenous vein and the branch varicosities should suffice in alleviating the symptomatology and minimize recurrence. There is no added benefit from performing additional procedures to treat these pathologic veins in this select population.

SUMMARY

All practitioners treating varicose veins should review the clinical practice guidelines on the care of patients with varicose veins as put forth by the Society for Vascular Surgery and the American Venous Forum.[9] This brief manuscript reviews the GRADE criteria for the creation of guidelines and then summarizes those important venous guidelines using it that may "change" practice and promote more evidence-based care. Patient advocates, health administrators, federal agencies, and insurers would also benefit from review as well in order to provide consistent messaging and care to patients afflicted with varicose veins.

REFERENCES

1. Kaplan RM, Criqui MH, Denenberg JO, et al. Quality of life in patients with chronic venous disease: San Diego population study. *J Vasc Surg*. 2003;37:1047–1053.
2. Bradbury A, Ruckley CV. Clinical presentation and assessment of patients with venous disease. In: Gloviczki P, editor. *Handbook of Venous Disorders*. 3rd ed. London: Edward Arnold, Ltd; 2009. pp. 331–341.

3. Smith JJ, Garrett AM, Guest M, et al. Evaluating and improving health-related quality of life in patients with varicose veins. *J Vasc Surg*. 1999;30:710–719.
4. Eklof B, Rutherford RB, Bergan JJ, et al. Revision of the CEAP classification for chronic venous disorders: consensus statement. *J Vasc Surg*. 2004;40:1248–1252.
5. Coleridge-Smith P, Labropoulos N, Parsch H, et al. Duplex ultrasound investigation of the veins in chronic venous disease of the lower limbs: UIP consensus document: part I. Basic principles. *Eur J Vasc Endovasc Surg*. 2006;31:83–92.
6. Luebke T, Gawenda M, Heckenkamp J, Brunkwall J. Meta-analysis of endovenous radio-frequency obliteration of the great saphenous vein in primary varicosis. *J Endovasc Ther*. 2008;15:213–223.
7. Coleridge-Smith P. Foam and liquid sclerotherapy for varicose veins. *Phlebology*. 2009;24 (suppl 1):62–72.
8. Vasquez MA, Rabe E, McLafferty RB, et al. Revision of the venous clinical severity score: venous outcomes consensus statement: special communication of the American Venous Forum Ad Hoc Outcomes Working Group. *J Vasc Surg*. 2010;52:1387–1396.
9. Gloviczki P, Comerota AJ, Dalsing MC, et al. The care of patients with varicose veins and associated chronic venous disease: Clinical practice guidelines of the Society for Vascular Surgery and the American Venous Forum. *J Vasc Surg*. 2011;53(suppl):1S–48S.
10. Guyatt G, Gutterman D, Baumann MH, et al. Grading strength of recommendations and quality of evidence in clinical guidelines: report from the American College of Chest Physicians task force. *Chest*. 2006;129:174–181.
11. Meissner MH, Eklof B, Lohr JM, et al. Acute and chronic venous disease. *J Vasc Surg*. 2007;46(suppl):1S–93S.
12. Henke P, Kistner B, Wakefield TW, et al. Reducing venous stasis ulcers by fifty percent in 10 years. *J Vasc Surg*. 2011;53(suppl):1S–85S.
13. Gloviczki P, editor. *Handbook of Venous Disorders: Guidelines of the American Venous Forum*. 3rd ed. London: Hodder Arnold; 2009.
14. Caggiati A, Bergan JJ, Gloviczki P, et al. Nomenclature of the veins of the lower limb: extentions, refinements, and clinical application. *J Vasc Surg*. 2005;41:719–724.
15. Vasquez MA, Rabe E, McLafferty RB, et al. Revision of the venous clinical severity score: venous outcomes consensus statement: special communication from the American Venous Forum Ad Hoc Outcomes Working Group. *J Vasc Surg*. 2010;52:1387–1396.
16. Barwell JR, Davies CE, Deacon J, et al. Comparison of surgery and compression with compression alone in chronic venous ulceration (ESCHAR study): randomized controlled trial. *Lancet*. 2004;363:1854–1859.
17. Gohel MS, Barwell JR, Taylor M, et al. Long term results of compression therapy alone versus compression plus surgery in chronic venous ulceration (ESCHAR): randomized controlled trial. *BMJ*. 2007;335:383.

19

Tips and Tricks for Successful Endovenous Ablation

Abby Wochinski, MD and Kellie R. Brown, MD

INTRODUCTION

The evolution of endovascular technology over the past decade has brought the treatment of chronic venous insufficiency into the forefront of vascular surgery. Surgical ligation and stripping are relatively invasive and have been notorious for recurrence rates as high as 30% after one year.[1] Therefore, minimally invasive techniques (endovenous ablation, microphlebectomy, and sclerotherapy) have moved ahead as primary treatment methods of varicose veins. These modalities not only improve patients' quality of life but also have fewer side effects, overall cost, and postoperative pain. However, as with any emerging technology, success rates heavily rely on operator experience. This chapter is meant to be a summary of how to approach these patients from an operative standpoint, including discussion of standard techniques, tips and tricks for avoiding complications, and trouble-shooting challenging patient anatomy and comorbidities.

PREOPERATIVE WORKUP

History and physical exam are the first important step in successful treatment planning. In addition to elucidating the patient's history of varicose veins and symptom occurrence, history of deep vein thrombosis, clotting disorders, bleeding episodes and ulceration are very important. Special attention must also be paid to anyone who states that they have had varicose veins since birth. This history necessitates further workup for congenital venous malformation.

Even in the standard patient, the importance of preoperative duplex ultrasound and marking with legs in a dependent position must not be underestimated. Ultrasound can not only identify potential locations for venous access but also can give an estimation of vein tortuosity and location and diameter of nearby tributaries or perforating veins (PVs). Even though intraoperative ultrasound can provide similar information, having marked the course of the vein preoperatively will give the surgeon a rough road map and help with preoperative planning. Additionally, it is very important to determine the presence and patency of the deep venous system, as ablation of the superficial system is contraindicated in cases of deep system obstruction.

STANDARD ABLATION TECHNIQUE

Standard therapy for treatment of reflux involving the greater saphenous vein (GSV) is relatively straightforward. The vein is accessed under direct ultrasound guidance, using the Seldinger technique with a 22-gauge micropuncture needle, typically just below the knee. The choice of a smaller needle size decreases local vasospasm as well as minimizes bleeding complications. At the level of the knee, the GSV consistently has a large diameter and relatively straight course, allowing for easier access. Initiating ablation at or just below the knee rather than above maximizes the length of vein available for ablation. There is also decreased risk of injury to the saphenous nerve at this location.[2] Once venous access is obtained, a 0.018-inch micropuncture wire is placed, followed by the micropuncture sheath. Through this sheath, a 0.038-inch guide wire is passed through the micropuncture sheath into the vein. This passage can be made difficult due to various factors, including venous tortuosity, small vessel diameter, and scarring/sclerosis. Dealing with these intraoperative challenges will be discussed later.

After successful placement of the guide wire, the micropuncture sheath is removed and a small incision made over the wire to allow passage of the introducer sheath. The 5Fr sheath is then advanced until the tip is at the saphenofemoral junction, at which time the guide wire is removed and the sheath is withdrawn to the proper location within the vein. Appropriate positioning of the sheath (1.5–2 cm distal to the saphenofemoral junction and below the superficial epigastric vein) is by far the most crucial step in the procedure. Excessive advancement increases the risk of injury to the deep venous system and subsequent DVT. This endovenous heat-induced thrombosis (EHIT) has an incidence of approximately 3%, but is a relatively preventable complication if one is vigilant about catheter tip location. On the other hand, insufficient advancement leaves a venous stump, which may increase recurrence of venous reflux and create a nidus for neovascularization. Once the sheath is appropriately placed, the thermal ablation catheter is inserted (either radiofrequency or laser) and position rechecked with ultrasound. For endovenous laser ablation (EVLA), the position of the laser tip can also be confirmed by transcutaneous visualization of the red standby light.

Tumescent anesthesia consisting of diluted lidocaine and bicarbonate is injected around the vein. Adequate tumescent anesthesia not only increases patient comfort but also acts as a heat sink and decreases damage to the surrounding tissues during ablation. It also has been shown to provide some external venous compression, increasing contact with the catheter and the vein wall.

Thermal ablation is then achieved by retraction of either the laser or radiofrequency catheter while activating the thermal generator. Each technology has its own specific parameters that improve success of ablation and minimize complications.

For EVLA, the amount of energy given, as measured by fluence (J/cm), is the most important variable in determining success of ablation.[3] This is calculated using the following calculation:

$$\text{Fluence} = \frac{\text{total wattage used per second duration of treatment}}{\text{estimated length of vein}}$$

Several studies have demonstrated that fluence of 60–100 J/cm is an independent predictor of durable GSV occlusion.[4] This increased success comes without increased local complications including nerve injury, micropuncture, or skin burn. There has been some data to support the use of higher wavelength lasers (1064–1470 nm) in the treatment of GSV >2 cm in diameter. These higher wavelength lasers have increased affinity to water and cause direct damage to the intima by evaporating the water within the vein wall. In contrast, the lower wavelength lasers (810–980 nm) target hemoglobin and create steam bubbles, which produce endothelial damage and thrombosis without direct contact. In addition to wavelength variation, lasers often have options for either pulsed or continuous mode. For pulsed mode, the vein is exposed to a fixed amount of energy at equal distances. Total energy delivered depends on multiple variables, including distance between pulses, pulse duration, and wattage. Lasers using continuous mode require the catheter to be pulled back at a constant, even speed. In this case, the total energy delivered relies only on the pullback speed and wattage.

Radiofrequency ablation (RFA) employs a catheter that treats continuous segments of vein up to 7 cm in length. The ClosureFAST catheter contains within it a coil that reaches a temperature of 120°C, which causes direct injury to the venous wall, resulting in collagen contraction and denaturation, followed by fibrosis and thrombosis of the vessel.[5,6] After ablating the initial segment just distal to the saphenofemoral junction (SFJ) with two 20-second treatment cycles, the catheter is withdrawn 6.5 cm to allow sufficient overlap of neighboring segments. Ultrasound compression during the treatment cycle along with adequate circumferential tumescent anesthesia ensures contact with the vein wall, which increases success of treatment. Once treatment is completed for the entire length of vein, great care is taken to remove the catheter without burning the skin.

Once ablation is completed, it is important to perform a completion ultrasound documenting patency of the common femoral vein. The patient's compression stocking is then placed before allowing the patient to stand. This external compression of the extremity is crucial in preventing the development of postoperative complications (e.g., phlebitis and bruising), as well as increasing immediate post-op discomfort. While it seems that nearly everyone uses postprocedure compression, there is no standard strength or length of therapy. The few studies that have been performed document better outcomes with higher pressure compression (>40 mm Hg while standing) but have little to no data on duration of treatment.[7] One group in particular investigated the use of eccentric compression using a cross-taped technique beneath compression stockings (35 mm Hg). After one-week post-op, they found both decreased presence of bruising and decreased pain medication use in the group that had the additional eccentric compression.[8] We use 30–40–mm Hg compression to cover the treated area for three weeks and have the patient keep them on without removal for the first three days.

ANATOMIC CHALLENGES

There are several anatomic variations that pose a challenge to the inexperienced surgeon and may lead to increased failure rates if not treated appropriately. Patients who have small vein diameter (due to either natural anatomy or venous spasm) are often difficult to access in spite of direct visualization with ultrasound. The easiest steps include placing the patient in reverse Trendelenburg position or applying a heat pack to increase venous dilation. Studies have also investigated the use of topical nitroglycerin ointment as an adjunctive therapy. One prospective, double-blinded randomized control trial (RCT) compared pretreatment with topical nitroglycerin with treadmill ambulation for endovascular access in patients with venous diameter <5 mm. They found that nitroglycerin ointment alone or used in combination with treadmill ambulation produced significant venodilation (69% and 51.7%, respectively) in comparison to ambulation alone (2.7%).[9] If these attempts are unsuccessful, one can perform venous cutdown and access the vein directly.

On the other hand, patients with enlarged vein diameters are also at increased risk for treatment failure. As previously discussed, successful ablation relies primarily on the energy density delivered during ablation (fluence). Therefore, if the same amount of energy is distributed across a larger venous cross section, the effective energy dose delivered to the intima may be insufficient to produce contraction and fibrosis. The first step in these cases with significant venous dilation (>1 cm) is to position the patient in Trendelenburg position to increase venous return. Several other technical options exist, which increase the total energy delivered, including use of a higher wavelength laser (1470 nm) or increasing wattage. However, these measures may increase the risk of paresthesias due to nerve damage. The surgeon can also apply manual pressure with the ultrasound probe to the vessel during catheter pullback to allow for better catheter–intima interface. Finally, the use of appropriately placed tumescent anesthesia also acts to externally compress the vein onto the catheter, decreasing the overall surface area of the vein. In cases of very large veins (>1.8 cm), another option is to perform a high ligation under tumescent anesthetic and then perform the ablation in standard fashion. This allows for better catheter–intima interface as well as decreased flow through the vein, thereby allowing for a higher success of ablation.

For veins that have significant scarring, sclerosis, or tortuosity, the most challenging aspect of ablation is often passage of the guide wire. Using excessive force can not only be quite painful for the patient but there is also increased risk of venous perforation. Reverse Trendelenberg positioning and the concurrent venous distention can make the tortuosities less extreme, allowing for easier passage. The assistant can stretch the skin to try to straighten out the vein. If the tortuosities are located near a joint space, repositioning the limb can also be helpful. If these physical maneuvers are unsuccessful, attempted passage of a hydrophilic or more flexible wire can make this step easier. Another option is to place the introducer sheath, remove the wire, and irrigate through the sheath while gently advancing. Extreme caution must be used with this maneuver, as there is no guide wire in place. If the guide wire and sheath cannot be advanced past a certain point despite these efforts, the safest way to achieve effective ablation is to access the vein at a second location just proximal to the lesion and perform separate ablation treatments.

The last anatomic variation we will discuss is dealing with superficial veins located just deep to the skin. In these cases, the heat caused by the ablation process puts the patient at significantly increased risk of superficial skin burns during treatment (1% incidence) or skin discoloration as the vein breaks down after treatment.[10] Injection of tumescent anesthesia into the subdermal area can create enough separation between the vein and the epidermis to provide protection from these complications. Generally, the vein must be 1 cm below the skin to safely ablate. If the vein is unable to be separated a safe distance away from the skin, one can perform a high ligation with phlebectomy of the GSV through micropuncture incisions. This can be done safely and effectively under tumescent anesthetic.

ENDOVENOUS HEAT-INDUCED THROMBOSIS

Incidence of EHIT of the deep system following ablation is about 3%, and if it goes unrecognized, it can progress to DVT.[11] As previously discussed, appropriate placement of the catheter 1.5–2 cm distal to the SFJ greatly reduces this risk. However, it is also important to encourage the patient to walk immediately after the procedure. Repeat postprocedure ultrasound should be performed within the first week after treatment to rule out EHIT. The treatment of EHIT is determined by the severity of the thrombosis, and the majority of cases resolve within four weeks without progression to DVT. Most studies recommend anticoagulation for patients with nonocclusive thrombosis extending into the deep system (>50% cross-sectional area) or complete occlusion of the deep venous system (EHIT class 3 or 4, respectively).[10] However, there is more variable data regarding treatment of EHIT class 2 (nonocclusive thrombus <50% cross-sectional area), with some studies supporting observation and others low-molecular-weight heparin (LMWH) therapy. Ultimately, no consensus has yet been reached regarding treatment of EHIT and further research is needed. Our typical approach for EHIT class 2 includes LMWH and weekly reimaging until the thrombus retracts into the GSV, which, in our experience, takes between—one and two weeks.

SMALL SAPHENOUS VEIN TREATMENT

Reflux involving the small saphenous vein (SSV) occurs in approximately 15% of patients with varicose veins.[12] As with the GSV, open ligation and stripping are associated with higher rates of failure and complications. This is seen to a greater extent in the SSV system due to varied anatomy of the saphenopopliteal junction (SPJ) as well as the proximity to the sural nerve. Therefore, endovascular ablation as a primary treatment modality has great potential for improving outcomes in these patients. Early data show significant improvements in comparison to surgical ligation, with both ablation success rates (96% vs. 72% at six weeks) and postoperative quality of life.[13]

The technique of SSV ablation is very similar to that of GSV ablation. Patients are typically placed in the prone, reverse Trendeleberg position and the vein identified through ultrasound. Due to the close relationship with the sural nerve, the access site for SSV ablation is critical in preventing postoperative paresthesias. The goal is to access the vein as distal as possible while remaining above the ankle. One study found significantly increased postoperative paresthesias in patients accessed near the lateral malleolus compared to the distal mid-calf (20% vs. 3%) without impact on success of ablation.[14] Therefore, it is best to access the SSV at the junction between the distal and middle third of the calf, where the belly of the gastrocnemius muscle joins the tendon. The position of the tip of the catheter is also important to avoid both DVT and nerve injury. Since the tibial and peroneal nerves lie below the fascia near the SPJ, it is best to position the catheter tip at or just below the fascia where the SSV dips below to join the popliteal vein. This is often 2 cm or so from the SPJ. If there is SSV reflux that extends into the thigh, the catheter can be passed into this segment of vein into the thigh. In addition, adequate use of tumescent anesthesia is critical to avoiding nerve and cutaneous injury. Trendelenberg positioning during ablation also helps separate the vein from the surrounding cutaneous and motor nerves. Again, appropriate positioning of the catheter 2 cm distal to the SPJ is crucial in the prevention of EHIT.

ANTERIOR ACCESSORY SAPHENOUS VEIN TREATMENT

Anterior accessory saphenous vein (AASV) reflux is commonly seen in conjunction with GSV reflux, and the majority of the data surrounding AASV ablation deals with concurrent GSV ablation or open ligation and stripping. However, isolated AASV incompetence is found in about 10% of patients. In addition, new onset AASV reflux can be a cause of recurrent varicose veins after successful GSV treatment. It has been demonstrated in smaller studies and case series that endovenous ablation of the AASV alone can be performed with preservation of the GSV. Access is obtained at the most distal point of significant venous reflux, usually the anterior mid-thigh, and ablation performed in the standard fashion. At one year follow-up, these patients have significant improvement in their symptoms without evidence of increased GSV reflux or recurrence due to neovascularization.[15]

RECURRENT VARICOSE VEIN TREATMENT

Recurrent venous insufficiency following surgical ligation and stripping has been seen in almost two-thirds of patients after five years.[16] Half of these patients go on to develop symptoms requiring additional interventions. The cause of recurrence may be due to insufficient surgical removal of the GSV, incorrect identification and ligation of the SFJ, duplication of the GSV system, or increased flow through surrounding tributaries. For patients who primarily underwent endovenous ablation, recurrence rates are significantly less after five years compared to surgical treatment (4%).[17] Even in the setting of successful above-knee GSV ablation, residual below-knee GSV incompetence can allow for recurrent venous insufficiency. In one study, 89% of patients with significant below-knee-GSV reflux required additional procedures.[18] Other potential causes for recurrence following ablation are spontaneous recanalization, the mechanism of which is thought to be similar to that following acute thrombosis and DVT, reflux in the AASV, perforator incompetence, and neovascularization.

Neovascularization is seen most commonly following primary surgical treatment. The positive predictive value of neovascularization on ultrasound at one year for clinically significant recurrence is 70%–100%.[1] It has been suggested that the tissue trauma and inflammation associated with vein stripping stimulates angiogenesis, allowing for reconnection between the deep and superficial systems.

Due to the high technical demands and failure rates of reoperation, endovenous ablation has become an increasingly common treatment modality for recurrent cases. The use of ultrasound to define the pattern of incompetence is critical in preoperative planning. Recurrences due to neovascularization often reveal a great deal of tortuosity and variable anatomy. Access should again be obtained at the most distal point of reflux as seen on ultrasound. Below the knee, one must be conscious of the proximity of the saphenous nerve with the GSV. Tumescent anesthesia is again used to provide separation between the two structures and decrease the risk of damage to the saphenous nerve. The passage of the wire in a recannalized segment may be difficult, and the aforementioned techniques described for primary treatment of tortuous veins can also be employed here for treatment of neovascularization or recanalization, provided there is a relatively straight segment. In those cases of multiple tortuous veins arising from the common femoral vein, or inability to pass the wire, either ultrasound-guided sclerotherapy or surgical ligation with concomitant phlebectomy or sclerotherapy is generally effective.

Residual varicosities following endovascular ablation can also be treated by phlebectomy or sclerotherapy. One study investigated the use of concomitant phlebectomy in the setting of EVLA. They found no significance with respect to postoperative pain or return to activity after the initial procedure. However, 66% of the group that did not have phlebectomy at the time of EVLA required subsequent procedures to eliminate symptoms of venous insufficiency, compared to 4% in the concurrent phlebectomy group.[17] For these patients, it took up to one year longer to see the same improvement in quality of life. Therefore, it is important for a surgeon to have an informed discussion with each patient regarding the risks/benefits of sequential versus concomitant phlebectomy at the time of endovenous ablation. Our typical practice is to stage axial venous ablation and phlebectomy or sclerotherapy in most cases. This allows us to perform the least amount of treatment for effective relief of symptoms.

PERFORATING VEIN TREATMENT

PVs create a unidirectional connection from the superficial to the deep venous system. When these valves become incompetent, reflux occurs back into the superficial system, increasing the severity of venous insufficiency. An incompetent perforator can be a cause of recurrent or residual varicose veins after treatment of the GSV, SSV, or AASV. Once again, preoperative ultrasound is very important in determining the role perforator incompetence plays in overall venous insufficiency. PVs >3.5 mm in diameter are assumed to be incompetent.[19] Access is obtained by ultrasound guidance using a slightly larger cannula (18-gauge) and the catheter tip advanced to the peri-fascial vein, at least 2 cm from the deep veins. This location is again important to prevent EHIT and preserve functioning of the deep and muscular veins. It is very important to distinguish between and avoid arterial perforators, which, if inadvertently treated, can cause localized muscle ischemia. If treating multiple perforators, hematomas and bruising can be minimized by working from the distal to proximal limb and placing a sterile compressive dressing as you progress. Successful ablation of perforator veins seems to be related to vein diameter, with >84% thrombosis and occlusion for veins <6 mm and 43% when the vein is >6 mm.[20]

PATIENTS ON SYSTEMIC ANTICOAGULATION

One group that requires special mention are those patients with medical comorbidities requiring anticoagulation with warfarin. When performing ligation and stripping, the current standard of care is to have patients hold their anticoagulation before surgery due to the increased risk of bleeding. This incurs a significant increase in cost to these patients, as they require bridging therapy, which may mean preprocedure hospital admission. However, for endovascular approaches, this may not be necessary. Several studies have investigated the success of ablation as well as postoperative complications (bleeding, bruising, hematoma formation, etc.) in patients who have remained on their anticoagulation therapy.[21] They found similar success rates with no significant difference in bleeding complications either intraoperatively or on follow-up. From these studies, it can be concluded that patients on wafarin can safely undergo endovascular ablation for venous disease without cessation of anticoagulation therapy.

SUMMARY

Endovenous ablation is now the primary mode of treatment for superficial venous reflux involving the GSV, SSV, AASV, and PVs. This is supplemented by phlebectomy and sclerotherapy techniques. These treatments are relatively straightforward, but do require a degree of expertise by the operator. With experience, successful treatment of all types of superficial reflux can be treated in a minimally invasive, office based, cosmetically acceptable manner with minimal discomfort and excellent results.

REFERENCES

1. Carradice D, Mekako AI, Mazari FA, et al. Clinical and technical outcomes from a randomized clinical trial of endovenous laser ablation compared with conventional surgery for great saphenous varicose veins. *Br J Surg.* 2011;98:1117–1123.
2. Van den Bos RR, Kockaert MA, Neumann HA, Nijsten T. Technical review of endovenous laser therapy for varicose veins. *Eur J Vasc Endovasc Surg.* 2008;35:88–95.
3. Theivacumar NS, Dellagrammaticas D, Beale RJ, et al. Factors influencing the effectiveness of endovenous laser ablation (EVLA) in the treatment of great saphenous vein reflux. *Eur J Vasc Endovasc Surg.* 2008;35:119–123.
4. Sadek M, Kabnick LS, Berland T, et al. Update of endovenous laser ablation: 2011. *Perspect Vasc Surg Endovasc Therapy.* 2011;23:233–237.
5. Gale SS, Lee JN, Walsh ME, et al. A randomized, controlled trial of endovenous thermal ablation using the 810-nm wavelength laser and the ClosurePLUS radiofrequency ablation methods for superficial venous insufficiency of the great saphenous vein. *J Vasc Surg.* 2010;52:645–650.
6. Lohr J, Kulwicki A. Radiofrequency ablation: evolution of a treatment. *Semin Vasc Surg.* 2010;23:90–100.
7. Mosti G. Post-treatment compression: duration and techniques. *Phlebology.* 2013;28:21–24.
8. Lugli M, Cogo A, Guerzoni S, et al. Effects of eccentric compression by a cross-tape technique after endovenous laser ablation of the great saphenous vein: a randomized study. *Phlebology.* 2009;24:151–156.

9. Hogue RS, Schul MW, Dando CF, Erdman BE. The effect of nitroglycerin ointment on great saphenous vein targeted venous access site diameter with endovenous laser treatment. *Phlebology.* 2008;23:222–226.

10. Dexter D, Kabnick L, Berland T, et al. Complications of endovenous lasers. *Phlebology.* 2012;27:40–45.

11. Sufian S, Arnez A, Labropoulos N, Lakhanpal S. Incidence, progression, and risk factors for endovenous heat-induced thrombosis after radiofrequency ablation. *J Vasc Surg: Venous and Lym Dis.* 2013;1:159–164.

12. Tellings SS, Ceulen RP, Sommer A. Surgery and endovenous techniques for the treatment of small saphenous varicose veins: a review of the literature. *Phlebology.* 2011;26:179–184.

13. Samuel N, Carradice D, Wallace T, et al. Randomized clinical trial of endovenous laser ablation versus conventional surgery for small saphenous varicose veins. *Ann Surg.* 2013;257:419–426.

14. Doganci S, Yildirim V, Demirkilic U. Does puncture site affect the rate of nerve injuries following endovenous laser ablation of the small saphenous veins? *Eur J Vasc Endovasc Surg.* 2011;41:400–405.

15. Theivacumar NS, Darwood RJ, Gough MJ. Endovenous laser ablation (EVLA) of the anterior accessory great saphenous vein (AAGSV): abolition of sapheno-femoral reflux with preservation of the great saphenous vein. *Eur J Vasc Endovasc Surg.* 2009;37:477–481.

16. Anchala PR, Wickman C, Chen R, et al. Endovenous laser ablation as a treatment for postsurgical recurrent saphenous insufficiency. *Cardiovasc Intervent Radiol.* 2010;33:983–988.

17. Carradice D, Mekako AI, Hatfield J, Chettner IC. Randomized clinical trial of concomitant or sequential phlebectomy after endovenous laser therapy for varicose veins. *Br J Surg.* 2009;96:369–375.

18. Theivacumar NS, Darwood RJ, Dellegrammaticas D, et al. The clinical significance of below-knee great saphenous vein reflux following endovenous laser ablation of above-knee great saphenous vein. *Phlebology.* 2009;24:17–20.

19. Gloviczki P, Comerota AJ, Dalsing MC, et al. The care of patients with varicose veins and associated chronic venous diseases: clinical practice guidelines of the society for vascular surgery and the American venous forum. *J Vasc Surg.* 2011;53:2S–48S.

20. Corcos L, Pontello D, De Anna D, et al. Endovenous 808-nm diode laser occlusion of perforating veins and varicose collaterals: a prospective study of 482 limbs. *Dermatol Surg.* 2011;37:1486–1498.

21. Riesenman PJ, De Fritas DJ, Konigsberg SG, Kasirajan K. Noninterruption of warfarin therapy is safe and does not compromise outcome in patients undergoing endovenous laser therapy (EVLT). *Vasc Endovasc Surg.* 2011;45:524–526.

20

Venous Aneurysms

Heron E. Rodriguez, MD

INTRODUCTION

Venous aneurysms are uncommon. They have been reported to occur in virtually every major vein.

Solitary primary venous aneurysms should be distinguished from secondary aneurysms. Secondary aneurysmal dilatation of veins is often observed in association with either high-flow states or congenital venous malformations.[1] Following the creation of an arteriovenous fistula, venous dilation occurs to accommodate the high shear forces. Eventually, venous aneurysms form. Such aneurysms are associated with arteriovenous fistula access for chronic hemodialysis and with trauma. Occasionally, venous aneurysms form proximal to a partial venous obstruction, presumably as a result of increased pressure.[2] Multiple venous aneurysms are also found in association with vascular malformations that do not have arteriovenous shunting.

Solitary venous aneurysms (those not associated with high-flow states, trauma, inflammation, or congenital malformations) are uncommon and they are the focus of this chapter. More extensive, comprehensive reviews of the topic have been published elsewhere.[3]

POPLITEAL ANEURYSMS

The popliteal vein is believed to be the most common site of venous aneurysms, with 147 cases reported in the literature.[4] The true prevalence of popliteal venous aneurysms and the frequency with which they cause symptoms are impossible to estimate. Most patients with venous aneurysms present with chest symptoms suggestive of pulmonary embolism or local symptoms in the popliteal fossa. Rupture has never been reported. Bilaterality can occur but is uncommon. Very often, associated symptoms of venous insufficiency are present.

The diagnosis can be accurately made with duplex ultrasonography. Operative plans can be made with US alone but most surgeons prefer the details of venography. CT-venograms and MR-venograms have virtually replaced ascending phlebography in our (and most) practices.

Given their frequent association with pulmonary embolism, popliteal venous aneurysms should undergo surgical treatment once the diagnosis is made. Anticoagulation alone has been associated with fatal outcomes.[5,6] The size of the aneurysm does not appear to correlate with the risk of thromboembolism.[7] The short-term results of surgical treatment at our institution[8,1] and those reported in the literature are excellent. Aneurysmectomy with lateral venography or patch angioplasty repair, resection with end-to-end anastomosis or bypass (using nonreversed great saphenous vein, internal jugular vein, saphenous panel composite, or spiral vein) appear to have similar results. The long-term patency rates of venous repairs remain poorly defined. Reported rates in the literature vary from 40% to 90%,[6] but very few studies report patency rates after 12 months. Some have suggested that even short-term patency may facilitate the development of collateral venous channels. Most aneurysms can be approached posteriorly (Fig. 20-1), and perioperative intravenous anticoagulation has been routinely used and frequently continued through the oral route for one to three months postoperatively.

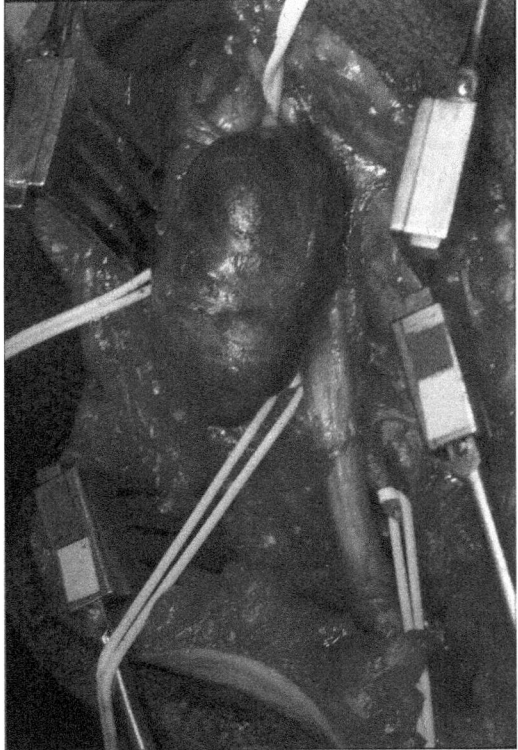

Figure 20-1. Popliteal vein aneurysm exposed through a posterior approach. The sural nerve is observed lateral to the venous aneurysm and the popliteal artery has been encircled with vessel loops medially.

OTHER VENOUS ANEURYSMS OF THE EXTREMITIES

Venous aneurysms of the extremities can develop in the superficial or in the deep venous system. Most superficial venous aneurysms of the extremities present as a soft, blue, compressible mass with few symptoms. Aneurysms of the saphenous vein are often associated with varicosities (Fig. 20-2). It is not uncommon for those aneurysms located in the upper thigh to be misdiagnosed as reducible inguinal or femoral hernias. If the aneurysm is located in the superficial venous system, engorgement causing expansion during inspiration (lower extremities) or expiration (upper extremities) is typical.

The risk of pulmonary embolism due to aneurysms in the superficial veins of the lower extremity is low and very likely null for those in the upper extremities. For these reasons, most superficial venous aneurysms should only be treated if symptoms occur (cosmesis, pain, and thrombosis). In the majority of cases, excision of the aneurysmal segment alone is the best management option. In cases when there is evidence of thrombosis or occlusion of the deep system, excision with reconstruction may be necessary.[9,10]

Deep venous aneurysms of the extremities usually present as an asymptomatic soft mass or are discovered incidentally during imaging studies performed for other reasons. Surgical repair of venous aneurysms of the extremities is determined by location. Venous aneurysms of the brachial or axillary veins (Fig. 20-3) are not associated with pulmonary embolism and should be treated only if symptoms occur (cosmetic and thrombosis). Iliac aneurysms (Fig. 20-4), although rare, appear to be associated with thromboembolic events in the majority of the reported cases[1,2,11] and thus should be treated surgically.

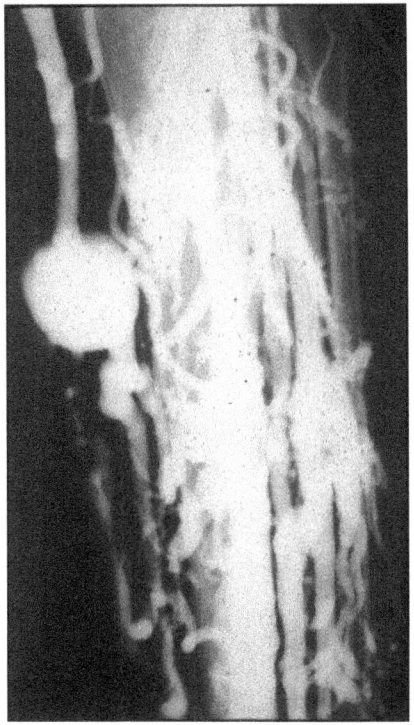

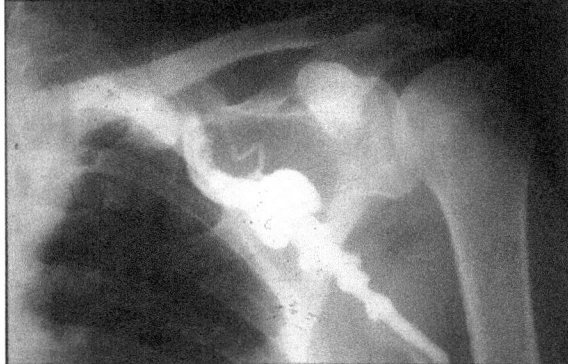

Figure 20-2. Lower extremity venogram showing a saphenous vein aneurysm in a patient with varicose veins.

Figure 20-3. Venogram showing a large left axillary vein aneurysm.

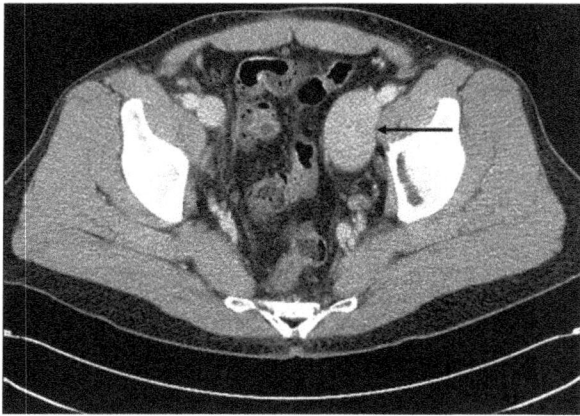

Figure 20-4. Large left external iliac vein aneurysm discovered incidentally in an asymptomatic patient undergoing a CT scan of the pelvis.

The same applies to femoral vein aneurysms. As with popliteal aneurysms, tangential excision with lateral venography or resections with reconstruction are viable options.

CERVICAL AND FACIAL VENOUS ANEURYSMS

Venous dilatations have been described in the facial vein, over the parotid gland and in the jugular system. Jugular aneurysms can be saccular or—more commonly—fusiform. The latter condition is more often seen in children and has been named jugular phlebectasia. Typically, a unilateral soft mass in the neck is discovered. It enlarges on straining, crying, coughing, and Valsalva maneuver. The mass is almost always asymptomatic, although some patients have described the feeling of constriction, sensation of chocking and giddiness, bluish discoloration of the neck, discomfort during physical activity, coughing, swallowing, and cessation of voice during reading or speaking out loud.[12] Phlebectasia occurs more commonly on the right internal jugular vein and bilaterality is uncommon. Duplex US is the diagnostic method of choice.

The management of jugular phlebectasia is controversial, especially in asymptomatic cases. Spontaneous rupture has never been described. The risk of thromboembolic complications appears to be very low. Spontaneous thrombosis has been reported in only six cases, all of them adults with external jugular vein aneurysms.[13–16] No instances of pulmonary embolism associated with jugular phlebectasia have been described. For these reasons, most authors strongly recommend conservative treatment, but others follow a more aggressive approach with liberal surgical repair. If surgical management is entertained, a choice is made between simply ligating the ectatic jugular vein versus the use of reconstructive techniques to maintain patency. Jugular vein ligation can result in head and neck edema.

THORACIC ANEURYSMS

Thoracic aneurysms can arise from the superior vena cava (SVC), the azygos vein system, or the innominate and subclavian veins.

SUPERIOR VENA CAVA ANEURYSMS

Most SVC aneurysms are found incidentally in asymptomatic patients undergoing imaging studies for other reasons or in patients with mild symptoms like cough, dyspnea, and chest discomfort.

Although the collective experience of surgical management of SVC reported in the literature is limited, it appears that surgical repair for fear of hemorrhage is unjustified, since only two cases of aneurysm rupture exist, and in both, the rupture was contained. One was treated surgically and the other one did well with observation alone. No cases of free rupture with hemodynamic collapse have ever been reported. Although thrombus was observed within several aneurysms on imaging studies or in surgical specimens, no cases of documented spontaneous pulmonary embolism and more importantly spontaneous fatal pulmonary embolism have been reported. On the other hand, pulmonary embolism has occurred with catastrophic consequences during venography and during surgery as well. It seems that a prudent approach to SVC aneurysms is justified, with noninvasive imaging follow-up using magnetic resonance venography and dynamic CT scans. In patients with progressive enlargement, severe symptoms, presence of thrombus, or evidence of pulmonary embolism, operative intervention should be considered.

AZYGOS VEIN ANEURYSMS

Azygos and hemiazygos vein aneurysms can be idiopathic but they are also associated with certain anatomic and hemodynamic abnormalities. These abnormalities include cirrhosis and portal hypertension, pulmonary sequestration, inferior vena cava (IVC) obstruction, azygos continuation syndrome (congenital anomaly consistent of failure of the right supracardinal vein to anastomose with the hepatic vein, resulting in drainage of blood from the distal IVC through the azygos vein into the SVC), Ehlers–Danlos syndrome, and lung cancer. Most aneurysms were discovered incidentally in asymptomatic patients or in patients complaining of mild chest discomfort, dyspnea, or cough. Chest radiographs showed mediastinal enlargement and nonspecific findings. Dynamic CT shows slight enhancement in the arterial phase and homogeneous enhancement in the late phase (Fig. 20-5). Respiratory and postural maneuvers induce changes in the size of the contrast enhancing mass. Other radiographic features include homogeneous enhancement of the aneurysm during gadolinium injection, compression of the right main stem bronchus or the SVC, and the presence of an anechoic mass during transesophageal echocardiography.[17] No instances of pulmonary embolism or rupture have been reported.

Given the very low incidence of thrombosis and the fact that no reported cases of pulmonary embolism or rupture exist, a conservative approach with imaging follow-up appears more reasonable for most patients with no symptoms. If obstruction of the right bronchus or SVC exists, if symptoms are present, or if follow-up studies show enlargement or thrombosis, surgical or interventional treatment may be indicated. Podbielski[18] and others[19] suggest that azygos vein aneurysms are ideal for video-assisted thoracoscopic excision. Alternatively, the creation of azygo-systemic shunts as described by D'Souza and colleagues can be considered by experienced endovascular specialists after careful definition of suitable anatomy.

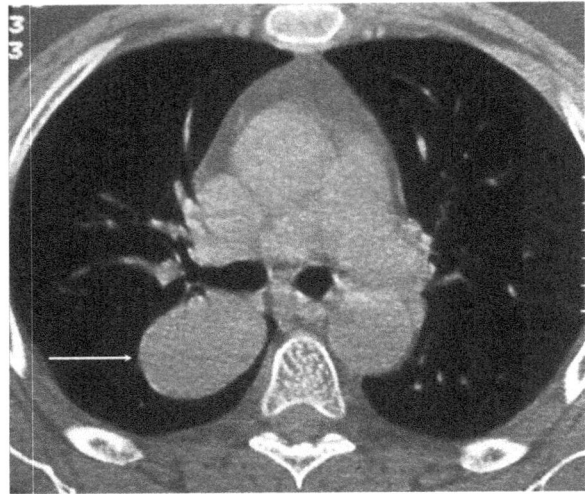

Figure 20-5. Azygous vein aneurysm. (Courtesy of Dr. Francis J. Podbielski.)

ABDOMINAL VENOUS ANEURYSMS

The majority of portal aneurysms are associated with liver cirrhosis and portal hypertension. Pancreatitis has also been linked to the development of splenic and superior mesenteric aneurysms, presumably due to the severe local inflammation.[20] Most aneurysms are found in the extrahepatic segment of the portal vein (Fig. 20-6), but aneurysms have been reported in the intrahepatic portal segment, the superior mesenteric vein, and the splenic vein. Small portal aneurysms are usually asymptomatic. Larger aneurysms can cause abdominal discomfort or compression of adjacent structures provoking jaundice (common bile duct), dyspepsia (duodenum), and even portal hypertension (as in one aneurysm of the superior mesenteric vein causing obstruction of the portal vein with no evidence of liver disease).

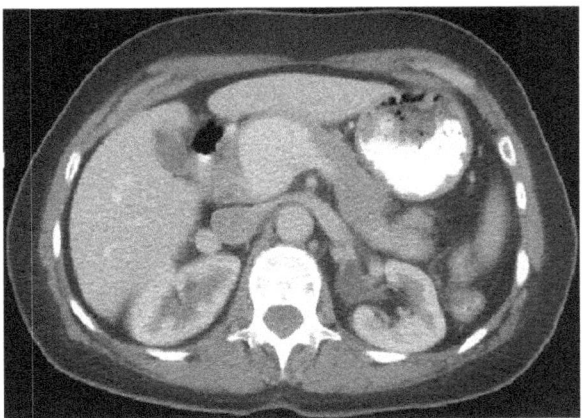

Figure 20-6. Large aneurysm of the portal vein discovered incidentally on an asymptomatic patient.

The natural history of these aneurysms has not been defined. Spontaneous thrombosis has been reported in at least a dozen cases and rupture in at least four.[21,22] The more common occurrence of gastrointestinal bleeding is almost always caused by portal hypertension and it is not a consequence of the aneurysm itself. It appears prudent to perform repeat imaging studies on asymptomatic patients with portal aneurysms. If gastrointestinal bleeding occurs, portosystemic shunts to alleviate portal hypertension should be considered. Patients presenting with thrombosis or symptoms related to compression of adjacent structures should be considered for aneurysm repair and those caused by portal hypertension for portal decompression. Surgical intervention can be selectively applied to average and low-risk patients and that observation can be used in elderly, high-risk subjects.

INFERIOR VENA CAVA ANEURYSMS

In most cases, IVC aneurysms are asymptomatic and discovered incidentally. Nevertheless, thrombosis, rupture, and pulmonary embolism have been reported. In cases of thrombosed IVC aneurysms, diagnosis may be difficult and the aneurysm can be confused with retroperitoneal tumors, renal carcinoma, lymphadenopathy, and IVC tumors.[23] In one report, an IVC aneurysm coexisted with a retroperitoneal ganglioneuroma. As with other venous aneurysms, the limited number of cases makes their natural history unclear and, thus, management recommendations are difficult to make. Since thrombosis, rupture, and embolism have been described, low-risk patients should be considered for operative repair. Simple resection, resection with primary repair, patch-angioplasty repair, and caval replacement have been described. Patients who cannot undergo surgical treatment can be considered for filter placement in the suprarenal segment of the IVC for the prevention of pulmonary embolism.

CONCLUSIONS

Venous aneurysms are uncommon. The presentation and management of these abnormalities depend on their location. Aneurysms of the deep veins in the lower extremities carry a significant risk of thrombosis and embolism and repair should be carried out once the diagnosis is made. Aneurysms of the lower extremity superficial system and those in the upper extremities—whether superficial or deep—are rarely associated with thromboembolism and repair is only indicated for cosmetic reasons or if thrombosis occurs. Aneurysms of the neck and face often present as visible, soft masses that change in size with respiration and straining. In children, jugular phlebectasia should be included in the differential diagnosis of neck masses that enlarge during the Valsalva maneuver. The management of this condition remains controversial.

Thoracic aneurysms are rarely associated with thromboembolism or hemorrhage and can be managed conservatively. When enlargement or complications occur, traditional surgical repair, thoracoscopic excision, and endovascular techniques are viable alternatives. Venous aneurysms in the abdomen are most frequently discovered incidentally during imaging exams. Management should be individualized with surgical treatment for low-risk patients and expectant management for asymptomatic patients who are poor candidates for surgery.

REFERENCES

1. Pearce WH, Winchester DJ, Yao JST. Venous aneurysms. In: Yao JST, Pearce WH, editors. *Aneurysms: New Findings and Treatment*. Norwalk, CT: Appleton and Lange, 1994:379–388.
2. Hurwitz RL, Gelabert H. Thrombosed iliac venous aneurysm: a rare cause of lower extremity venous obstruction. *J Vasc Surg*. 1989;9:822–824.
3. Rodriguez HE, Pearce WH. The management of venous aneurysms. In: Gloviczki P, editor. *Handbook of Venous Disorders. Guidelines of the American Venous Forum*. 3rd ed. London: Arnold Hodder; 2009. pp. 604–616.
4. Bergqvist D, Bjorck M, Ljungman C. Popliteal venous aneurysm—a systematic review. *World J Surg*. 2006;30(3):273–279.
5. Greenwood LH, Yrizarry JM, Hallett JW. Peripheral venous aneurysm with recurrent pulmonary embolism: report of a case and review of the literature. *Cardiovasc Intervent Radiol*. 1982;5:43–45.
6. Donald IP, Edwards RC. Fatal outcome from popliteal venous aneurysm associated with pulmonary embolism. *Br J Radiol*. 1982;55:930–931.
7. Sessa C, Nicolini P, Perrin M, et al. Management of symptomatic and asymptomatic popliteal venous aneurysms: a retrospective analysis of 25 patients and review of the literature. *J Vasc Surg*. 2000;32(5):902–912.
8. Winchester D, Pearce WH, McCarthy WJ, et al. Popliteal venous aneurysms. *Surgery*. 1993;114(3):600–607.
9. Ranero-Juarez GA, Sanchez-Gomez RH, Loza-Jalil SE, Cano-Valdez AM. Venous aneurysms of the extremities—report of 4 cases and review of literature. *Angiology*. 2005;56(4):475–481.
10. Gillespie DL, Villavicencio JL, Gallagher C, et al. Presentation and management of venous aneurysms. *J Vasc Surg*. 1997;26(5):845–852.
11. Banno H, Yamanouchi D, Fujita H, et al. External iliac venous aneurysm in a pregnant woman: a case report. *J Vasc Surg*. 2004;40(1):174–178.
12. Calligaro KD, Ahmed S, Dandora R, et al. Congenital aneurysm of the internal jugular vein in a pregnant woman. *Cardiovasc Surg*. 1995;3(1):63–64.
13. Porcellini M, Selvetella L, Bernardo B, et al. Aneurysms of the external jugular vein. *G Chir*. 1996;17(5):238–241.
14. Beale TJ, Smedley FH, Knee G. Thrombosis within an external jugular venous aneurysm. *J R Coll Surg Edinb*. 1996;41(3):181–182.
15. Andreev A, Petkov D, Kavrakov T, Penkov P. Jugular venous aneurysms: when and how to operate. *Int Angiol*. 1998;17(4):272–275.
16. Uematsu M, Okada M. Primary venous aneurysms—case reports. *Angiology*. 1999;50(3):239–244.
17. Léna H, Desrues B, Heresbach D, et al. Azygos vein aneurysm: contribution of transesophageal echography. *Ann Thorac Surg*. 1996;61:1253–1255.
18. Podbielski FJ, Sam AD, II., Halldorsson AO, et al. Giant azygos vein varix. *Ann Thorac Surg*. 1997;63:1167–1169.
19. Watanabe A, Kusajima K, Aisaka N, et al. Idiopathic saccular azygos vein aneurysm. *Ann Thorac Surg*. 1998;65:1459–1461.
20. Lopez-Rasines GJ, Alonso JR, Longo JM, Pagola MA. Aneurysmal dilatation of the superior mesenteric vein: CT findings. *J Comput Assist Tomogr*. 1985;9(4):830–832.
21. Ohnami Y, Ishida H, Konno K, et al. Portal vein aneurysm: report of six cases and review of the literature. *Abdom Imaging*. 1997;22:281–286.
22. Okur N, Inal M, Akgul E. Demircan O. Spontaneous rupture and thrombosis of an intrahepatic portal vein aneurysm. *Abdom Imaging*. 2003;28(5):675–677.
23. DeBree E, Klaase JM, Schultze Kool LJ, van Coevorden F. Case report. Aneurysm of the inferior vena cava complicated by thrombosis mimicking a retroperitoneal neoplasm. *Eur J Vasc Endovasc Surg*. 2000;20:305–307.

Lower Extremity Arterial Disease

21

Impact of Failed Superficial Femoral Artery Intervention for Advanced Infrainguinal Occlusive Disease

Omar Al-Nouri, DO, MS and Ross Milner, MD

INTRODUCTION

Peripheral arterial disease (PAD) is highly prevalent in the western world affecting nearly 10 million Americans. In its most advanced form, PAD from infrainguinal occlusive disease results in critical limb ischemia (CLI), which carries significant morbidity and mortality for many aging Americans. CLI, defined as chronic ischemic rest pain, ulcers, or gangrene, has challenged vascular specialists for decades.[1]

CLI represents the most advanced form of PAD; however, many more people are affected by lesser degrees of infrainguinal occlusive disease, namely, claudication. Evaluation of leg pain serves as one of the most common reasons referrals are made to vascular specialists. PAD is also a marker for systemic atherosclerotic disease and the vascular specialist needs to be well versed in all aspects of diagnosis to prevent morbidity and mortality in vascular patients not only from CLI but also from ischemic stroke and myocardial infarction (MI).

INFRAINGUINAL OCCLUSIVE DISEASE: GENERAL CONSIDERATIONS

Claudication and CLI represent the two major forms of symptomatic PAD. Patients who are significantly disabled by claudication, such as those unable to work or cannot comfortably carry out the activities of daily living, are candidates for intervention with either open or endovascular techniques. Medical therapy is recommended for those patients with stable claudication that consists of a trial of smoking cessation, exercise, risk factor modification, and medical treatment with pletal or similar agent.

Most patients with CLI will require some form of intervention. Most of these patients are classified into Rutherford 4–6 categories (Table 21-1). Traditionally, the mainstay treatment strategy for limb revascularization in this patient population has been open surgical bypass. However, since the advent of balloon angioplasty 30 years ago,[2] there has been a large increase in endovascular treatment of lower extremity atherosclerotic disease. In the past decade, there has been a threefold increase in endovascular treatment of lower extremity atherosclerotic disease with a simultaneous 42% decrease in open surgical bypass.[3]

The Transatlantic Intersocietal Consensus (TASC) reported recommendations both in 2000 and in 2007 (Fig. 21-1). Lesions defined as TASC A should undergo

TABLE 21-1. RUTHERFORD CLASSIFICATION FOR ACUTE LIMB ISCHEMIA

Category	Patient Presentation
0	Asymptomatic
1	Mild claudication
2	Moderate claudication
3	Severe claudication
4	Ischemic rest pain
5	Minor tissue loss
6	Major tissue loss

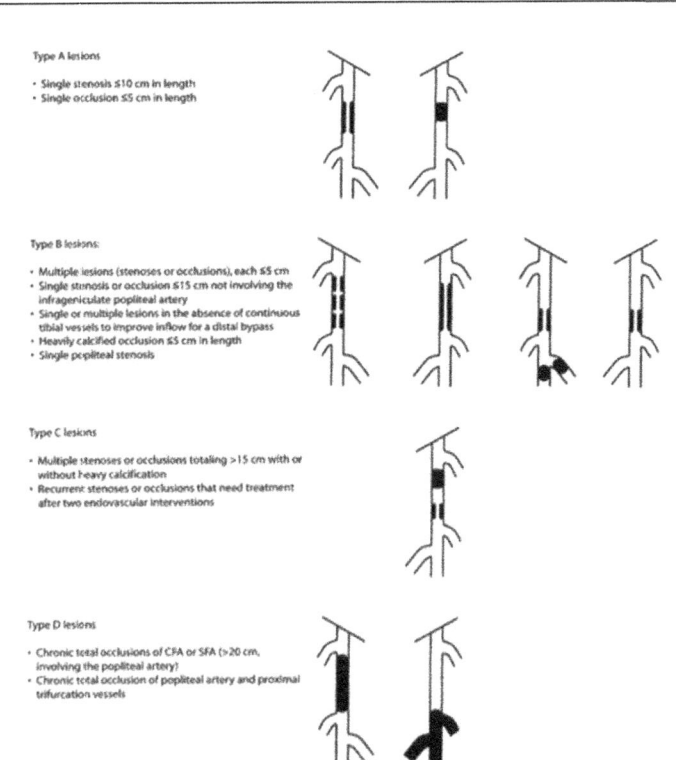

Type A lesions

· Single stenosis ≤10 cm in length
· Single occlusion ≤5 cm in length

Type B lesions:

· Multiple lesions (stenoses or occlusions), each ≤5 cm
· Single stenosis or occlusion ≤15 cm not involving the infrageniculate popliteal artery
· Single or multiple lesions in the absence of continuous tibial vessels to improve inflow for a distal bypass
· Heavily calcified occlusion ≤5 cm in length
· Single popliteal stenosis

Type C lesions

· Multiple stenoses or occlusions totaling >15 cm with or without heavy calcification
· Recurrent stenoses or occlusions that need treatment after two endovascular interventions

Type D lesions

· Chronic total occlusions of CFA or SFA (>20 cm, involving the popliteal artery)
· Chronic total occlusion of popliteal artery and proximal trifurcation vessels

Figure 21-1. TransAtlantic Inter-Society Consensus II classification.

endovascular treatment as the first-line therapy, whereas lesions defined as TASC D should undergo traditional open surgical bypass. It was unclear about the ideal treatment strategy for TASC B and C lesions, but the consensus was that most TASC B lesions underwent endovascular treatment and most TASC C lesions underwent open surgical bypass.[4]

OPEN VERSUS ENDOVASCULAR TREATMENT OF SFA OCCLUSIVE DISEASE

Endovascular treatment of superficial femoral artery (SFA) occlusive disease includes use of balloon angioplasty, stenting, and atherectomy. Advancement in endovascular technology and skill, namely, use of subintimal angioplasty, has sparked tremendous interest in endovascular treatment of advanced infrainguinal occlusive disease. These minimally invasive techniques have dramatically reduced morbidity and mortality in a high-risk group of patients. At the same time, multiple studies have demonstrated similar short and mid-term results with open surgical bypass. These reports on the successful treatment of advanced infrainguinal disease with endovascular means are described in various terms of the clinical response seen, technical success, hemodynamic success, and patency rates. Clinical response is defined as resolution of claudication or rest pain symptoms, wound healing, freedom from gangrene, and limb salvage. Objective means to measure clinical response included improvement in ankle brachial index (ABI) of 0.15 or greater and increase of at least 1 point on the Rutherford scale.[4] Technical success following an endovascular intervention is defined as the presence of antegrade flow through the treated lesion. It is our general practice to define a successful endovascular intervention when <30% residual stenosis is present on completion angiography. Some centers use duplex ultrasound at completion of intervention to define technical success, with a successful intervention defined as a peak systolic velocity (PSV) <180 or PSV ratio of 2 or less.[5]

Endovascular treatment of advanced femoropopliteal disease (e.g., TASC D) in some studies has been shown to be as effective as open surgical bypass. Baril et al.[6] reviewed their institutional experience in treatment of femoropopliteal occlusive disease with endovascular means over a five-year span. 79 TASC D limbs in 74 patients were identified that were treated from 2004 to 2009. Seventy one percent of patients had CLI and 53% patients had tissue loss. Endovascular treatment consisted of recanalization of the SFA and balloon angioplasty with noncompliant balloon. Stents were implanted following balloon angioplasty for the treatment of flow-limiting dissections or residual stenosis of >30% after angioplasty or at the discretion of the operating surgeon. All stents utilized were nitinol self-expanding stents. Follow-up was available for 74 limbs at a mean of only 10.7 months. Technical success rate for endovascular procedures was 89%. Primary, assisted-primary, and secondary patency rates at 12 and 24 months were 52.2%, 88.4%, 92.6% and 27.5%, 74.2%, and 88.9%, respectively. No patient required a major amputation during follow-up. Twenty-one limbs (26.6%) experienced restenosis and nine limbs (11.4%) experienced occlusion. Twenty-nine limbs underwent reintervention during the follow-up time, including nine that underwent multiple reinterventions. Excellent hemodynamic improvement and limb salvage rates were accomplished by endovascular treatment of TASC II D lesions. However, there was a high failure and reintervention rate and with the short follow-up, thus not much is known of the negative impact these failed interventions may have.

McQuade et al.[7] performed a prospective randomized trial comparing 50 above-knee prosthetic femoral popliteal bypass extremities, in which saphenous vein was either absent or unsuitable with 50 limbs treated with percutaneous SFA stenting with Viabahn stent grafts (Gore, Flagstaff, AZ) for treatment of SFA occlusive disease. The two groups were similar in terms of level of CLI according to Rutherford classification and TASC II lesions. Technical success rate was 100%. Primary patency rate for the stent graft group at 12, 24, 36, and 48 months was 72%, 63%, 63%, and 59%, respectively, while the primary patency for the surgical bypass group was 76%, 63%, 63%, and 58%, respectively. During the follow-up period, a total of 18, the stent grafts failed (36%). Eleven out of the 18 thrombosed grafts were unable to be recanalized requiring open surgical bypass. Seven out of the 11 were able to have above-knee popliteal bypass; in four limbs, infrageniculate bypasses were needed. Despite similar patency rates between endovascular treatment and open surgical treatment, these above studies fail to look at the impact of a failed SFA intervention on limb salvage and subsequent patency of an open surgical intervention.

IMPACT OF FAILED SFA INTERVENTION

A paucity of literature exists regarding the impact that failed SFA interventions have on subsequent infrainguinal revascularization and limb salvage. A recent retrospective review by Gur et al.[8] examined their five-year experience with endovascular treatment of SFA lesions. In their report, they found that lesions classified as TASC C or D were more likely to fail with occlusion, lose runoff vessels, and alter the site of subsequent open operation than their TASC A or B counterparts. The authors concluded that a failed SFA intervention in advanced infrainguinal occlusive disease might negatively impact later attempts at revascularization.

We performed a retrospective study of our institution's experience with endovascular stenting of SFA lesions to identify those patients at risk for SFA stent failure and the negative impact, if any, that occurs with SFA stent failure. From 2007 to 2010, we performed 42 endovascular stenting procedures on 39 limbs. Mean patient age was 68 years (range 43–88). Patient's comorbidities are listed in Table 21-2. Of the 42 stents placed, 19 (45%) were placed for tissue loss, 15 (36%) for claudication, and seven (17%) for rest pain. Technical success rate was 100%. At one year, follow-up was available for 34 limbs with a mean of 14.9 months (range 1–42). Fifteen lesions were classified as TASC A (36%), nine were TASC B (21%), five were TASC C (12%), and 13 were TASC D (31%).

TABLE 21-2. PATIENT CO-MORBIDITIES AND RISK FACTORS

Risk Factors	Number of Patients (n = 39)	Percentage
Coronary artery disease	19	49
Myocardial infarction	9	23
Hypertension	36	92
Diabetes	19	49
Hypercholesterolemia	29	74
End-stage renal disease	6	15
Warfarin anticoagulation	5	11
Smoking history	30	77

Overall, primary patency, primary-assisted, and secondary patency rates at one year were 24%, 44%, and 51%, respectively (Fig. 21-2). Primary, primary-assisted, and secondary patency rates at one year for TASC A lesions were 47%, 66%, and 72%, respectively; for TASC B, 13%, 33%, and 33% respectively; for TASC C, 40%, 40%, and 40% respectively; for TASC D, 0%, 32%, and 46%, respectively (Fig. 21-3). In univariate analysis, history of hypercholesterolemia and smoking had a negative impact on primary patency. Seventeen interventions failed (40%) at one year. SFA failure was evenly distributed among TASC classifications, with five classified as TASC A, four as TASC B, three as TASC C, and five as TASC D. During follow-up, of the 17 failed SFA interventions, three went on to open bypass for limb salvage and three went on to major amputation (one following a failed bypass). The six limbs requiring either bypass or major amputation were TASC C or D lesions (Table 21-3).

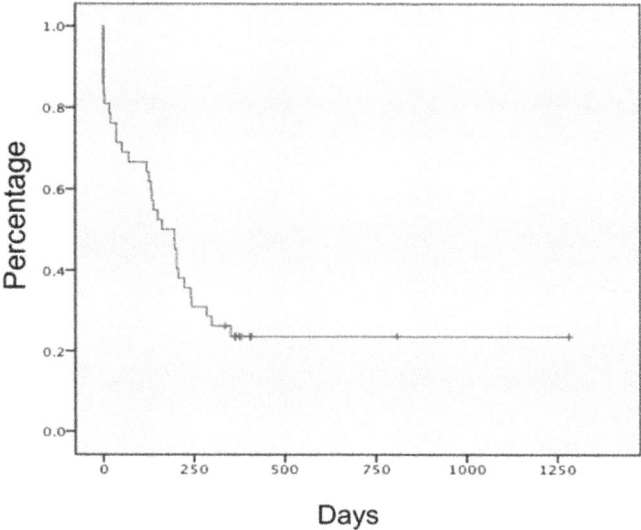

Figure 21-2. Overall primary patency rates at one year.

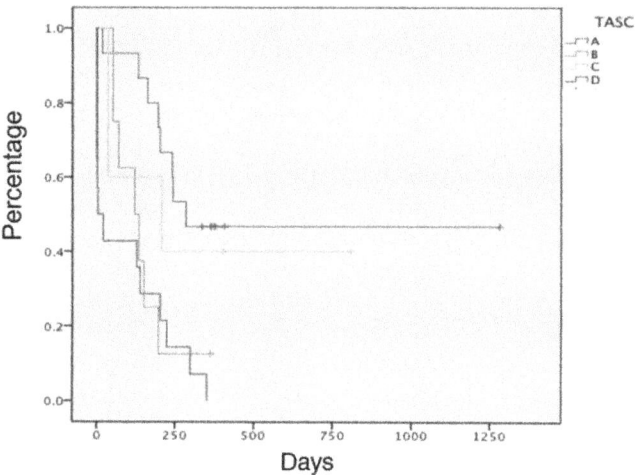

Figure 21-3. One-year primary patency by TransAtlantic Inter-Society Consensus (TASC) classification.

TABLE 21-3. OUTCOMES OF FAILED SFA INTERVENTION BY TASC CLASSIFICATION

Event	TASC A (N = 15)	TASC B (N = 9)	TASC C (N = 5)	TASC D (N = 13)
Stent failure	5	4	3	5
Loss of runoff vessels	0	0	0	2
Open revascularization	0	0	1	2
Major amputation	0	0	2	1

SFA stenting performed for TASC C or D lesions was more likely to fail and more likely to lead to bypass or amputation when compared to TASC A or B lesions. When an SFA intervention failed with stent occlusion in TASC C or D lesions, they were more likely to undergo major amputation. None of the patients in our study with TASC A or B lesions and with loss of patency required any further intervention. Patients that were intervened for claudication, despite having a hemodynamically significant stenosis or occlusion, were more likely to be either asymptomatic or have tolerable claudication and not require a bypass or amputation. Whereas patients intervened for CLI that had a failed SFA intervention were more likely to lead to multiple attempts at open revascularization and major amputation. The higher amputation rate seen in our study in more advanced TASC C/D lesions compared to TASC A/B lesions may just represent the extent of disease. Several authors[8,9] have found that failed SFA interventions in advanced TASC C/D lesions affect subsequent distal bypass procedures. When performing endovascular stenting of advanced TASC C/D lesions with use of angioplasty in the subintimal plane, loss of collateral circulation can occur. Without this circulation in place, if stent failure occurs, patients may progress to more advanced clinical disease. Furthermore, with the lack of collateral circulation in place, there is a theoretic risk of stent thrombosis propagating to runoff vessels and affecting limb salvage.

In our series, six patients with failed SFA interventions went on to undergo major amputation or bypass. Four patients required open surgical bypass, one of them failed and required a below the knee ampuation (BKA). Of the three remaining bypasses, two of them required further secondary balloon angioplasty for anastomotic stenosis and one of them required an open surgical revision. None of the amputations occurred in the face of patent stents. Similar to findings in the Bypass versus Angioplasty in Severe Ischaemia of the Leg (BASIL) trial,[9] four of the six failed SFA interventions had significant negative impact on patency of bypass grafts and limb salvage. It appears that the stenting first with no consequence adage can be detrimental to both limb salvage and further attempts at revascularization.

Patients with advanced infrainguinal occlusive disease with CLI (TASC C/D lesions) would likely benefit from open surgical bypass over endovascular stenting. However, many of these patients are not appropriate surgical candidates and endovascular therapy is the only option. These patients present a difficult treatment dilemma for vascular surgeons. Based on our study, patients with CLI that undergo a failed percutaneous SFA intervention have a higher likelihood of amputation. Furthermore, stent thrombosis may have a negative impact on bypass patency. The higher amputation rates seen in patients with TASC C or D lesions compared to TASC A or B lesions again may just represent extension of disease. Randomized control trials comparing stenting versus open bypass in advanced TASC C and D lesions with limb salvage as the primary outcome would shed some light on the subject. Patients with advanced TASC C or D lesions that undergo stenting for claudication are more likely to fail than their TASC A or B counterparts, but a failed SFA intervention in these patients does not necessarily lead to amputation or bypass. Based on this experience, patients with lifestyle-limiting claudication with TASC C and D lesions that are appropriate surgical candidates and have adequate autogenous vein available should undergo open surgical bypass as opposed to endovascular therapy.[10]

REFERENCES

1. Mills JL. Infrainguinal disease: surgical treatment. In Cronenwett JL, Johnston KW, editors. *Rutherford Vascular Surgery*. 7th ed. Philadelphia, PA: Elsevier, 2010.
2. Gruntzig A, Hopff H. Percutaneous recanalization after chronic arterial occlusion with a new dilator-catheter (modification of the Dotter technique). *Dtsch Med Wochenschr.* 1974;99:2502–2511.
3. Goodney PP, Beck AW, Nagle J, et al. National trends in lower extremity bypass surgery, endovascular interventions, and major amputations. *J Vasc Surg.* 2009;50(1):54–60.
4. Rutherford RB, Baker JD, Ernst C, et al. Recommended standards for reports dealing with lower extremity ischemia: revised version. *J Vasc Surg.* 1997;26:517–538.
5. Myers KA. Reporting standards and statistics for evaluating intervention. *Cardiovasc Surg.* 1995;3:455–461.
6. Baril DT, Chaer RA, Rhee RY, et al. Endovascular intervention for TASC II D femoropopliteal lesions. *J Vasc Surg.* June, 2010;51(6):1406–1412.
7. McQuade K, Gable D, Pearl G, et al. Four-year randomized prospective comparison of percutaneous ePTFE/nitinol self-expanding stent graft versus prosthetic femoral-popliteal bypass in the treatment of superficial femoral artery occlusive disease. *J Vasc Surg.* Sep, 2010;52(3):584–591.
8. Gur I, Lee W, Akopian G, et al. Clinical outcomes and implications of failed infrainguinal endovascular stents. *J Vasc Surg.* Mar, 2011;53(3):658–666.
9. Bradbury AW, Adam DJ, Bell J, et al. Bypass versus Angioplasty in Severe Ischaemia of the Leg (BASIL) trial: An intention-to-treat analysis of amputation-free and overall survival in patients randomized to a bypass surgery-first or a balloon angioplasty-first revascularization strategy. *J Vasc Surg.* May, 2010;51(suppl 5):5S–17S.
10. Al-Nouri O, Krezalek M, Hershberger R, et al. Failed superficial femoral artery intervention for advanced infrainguinal occlusive disease has a significant negative impact on limb salvage. *J Vasc Surg.* Jul, 2012;56(1):106–110.

22

Tibial Artery Bypass: Heparin-Bonded Expanded Polytetrafluoroethylene versus Saphenous Vein Graft

Richard F. Neville, MD

INTRODUCTION

There remains a continued role for surgical bypass in patients suffering from critical limb ischemia. This may be especially true for those patients with significant tissue loss in need of pulsatile flow directly to a specific angiosome to heal significant tissue loss in the lower extremity.[1] Although most vascular surgeons continue to favor autogenous vein as the favored conduit for below-knee bypass, results with grafts constructed using heparin-bonded expanded polytetrafluoroethylene (HePTFE) (GORE® PROPATEN® Vascular Graft, WL Gore & Associates, Flagstaff, AZ), have challenged this concept. Heparin bonding to medical devices has been used in other applications. The HePTFE graft takes advantage of a covalent bonding of heparin to the inner surface of an expanded polytetrafluoroethylene (ePTFE) graft thereby maintaining heparin activity.[2] The heparin bonding has been demonstrated to improve graft performance in animal models and human experience by decreasing acute and chronic graft failure through a reduction in platelet adhesion,[3] graft thrombogenicity,[4] and the formation of myointimal hyperplasia.[5] Clinical results have reflected these improvements, although most trials are nonrandomized and retrospective. However, the trials have shown encouraging results for below-knee bypass that may challenge routine use of autogenous vein as the primary conduit. We examined our own outcomes comparing HePTFE to saphenous vein for tibial bypass over a contemporaneous time period as well as the available literature.

VEIN BYPASS

Autogenous vein remains the ideal conduit for lower extremity bypass. The greater saphenous vein results in a durable reconstruction no matter which configuration is favored by the surgeon: in situ, reversed, or translocated. However, the lack of saphenous vein is becoming a common clinical scenario due to previous bypass, coronary surgery, thrombophlebitis, or poor quality vein, with as many as 30% of patients in need of bypass lacking suitable saphenous vein. This number increases to 50% in those patients requiring a second bypass procedure. This has led to innovative approaches to alternative autogenous and prosthetic conduits.

Alternative autogenous conduits include lesser saphenous vein, arm vein, composite veins, umbilical vein, and cryopreserved vein. Because arm and lesser saphenous segments may not be long enough to reach a distal tibial artery, composite vein configurations are often required.[6] Cryopreserved vein and human umbilical vein are other alternative conduits that are biologic in their properties and therefore have an intrinsic appeal for distal reconstruction. These conduits have met with limited success when used for tibial bypass.[7,8] The use of cryopreserved vein may be best limited to bypasses that must traverse infected fields in the absence of other autogenous conduit.[9] McPhee and colleagues have reported similar patency rate for current prosthetic conduits compared to alternative venous grafts to the below-knee popliteal artery.[10]

However, consideration would be given to these alternate autogenous conduits in a relatively younger patient with a longer anticipated life span or the patient with any documented hypercoagulability.

INNOVATIONS IN PROSTHETIC BYPASS

Historically, prosthetic grafts have not performed well for distal revascularization.[11] Past results were discouraging enough to consider primary amputation in certain patient subgroups.[12] Innovative techniques were required to improve the performance of prosthetic graft for bypass. These innovations include improvements in graft biology such as the interposition of venous tissue at the distal anastomosis and heparin bonding the inner surface of the graft. The interposition of venous tissue between a prosthetic graft and the recipient artery attempts to improve graft performance in several ways. The venous tissue may reduce the hyperplastic response and improve graft patency by creation of a biologic "buffer zone" by the endothelium of the venous segment. The interposed venous tissue makes the bypass less technically demanding by suturing vein to the diseased tibial artery, and there may be an effect on thrombogenicity at the interface between the high resistance outflow artery and prosthetic material. In 1984, Miller described a vein cuff to improve prosthetic graft patency.[13] The Miller technique involved the construction of an oval venous cuff sutured to the recipient artery. The prosthetic graft was then sutured directly to the vein cuff. Miller reported on 114 bypasses with 72% patency rate at 18 months but had only 21 distal bypasses in the series. Taylor described a vein interposition technique in an effort to address these concerns.[14] Taylor's technique required a vein patch four to five times the diameter of the prosthetic conduit. A U-shaped slit was made on the underside of the graft with minimal angulation to ensure that the graft lay parallel to the artery. The heel of the graft was then sutured directly to the artery with vein used to close the anterior elliptical defect. Taylor reported on 256 grafts with one-, three-, and five-year patency rates of 74%, 58%, and 54%, respectively.

Our distal vein patch (DVP) technique utilizes a technique familiar to vascular surgeons and requires a shorter arteriotomy, thereby decreasing the amount of venous tissue required for the procedure[15] (Fig. 22-1). A two- to three-centimeter segment of tissue is suitable and can include saphenous vein remnants, arm vein harvested under local anesthesia, or superficial femoral vein. After the patch is sewn in place, a longitudinal cut is made in the proximal two-thirds of the patch and the graft is sutured to the patch. The anastomosis is constructed to maintain a rim of venous tissue interposed between the graft and the entire circumference of the arterial wall. Because the venotomy is made in the proximal two-thirds of the patch, more venous tissue is left interposed at the toe of the anastomosis that is often a problem area for future hyperplasia. Experience with this technique was reported in 270 bypasses with primary graft patency at one and four years of 79.8% and 51.2%, respectively. Corresponding limb salvage rates were 80.6% and 67.5%.[16]

HEPARIN BONDED ePTFE

The reasons for poor prosthetic graft performance in the past have been technical, biologic, and hemodynamic. These factors are especially important for bypass to the small tibial arteries below the knee. Technically, the anastomosis may be difficult with a prosthetic graft being sutured to small, calcified arteries, and in this regard a venous adjunct such as a

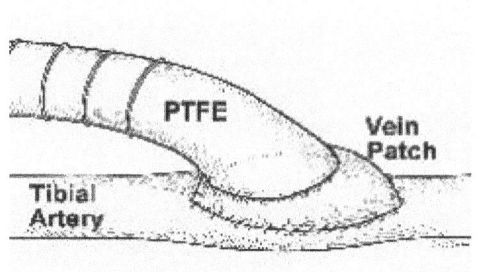

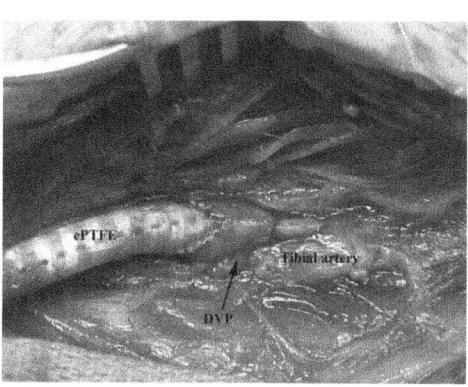

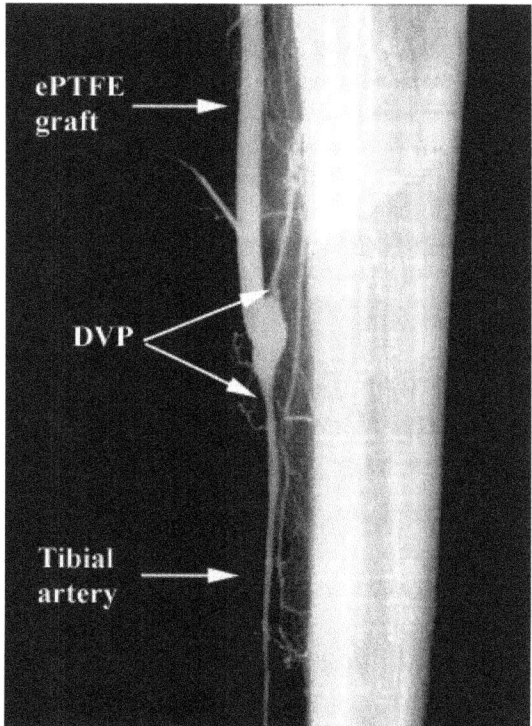

Figure 22-1. Distal vein patch anastomotic configuration to improve the performance of tibial bypass with ePTFE.

DVP may be of some benefit. In a biological sense, prosthetic grafts are more thrombogenic with increased platelet adhesion and activation of the coagulation cascade. This increased thrombogenicity may be especially important when blood flow rates drop below the critical thrombotic threshold as may occur in tibial bypass with high resistance. Myointimal hyperplasia also can occur especially at the distal anastomosis in these prosthetic grafts. Heparin bonding using the Carmeda bioactive surface technology (CBAS, Carmeda, Upplands Vasby, Sweden) allows binding of the heparin molecule to the luminal surface of ePTFE grafts while maintaining the morphology of the heparin molecule and hence its bioactivity for at least 16 weeks.[2] The generation of heparin antibodies leading to heparin-induced thrombocytopenia does not seem to be an important clinical concern,[17] although the question has been raised.[18] The heparin bonding process does lead to a reduction in platelet deposition on the graft surface in animal and human models. Heparin bonding also has reduced thrombus formation on the surface of the graft with a subsequent decrease in graft thrombogenicity in acute and chronic models.[5] A reduction in myointimal hyperplasia at the anastomotic site has also been demonstrated with heparin-bonded biomaterial surfaces. Decreased platelet adherence, thrombus formation, and inhibition of myointimal hyperplasia could be hypothesized to decrease both early and late graft failures.

HEPARIN-BONDED VS. VEIN GRAFTS

To examine the effect of heparin-bonded ePTFE, a retrospective analysis of prospectively collected data was performed to include all patients having a tibial artery bypass using large saphenous vein or heparin-bonded PTFE over a contemporaneous time period. The analysis was performed with investigational review board protocol approval for medical record review. The series included all patients during the study period having a tibial bypass using single segment large saphenous vein from the ipsilateral or contralateral extremity of a Propaten graft as the conduit. Bypasses performed with arm vein, short saphenous vein, or composite grafts were excluded from the analysis.[19]

All patients were evaluated for available ipsilateral or contralateral great saphenous vein by physical exam, duplex ultrasound imaging in an accredited vascular lab, and intraoperative evaluation with gentle hydrostatic dilation if there was any question as to vein utility. The vein was used for bypass if the diameter was greater than 2 mm. Vein bypasses were performed with 45 ipsilateral and five contralateral large saphenous veins. All vein conduits were single segments with no composite grafts included in the analysis. The vein graft configuration was translocated in 80% with 20% reversed vein conduits. All saphenous vein grafts were taking aspirin preoperatively, and this was continued postoperatively with no postoperative heparinization used. The HePTFE grafts (Propaten) were 6 mm and externally reinforced. All Propaten patients received intravenous heparin postoperatively with conversion to warfarin if there was no contraindication to long-term anticoagulation. If the patient did have a bleeding history or some other factor preventing him from chronic warfarin, then Clopidogrel (Plavix) was administered. This occurred in 16% of the HePTFE grafts.

All patients were followed with a routine graft surveillance program involving pulse examination, ankle brachial index measurement, and duplex ultrasound scans at one month, three months, six months, and 12 months. If the pulse exam changed, the ankle brachial index dropped (>0.15), or the duplex ultrasound indicated possible graft stenosis based on velocities or B mode images, an arteriogram was performed with appropriate intervention for any hemodynamic lesions that were discovered. Secondary intervention was considered a failure of primary patency. All bypass in this analysis had follow-up data to at least a 12-month interval and/or documentation of any etiology of exclusion from the analysis by graft thrombosis or death.

The series cohort included 112 bypasses, 62 HePTFE (with a DVP), and 50 saphenous vein (Table 22-1). Mean follow-up was 417 days (range 369–963). Indication for revascularization was similar between the two groups with claudication being the indication in 10% and the remaining 90% being rest pain or tissue loss. There was a statistically significant difference in a history of prior attempts at bypass with 43% of the HePTFE patients having had a prior attempt at revascularization while only 18% of the vein conduit patients had a prior attempt at revascularization (Table 22-2). The mean preoperative Ankle Brachial Index in the vein bypass group was 0.43, rising to 0.94 postoperatively. The HePTFE group started with a mean ABI of 0.39 increasing to 0.83 postoperatively.

All bypasses in both groups were to tibial arteries with no femoral below-knee popliteal bypasses included in the analysis. The HePTFE group had a higher number of proximal anastomoses originating from the external iliac artery given the fact that length was not a factor in choice of inflow site; 21% with 4% in the vein group. This allowed HePTFE bypasses to avoid hostile, scarred, reoperative groin dissections by moving up onto external iliac artery through a small retroperitoneal incision. Conversely, 15% of the vein bypasses used the popliteal artery (10%) or the profunda femoris artery (5%) to conserve conduit length. The tibial outflow bypass anatomy was similar in both groups with grafts divided between the anterior tibial, posterior tibial, and peroneal artery. There were slightly more anterior bypasses than peroneal bypasses in the vein group, possibly reflecting the higher incidence of prior revascularizations in the HePTFE group leaving the peroneal artery as the only outflow

TABLE 22-1. CHARACTERISTICS OF COMPARATIVE STUDY COHORT; HePTFE VERSUS VEIN GRAFTS; DEMOGRAPHICS

Characteristics	HePTFE (*N* = 62)	Vein (*N* = 50)	*P*
Age			.428[a]
Mean	70.7	63	
Standard dev	13.7	11.0	
Sex			.647[b]
Male	64.5% (*n* = 40)	62.0% (*n* = 31)	
Female	35.5% (*n* = 22)	38.0% (*n* = 19)	
Race			.425[c]
Caucasian	46.8% (*n* = 29)	44.0% (*n* = 22)	
African American	51.6% (*n* = 32)	52.0% (*n* = 26)	
Other	1.6% (*n* = 1)	4.0% (*n* = 2)	

[a]*P* from two-tailed *t*-test.
[b]*P* from Fisher's exact test two-tailed.
[c]*P* from Fisher's generalized exact test.

TABLE 22-2. CHARACTERISTICS OF COMPARATIVE STUDY COHORT; HePTFE VERSUS VEIN
GRAFTS; COMORBIDITIES AND INDICATIONS FOR REVASCULARIZATION

	HePTFE (N = 62)	Vein (N = 50)	P
Hypertension	72.6% (n = 45)	62.0% (n = 31)	.177
Diabetes mellitus	46.8% (n = 29)	60.0% (n = 30)	.150
End Stage Renal Disease	12.9% (n = 8)	18.0% (n = 9)	.454
Claudication	8.1% (n = 5)	10.0% (n = 5)	.133
Rest pain	27.4% (n = 17)	20.0% (n = 10)	.283
Nonhealing ulcer	48.4% (n = 30)	44.0% (n = 22)	.075
Gangrene	16.1% (n = 10)	26.0% (n = 13)	.029
Tissue loss	64.5%	70.0%	
Prior bypass	43.5% (n = 27)	18.0% (n = 9)	.016

Note: P from Fisher's two-sided exact test.

option. A pedal bypass (dorsalis pedis or plantaris pedis) was performed in 6% of the
HePTFE group and 10% of the vein conduit group.

Perioperative complications included one groin hematoma requiring drainage in
the HePTFE group due to the postoperative heparinization and two vein graft patients
requiring operative debridement of the vein harvest incision. During the follow-up
interval, two vein grafts and six Propaten grafts underwent arteriography for hemodynamically significant lesions based on routine graft surveillance. All of these grafts had
a secondary intervention to maintain patency with the six HePTFE grafts undergoing
surgical patch angioplasty and the two vein grafts undergoing percutaneous angioplasty with a cutting balloon.

Analysis based on conduit revealed that graft thrombosis occurred in 12 HePTFE
grafts and seven vein grafts resulting in a primary patency at one year of 75.4% for
the HePTFE group and 86.0% for the vein group (Fig. 22-2). This was not a statistically significant difference. There were mortalities in the follow-up interval. Subgroup
analysis demonstrated significance for decreased graft survival function with end state
renal disease and nonhealing ulceration as an indication for revascularization. Patients
with renal failure had an 86% higher risk of death and graft thrombosis with nonhealing ulceration carrying an increased risk of 56%. There was no significant difference
in primary patency based on gender, race, or diabetes mellitus. Primary patency was
highest for the claudicant patients compared to those with rest pain or tissue loss.
There were four graft infections in the follow-up interval (6.5%). These graft infections occurred in HePTFE patients at 3, 4, 9, and 12 months postoperatively. In all of
these patients, the indication for surgery was an open, nonhealing wound with all
four receiving extended perioperative antibiotics after the bypass. Of the four infected
grafts, three were excised resulting in two major amputations. The other patient with
an excised graft did not require amputation as wound healing had occurred at the
point at which the graft became infected and was excised. The fourth infected graft
was treated with aggressive wound care, debridement, and a sartorius muscle flap
for graft coverage and this was successful. No vein conduits were impacted by graft
infection. Amputations were required in 16 patients (14%) during the follow-up period
at a mean postoperative interval of 4.9 months. Amputation rate was not statistically
dependent on conduit type.

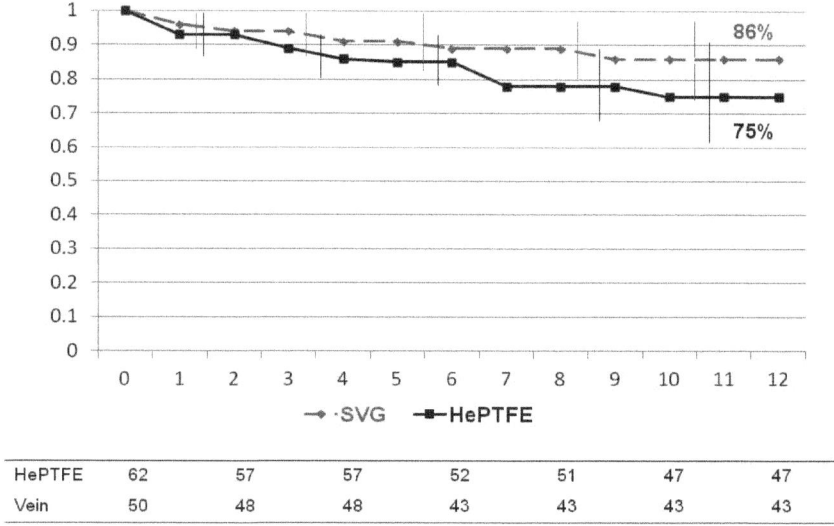

HePTFE	62	57	57	52	51	47	47
Vein	50	48	48	43	43	43	43

Figure 22-2. Primary patency rates for tibial bypass performed using heparin-bonded ePTFE (HePTFE) and single segment large saphenous vein (vein); no statistically significant difference noted.

There was a higher one-year patency for vein grafts in the setting of tibial bypass. However, we could not demonstrate a statistically significant difference in patency and believe that this data indicates that a HePTFE conduit can result in acceptable tibial patency at the one-year interval. There was no difference in amputations based on conduit type and the rate of infection in the prosthetic grafts was not prohibitive, although not insignificant. We would advocate aggressive debridement and rapid wound closure for those patients who have a heparin-bonded PTFE graft with the indication being a chronic nonhealing wound. This may be important to prevent graft infection in the future. It was also interesting to note that diabetes did not affect results, although patency rates were decreased in those patients on hemodialysis. Patients on hemodialysis may benefit from an aggressive approach with autologous conduit; however, these are often the very patients in whom there is no arm vein available, so it is in these challenging patients where heparin-bonded graft may be required despite some reduction in one-year patency.

OTHER EXPERIENCE

HePTFE has been clinically used for over 10 years, with the first human implant in 2001 with more than 80,000 of these prostheses implanted. Clinical trials have generated data regarding HePTFE graft performance in lower extremity bypasses for patients with significant peripheral arterial disease. However, the initial clinical trials using HePTFE grafts included a limited number of tibial bypasses that are often required in limb salvage cases. Peeters et al. demonstrated 69% two-year patency for tibial bypass in a series of below-knee bypasses using HePTFE.[20] Similarly, Lösel-Sadée and Alefelder reported tibial bypass patency with HePTFE of 64% at one year.[21] A large, multicenter trial from the Italian Registry was reported by Pulli et al. with HePTFE tibial bypass patency at one year of 66% and 52% at three years.[22]

Comparative trials of HePTFE and vein for below-knee bypass have been advocated to assess the efficacy of the heparin-bonded conduit for distal bypass. Battaglia found vein graft patency to be better than HePTFE, especially in those patients with single artery runoff and more severe symptoms at initial presentation.[23] However, Daenens and Nevelsteen compared 240 HePTFE to 110 vein bypasses and actually found a trend toward higher patency for the HePTFE grafts versus vein grafts for below-knee bypass.[24] Primary patency for tibial bypass at one and two years was 79/69% for HePTFE and 69/64% for vein grafts. These authors concluded that HePTFE should be routinely considered for below-knee bypass. In a comparison of primary patency for in situ vein, standard PTFE, and HePTFE, Dorigo et al. found HePTFE more effective than standard PTFE, but not as good as vein in a below-knee experience.[25] There was a 57% reduction in early graft thrombosis when using HePTFE compared to standard ePTFE, but HePTFE remained inferior compared to saphenous vein. Another analysis from the Italian Registry focused on the diabetic patient population, which is often the recipient of a tibial bypass for limb preservation. This report was a comparison between HePTFE and vein grafts including a subgroup of tibial bypasses (48 HePTFE and 88 venous) with long-term primary patency at four years of 45% for HePTFE and 58% for vein grafts.[26]

SUMMARY

Our experience with HePTFE grafts for solely tibial artery bypass yielded patency and limb salvage rates that are comparable to intact greater saphenous vein. We currently use a DVP with all our HePTFE grafts for tibial bypass. Our data shares those limitations found in similar nonrandomized, retrospective investigations and is further limited by its short observation period. However, this is a relatively large comparison of exclusively tibial bypasses and some insights may be possible. We believe that a quality saphenous vein remains the idea conduit for tibial bypass, although HePTFE should be considered when intact ipsilateral or contralateral vein is not available. The decreased graft patency noted for patients on hemodialysis would also suggest strong consideration for an autogenous conduit in patients with renal failure. However, HePTFE has emerged as our choice over arm vein even in the renal failure patient who may need the upper extremity veins for dialysis access. We would also choose HePTFE over composite lesser saphenous vein given the increased dissection required and lack of adequate length of conduit. In our patients, diabetes did not impact patency, and, therefore, we do not exclude diabetic patients from prosthetic revascularization for limb salvage. However, we would advise extra efforts to use vein for tibial bypass in diabetics and those with a chronic nonhealing wound.

REFERENCES

1. Neville RF, Attinger C, Bulan E, et al. Revascularization of a specific angiosome for limb salvage: does the target artery matter? *Ann Vasc Surg.* 2009;23(3):367–373.
2. Begovac PC, Thomson RC, Fisher JL, et al. Improvements in Gore-Tex vascular graft performance by Carmeda bioactive surface heparin immobilization. *Eur J Vasc Endovasc Surg.* 2003;25:432–437.

3. Lin PH, Chen C, Bush RL, et al. Small caliber heparin coated ePTFE grafts reduce platelet deposition and neointimal hyperplasia in a baboon model. *J Vasc Surg.* 2004;39:1322–1328.

4. Heyligers JM, Verhagen HJ, Rotmans JI, et al. Heparin immobilization reduces thrombogenicity of small-caliber expanded polytetrafluoroethylene grafts. *J Vasc Surg.* 2006;43:587–591.

5. Pederson G, Laxdal E, Ellensen V, et al. Improved patency and reduced intimal hyperplasia in PTFE grafts with luminal immobilized heparin compared with standard PTFE grafts at six months in a sheep model. *J Cardiovasc Surg.* 2010;5:435–442.

6. Calligaro KD, Syrek JR, Dougherty MJ, et al. Use of arm and lesser saphenous vein compared with prosthetic grafts for infrapopliteal bypass: are they worth the effort? *J Vasc Surg.* 1997;26:919–927.

7. Anderson LI, Nielsen OM, Hansen HJB. Umbilical vein bypass in patients with severe lower limb ischemia: a report of 121 consecutive cases. *Surgery.* 1985;97:294–298.

8. Bannazadeh M, Sarac T, Bena J, et al. Reoperative lower extremity revascularization with cadaver vein for limb salvage. *Ann Vasc Surg.* 2009;23:24–31.

9. Castier Y, Francis F, Cerceau F, et al. Cryopreserved arterial allograft reconstruction for peripheral graft infection. *J Vasc Surg.* 2005;41:30–37.

10. McPhee JT, Barshes N, Ozaki CK, et al. Optimal conduit choice in the absence of single-segment great saphenous vein for below-knee popliteal bypass. *J Vasc Surg.* 2012;55:1008–1014.

11. Albers M, Battistella VM, Romiti M, et al. Metaanalysis of polytetrafluoroethylene bypass grafts to infrapopliteal arteries. *J Vasc Surg.* 2003;37:1263–1269.

12. Bell PR. Are distal vascular procedures worthwhile? *Br J Surg.* 1985;72:335.

13. Miller JH, Foreman RK, Ferguson L, Faris A. Interposition vein cuff for anastomosis of prostheses to small arteries. *Aust NZ J Surg.* 1984;54:283–285.

14. Taylor RS, Loh A, McFarland RJ, et al. Improved technique for polytetrafluoroethylene bypass grafting: long-term results using anastomotic vein patches. *Br J Surg.* 1992;79:348–354.

15. Neville RF, Tempesta B, Sidway AN. Tibial bypass for limb salvage using polytetrafluoroethylene with a distal vein patch. *J Vasc Surg.* 2001;33:266–272.

16. Neville RF, Lid sky M, Capone A, et al. An expanded series of distal bypass using the distal vein patch technique to improve prosthetic graft performance in critical limb ischemia. *Eur J Vasc Endovasc Surg.* 2012;44:177–182.

17. Heyligers J, Lisman T. Verhagen HFM, et al. A heparin-bonded vascular graft generates no systemic effect on markers of hemostasis activation or detectable heparin-induced thrombocytopenia-associated antibodies in humans. *J Vasc Surg.* 2008;47:324–329.

18. Thakur S, Pigott J, Comerota A. Heparin-induced thrombocytopenia after implantation of a heparin-bonded polytetrafluoroethylene lower extremity bypass graft: A case report and plan for management. *J Vasc Surg.* 2009;49:1037–1040.

19. Neville RF, Capone A, Amdur R, et al. A comparison of tibial artery bypass performed with heparin bonded ePTFE and great saphenous vein to treat critical limb ischemia. *J Vasc Surg.* 2012;54(4):1008–1014.

20. Peeters P, Verbist J, Deloose K, Bosiers M. Results with heparin bonded polytetrafluoroethylene grafts for femorodistal bypasses. *J Cardiovasc Surg.* 2006;47:407–413.

21. Lösel-Sadée H, Alefelder C. Heparin bonded expanded polytetrafluoroethylene graft for infragenicular bypass: five year results. *J Cardiovas Surg.* 2009;50:339–343.

22. Pulli R, Dorigo W, Castelli P, et al. Midterm results from a multicenter registry on the treatment of infrainguinal critical limb ischemuia using a heparin bonded ePTFE graft. *J Vasc Surg.* 2010;51:1167–1177.

23. Battaglia G, Tringale R, Monaca V. Retrospective comparison of a heparin bonded ePTFE graft with saphenous vein for infragenicular bypass: implication for standard treatment protocol. *J Cardiovasc Surg.* 2006;47:41.

24. Daenens K, Schepers S, Fourneau I, et al. Heparin bonded ePTFE grafts compared with vein grafts in femoropopliteal and femorocrural bypasses: 1 and 2 year results. *J Vasc Surg.* 2009;49:1210–1216.

25. Dorigo W, Di Carlo F, Troisi N, et al. Lower limb revascularization with a new bioactive prosthetic graft: early and late results. *Ann Vasc Surg.* 2008;22:79–87.
26. Dorigo W, Pulli R, Castelli P, et al. A multicenter comparison between autologous saphenous vein and heparin-bonded expanded polytetrafluoroethylene (ePTFE) graft in the treatment of critical limb ischemia in diabetics. *J Vasc Surg.* 2011;54:1332–1338.

23

Outcomes of Endovascular Repair for Popliteal Artery Aneurysms

Neal S. Cayne, MD and Glenn Jacobowitz, MD

INTRODUCTION

The popliteal artery extends from the adductor canal above the knee joint to the origin of the anterior tibial artery below the knee. It is unique due to its location behind the knee joint and the associated high degree of flexion as compared to other arteries in the lower extremity. The normal caliber of the popliteal artery ranges from approximately 0.7 to 1.1 cm.[1,2] When the diameter of the popliteal artery is greater than 150% of its normal diameter, it is considered aneurysmal.[3] This chapter will review the topic of popliteal artery aneurysms (PAAs) and focus on the outcomes of endovascular repair.

EPIDEMIOLOGY AND PATHOGENESIS OF POPLITEAL ARTERY ANEURYSMS

PAAs are found almost exclusively in males. While they are relatively rare in the general population, they are the most common peripheral artery aneurysm and constitute at least 70% of all peripheral artery aneurysms.[4] The incidence of femoral or PAAs is much more common in males and was identified to be 7.4 per 100,000 males and only 1.0 per 100,000 females[4] in a study of hospitalized patients. Bilateral PAAs are found in 50% of patients and 30%–50% of patients may have an associated abdominal aortic aneurysm (AAA).[5,6] On the contrary, less than 15% of all AAA patients have a coexisting PAA.[7]

The majority of PAAs are considered to be true aneurysms, involving all layers of the arterial wall. While many authors in the past considered PAAs as atherosclerotic, most PAAs are degenerative. Jacob et al.[8] identified disruption and fragmentation of the elastic lamellae in the walls of PAA specimens when compared to normal popliteal arteries. In addition, they identified decreased number of vascular smooth muscle cells in the walls and an increased expression of molecules linked to apoptosis. They attribute the aneurysm formation to a loss of the mechanical integrity of the popliteal artery wall and the altered balance between the production and degradation of the vascular wall constituents.

The anatomic location of the popliteal artery at a high flexion point and the encountered repetitive stresses of the artery in this location may be an additional causative factor for development PAAs.

NATURAL HISTORY OF POPLITEAL ARTERY ANEURYSMS

In contrast to AAAs, PAAs rarely rupture, with a reported incidence in the literature only around 2.5%.[9] The mean growth rate is 1.5 mm/year for PAAs less than 20 mm, 3 mm/year for PAAs 20-30 mm and 3.7 mm/y at sizes greater than 30 mm. The most common risk factor associated with PAA growth identified was hypertension.[10] When PAAs present with symptoms, it is typically acute or chronic ischemia due to distal embolization or thrombosis. While the actual percentage of PAA patients that become symptomatic over time may be difficult to determine, several series of observed PAA patients report a high incidence of thromboembolic complications. Dawson et al. reviewed 71 PAAs, 25 of which were initially treated nonsurgically. Complications developed in 12 of the 21 asymptomatic popliteal aneurysms (57%) and in two of the four symptomatic PAAs (50%). The probability of developing complications increased with time to 74% within five years. Szilagyi et al. reported that over a five-year period, only 32% of observed (nonoperated) PAA patients remained without lower extremity complications.[11]

CLINICAL PRESENTATION AND DIAGNOSIS OF PAAs

Patients with a PAA may present with an asymptomatic pulsatile mass in the popliteal fossa. More than half of patients, however, typically present with symptoms or evidence of embolization.[12–15] Lower extremity ischemia is the most common presenting symptom. The ischemia can be due to embolization or thrombosis and patient's symptoms can range from being essentially asymptomatic or having minimal claudication to acute limb threatening ischemia. Patients may present with chronic ischemic symptoms similar to that of atherosclerotic occlusive disease. It is not uncommon for patients to have occlusion of multiple tibial vessels secondary to chronic emboli.

Patients can less often present with compressive symptoms, including vein (leg swelling and deep venous thrombosis) or nerve compression. Lastly, PAAs can present with the rare complication of rupture.

The diagnosis of PAA is suspected anytime there is a prominent or widened popliteal artery pulse felt on physical exam. This is especially true when a popliteal artery pulse can be easily felt with one hand. Special attention should be given to detecting possible PAAs in males with a known AAA, femoral aneurysm, or contralateral PAA as the incidence is higher. Likewise, a prominent popliteal pulse with gangrene of the ipsilateral foot in a nondiabetic male should trigger the possible diagnosis of possible PAA. A nonpulsating popliteal mass in a patient with ischemic symptoms should lead one to suspect a possible thrombosed PAA. Ideally, the diagnosis of PAA should be made before the onset of limb-threatening complications. The outcomes of surgical or endovascular treatment are best in asymptomatic patients and progressively worse in those with either chronic ischemic symptoms or acute, critical limb ischemia.[5]

Radiographic Detection of PAAs

The main radiologic modalities used for the diagnosis of PAA are duplex ultrasound (DU), magnetic resonance angiography (MRA), and computed tomography angiography (CTA). Occasionally PAAs can be seen on a plain radiograph by a radiopaque calcified enlarged aneurysm perimeter behind the knee.

DU has the advantage of not needing ionizing radiation or contrast agents. It can be accurate in detecting PAA, thrombus burden, and patency of outflow vessels.[16,17] DU is also useful in detecting PAAs when DSA reveals an occluded popliteal artery and PAA is suspected.

MRA has the advantage of not utilizing radiation and is also a very accurate imaging modality for PAA. It is limited to those patients without pacemakers and somewhat limited to those with advanced renal failure. MRA can give good information on the inflow and outflow vessels as well as the thrombus burden as long as the cross-sectional images are evaluated.

CTA is a very useful and accurate imaging modality for the diagnosis and evaluation of PAAs. Disadvantages include the use of ionizing radiation and intravenous contrast administration, which limits its use in patients with renal insufficiency and severe contrast allergy. CTA can accurately demonstrate the size, thrombus burden, and inflow and outflow vessels. It can be extremely helpful when planning for both open and endovascular repair of PAAs.

While digital subtraction angiography (DSA) may help identify a PAA, its use can be misleading in the diagnosis due to nonvisualization of either mural thrombus or a thrombosed PAA. DSA, however, can be very useful for planning revascularization once the diagnosis is confirmed. DSA is used in conjunction with the aforementioned radiologic exams to determine inflow and outflow vessel patency and for operative planning. It is the gold standard for determining the status of the outflow vessels. In most institutions, the quality of CTA and MRA, particularly with three-dimensional reconstructions, may provide very accurate information about the runoff vessels. However, if there is any question concerning the outflow or perfusion, DSA should be obtained before any intervention.

TREATMENT OF PAAs

While it is generally accepted that PAAs ≥ 2.0 cm and all symptomatic patients should be considered for treatment in medically suitable candidates, some controversy exists. The rationale for treating asymptomatic patients with PAAs ≥ 2.0 cm is that these patients have a 30%–40% risk of developing acute ischemic complications that are associated with a high risk of limb loss.[11,18–20] Some authors suggest that all popliteal aneurysms should be repaired once found, regardless of size, due to the high complication and limb loss rate.[20–22] Ascher et al. suggested in a review of 34 popliteal aneurysms that there may be a higher incidence of embolic/thrombotic complications associated with smaller PAAs. Those that advocate repairing almost all PAAs regardless of size before limb-threatening symptoms develop quote high limb salvage and patency rates and low operative mortality for smaller, asymptomatic aneurysms.[15,23,24] Critical limb ischemia before intervention is associated with up to three to four times higher perioperative mortality and considerably higher rates of limb loss.[12–14]

The decision to treat a patient with a PAA must be individualized. As with any decision in medicine, one must weigh the risks and benefits of treating or observing. Treatment should generally be offered to medically fit patients that have a symptomatic PAA or who are asymptomatic, but have a PAA at least 2.0–2.5 cm that contains thrombus. In older patients with multiple comorbidities, observation of even a larger aneurysm may be warranted, but extensive thrombus or asymptomatic occlusion of tibial vessels may be indications for intervention. Chronically thrombosed PAAs associated with lifestyle limiting claudication or limb threatening ischemia may need revascularization similarly to patients with chronic arterial occlusive disease.

Elective Treatment

Once the decision has been made to treat the patient, the preoperative evaluation involves making sure that the patient is medically optimized and determining the operative approach. If indicated, B-blockers should be considered and statins should be added, ideally at least one month before the procedure.[25] The patient should be on aspirin or some other antiplatelet agent.

Planning for surgery and deciding on proceeding with an endovascular, open, or hybrid approach will depend on the patient's anatomy, age, and comorbidities. The patient's circulation should be imaged from the abdominal aorta down to the pedal vessels. If the preoperative imaging is not of sufficient quality, an angiogram should be performed. Options for elective repair of PAAs include an endovascular approach (purely percutaneous or hybrid with exposure of the femoral artery) utilizing an intraluminal stent graft or an open approach utilizing an arterial bypass. It should be stated here that although endovascular repair of PAAs is being widely performed and reported on, there is not yet approval of devices and endografts by the Food and Drug Administration (FDA) in the United States for this particular procedure. Endovascular repair of PAAs is therefore considered an off-label use of a stent graft.

Endovascular/Hybrid Approach

An endovascular approach has the benefit of not requiring general or regional anesthesia and therefore a theoretical advantage of decreasing cardiac risk. The procedure can be performed either through a percutaneous puncture or through small cutdown to expose either the superficial femoral artery (SFA) or common femoral artery (CFA). If a cutdown is to be performed, the preferred exposure is of the SFA because it is an easy dissection, the artery is usually fairly large in PAA patients, and direct access avoids an extra step of having to direct a wire into the vessel from the CFA. Anatomic selection criteria for endovascular repair of PAA include an adequate proximal and distal landing zone of at least 2 cm (without a large discrepancy in size between proximal and distal landing zones), lack of extensive vessel tortuosity, and lack of a large voluminous aneurysm that would make a stent graft prone to kinking and displacement. Patients who frequently flex their knee >90 degrees such as a carpenter or one who gardens are usually excluded due to the risk of stent deformation and thrombosis. In addition, if antiplatelet therapy is contraindicated, an endovascular approach is not recommended. All patients are loaded with and maintained on Plavix clopidogrel, because it has been shown to be a predictor of success in endovascular PAA repair.[26] If there is no contraindication in prolonged use, clopidogrel is maintained indefinitely. A minimum of four to six weeks of antiplatelet therapy is recommended in all cases. Unless there is a known hypercoagulable state, anticoagulation with Coumadin is not routinely used.

Procedure

For an endovascular approach, the Viabahn (W.L. Gore, Tempe, AZ) endoprosthesis has been useful. It is made of polytetrafluoroethylene (PTFE) with a nitinol exoskeleton. Viabahn is approved by the FDA for treating occlusive disease rather than PAA. The device is usually oversized about 10%–15%, based on the internal diameter of the popliteal vessel above and below the aneurysm. It is not recommended to oversize the graft much greater than 15%. There is a case report of graft infolding and operative occlusion related to oversizing that required conversion to an open femoral to popliteal bypass.[27] The vessel measurements can be based on preoperative imaging and checked using the intraoperative angiogram. As the profile of the device has decreased, up to an 8-mm graft can be delivered through a 7 French sheath using a .018″ wire. Therefore, in most cases, percutaneous common femoral access through an ipsilateral prograde or contralateral retrograde approach (over the iliac bifurcation) can usually be used. If a larger sheath is required (9-13 mm device requires a 9-12 French sheath, .035″ system), or if direct vessel exposure is desired, the superficial femoral artery can be easily exposed under local anesthesia. Once vascular access is obtained and the appropriate sheath is placed, an angiogram is performed. The proximal and distal landing zones as well as the runoff vessels are confirmed. The patient is systemically heparinized to an activated clotting time of over 250 seconds. The PAA can then be carefully crossed and the correct devices can be chosen based on the preoperative imaging and the intraoperative angiogram. A maximum of no more than 1 mm size differential between grafts is suggested if more than one graft is required due to a discrepancy in proximal and distal landing zones. It is preferable to avoid landing the distal end of the graft at the bend of the popliteal artery. This bend in the artery is usually a few centimeters above the actual knee joint and can be located by performing an angiogram with the knee bent. The grafts are deployed from small to large if multiple grafts are needed. Usually at least 2–3 cm of normal artery on either side of the aneurysm are preferable for landing zones. If more than one graft is required, a minimum of 2–3 cm overlap between grafts is preferred. The grafts are always molded with a balloon about the size of the graft. The balloon is inflated inside of the graft and not in native artery to avoid arterial dissection. A completion angiogram is performed and runoff is assessed. An angiogram is performed again with the knee bent. If the graft ends on the bend of the popliteal artery, it is usually extended. The access site is either repaired open or using access closure devices or direct manual pressure is held on the puncture site for 20–30 minutes after the activated clotting time (ACT) is normalized.

The detail on purely open approaches for the repair of PAAs is beyond the scope of this chapter and will not be discussed.

Urgent/Emergent Repair

When patients present with acute occlusion or symptomatic embolization, there is a high rate of limb loss.[12–14] In an acutely symptomatic PAA patient without motor or sensory deficits, preoperative imaging can be very useful. The patient should be admitted to the hospital and systemically heparinized. Either CTA or MRA can be used to evaluate the perfusion of the affected extremity and the outflow vessels. Angiography can be used in place of either of these tests if the diagnosis of PAA is already made and can give additional information about the status of the runoff vessels. It is still considered the gold standard to evaluate the outflow vessels. Based on the symptoms and the preoperative imaging, a treatment strategy can be formulated. If there are no motor or sensory deficits, treatment can be delayed for imaging and preoperative planning. The patient with neurosensory deficits should be taken directly to the operating room, ideally to a hybrid operating room/angiosuite for thrombectomy and/or bypass to restore perfusion as soon as possible. If there have been neurosensory deficits for more than six hours before reperfusion, fasciotomy should be considered. The most urgent and difficult scenario is when not only the PAA thromboses but the tibial outflow vessels are also occluded. In this scenario, preoperative lysis is associated with improved limb salvage rates and graft patency rates when compared to surgery alone.[5,13,28] Lytic therapy can not only open the occluded vessel, but maybe more importantly, can open the out flow vessels if they are not chronically occluded. Traditional lysis is usually performed through a 6 French sheath placed in the contralateral CFA and over the aortic bifurcation and into the affected leg. If the thrombus can be traversed, this is one of the best predictors of the success of lytic therapy. A 5 French lytic catheter can be placed in the thrombosed popliteal artery and a lytic wire can be placed through the lytic catheter and into one of the tibial outflow vessels. Direct intra-arterial lytic therapy can be begun with tissue plasminogen activator (tPA) or other thrombolytics at equivalent doses. The patient is placed in a monitored setting (ICU or PACU) during the infusion for careful monitoring. Infusion rates are typically 2 mg/h of tPA or less, administered through the catheter and wire combined. Five hundred units of heparin are given through the 6 French sheath to prevent thrombosis around the catheter. The tPA is diluted to 25 mg in 500 cc to ensure sufficient volume through the catheters (20 cc/h = 1 mg/h). Partial thromboplastic time (PTT) and fibrinogen are checked every three to four hours. The PTT should be less than therapeutic to prevent bleeding complications (PTT < 50). As long as the fibrinogen is above 200 mg/dL, lytic therapy is continued. If it drops below 200 mg/dL, the dose is halved and the drip is held when the fibrinogen drops below 150 mg/dL. Repeat angiogram is performed within 6–18 hours or before if required. Based on the angiographic findings and clinical scenario, either a bypass can be performed if a target vessel opens, lytic therapy can be continued, or the patient can undergo attempt at urgent thrombectomy/bypass if the leg is acutely threatened. Alternatively, if the thrombus lyses and anatomy permits (as described earlier), and there is more than one outflow vessel, an endovascular stent graft can be placed as previously described. As previously reported, PAA patients with single vessel outflow that are treated with an endovascular stent graft have inferior patency rates.[29] A rheolytic percutaneous thrombectomy catheter may also be used to spray tPA (10 mg tPA in 100 cc) directly using the Power Pulse technique (10 mg tPA in 100 cc) into thrombus and the catheter can help to debulk the thrombus before beginning a lytic drip as described above.

Hybrid Approach for Urgent/Emergent Repair

It is not uncommon for a combination of the aforementioned endovascular and open techniques to be used for emergent cases, which should ideally be performed in a hybrid operating room with optimal angiographic equipment and operative capability. Open thrombectomy can be performed through the below-knee popliteal artery if intraoperative lysis is not successful and the patient's symptoms will not allow for the time that it takes for the lytic therapy to work. Likewise, if open thrombectomy is not successful, intraoperative lytic therapy and pharmacomechanical thrombectomy can be attempted.

If there is remaining distal tibial thrombus after open thrombectomy and the below-knee popliteal artery is patent, a below-knee bypass can be performed and a 4 French sheath can be placed percutaneously and then into the bypass graft. A lytic wire can be left in the tibial outflow vessel for further lytic therapy. The TPA dose is kept fairly low in this circumstance as bleeding can be encountered from the surgical sites. The patient is taken back to the operating room for repeat angiogram and removal of the catheter/repair of the graft.

OUTCOMES OF PAA REPAIR

The results of both open and endovascular repair of PAAs are somewhat dependent on the severity of the patient's symptoms upon presentation with the most symptomatic having the worst outcomes.[12–14]

Endovascular repair of PAAs overall has been shown to be relatively safe with patency rates approaching that of open repair in patients that have appropriate anatomy. We earlier reported on the endovascular treatment of PAA on 26 limbs in 21 patients utilizing the Viabahn endoprosthesis.[29] Primary and secondary patency rates were both 91% at one year and 86% and 91% at two years. Single vessel runoff was the only significant predictor of graft failure. Mohan et al.[30] reviewed 35 PAAs treated with endovascular grafts. They found three-year primary and secondary patency to be 75% and 83%. In a review of 73 PAAs treated with an endovascular graft, a follow-up paper by Tielliu et al.[31] to their earlier study found five-year primary and secondary patency rates of 70% and 76%. When analyzing the later cases, they found that with more experience and the addition of clopidogrel, the five-year primary patency increased to 80%. Jung et al.[32] performed a retrospective review of 15 PAAs treated with an endovascular grafts that had long-term follow-up (mean, 54 months). Primary and secondary patency rates were 85% and 100%, respectively. Two patients developed endoleaks that were successfully treated with additional endovascular grafts. Both amputation-free survival and overall survival were 86% by Kaplan–Meier analysis. Thakar et al.[33] reported on one of the first experiences with the use of a multilayer stent in the endovascular treatment of six PAAs in the United Kingdom. Their results were quite poor utilizing this noncovered multilayer stent, reporting a 50% stent occlusion rate within a six-week time period.

Antonello et al.[34] reported one of the first prospective randomized trials comparing open and endovascular PAA repair; however, it only included 30 patients, 15 in each group. They did not find a statistically significant difference in patency or limb salvage rates at a follow-up of up to four years. As would be expected, they did find a statistically significant decrease in operative time and length of stay in the hospital with the endovascular group. Lovegrove et al.[35] in a meta-analysis comparing open versus endovascular repair of PAAs had similar results with no significant difference in long-term patency rates; however, patients who underwent endovascular repair were more likely to have graft thrombosis and reintervention at 30 days than open repair. They also found significantly shorter length of stay and operative times for the endovascular patients.

A retrospective review by Curi et al.[36] of 56 PAA repairs comparing open versus endovascular treatment demonstrated no significant difference in primary patency, secondary patency, or survival between the two groups. All urgent cases, however, were treated with open repair and 20% of the endovascular patients developed endoleaks.

CONCLUSION

Although PAA is a relatively infrequent disease, its presence has the potential to place the limb at risk. Once suspected, it should be fully evaluated PAAs larger than 2–2.5 cm and symptomatic in any way should be considered for repair in a medically fit patient. While endovascular repair of PAAs have been shown to decrease length of stay and operative morbidity, data is somewhat varied as to its durability compared with open repair. In addition, endovascular devices for PAA repair are yet to be approved by the FDA. Based on current literature, endovascular repair in general should be reserved for patients with good anatomy (as described earlier), patients that do not frequently bend their knee greater than 90 degrees, and patients that can take clopidogrel for a minimum of four to six weeks. However, the decision to perform open or endovascular repair should be individualized to the patient and clearly deserves a discussion between the treating physician and the patient.

REFERENCES

1. Wolf YG, Kobzantsev Z, Zelmanovich L. Size of normal and aneurysmal popliteal arteries: a duplex ultrasound study. *J Vasc Surg*. 2006;43:488–492.
2. Davis RP, Neiman HL, Yao JS, Bergan JJ. Ultrasound scan in diagnosis of peripheral aneurysms. *Arch Surg*. 1977;112:55–58.
3. Johnston KW, Rutherford RB, Tilson MD, et al. Suggested standards for reporting on arterial aneurysms. Subcommittee on reporting standards for arterial aneurysms, ad hoc committee on reporting standards, society for vascular surgery and North American chapter, international society for cardiovascular surgery. *J Vasc Surg*. 1991;13:452–458.
4. Lawrence PF, Lorenzo-Rivero S, Lyon JL. The incidence of iliac, femoral, and popliteal artery aneurysms in hospitalized patients. *J Vasc Surg*. 1995;22:409–415; discussion 15–16.
5. Huang Y, Gloviczki P, Noel AA, et al. Early complications and long-term outcome after open surgical treatment of popliteal artery aneurysms: is exclusion with saphenous vein bypass still the gold standard? *J Vasc Surg*. 2007;45:706–713; discussion 13–15.
6. Dawson I. Management of popliteal aneurysm (*Br J Surg*. 2002;89:1382–1385). *Br J Surg*. 2003;90:249–250.
7. Diwan A, Sarkar R, Stanley JC, et al. Incidence of femoral and popliteal artery aneurysms in patients with abdominal aortic aneurysms. *J Vasc Surg*. 2000;31:863–869.
8. Jacob T, Hingorani A, Ascher E. Examination of the apoptotic pathway and proteolysis in the pathogenesis of popliteal artery aneurysms. *Eur J Vasc Endovasc Surg*. 2001;22:77–85.
9. Sie RB, Dawson I, van Baalen JM, et al. Ruptured popliteal artery aneurysm. An insidious complication. *Eur J Vasc Endovasc Surg*. 1997;13:432–438.
10. Pittathankal AA, Dattani R, Magee TR, Galland RB. Expansion rates of asymptomatic popliteal artery aneurysms. *Eur J Vasc Endovasc Surg*. 2004;27:382–384.
11. Szilagyi DE, Schwartz RL, Reddy DJ. Popliteal arterial aneurysms. Their natural history and management. *Arch Surg*. 1981;116:724–728.
12. Shortell CK, DeWeese JA, Ouriel K, Green RM. Popliteal artery aneurysms: a 25-year surgical experience. *J Vasc Surg*. 1991;14:771–776; discussion 6–9.
13. Carpenter JP, Barker CF, Roberts B, et al. Popliteal artery aneurysms: current management and outcome. *J Vasc Surg*. 1994;19:65–72; discussion 72–73.
14. Reilly MK, Abbott WM, Darling RC. Aggressive surgical management of popliteal artery aneurysms. *Am J Surg*. 1983;145:498–502.

15. Varga ZA, Locke-Edmunds JC, Baird RN. A multicenter study of popliteal aneurysms. Joint Vascular Research Group. *J Vasc Surg.* 1994;20:171–177.

16. Turnipseed WD, Acher CW, Detmer DE, et al. Digital subtraction angiography and B-mode ultrasonography for abdominal and peripheral aneurysms. *Surgery.* 1982;92:619–626.

17. Kallakuri S, Ascher E, Hingorani A, et al. Effect of duplex arteriography in the management of acute limb-threatening ischemia from thrombosed popliteal aneurysms. *Angiology.* Epub, April 29, 2008. DOI: 10.1177/0003319708316009.

18. Dawson I, Sie RB, van Bockel JH. Atherosclerotic popliteal aneurysm. *Br J Surg.* 1997;84:293–299.

19. Vermilion BD, Kimmins SA, Pace WG, Evans WE. A review of one hundred forty-seven popliteal aneurysms with long-term follow-up. *Surgery.* 1981;90:1009–1014.

20. Ascher E, Markevich N, Schutzer RW, et al. Small popliteal artery aneurysms: are they clinically significant? *J Vasc Surg.* 2003;37:755–760.

21. Poirier NC, Verdant A, Page A. [Popliteal aneurysm: surgical treatment is mandatory before complications occur]. *Ann Chir.* 1996;50:613–618.

22. Cross JE, Galland RB, Hingorani A, Ascher E. Nonoperative versus surgical management of small (less than 3 cm), asymptomatic popliteal artery aneurysms. *J Vasc Surg.* 2011;53:1145–1148.

23. Whitehouse WM, Jr., Wakefield TW, Graham LM, et al. Limb-threatening potential of arteriosclerotic popliteal artery aneurysms. *Surgery.* 1983;93:694–699.

24. Lowell RC, Gloviczki P, Hallett JW, Jr., et al. Popliteal artery aneurysms: the risk of non-operative management. *Ann Vasc Surg.* 1994;8:14–23.

25. Bauer SM, Cayne NS, Veith FJ. New developments in the preoperative evaluation and perioperative management of coronary artery disease in patients undergoing vascular surgery. *J Vasc Surg.* 2010;51:242–251.

26. Tielliu IF, Verhoeven EL, Zeebregts CJ, et al. Endovascular treatment of popliteal artery aneurysms: results of a prospective cohort study. *J Vasc Surg.* 2005;41:561–567.

27. Ranson ME, Adelman MA, Cayne NS, et al. Total Viabahn endoprosthesis collapse. *J Vasc Surg.* 2008;47:454–456.

28. Dorigo W, Pulli R, Turini F, et al. Acute leg ischaemia from thrombosed popliteal artery aneurysms: role of preoperative thrombolysis. *Eur J Vasc Endovasc Surg.* 2002;23:251–254.

29. Garg K, Rockman CB, Kim BJ, et al. Outcome of endovascular repair of popliteal artery aneurysm using the Viabahn endoprosthesis. *J Vasc Surg.* 2012;55:1647–1653.

30. Mohan IV, Bray PJ, Harris JP, et al. Endovascular popliteal aneurysm repair: are the results comparable to open surgery? *Eur J Vasc Endovasc Surg.* 2006;32:149–154.

31. Tielliu IF, Verhoeven EL, Zeebregts CJ, et al. Endovascular treatment of popliteal artery aneurysms: is the technique a valid alternative to open surgery? *J Cardiovasc Surg.* (Torino) 2007;48:275–279.

32. Jung E, Jim J, Rubin BG, et al. Long-term outcome of endovascular popliteal artery aneurysm repair. *Ann Vasc Surg.* 2010;24:871–875.

33. Thakar T, Chaudhuri A. Early experience with the multilayer aneurysm repair stent in the endovascular treatment of trans/infragenicular popliteal artery aneurysms: a mixed bag. *J Endovasc Ther.* 2013;20:381–388.

34. Antonello M, Frigatti P, Battocchio P, et al. Open repair versus endovascular treatment for asymptomatic popliteal artery aneurysm: results of a prospective randomized study. *J Vasc Surg.* 2005;42:185–193.

35. Lovegrove RE, Javid M, Magee TR, Galland RB. Endovascular and open approaches to non-thrombosed popliteal aneurysm repair: a meta-analysis. *Eur J Vasc Endovasc Surg.* 2008;36:96100.

36. Curi MA, Geraghty PJ, Merino OA, et al. Mid-term outcomes of endovascular popliteal artery aneurysm repair. *J Vasc Surg.* 2007;45:505–510.

24

Will Drug-Eluting Superficial Femoral Artery Stents Replace All Other Interventions?

H. Bob Smouse, MD; Caroline Cusack, BS; and Katherine Cusack, BS

BACKGROUND

Lower Extremity Peripheral Arterial Disease

An estimated 27 million people in North America and Europe are affected by peripheral arterial disease (PAD), of whom 88,000 are currently hospitalized for lesions involving the lower extremities. Since increasing age is a risk factor for developing PAD, this number will grow as our population ages. In patients above 70 years of age, the incidence of PAD is 15%–20%. There are other risk factors associated with PAD including smoking, diabetes, hypertension, hyperlipidemia, family history, and male gender. Presence of PAD is a strong predictor of cerebrovascular and cardiovascular health, and patients who suffer from PAD have—four to five times greater risk of dying from a cardiovascular event. Annually, approximately 10% of cerebrovascular and cardiovascular events can be attributed to PAD progression.[1]

Although PAD is associated with great morbidity and mortality, only 25% of affected patients have attained treatment. PAD remains asymptomatic for years and only presents when at least 50% narrowing of the vessels has occurred. The degree of stenosis in the vessel dictates the severity of the symptoms. Pain caused by PAD is a discomfort experienced anywhere between the buttock and the foot that is relieved by rest, an event known as claudication. Calf claudication is most commonly described by patients. Superficial femoral artery (SFA) lesions usually cause pain in the upper two-thirds of the calf while popliteal lesions cause pain in the lower one-third. Very severe PAD can lead to ischemic rest pain, which is characterized by pain at rest, usually at night, occurring in the foot and toes. If PAD persists untreated, ischemia will damage nerves and lead to a burning pain in the foot, or a pain that seems to shoot up the leg.[1]

Once a patient presents with symptoms, the diagnosis of PAD is relatively simple. The most commonly used measure of PAD is the ankle brachial index (ABI). This is a ratio of the highest blood pressure measured in the ankle to the highest blood pressure measured in the arm. When an abnormal ABI is detected, Doppler ultrasonography can be used to evaluate flow in the vessels and further assess the severity of stenosis. Some physicians also use CT angiography (CTA) and MR angiography (MRA) as noninvasive measures to diagnose PAD. The gold standard for definitive diagnosis of PAD is angiography. This allows the physician to pinpoint the exact location of the lesion and better evaluate the degree of stenosis.[1]

FEMOROPOPLITEAL SEGMENT

The vessels most affected by PAD in the lower extremity can be divided into three categories: aortoiliac, femoropopliteal, and infrapopliteal. The SFA in the femoropopliteal segment of the lower extremity is the artery that is most commonly affected by PAD. The SFA is a very long vessel with complex anatomy. The bones and muscles that surround the SFA cause it to undergo a unique set of mechanical forces including extension, contraction, torsion, compression, and flexion. These forces are especially imposed where the SFA runs through the adductor canal, between the quadriceps, adductor, and sartorius muscles. Since this artery spirals down the canal, blood flowing through the artery begins to flow in a helical pattern. This pattern is especially prominent on the inner curvature of the vessel, which makes this area most susceptible to atherosclerosis.[2]

Classification of femoropopliteal disease can be accomplished by lesion morphology with the Trans Atlantic Inter-Society Consensus (TASC II) guidelines. These classify lesions according to anatomic distribution and number and nature of lesions. Lesions are graded as type A, B, C, or D. Type A lesions are the least severe. As a patient acquires longer lesions, lesions that are heavily calcified, multiple lesions, lesions involving the popliteal artery, or lesions that are refractory to treatment, their TASC II classification increases to a higher grade. Generally endovascular treatments are used for type A and most type B lesions. Surgery is the treatment of choice for type D lesion and is the preferred treatment for good risk patients with type C lesions.[3]

SURGERY AS GOLD STANDARD

Historically, surgery has been the gold standard for treating SFA occlusions. Jean Kunlin performed the first successful femoropopliteal bypass in 1948 using an autologous vein graft. Several prosthetic materials have been introduced as grafts to replace the saphenous vein since then. Because of this, one of the main factors that can modify the result of the procedure is the type of the conduit used. When comparing autologous vein grafts with prosthetic conduits, immediate and long-term patency rates are superior in the autologous group for both above-the-knee and below-the-knee (BTK) bypasses. When using polytetrafluoroethylene (PTFE) grafts, autologous vein conduit has a significantly higher primary patency at five years.[4] However, the introduction of heparin-bonded Dacron grafts improved the midterm primary patency compared to PTFE grafts in above-the-knee bypasses.[5] Overall, the five-year patency rates of femoropopliteal bypass grafts are reported as 80% for vein grafts, 75%

for above-the-knee synthetic grafts, and 65% for BTK synthetic grafts.[6] Antiplatelet therapy must be added to the postoperative treatments when using synthetic grafts.

Remote SFA endarterectomy (RSFAE) was introduced in 1994. This allows a less invasive surgical alternative to bypass. When compared to venous bypass, the primary patency rate of the RSFAE at three years is inferior. However, when compared to synthetic bypass, patency rates are comparable. The advantages with RSFAE include a shorter hospital stay and avoidance of prosthetic materials. Although thought to be a safer procedure, there is no demonstration of a decrease in early postoperative complications with RSFAE compared to bypass.[7]

Surgery is indicated for patients with claudication and significant functional disability or critical limb ischemia (CLI). In real-world practice, surgery is most often employed after failure of conservative or endovascular therapy and if there is a reasonable likelihood of symptomatic improvement. In addition, patients must have favorable limb arterial anatomy and low cardiovascular risk for surgical revascularization.[8] Currently, surgery is recommended for task D lesions.

ENDOVASCULAR TREATMENT

There are many advantages in the use of endovascular treatment when compared to invasive surgical approaches. Morbidity and mortality is lowered with the use of percutaneous treatments. Endovascular treatment does not require general anesthesia and is therefore suitable for patients with comorbidities who are poor surgical candidates. After an uncomplicated procedure, patients who undergo endovascular treatment have the ability to return to normal activities within—one to two days.

Atherosclerotic disease in the SFA is usually characterized by diffuse lesions with heavy calcifications. Due to the increased amount of smooth muscle cells, this segment of the artery responds to stress and injury with extensive scar formation, which can lead to restenosis. This response to injury is responsible for balloon angioplasty failure in up to 70% of cases. Stent implantation avoids the problems of elastic recoil, flow-limiting dissection, and residual stenosis. Over two decades ago, the first stent was placed in the femoropopliteal segment. These first procedures used stainless steel stents in short lesions. Five randomly controlled trials failed to show improved results when comparing stent placement to angioplasty in the femoropopliteal segment. The use of self-expanding Elgiloy Wallstents (Boston Scientific Corporation) showed promising initial results, but were abandoned when it was found that they had a high rate of stent fracture and low midterm patency. Covered stents (stent grafts) were evaluated and showed unacceptable rates of stent thrombosis and morbidity. For more than a decade, stent placement remained a bailout procedure for failed angioplasty and was not recommended as a first-line therapy by TASC guidelines due to the lack of long-term benefits.[9]

The creation of self-expanding nitinol stents with improved strength and flexibility decreased the amount of stent fractures, allowed precise stent placement, and increased patency rates. In the Vienna Absolute trial, balloon angioplasty was compared with nitinol stents in 104 patients with a primary end point of binary angiographic restenosis at six months. Average lengths were 132 ± 71 and 127 ± 55 mm for the stent and balloon angioplasty groups, respectively. At 12 months, restenosis rates were 36.7% and 63.5% for stent placement and angioplasty, respectively. A two-year follow-up confirmed improved results in the stent group.[10] During this time, the Femoral Artery Stenting Trial trial was also completed comparing plain angioplasty with primary nitinol stent placement in lesions between 1 and 10 cm. At 12 months, restenosis rates were 32% and 39% for stent placement and angioplasty, respectively, and the authors concluded that there was no benefit in stent placement for lesions <10 cm in the femoropopliteal segment.[11] The RESILIENT trial (A randomized study comparing the Edwards self-expanding LifeStent versus angioplasty alone in lesions involving the superficial femoral artery and/or proximal popliteal artery) compared angioplasty and nitinol stent placement in 206 patients in lesions with a median length of 6.5 cm and found that nitinol stent placement was superior when comparing 12-month restenosis rates (80% vs. 38%).[12] Finally, the ASTRON trial (Angioplasty versus stenting for superficial femoral artery lesions), which involved 73 patients, found a significantly lower restenosis rate with primary stenting when compared to angioplasty alone in a average lesion length of 8.4 cm (34.4% vs. 61.1%).[13]

Despite the success that was found with stent placement over angioplasty, there were still obstacles to overcome with stents. In the SIROCCO drug-eluting stent trials (Sirolimus-eluting versus bare nitinol stent for obstructive superficial femoral artery disease), one secondary end point was to evaluate stent fractures in the SFA. In the first trial, fractures were found in 31% of patients and this number was reduced to 11% in the second trial by limiting maximum stent placement to two and thereby decreasing stent overlap. Furthermore, impressive fracture differences were seen between different commercially available nitinol stents and this prompted continued improvement in stent design. However, despite improvements in strut and cell design, the main obstacle of the restenosis caused by neointimal hyperplasia (NIH) remained a problem. Placing drug-eluting stents in the femoropopliteal segment aimed to ameliorate this problem.[9]

There is some evidence to suggest that plaque-debulking techniques may yield similar results when comparing midterm and long-term patency rates with PTA. These techniques include remote endarterectomy, directional, rotational, orbital, and laser-guided atherectomy. Although newer devices created in the past decade may have improved debulking results, they have failed to show a higher rate of long-term primary and secondary patency. RCTs evaluating available devices and debulking techniques are expected in the near future.[14]

DRUG-ELUTING STENTS

Coronary Drug-Eluting Data

Drug-eluting stents have been extremely successful in the coronary arteries. Percutaneous coronary intervention was first pioneered in 1977 and has become the most frequently performed therapeutic procedure in medicine. Due to the introduction of drug-eluting stents with controlled release of antiproliferative agents, the risk of NIH and repeat revascularization has decreased.[15]

Coronary drug-eluting stents have changed over the years. These DES have three components: the metallic stent platform, a polymer coating, and an antiproliferative agent. Platforms are made of stainless steel, cobalt-chromium, or platinum-chromium. Cobalt-chromium and platinum-chromium stents have improved radial strength allowing for greater deliverability with thinner struts when compared to stainless steel. These thinner struts may also result in less arterial injury and decrease the thrombogenicity of the stents. The polymer coatings contain the drug and permit a controlled release. The biocompatibility of the polymers is very important to decrease local inflammatory reactions and thrombosis.[15]

As stents have moved from stainless steel platforms to cobalt-chromium platforms and more biocompatible durable coatings, the antiproliferative agents have shifted as well. Early generation stents released sirolimus or paclitaxel, whereas new generation stents release everolimus or zotarolimus. In a meta-analysis involving 38 trials and more than 18,000 patients, there was marked reduction in the rate of repeat revascularization with both sirolimus-eluting stents and paclitaxel-eluting stents, as compared to bare metal stents.[16] Although the risks of death and myocardial infarction (MI) with sirolimus-eluting and paclitaxel-eluting stents were similar to bare metal stents, these DES were associated with an increased risk of very late stent thrombosis. After this, randomized trials showed that everolimus-eluting stents improved clinical outcomes as compared with paclitaxel-eluting stents, reducing the risks of repeat revascularization, MI, and stent thrombosis. The Endeavor zotarolimus-eluting stent has also been shown to reduce the risk of MI without compromising effectiveness as compared with paclitaxel-eluting stents. When comparing the Endeaver zotarolimus-eluting stents with sirolimus-eluting stents, there was no difference in thrombosis at three years. However, it was shown that a higher risk of repeat revascularization was seen among patients treated with Endeavor zotarolimus-eluting stents and patients treated with sirolimus-eluting stents had a higher risk of very late stent thrombosis.[15]

Stent restenosis and thrombosis are the major complications with coronary stents. This occurs most frequently in the first year after percutaneous coronary interventions and may present as MI. Due to this, almost all patients receiving coronary stents are prescribed a combination of aspirin and another antiplatelet agent for some time after stenting. This is referred to as dual antiplatelet therapy (DAPT). To determine which antithrombotic drug regimen was best, the STARS trial (stent anticoagulation restenosis trial) compared three different regimens after coronary stenting with bare metal stents. In this study, 1653 patients were treated with aspirin alone, aspirin and warfarin, or aspirin and ticlopidine. The primary end point included all events reflecting stent thrombosis within 30 days such as death, revascularization of the target lesion, angiographically documented thrombosis, or MI. The incidence of the primary endpoint was 3.6% in the aspirin-alone group, 2.7% in the aspirin and warfarin group, and only 0.5% in the aspirin and ticlopidine group showing that overall treatment with combination aspirin and ticlopidine resulted in a lower rate of stent thrombosis.[17] Because of side effects such as skin disorders, gastrointestinal symptoms, and allergic adverse events with ticlopidine, clopidogrel has been adopted as an equally effective medication to be used in combination with aspirin.[18]

When comparing antiplatelet therapy with BMS and DES, DES requires longer treatment times. Stent thrombosis most commonly occurs during the period of time that the stent is exposed to circulating blood. When the stent has been endothelialized, the risk of thrombosis falls. Most BMS are significantly endothelialized by one month and completely endothelialized by six months. From autopsies of patients who had recently received DES, evidence shows that it may take much longer than six months to completely endothelialize the stents.[19] For this reason, DAPT is prescribed for at least 12 months in stable patients receiving DES.

Due to the decreased risk of restenosis, DES represent an important advancement in treatment of coronary artery disease. These stents have evolved to stronger, thinner, less thrombogenic devices with more durable polymers and more effective antiproliferative agents. Exploring the use of these DES in other vascular areas could reveal more cost-effective permanent solutions to PAD.

Peripheral Drug-Eluting Stents

Although DES were successful in the coronary arteries, initial trials of peripheral DES were less successful. When treating SFA occlusions, restenosis is an especially important complication to consider. Although a stent can act as a scaffold to keep vessels open in the short term, stents alone cannot prevent NIH and may actually promote NIH due to stent vessel interaction. As already discussed, drug-eluting stents have been very successful in preventing NIH in the coronary arteries. To evaluate the safety of using drug-eluting stents in the SFA, the SIROCCO II trial randomized 57 patients to receive a S.M.A.R.T.® Nitinol Self-expanding stent (Cordis Corporation, Miami Lakes, FL) or a bare metal stent in the SFA. The eligible patients were at least 30 years of age with symptomatic peripheral artery disease classified as Rutherford stages 1–4 (Table 24-1).

They all had obstructive, native, de novo, or restenotic lesions with a diameter stenosis of at least 70% in the SFA. S.M.A.R.T.® Nitinol Self-expanding stents were used. The S.M.A.R.T® stent coating had a thickness of ≈5 μm and was composed of an elastic copolymer combined with sirolimus in a 30:70 drug:copolymer weight ratio. The amount of drug per vessel area is equivalent to that used in the coronary applications (90 μg/cm²). All stents were 80 mm in length and 6–7 mm in diameter. Angiograms were then obtained at baseline and at the six-month follow-up visit. Restenosis was defined as a diameter stenosis of at least 50% within the treated segment at follow-up. Of the 57 patients enrolled in the study, eligible angiographic data was available on 50. All analyses were performed on an intent-to-treat basis. There was no statistically significant difference in the primary end point of final in-stent mean lumen diameter between the groups. There were two stent fractures in each group. There was no significant difference in other adverse effects in each group.[20]

The first-in-human Superficial Femoral Artery Treatment with Drug-Eluting Stents (STRIDES) trial was then designed to help address some of these shortcomings. This trial provided a higher level of drug delivery to target tissue, longer profile of elution, and a more flexible design to prevent stent fractures. The trial enrolled 104 patients in a prospective, nonrandomized, single-arm trial. Patients were eligible for enrollment if they had symptomatic PAD due to a single de novo or restenotic lesion of the SFA or proximal popliteal artery. Lesions had to have at least 50% stenosis. An everolimus-eluting peripheral stent was composed of three components: the Dynalink® nitinol self-expanding stent (Abbot Vascular, Abbott Park, IL), the antiproliferative drug everolimus, and an ethylene vinyl alcohol copolymer. This combination is referred to as the "Dynalink-E" stent. This stent system was designed with a relatively high drug load of 225 ug/cm² and long elution profile. Following diagnostic arteriography and systemic anticoagulation, drug-eluting stents in lengths of 28, 80, and 100 mm were implanted in the SFA. Clinical improvement, defined as a sustained decrease in Rutherford–Becker clinical category (Table 24-1), was achieved in 80% of patients. Primary patency was 94% ± 2.3% and 68% ± 4.6% at 6 and 12 months, respectively. There was no evidence for stent fracture in plain radiographic examination of 122 implanted devices. This 68% primary patency rate at 12 months is only a modest improvement in outcomes compared with previous trials of bare metal stents.[21]

TABLE 24-1. PERIPHERAL DES TRIALS

Study	Description	Patency Rates
Zilver PTX single arm study. *The Journal of Cardiovascular Surgery.* 2013. 54(1):115–122	12-month results of the Zilver® PTX® Single-Arm Study for TASC C/D de novo lesion subgroup in above-the-knee femoropopliteal artery	77.6% primary patency rate, an 84.7% event-free survival rate, and an 85.4% rate of freedom from target lesion revascularization
Randomized comparison of everolimus-eluting versus bare-metal stents in patients with critical limb ischemia and infrapopliteal arterial occlusive disease. *Journal of Vascular Surgery.* 2012. 55(2):390–398	74 patients were treated with Xience V DES and 66 patients were treated with Vision BMS in the infrapopliteal arteries	After 12 months, the primary patency rate after treatment with Xience V was 85% compared with 54% after treatment with Vision
Paclitaxcel-coated balloon plus bare metal stent vs. sirolimus-eluting stent in de novo lesions: an IVUS study. *European Society of Cardiology.* 2012. 8(4):450–455	IVUS study, nine-month follow-up 26 patients were treated with Cypher(®) DES and 29 patients with DCB/BMS in peripheral arteries	Significantly higher in-stent restenosis in the DCB/BMS group (19.7 vs. 11 %, $P < .01$)
Sirolimus-eluting stents for treatment of infrapopliteal arteries reduce clinical event rate compared to bare-metal stents. *Journal of the American College of Cardiology.* 2012. 60(7):587–591	Follow-up of prospective, randomized, multicenter, double-blind trial comparing polymer-free SES with placebo-coated BMS in the treatment of focal infrapopliteal de novo lesions, 161 patients	Target vessel revascularization rates at about 34 months were 9.2% in the SES group and 20% in the BMS group ($P = .06$)
ACHILLES trial, 1 year results. *Journal of the American College of Cardiology.* 2012. 60(22):2290–2295	200 patients were randomized to infrapopliteal serolimus eluting stent placement or PTA	At one year, there were lower angiographic restenosis rates (22.4% vs. 41.9%, $P = .019$) and greater vessel patency (75.0% vs. 57.1%, $P = .025$) in the SES group
Sirolimus-eluting stents for the treatment of infrapopliteal arteries in chronic limb ischemia: long-term clinical and angiographic follow-up. *Journal of Endovascular Therapy: An Official Journal of the International Society of Endovascular Specialists.* 2012. 19(1):12–19	2004–2009, 158 patients with chronic lower limb ischemia (Rutherford categories 3–6) underwent primary SES placement in focal infrapopliteal lesions	The primary patency rates were 97.0% after six months, 87.0% after 12 months, and 83.8% at 60 months
Sirolimus-eluting versus bare nitinol stent for obstructive superficial femoral artery disease: the SIROCCO II trial. *Journal of Vascular and Interventional Radiology.* 2005 Mar;16(3):331–338	Randomized, double-blind study involved 57 patients (29 in the sirolimus-eluting stent group and 28 in the bare stent group) with chronic limb ischemia and SFA occlusions or stenoses	There was no statistically significant difference between treatment groups in the in-stent mean lumen diameter at six months

Study	Description	Patency Rates
Paclitaxel-eluting stents show superiority to balloon angioplasty and bare metal stents in femoropopliteal disease: twelve-month Zilver PTX randomized study results. *Circulation. Cardiovascular Interventions.* 2011. 4(5):495–504	Patients were randomly assigned to primary DES implantation ($n = 236$) or PTA ($n = 238$) in femoropopliteal arteries	Compared with the PTA group, the primary DES group exhibited superior 12-month event-free survival (90.4% vs. 82.6%; $P = .004$) and primary patency (83.1% vs. 32.8%; $P < .001$)
Nitinol stents with polymer-free paclitaxel coating for lesions in the superficial femoral and popliteal arteries above the knee: twelve-month safety and effectiveness results from the Zilver PTX single-arm clinical study. *Journal of Endovascular Therapy.* 2011. 18(5):613–23.	787 patients enrolled in a prospective, single-arm, multicenter clinical study evaluating the Zilver® PTX® drug-eluting stent for treating the above-the-knee femoropopliteal segment	The 12-month Kaplan–Meier estimates included an 89.0% event-free survival rate, an 86.2% primary patency rate, and a 90.5% rate of freedom from target lesion revascularization
Primary everolimus-eluting stenting versus balloon angioplasty with bailout bare metal stenting of long infrapopliteal lesions for treatment of critical limb ischemia. *Journal of Endovascular Therapy: An Official Journal of the International Society of Endovascular Specialists.* 2011. 18(1):1–12	81 patients evaluated for long-term outcomes of a single-center prospective study investigating primary placement of everolimus-eluting metal stents for recanalization of long infrapopliteal lesions compared to a matched historical control group treated with plain balloon angioplasty and provisional placement of bare metal stents in a bailout manner	Up to three years, lesions fully covered with everolimus-eluting stents were associated with significantly higher primary patency hazard ratio (HR) 7.98, 95% CI 3.69–17.25, $P < .0001$], reduced binary restenosis (HR 2.94, 95% CI 1.74–4.99, $P < .0001$), and improved overall event-free survival (HR 2.19, 95% CI 1.16–.13, $P = .015$)
First clinical trial of nitinol self-expanding everolimus-eluting stent implantation for peripheral arterial occlusive disease. *Journal of Vascular Surgery.* 2011. 54(2):394–401	104 patients with symptomatic superficial femoral and proximal popliteal arterial occlusive disease received a novel self-expanding drug-eluting stent designed to slowly release everolimus to prevent restenosis following peripheral arterial intervention	Primary patency (freedom from ≥50% in-stent restenosis) was 94 ± 2.3% and 68 ± 4.6% at 6 and 12 months, respectively
Preventing leg amputations in critical limb ischemia with below-the-knee drug-eluting stents: the PaRADISE trial. *Journal of the American College of Cardiology.* 2010. 55(15):1580–1589	106 patients (118 limbs) were treated with DES in a prospective, nonrandomized trial	Target limb revascularization occurred in 15% of patients, and repeat angiography in 35% of patients revealed a binary restenosis in 12%. The three-year cumulative incidence of amputation was 6 ± 2%, survival was 71 ± 5%, and amputation-free-survival was 68 ± 5%
Primary use of sirolimus-eluting stents in the infrapopliteal arteries. *Journal of Endovascular Therapy: An Official Journal of the International Society of Endovascular Specialists.* 2010. 17(4):480–487	A prospective single-center study was conducted involving 146 consecutive patients with Rutherford–Becker categories 2–5 lower limb ischemia who underwent SES placement in the infrapopliteal arteries	104 patients were evaluated at the 6- and 12-month follow-up examinations. After six months and one year, the primary patency rates were 88.5% and 83.7%, respectively. The mean ABI increased from 0.6 ± 0.4 at baseline to 0.8 ± 0.2 after six months and remained significantly improved during one-year follow-up ($P < .0001$). The mean Rutherford–Becker classification decreased from 3.3 ± 0.8 at baseline to 0.9 ± 1.1 ($P < .0001$) after one year

Study	Description	Patency Rates
Drug-eluting tibial stents: objective patency determination. *Journal of Vascular and Interventional Radiology.* 2010. 21(12):1825–1829	Reviewed medical records of 240 patients who underwent 283 tibial angioplasty procedures to treat limb-threatening ischemia during the four-year period. Balloon-expandable paclitaxel-eluting stents were used in all patients	Target lesion patency of the drug-eluting tibial stent was 73% at 24 months (SE < 10%). Limb salvage rate in patients treated with drug-eluting tibial stents was 86% at 26 months (SE < 10%), and the survival rate was 65% at 24 months (SE < 10%)
The evaluation of primary stenting of sirolimus-eluting versus bare-metal stents in the treatment of atherosclerotic lesions of crural arteries. *European Radiology.* 2009. 19(4):966–974	Patients were randomly divided into two groups: (1) patients treated with sirolimus-eluting stents and (2) patients treated with bare stents. Each group consisted of 25 patients, and every patient had one stent implanted	The follow-up angiographic examination demonstrated a significantly lower rate of restenosis among the sirolimus-eluting stent group (4, 16%) vs. the bare stent group (19, 76%) ($P < .001$), with lower target lesion revascularization in three (12%) vs. 14 (56%) ($P < .05$), respectively
Infrapopliteal application of sirolimus-eluting versus bare metal stents for critical limb ischemia: analysis of long-term angiographic and clinical outcome. *Journal of Vascular and Interventional Radiology.* 2009. 20(9):1141–1150	A single-center double-arm prospective registry included patients with CLI who underwent infrapopliteal revascularization with angioplasty and "bailout" use of an SES or BMS. 103 patients were included in the analysis; 41 (75.6% with diabetes) were treated with a BMS (47 limbs; 77 lesions) and 62 (87.1% with diabetes) with an SES (75 limbs; 153 lesions)	At three years, SES-treated lesions were associated with significantly better primary patency (hazard ratio HR], 4.81; 95% CI, 2.91–7.94; $P < .001$), reduced binary restenosis (HR, 0.38; 95% CI, 0.25–0.58; $P < .001$), and better repeat intervention-free survival (HR, 2.56; 95% CI, 1.30–5.00; $P = .006$) vs. BMS-treated ones
Sirolimus-eluting stents for the treatment of obstructive superficial femoral artery disease: six-month results. *Circulation.* 2002 Sep 17;106(12):1505–1509	36 patients were recruited for this double-blind, randomized, prospective trial. 18 patients received sirolimus-eluting SMART stents and 18 patients received uncoated SMART stents	The in-stent mean percent diameter stenosis was 22.6% in the sirolimus-eluting stent group vs. 30.9% in the uncoated stent group ($P = .294$). The in-stent mean lumen diameter was significantly larger in the sirolimus-eluting stent group (4.95 vs. 4.31 mm in the uncoated stent group; $P = .294$)

Current Drug-Eluting Stents

Nonabsorbable: Nitonol and Biocompatible Polymers

As discussed above, sirolimus-eluting SFA stents showed a lack of significant benefit at 12-month follow-up. To investigate other methods of preventing NIH, the Zilver® PTX® Randomized Clinical Trial and Zilver® PTX® Single-Arm Study were designed. This trial investigated the safety and effectiveness of a paclitaxel-coated DES for treating femoropopliteal disease. The DES evaluated was the Zilver® PTX® nitinol stent, (Cook Inc. Bloomington, IN), which incorporates self-expanding, flexible nitinol stent platform with a 3-ug/mm^2 polymer coating of paclitaxel on its outer surface. The inclusion criteria for the randomized trial included Rutherford category ≥2 (Table 24-1), ≥50% diameter stenosis, reference vessel diameter 4–9 mm, lesion length up to 14 cm and at least one patent runoff vessel with <50% stenosis of the inflow tract and no previous target vessel stenting. The randomized trial included 238 patients randomized to PTA and 236 patients randomized to primary DES treatment. Then, 120 patients with acute PTA failure were subsequently randomized to provisional DES or provisional BMS placement. For the single-arm study, 787 patients enrolled were treated with the DES leaving 1084 total patients receiving the DES. Rutherford classification (Table 24-1), ABI, and Walking Impairment Questionnaire (WIQ) were assessed preprocedure. Stents were placed at least 1 cm below the SFA origin and above the medial femoral epicondyle to fully cover the target lesion. Procedural success was defined as <30% residual stenosis. For two-year follow-up, patients underwent clinical assessment for Rutherford classification, ABI, and WIQ. Of the 1261 patients enrolled in the complementary studies, 908 patients were eligible for two-year follow-up with data available for 781 patients. The rate of event-free survival (EFS) through the two-year follow-up period was statistically significantly superior for the DES group (86.6% vs. 77.9%). In the primary analysis for the randomized trial, the two-year primary patency rate of 74.8% for the primary DES group was significantly superior to the 26.5% for the long-term PTA subgroup. No adverse effects or reactions associated with the paclitaxel coating were observed through two years in either study. This long-term benefit after DES placement in femoropopliteal arteries has not been demonstrated previously.[22]

Absorbable: Abbott and ABSORB

There are many advantages bioabsorbable stents offer in comparison to bare metal stents. Metallic stents have the potential to develop late stent thrombosis if endothelialization is incomplete because blood will still be exposed to a foreign body. A bioabsorbable stent may have less potential for late thrombosis for this reason. Without a foreign body in the vessel, patients require a shorter duration of antiplatelet therapy. Furthermore, a metal stent might complicate future surgical approaches. Metal stents may also inhibit the artery's natural vasomotion and impair the ability of noninvasive imaging modalities such as CT and MRI to evaluate restenosis. A potential advantage of bioabsorbable stents is that they do not eliminate the potential for other drug applications such as angiogenesis and gene transfer. A bioabsorbable drug-eluting stent has the potential to provide the vessel with support and structure while avoiding the complications a bare metal stent poses and providing additional advantages.[23] It is important to weigh these potential long-term advantages of biodegradable stents with their limitations, which include lower radial strength, a relatively poor crossing profile, and their radiolucency on imaging placement.

The ABSORB family of trials (A bioabsorbable everolimus-eluting coronary stent system for patients with single de-novo coronary artery lesions) evaluates the bioresorbable everolimus-eluting vascular scaffold (BVS) in the treatment of coronary artery disease. Cohort A evaluates safety and performance in 30 patients at four sites with a single de novo lesion. Patients are evaluated at two-month, two-year, and five-year intervals. Cohort B of the ABSORB trial involves 101 patients at 12 sites with up to two de novo lesions with follow-up at two years. Patients are currently being enrolled in an extended trial to continue to assess safety and performance of the BVS stent at 100 sites.

For the first phase of the study, ABSORB A, 30 patients were enrolled at four sites in 2006 between March 7 and July 18. All patients had been diagnosed with stable angina, unstable angina, or silent ischemia. Vessels were 3.0 mm in diameter and all lesions were less than 14 mm in length, with the lesions less than 8 mm receiving a 12-mm stent. All arteries had stenoses of greater than 50%, but less than 100% stenosis. The BVS stent has a backbone made of Poly-L-Lactide Acid coated with poly-D lactide (PDLLA). This PDLLA contains everolimus and releases it in a controlled fashion. The stent material is slowly phagocytized by macrophages and by-products of degradation are metabolized by the citric acid cycle. All patients participating in the ABSORB trial were required to take aspirin (>75 mg) and clopidogrel (75 mg) for a minimum of six months.[23]

Stent sites were evaluated with quantitative coronary angiography (QCA), and minimal luminal diameter, reference lumen diameter, and binary restenosis values were obtained. Vasomotion was evaluated by recording mean lumen diameters using QCA after injection of either acetylcholine or methergin. Lumen stenosis was also evaluated with several other imaging techniques including multislice CT (MSCT) and phased-array intravascular ultrasound catheters.

After two years of follow-up, there was only one non-Q-wave MI related to non-flow-limiting stenosis. There were no incidences of stent thrombosis, all stents were qualitatively patent and calculated mean diameter stenosis was 19%. A significant decrease in minimal lumen diameter, reference luminal diameter, and luminal area was recorded at six months and remained significant at two years. Vasomotor studies conducted with methergin, acetylcholine, and nitroglycerin demonstrated vasomotor function remained intact. Between six months and two years, a significant increase in lumen diameter with a decrease in plaque diameter was recorded with grayscale intravascular ultrasound (IVUS). Optical Coherence Tomography (OCT) images showed homogeneous vessel walls, which indicates adequate healing of the artery. These results prove that the BVS is clinically safe for use.[23]

Although the BVS stent showed promising results in its first clinical trial, the polymeric scaffolds did show sign of late recoil, which resulted in late luminal loss within the first four months of use. The average late luminal loss was .44 mm, which is an intermediate length between the Xience V everolimus-eluting metallic stent and a bare metal stent. In order to address the late lumen loss, a second generation of BVS stents was manufactured with changes made to the stent platform. The new goal was to have an unchanged scaffold area (SA) without significant loss in lumen area. The new design uses zigzag hoops linked by bridges. This adjustment is designed to promote more uniform strut distribution, to reduce the amount of surface area in the vessel that is unsupported, and to provide uniform drug transfer. The new polymer has also been designed to degrade at a slower rate. This provides the vessel with support for a longer amount of time.[23]

The ABSORB Cohort B trial assessed the safety and efficacy of the second-generation BVS stent. In this trial, 101 patients with a maximum of two de novo coronary lesions were treated. In each patient, the stented segments were analyzed by QCA, IVUS, grayscale IVUS and vasomotion was assessed with nitrate. In three cases, additional drug-eluting stents were implanted due to a proximal stenotic lesion or to seal edge dissections that were caused by stent implantation. One patient received repeat revascularization due to recurrent atypical angina 42 days after BVS stent placement. At six months, planned angiography showed significant stenosis in the proximal end of the BVS stent in one patient. This was thought to be due to iatrogenic causes due to the location of the catheter at stent placement. Finally, one patient who underwent angiography at six months displayed proximal restenosis attributed to balloon miss on predilation during the placement procedure. There were three non-Q-wave MIs and six ischemic-driven target lesion revascularizations (TLRs).

The results from IVUS in the ABSORB COHORT B trial showed an increase in mean vessel area, total plaque area, and plaque area behind the struts. No compromise of the lumen was documented between 6 and 24 months. Significant enlargement of the mean SA was confirmed with OCT. The mean lumen area and flow showed additional decrease between six months and two years. The first-generation BVS stent used in the Cohort A trials showed a late loss of 0.44 mm at 6 months and 0.46 mm at 2 years. Late luminal loss in the COHORT B trial was significantly less with 0.19 mm at 6 months and 0.27 mm at 2 years. The new device also allowed vasomotion to be restored within the first year, but there was a significant increase in plaque media behind the struts evidenced by IVUS at two-year follow-up. The second-generation scaffold is also detectable at two years by various imaging modalities.

Abbott vascular has announced in a press release that they are currently evaluating the use of the BVS stent in BTK lesions in the ABSORB BTK study. This study involves 90 patients with CLI at 10 different sites in Europe and New Zealand. The study evaluates the treatment of de novo lesions <24 mm in length in the tibial arteries. The ABSORB 3.0 × 28 mm BVS system will be used. Patients will be assessed by duplex, angiography, OCT and MSCT, and MRI with a primary end point of freedom from major adverse events occurring within one year or periprocedural death.

Abbott vascular has also created an Esprit drug-eluting BVS specifically designed for use in peripheral arteries. The Esprit stent uses the same polymer that the Absorb BVS stent uses and delivers the same antiproliferative drug, everolimus. The Esprit stent has a different scaffold design however and comes in longer lengths to provide optimal treatment of lesions in the lower extremities. ESPIRIT I (A clinical evaluation of the Abbott vascular ESPRIT BVS [bioresorbable vascular scaffold] system for the treatment of subjects with symptomatic claudication from occlusive vascular disease of the superficial femoral [SFA] or common or external iliac arteries) is a single-arm, multicenter trial evaluating the treatment of one target lesion in the iliac arteries or SFA with a single 6.0 × 58 mm Esprit stent in 30 patients with symptomatic claudication. Subjects will be evaluated using duplex, angiograhy, IVUS or OCT, MSCT and MRI, and pharmacokinetic (PK) sub-study.

Treating lesions in the SFA has proven to be very difficult due to the unique forces that are exerted on the artery as it spirals down the leg. These distinctive biomechanical forces create a hostile environment for stents and predispose stents to restenosis. Bioabsorbable stents that do not leave a permanent prosthesis behind to promote restenosis will be especially important when treating lesions in the SFA. These stents have the potential to provide the same mechanical support to a vessel while allowing full recovery of endothelial function, clear assessment of stenosis with CTA and MRI, and shorter duration of antiplatelet therapy in addition to providing lower rates of restenosis than permanent stents. These characteristics of bioabsorbable drug-eluting stents may prove particularly important when treating vascular occlusive disease in the SFA.

SUMMARY

PAD affects millions of people around the globe. Although it is associated with great morbidity and mortality, a small percentage of affected patients have received the treatment that they need. With an aging population, we can only expect this patient population to grow. Since symptoms of PAD do not present until there is at least 50% narrowing of the vessel, significant stenosis and damage can progress fairly quickly after diagnosis. After a patient presents with symptoms of PAD, an abnormal ABI should lead to Doppler ultrasonography to confirm the diagnosis. The artery most commonly affected by PAD is the SFA. After diagnosis, the lesion can be classified and treatment can be decided based on the TASC II guidelines.

Although surgery was once the mainstay of treatment for SFA disease, surgery is now only indicated for very severe cases of PAD. Femoropopliteal bypass procedures have shown improved patency rates with autologous saphenous vein transplants compared to synthetic grafts. RSFAE was introduced as a less invasive surgical alternative to traditional bypass procedures but primary patency rates are inferior and there is no demonstration of a decrease in early postoperative complications. Due to these complications, endovascular treatment strategies have been gaining ground. Morbidity and mortality are lowered and only local anesthesia is necessary for these procedures.

Endovascular treatment offers many advantages over surgical approaches such as the use of local anesthesia and the ability of patients to return to their daily activities after only a couple of days in the hospital. Lesions in the SFA are characterized by intense calcification and scar formation. These properties cause angioplasty failure at rates of 70% and stent implantation was aimed at preventing this restenosis. Many RCTs failed to show improvement and stent placement was not recommended as a primary therapy for over a decade. The creation of nitinol stents with improved strength and flexibility finally showed improved results when compared to angioplasty alone. Impressive differences were noted between different types of commercially available stents and these prompted continued improvements in stent design. New drug-eluting stents hope to overcome the NIH that causes nitinol stents to become restenotic.

Drug-eluting stents were first introduced in the coronary arteries and were very successful. To avoid stent restenosis and thrombosis, a variety of stent platforms have been combined with different antiproliferative agents and coatings over the years. Since DES take a longer time to endothelialize compared to BMS, proper antithrombotic therapy is critical to prevent thrombosis. The use of DAPT for an extended duration of time has helped improve patency rates. The success of DES in the coronaries led to many trials of DES in the peripheral arteries, especially the SFA. Initially these trials did not show the same success rates that were shown in the coronary arteries. The Sirocco trials (Sirocco I & II) compared primary patency rates of S.M.A.R.T.® Nitinol Self-expanding stents and bare metal stents in the SFA and found no statistically significant difference in the primary end point of final in-stent mean lumen diameter between the groups. The STRIDES trial compared the Dynalink-E stent system in the SFA with BMS and displayed only a modest improvement in outcomes.

Next, the Zilver® PTX® Randomized Clinical Trial and Zilver® PTX® Single-Arm Study were designed to investigate the safety and effectiveness of a paclitaxel-coated DES for treating femoropopliteal disease. Here, there was a statistically significant improvement in primary patency rates for the DES after two years. The success of this study should lead to many more investigations into the possibility of using DES in the peripheral arteries.

Bioabsorbable, drug-eluting stents offer many advantages including less potential for late stent thrombosis, shorter duration of antiplatelet therapy and restoration of the artery's natural vasomotion. The BVS stent was evaluated in the ABSORB family of trials. Cohort A found no incidence of stent thrombosis and no decrease in vasomotor function, proving that the BVS stent is safe for use. However, a late average luminal loss of .44 mm was discovered, which prompted improvement in the BVS stent. The second-generation stent polymer degrades at a slower rate and is designed to provide more uniform structure and drug distribution. Late luminal loss was significantly decreased with the second-generation BVS stent. Due to the success of these trials, Abbott vascular is currently reviewing the use of the BVS stent in BTK lesions in the ABSORB BTK study. They have also created a new Esprit stent specifically designed to treat lesions in the lower extremities. Due to the unique, hostile environment of the SFA, bioabsorbable, drug-eluting stents may become a promising treatment option for lesions in this artery.

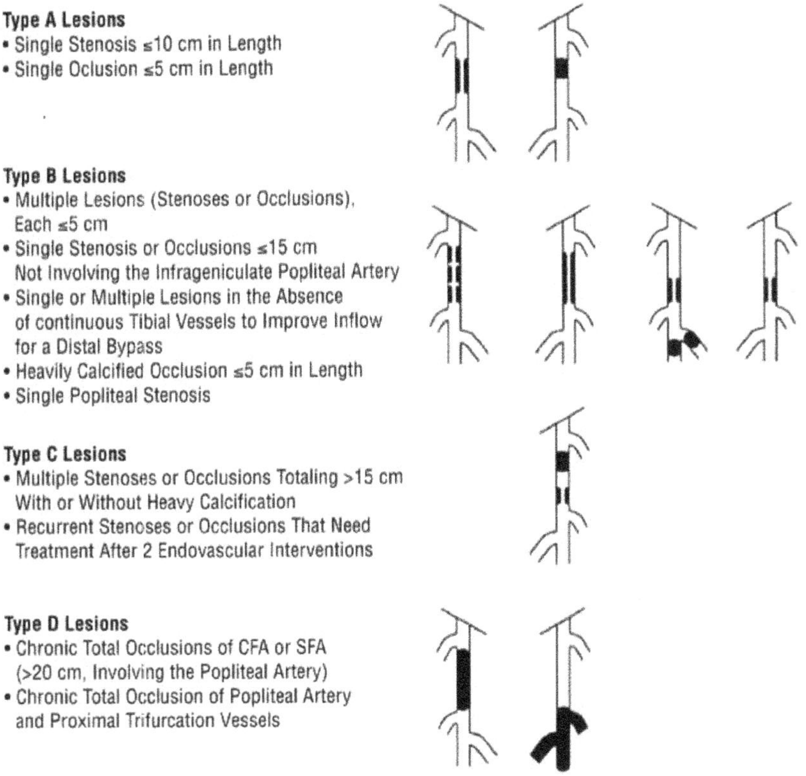

Type A Lesions
- Single Stenosis ≤10 cm in Length
- Single Oclusion ≤5 cm in Length

Type B Lesions
- Multiple Lesions (Stenoses or Occlusions), Each ≤5 cm
- Single Stenosis or Occlusions ≤15 cm Not Involving the Infrageniculate Popliteal Artery
- Single or Multiple Lesions in the Absence of continuous Tibial Vessels to Improve Inflow for a Distal Bypass
- Heavily Calcified Occlusion ≤5 cm in Length
- Single Popliteal Stenosis

Type C Lesions
- Multiple Stenoses or Occlusions Totaling >15 cm With or Without Heavy Calcification
- Recurrent Stenoses or Occlusions That Need Treatment After 2 Endovascular Interventions

Type D Lesions
- Chronic Total Occlusions of CFA or SFA (>20 cm, Involving the Popliteal Artery)
- Chronic Total Occlusion of Popliteal Artery and Proximal Trifurcation Vessels

Figure 24-1. Classification of femoropopliteal disease can be accomplished by lesion morphology with the Trans Atlantic Inter-Society Consensus (TASC II) guidelines.[3]

CONCLUSION

The evolution of nitinol stenting has facilitated important improvements in clinical outcomes following infrainguinal intervention. Further improvements may be forthcoming through new stent designs, more informed stent selection, and deployment, perhaps individually optimized through intravascular imaging. Assistance from drug elution will help achieve our realistic performance expectation, and combined with further evolution in stent design, whether permanent, bioresorbable, or biodegradable, we should be able to mobilize the required incremental performance enhancement to improve treatment cost-effectiveness and quality of life for patients with intermittent claudication. And if that is truly the case, then DES will replace most other types of interventions for PAD.

REFERENCES

1. Health Quality Ontario. Stenting for peripheral artery disease of the lower extremities: an evidence based analysis. *Ont Health Technol Assess Ser*. 2012;10(18):1–88. Epub 2010 Sep 1. http://www.ncbi.nlm.nih.gov/pmc/articles/PMC3377569.
2. Otsuka F, Nakano M, Sakakura K, et al. Unique demands of the femoral anatomy and pathology and the need for unique interventions. *J Cardiovasc Surg*. 2013;54(2):191–210.

3. Norgren L, Hiatt WR, Dormandy JA, et al. Inter-Society Consensus for the Management of Peripheral Arterial Disease (TASC II). *J Vasc Surg.* 2007;45(Suppl S):S5-67.
4. Klinkert P, van Dijk PJ. Polytetrafluorethylene femorotibial bypass grafting: 5 year patency and limb salvage. *Ann Vasc Surg.* 2003;17:486–491.
5. Devine C, McCollum C. Heparin-bonded, Dacron or polytetrafluorethylene for femoropopliteal bypass: five year results of a prospective randomized multicentre clinical trial. *J Vasc Surg.* 2004;40:924–931
6. Hunink MG, Wong JB, Donaldson MC, et al. Patency results of percutaneous and surgical revascularization for femoropopliteal arterial disease. *Med Decis Making.* 1994;14:71–81.
7. Gisbertz SS, Tutein Nolthenius RP, de Vries JP. Remote endarterectomy vs supragenicular bypass surgery for long occlusions of the SFA: medium term results of a randomized controlled trial (the REVAS trial). *Ann Vasc Surg.* 2010;24:1015–1023
8. Hirsch AT, Haskal ZJ, Hertzer NR, et al. ACC/AHA 2005 Practice Guidelines for the management of patients with peripheral arterial disease (lower extremity, renal, mesenteric, and abdominal aortic): a collaborative report from the American Association for Vascular Surgery/Society for Vascular Surgery, Society for Cardiovascular Angiography and Interventions, Society for Vascular Medicine and Biology, Society of Interventional Radiology, and the ACC/AHA Task Force on Practice Guidelines (Writing Committee to Develop Guidelines for the Management of Patients With Peripheral Arterial Disease): endorsed by the American Association of Cardiovascular and Pulmonary Rehabilitation; National Heart, Lung, and Blood Institute; Society for Vascular Nursing; TransAtlantic Inter-Society Consensus; and Vascular Disease Foundation. *Circulation.* 2006;113:e463-e654.
9. Schillinger M, Minar E. Past, present and future of femoropopliteal stenting. *J Cardiovasc Surg.* (Torino). February 2013;54(1 Suppl 1):141–149.
10. Schillinger M., Sabeti S, Dick P, et al. Sustained benefit at 2 years of primary femoropopliteal stenting compared with balloon angioplasty with optional stenting. *Circulation.* May 29, 2007;115(21):2745–2749. Epub 2007 May 14.
11. Rastan A, Krankenberg H, Baumgartner I, et al. Stent placement versus balloon angioplasty for the treatment of obstructive lesions of the popliteal artery: a prospective, multi-centre randomized trial. *Circulation.* June 25, 2013;127(25):2535–2541.
12. Laird JR, Katzen BT, Scheinert D, et al. Nitinol stent implantation versus balloon angioplasty for lesions in the superficial femoral artery and proximal popliteal artery: twelve-month results from the RESILIENT randomized trial. *Circ Cardiovasc Interv.* 2010;3(3):267–276.
13. Dick P, Wallner H, Sabeti S, et al. Balloon angioplasty versus stenting with nitinol stents in intermediate length superficial femoral artery lesions. *Catheter Cardiovasc Interv.* 2009;74(7):1090–1095.
14. Lenti M, Marucchini A, Isernia G, et al. Plaque debulking for femoro-popliteal occlusions: techniques and results. Source Unit of Vascular and Endovascular Surgery. *J Cardiovasc Surg (Torino).* February 2013;54(1 Suppl 1):141–149.
15. Stefanini GG, Holmes DR, Jr. Drug-eluting coronary-artery stents. *N Engl J Med.* 2013;368:254–265.
16. Stettler C, Wandel S, Allemann S, et al. Outcomes associated with drug-eluting and bare-metal stents: a collaborative network meta-analysis. *Lancet.* September 15, 2007;370 (9591):937–948.
17. Leon MB, Baim DS, Popma JJ, et al. A clinical trial comparing three antithrombotic-drug regimens after coronary-artery stenting. Stent Anticoagulation Restenosis Study Investigators. *N Engl J Med.* 1998;339:1665.
18. Bertrand ME, Rupprecht HJ, Urban P, et al. Double-blind study of the safety of clopidogrel with and without a loading dose in combination with aspirin compared with ticlopidine in combination with aspirin after coronary stenting : the clopidogrel aspirin stent international cooperative study (CLASSICS). *Circulation.* 2000;102:624.

19. Finn AV, Joner M, Nakazawa G, et al. Pathological correlates of late drug-eluting stent thrombosis: strut coverage as a marker of endothelialization. *Circulation*. 2007;115:2435.

20. Duda SH, Bosiers M, Lammer J, et al. Sirolimus-eluting versus bare nitinol stent for obstructive superficial femoral artery disease: the SIROCCO II trial. *J Vasc Interv Radiol*. 2005;16(3):331–338.

21. Lammer J, Bosiers M, Zeller T, et al. First clinical trial of nitinol self-expanding everolimus-eluting stent implantation for peripheral arterial occlusive disease. *J Vasc Surg*. 2011;54(2):394–401.

22. Dake MD, Ansel GM, Jaff MR, et al. Sustained safety and effectiveness of paclitacel-eluting stents for femoropopliteal lesions: two year follow up from the Zilver PTX randomized and single arm clinical studies. *J Am Coll Cardiol*. June 18, 2013;61(24):2417–2427. doi: 10.1016/j.jacc.2013.03.034. Epub 2013 April 10.

23. Ormiston JA., Serruys PW, Regar E, et al. A bioabsorbable everolimus-eluting coronary stent system for patients with single de-novo coronary artery lesions (ABSORB): a prospective open-label trial. *Lancet*. 2008;371(9616):899–907.

25

Reconstructive Options for Complex Groin Wounds

Claudia Chavez-Munoz, MD, PhD and Robert D. Galiano, MD

BACKGROUND

Complex groin wounds pose a serious challenge to patients and surgeons. They can occur in many patient populations across various surgical subspecialties, including those patients undergoing infrainguinal bypass,[1] femoral cannulation for cardiac and transplant surgery, and lymphadenectomies for urologic, gynecologic, or lower extremity malignancies.

The groin represents the most frequent site for vascular graft infections.[2,3] Groin wound infections complicate approximately 0.7%–7% of the lower extremity revascularization procedures that utilize open approaches.[1,3–6] Although the exact pathogenesis of a groin wound infection may be unclear, possible etiologies include the disruption of lymphatic channels and resultant seroma formation, moisture accumulation and skin maceration in intertriginous creases, and proximity to the genitalia and perineum, which are known to harbor various bacterial and fungal species.[1–3] Historically, the standard treatment for vascular graft infections in the groin was total graft excision with or without subsequent extra-anatomic reconstruction.[2–3] Such procedures resulted in limb loss and mortality rates of 10%–79% and 9%–58%, respectively.[2,3,7,8] Subsequently, with a better understanding of the blood supply to the muscles around the groin, muscle transposition flaps grew in popularity as an adjunctive measure in the management of groin infections. Among many advantages, muscle transposition flaps eliminate dead space and cover exposed grafts and prosthetic materials, thereby allowing for more thorough debridement of infected graft beds. Flaps have also been shown to increase local oxygen tension, augment immune cell and antibiotic delivery, and shorten hospital stay.[2,3,5] As a result of their more frequent application, both mortality and limb loss rates resulting from groin infections following lower extremity revascularization procedures have fallen dramatically (to 0%–14% and 0%–30%, respectively).[2,3] In addition, although less often described, muscle transposition flaps have been successfully used in the treatment of persistent lymphoceles.[7]

TABLE 25-1. POTENTIAL REASONS FOR GROIN WOUND COMPLICATIONS

Age

Immunosuppression

Obesity

Edema

Lymphedema

Hematoma

Anticoagulation

Lymphatic leak

Diabetes

Radiation

Renal failure

Re-operative procedure

ETIOLOGY AND INDICATIONS

There are many causes for groin wound infections and dehiscences (Table 25-1). In addition to being in a challenging anatomic area in terms of hygiene, most infections occur in patients who have underlying medical comorbidities including diabetes, renal insufficiency/failure, malignancies, or are obese, all of which can result in higher susceptibility to microbial infections. Obesity in particular is an underappreciated contributor to local wound complications, especially in patients with an abdominal pannus that overhangs the surgical incision. Meticulous protection of the groin incision in the postoperative period is a prudent measure to minimize maceration and chafing that can decrease skin barrier capabilities. Consideration should be given to use of advanced dressings including composite dressings designed for use on fresh incisions. These dressings combine an antimicrobial-coated foam dressing and a waterproof film barrier and can be very useful to decrease postoperative incisional complications.[9] There is also accumulating evidence that incisional negative pressure dressings may protect the surgical site in these vulnerable patients.[10,11]

TREATMENT OPTIONS

An evaluation of the patient as a whole allows treatment to be planned within the context of coexisting morbidities, socioeconomic considerations, and rehabilitative potential. It is prudent to select the initial procedure that delivers the best chance of success and minimizes iatrogenic morbidity. Our current algorithm for treating complex groin wounds is depicted in Figure 25-1.

DEBRIDEMENT AND NEGATIVE PRESSURE THERAPY

The first step in managing a complex groin wound is clearing the wound of devitalized and infected tissues and materials. Most commonly, affected patients present with a draining groin incision or local erythema, often with a fluid collection visualized on

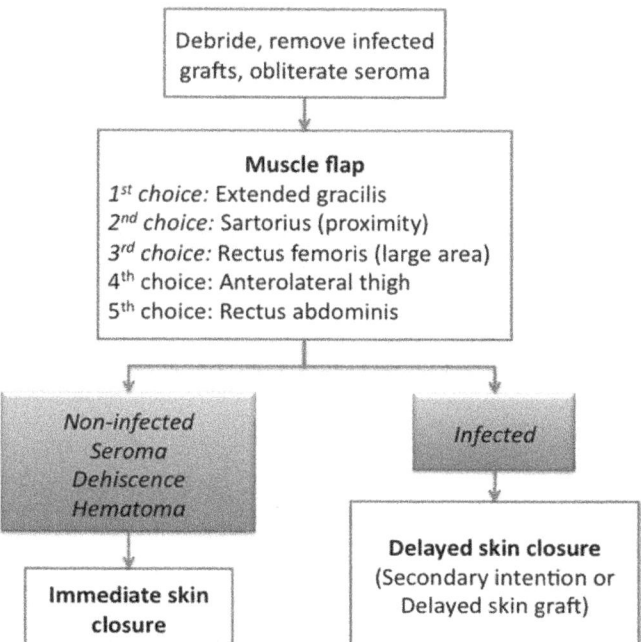

Figure 25-1. Algorithm for debriding and closing a complex groin wound.

radiographic imaging. Imaging is useful in delineating whether a fluid collection is present around a vascular graft or is located more superficially; this knowledge can be useful in planning the urgency and extent of surgical intervention. If synthetic vascular conduits have been utilized, prompt surgical exploration should be undertaken. The goals of surgical exploration should include—in addition to debridement—obtainment of tissue for culture and guidance of long-term antibiotic use; determination of the potential need for revision of the vascular graft or patch; and planning for soft tissue closure. Therefore, close cooperation between the vascular and plastic surgery teams is mandatory, particularly since the extent of contamination may not be apparent on clinical examination.

If the contamination is severe, it may be worthwhile to stage the closure to allow intravenous antibiotics and inpatient wound care with frequent dressing changes to decrease the bioburden before definitive reconstruction. This option, although prudent, must be balanced with the need to cover a vascular bypass graft to prevent catastrophic complications such as blow-out and anastomotic leaks. Clinical judgment and culture-guided antibiotics are the cornerstone of management of these difficult cases.

A valuable adjunct to the management of an open groin incision is negative pressure wound therapy (NPWT). NPWT is beneficial for decreasing lymphatic leak, reducing edema, clearing bacteria, and augmenting blood flow.[12] The sum effect is one conducive to healing, and since the dressings are impermeable, one can consider this a semi-closed dressing that minimizes environmental exposure of any underlying vascular grafts or repair sites. Several studies have demonstrated utility in bridging the complex wound between debridement and definitive closure and, in select cases, can be utilized for complete closure.[13,14]

A reasonable compromise in situations of infected wounds is to attain soft tissue coverage with a local flap but not to close the overlying skin incision. The benefits of this are that a drain can be placed underneath the muscle flap and then negative-pressure wound therapy can be placed on top of the exposed portion of the muscle flap, which serves as a "window" to allow edema fluid and exudate to be wicked away from the wound edges, while still ensuring coverage of the vascular graft or patch with a vascularized tissue bed. Definitive coverage is achieved in a delayed fashion with a skin graft or, if the area of exposed muscle is small enough, with closure by secondary intent.

STRATEGIES FOR CLOSURE UTILIZING MUSCLE FLAPS

The use of a muscle flap to cover exposed native vessels or to salvage prosthetic materials used in arterial reconstruction has proven beneficial.[2,15–17] As mentioned throughout this chapter, the goals of mobilizing a muscle flap are to achieve adequate coverage of any underlying vessel or prosthetic graft material and to eliminate or control infection in a single procedure that includes definitive closure of the muscle donor site. The transported muscle provides well-vascularized tissue, increases local oxygen tension in the area and enhances the ability of macrophages to combat infection. Furthermore, the overlaying muscle provides an ideal base for a skin graft, if required once deeper healing has occurred.[2] Our group prefers more definitive operations when possible, for example, graft removal and extra-anatomic bypass, or *in-situ* reconstruction with autologous or cadaveric homograft tissue, and muscle flaps are a useful adjunctive measure to enable these salvage procedures.

MUSCLE FLAPS

The option most commonly utilized for coverage of groin wounds is the sartorius muscle flap (Fig. 25-2). The sartorius muscle flap is a type IV flap according to the Mathes/Nahai classification system, meaning that the blood supply is derived in a segmental fashion. It has 6–10 segmental pedicles, but the ones that are pertinent are the first four. Most authors suggest that the first two to three can be ligated to allow the proximal part of the muscle to be dis-originated and transposed into the groin wound. The muscle can either be transposed for larger defects or simply flipped over for smaller defects. Benefits of this flap include its reliability, ease of dissection, and proximity to the defect. However, in many instances it may not be of adequate size or depth to reliably close off dead space and in addition does not reach more cephalic wounds extending above the inguinal ligament. For these reasons, our group at Northwestern prefers the use of the pedicled gracilis muscle flap for coverage of groin wounds after vascular surgery (Fig. 25-3).[6] Although the flap harvest technique can be a bit more challenging than that used to harvest a sartorius muscle flap, there are a number of advantages to the use of gracilis muscle compared with the more conventional rotational muscle flaps. First, patients with vascular disease may have an occluded superficial femoral artery (the vessel that supplies the sartorius muscle) so perfusion to the segmentally supplied sartorius muscle may be compromised in these patients. The segmental pattern is also an important consideration when three or more of the segmental pedicles must be ligated to create mobilization of the sartorius flap for

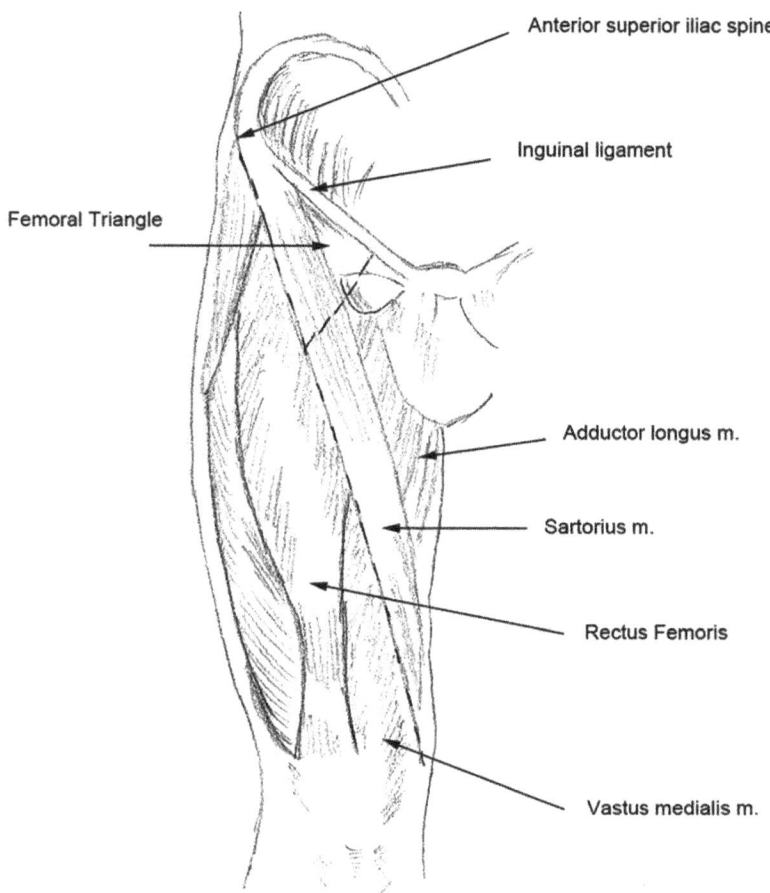

Figure 25-2. The sartorius muscle flap. This is traditionally considered the first choice for coverage of moderate size defects or wounds in the groin. Disorigination off the iliac spine and transposition of the proximal portion of the muscle to cover contents within the femoral triangle is readily achieved.

covering a larger area. Conversely, the blood supply to the gracilis muscle is derived from a single branch of the profunda femoris artery, which is more likely to be spared from atherosclerosis than is the superficial femoral artery. Second, the gracilis is a muscle that is located distant to the site of infection, from the bypass conduits and in an area that is simple to close primarily after harvest. Third, morbidity and functional deficits are fewer with use of a gracilis muscle compared with use of a rectus femoris or rectus abdominis flap, which are two other choices described for reconstruction of the infected groin.

However, the use of gracilis muscle for groin wound coverage has not been widely accepted, largely because of perceived difficulties involved with flap harvest and muscle flap. This misconception regarding flap harvest likely stems from the muscle's relatively remote location medial to the adductors and because of relative unfamiliarity with the dissection. In fact, isolation of the gracilis muscle by traditional methods may not provide adequate pedicle length to safely reach the groin. We circumvent this difficulty by using an extended harvest technique similar to methods previously described for other pedicled muscle flaps.[18]

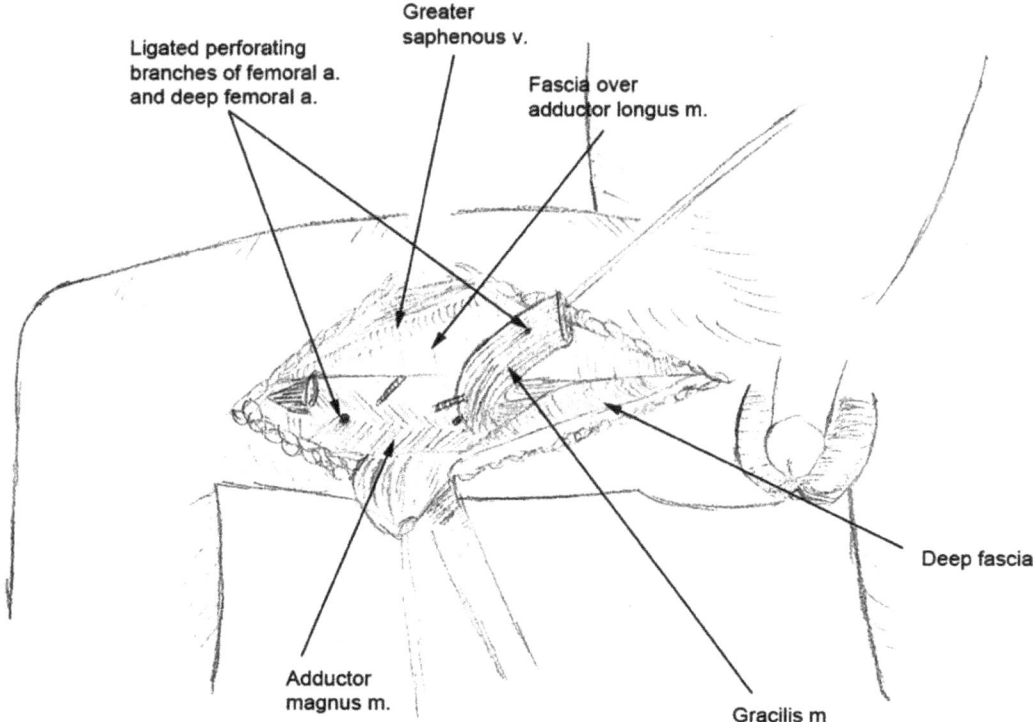

Figure 25-3. The gracilis muscle flap. This diagram shows the dissection of the gracilis muscle before being tunneled into the groin. The vascular medical (medial circumflex artery) is situated proximally (not visible). The length of the muscle allows it to reach proximally situated wounds in the groin; it can be tunneled subcutaneously or under the adductor longus muscle to decrease tension on the pedicle, particularly when the origin of the muscle is divided as well (the extended gracilis flap).

EXTENDED GRACILIS FLAP

The gracilis muscle has been widely utilized in reconstructive surgical procedures. The gracilis muscle is the most superficial and medial of the adductor group. It originates from the pubic tubercle and inserts on the medial femoral condyle. The dominant vascular pedicle comes from the profunda system, either as a direct branch or as the terminal branch of the medial femoral circumflex artery. The dominant pedicle can be observed entering the muscle on its medial surface, 5–10 cm distal to the pubic tubercle, as it passes in a fascial cleft between the adductor longus and the adductor magnus.[19–21] The advantage of extended harvest is that there is no tension on the vascular pedicle after the muscle is passed beneath the adductor muscle and positioned in the groin. In most cases, with extended harvest the flap will reach as high as the lower quadrant of the abdomen onto the external iliac artery. With extended harvest techniques the widest aspect of the gracilis muscle rests directly in the femoral triangle. Thus, this muscle can fill a fairly large defect. Liberal dissection of both sides of the adductor provides a full circumferential view of the gracilis' vascular pedicle. If this important step is not completed, pedicle tension and flap ischemia can occur.[22] Other local options, less frequently utilized, include the rectus femoris flap (Fig. 25-4), the rectus abdominus flap, and the anterolateral thigh (ALT) adipofasciocutaneous perforator flap (Fig. 25-5).[5,23–25]

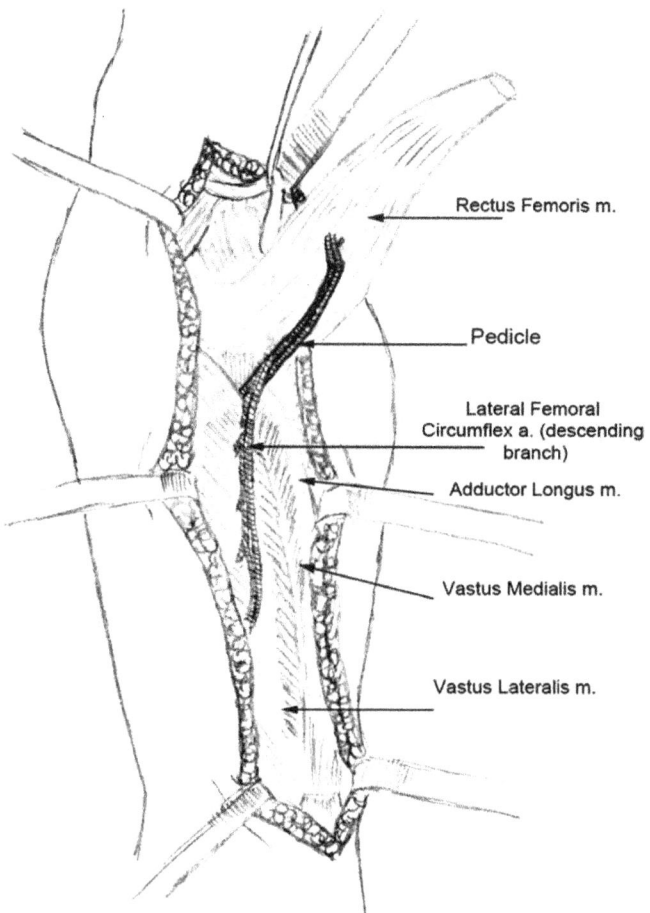

Rectus Femoris m.

Pedicle

Lateral Femoral Circumflex a. (descending branch)

Adductor Longus m.

Vastus Medialis m.

Vastus Lateralis m.

Figure 25-4. The rectus femoris muscle flap. This flap that is based off the lateral circumflex artery has the benefit of being a wide flap that is straightforward to dissect; it is most often used as a turnover flap. It has a thick fascial sheath on the undersurface which is removed by the authors before placing a skin graft.

PROPHYLACTIC MUSCLE FLAPS

Complex groin wounds are prone to myriad complications, including superficial cellulitis, lymphatic leak, deep wound infection, graft sepsis and even limb loss. These complications have been reported to occur in between 10% and 44% of inguinal procedures.[26] Patient characteristics such as obesity, smoking history, prior surgical procedures in the groin, radiation, and diabetes have shown to increase the risk of surgical site infections.[27] Additionally patients with surgical site infections or groin complications, in the setting of graft or prosthetic reconstruction, are at a fivefold greater risk for graft site infection.[28] These complications translate into increased patient morbidity and health care costs. The added cost of surgical site infection as of 2010 has been found to be between $4000 and $7000 per patient.[29]

In the effort to avert the morbidity and cost of these complications, it has been suggested to advocate aggressive, early, and—for the high-risk patient—prophylactic

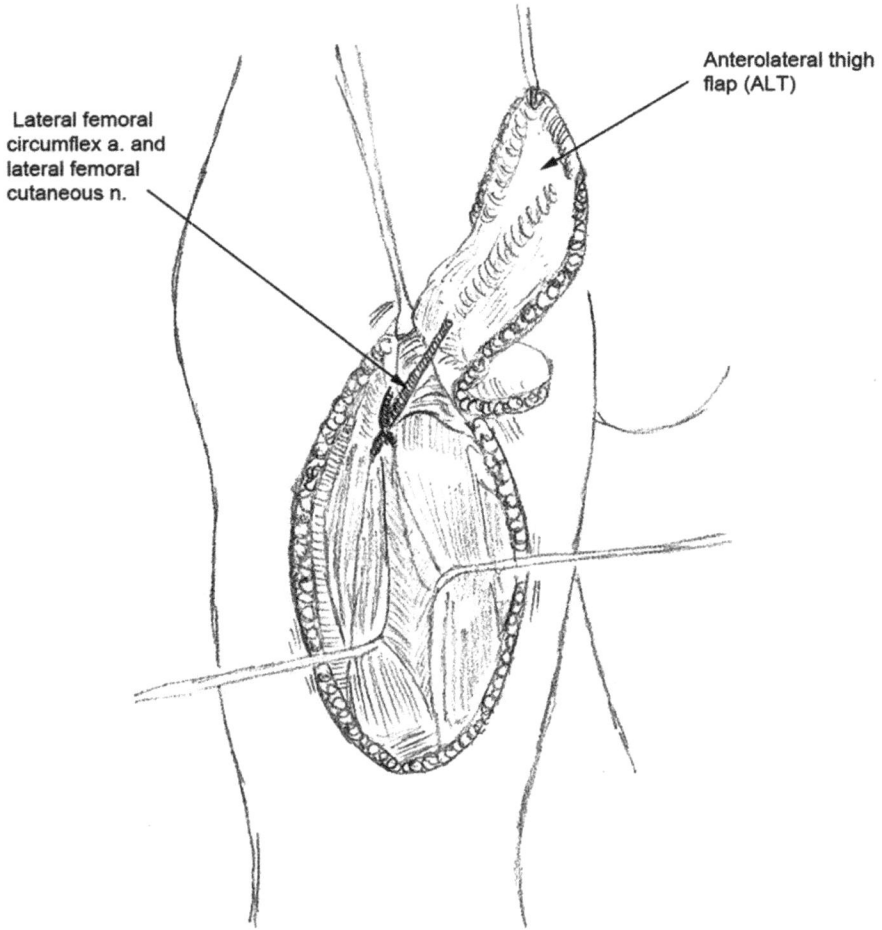

Figure 25-5. The anterolateral thigh (ALT) perforator flap. The blood supply to this flap usually comes off the descending or transverse branch of the lateral circumflex artery. This flap has the benefit of sparing all muscle, being a strictly adipofasciocutaneous flap. Although the dissection can therefore be quite tedious, it has the benefit of being a very large flap most often utilized by the senior author for sizable groin defects.

measures. A prophylactic muscle flap is defined as a flap that is utilized at the time of the initial procedure in a patient thought to be at high risk for regional groin complications following vascular surgery and is placed to "protect" the vascular graft or anastomosis from potential bacterial seeding from a skin wound dehiscence or infection. It has been demonstrated that prophylactic flaps exhibit protective effects by augmenting wound and deep tissue perfusion, reducing bacterial load, and obliterating dead space. Specifically musculocutaneous flaps have been shown in animal studies to reduce bacterial inoculum, inhibit bacterial growth, and optimize collagen deposition.[30] Prophylactic flaps may suppress bacterial colonization of groin beds through up-regulated blood flow through enhanced bacterial suppression in the first 24 hours of surgery, therefore reducing infectious complications. Our current algorithm for the use of prophylactic muscle flaps is depicted in Figure 25-6. The sartorius muscle flap has been established as an effective muscle flap and in most centers is the flap of first choice. In wounds with a significant volume of potential dead space following

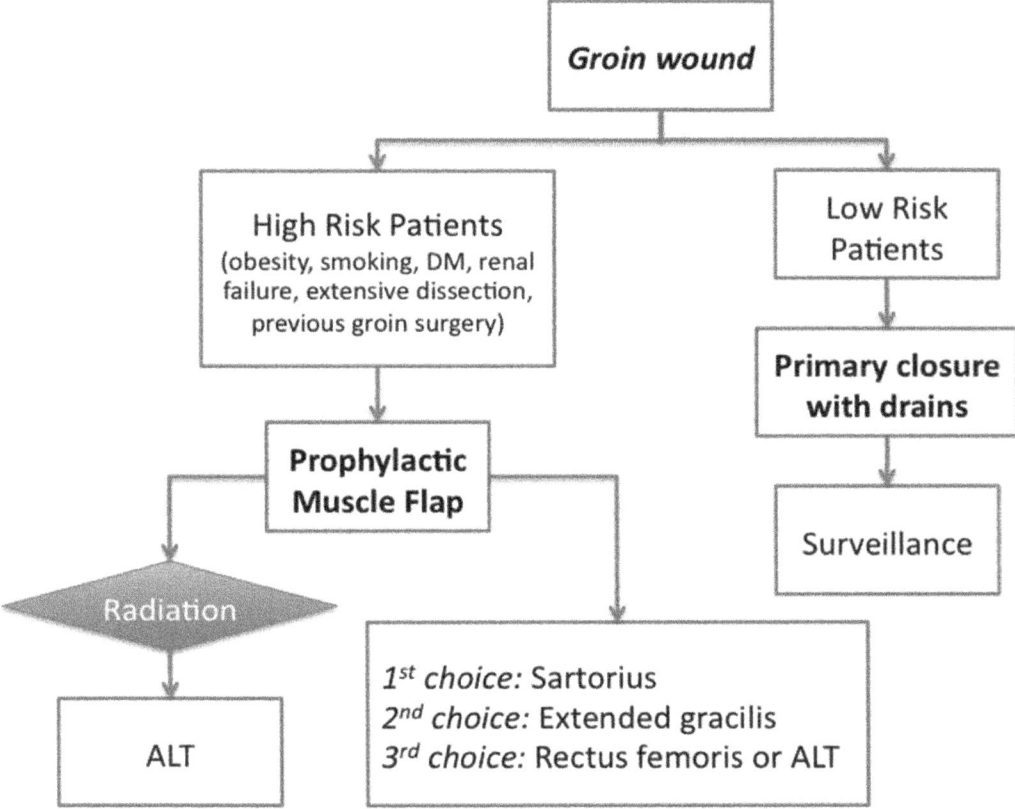

Figure 25-6. Algorithm for use of prophylactic muscle or local perforator flaps.

vascular intervention, our group prefers to use the extended gracilis flap due to its greater size and favorable patient outcomes. As a third choice, our group suggests the use of the rectus femoris muscle flap, which has not been shown to result in any significant functional deficit after muscle harvest.[25] Finally, the ALT flap is an excellent choice for large resections following oncologic surgery or when dealing with a large wound in an irradiated area.

In conclusion, performing prophylactic muscle flaps at the initial surgery in selected high-risk patients, such as reoperative prosthetic bypasses, has the potential to significantly reduce graft-associated complications and overall morbidity. The sartorius flap is an ideal prophylactic flap in high-risk groin surgery patients because of its proximity, easy mobility, effectiveness and low complication rate.

CONCLUSION

Close cooperation between vascular and plastic surgeons has led to increased rates of vascular graft salvage and ultimately limb salvage in a very challenging patient population. Muscle flaps have been demonstrated to reduce local complications, clear infections, and reduce overall morbidity and even mortality. In fact, muscle flaps are associated with sufficiently low morbidity that they should be utilized in a prophylactic fashion in patients at high risk for wound-associated complications. Further research to define and stratify at-risk patients will hopefully result in even higher rates of limb and graft salvage, which will be challenging to otherwise achieve as the incidence of obesity, diabetes, aging, and their related vascular complications continues to increase at epidemic rates.

REFERENCES

1. Szilagyi DE, Smith RF, Elliott JP, Vrandecic MP. Infection in arterial reconstruction with synthetic grafts. *Ann Surg*. 1972;176(3):321–333.
2. Graham RG, Omotoso PO, Hudson DA. The effectiveness of muscle flaps for the treatment of prosthetic graft sepsis. *Plast Reconstr Surg*. 2002;109(1):108–113; discussion 114–115.
3. Seify H, Moyer HR, Jones GE, et al. The role of muscle flaps in wound salvage after vascular graft infections: the Emory experience. *Plast Reconstr Surg*. 2006;117(4):1325–1333.
4. Dosluoglu HH, Schimpf DK, Schultz R, Cherr GS. Preservation of infected and exposed vascular grafts using vacuum assisted closure without muscle flap coverage. *J Vasc Surg*. 2005;42(5):989–992.
5. Illig KA, Alkon JE, Smith A, et al. Rotational muscle flap closure for acute groin wound infections following vascular surgery. *Ann Vasc Surg*. 2004;18(6):661–668.
6. Morasch MD, Sam AD 2nd, Kibbe MR, et al. Early results with use of gracilis muscle flap coverage of infected groin wounds after vascular surgery. *J Vasc Surg*. 2004;39(6):1277–1283.
7. Armstrong PA, Back MR, Bandyk DF, et al. Selective application of sartorius muscle flaps and aggressive staged surgical debridement can influence long-term outcomes of complex prosthetic graft infections. *J Vasc Surg*. 2007;46(1):71–78.
8. Calligaro KD, Veith FJ, Schwartz ML, et al. Selective preservation of infected prosthetic arterial grafts. Analysis of a 20-year experience with 120 extracavitary-infected grafts. *Ann Surg*. 1994;220(4):461–469; discussion 469–471.
9. Childress BB, Berceli SA, Nelson PR, et al. Impact of an absorbent silver-eluting dressing system on lower extremity revascularization wound complications. *Ann Vasc Surg*. 2007;21(5):598–602.
10. Blackham AU, Farrah JP, McCoy TP, et al. Prevention of surgical site infections in high-risk patients with laparotomy incisions using negative-pressure therapy. *Am J Surg*. 2013;205(6):647–654.
11. Conde-Green A, Chung TL, Holton LH 3rd, et al. Incisional negative-pressure wound therapy versus conventional dressings following abdominal wall reconstruction: a comparative study. *Ann Plast Surg*. August 3, 2012. Epub ahead of print.
12. Matatov T, Reddy KN, Doucet LD, et al. Experience with a new negative pressure incision management system in prevention of groin wound infection in vascular surgery patients. *J Vasc Surg*. 2013;57(3):791–795.
13. Colwell AS, Donaldson MC, Belkin M, Orgill DP. Management of early groin vascular bypass graft infections with sartorius and rectus femoris flaps. *Ann Plast Surg*. 2004;52(1):49–53.
14. Sumpio BE, Allie DE, Horvath KA, et al. Role of negative pressure wound therapy in treating peripheral vascular graft infections. *Vascular*. 2008;16(4):194–200.
15. Maser B, Vedder N, Rodriguez D, Johansen K. Sartorius myoplasty for infected vascular grafts in the groin. Safe, durable, and effective. *Arch Surg*. 1997;132(5):522–525; discussion 525–526.
16. Meyer JP, Durham JR, Schwarcz TH, et al. The use of sartorius muscle rotation-transfer in the management of wound complications after infrainguinal vein bypass: a report of eight cases and description of the technique. *J Vasc Surg*. 1989;9(5):731–735.
17. Thomas WO 3rd, Parry SW, Powell RW, et al. Management of exposed inguinofemoral arterial conduits by skeletal muscular rotational flaps. *Am Surg*. 1994;60(11): 872–880.

18. Moffett TR, Madison SA, Derr JW Jr, Acland RD. An extended approach for the vascular pedicle of the lateral arm free flap. *Plast Reconstr Surg.* 1992;89(2):259–267.
19. Giordano PA, Abbes M, Pequignot JP. Gracilis blood supply: anatomical and clinical re-evaluation. *Br J Plast Surg.* 1990;43(3):266–272.
20. Juricic M, Vaysse P, Guitard J, et al. Anatomic basis for use of a gracilis muscle flap. *Surg Radiol Anat.* 1993;15(3):163–168.
21. Lin CH, Wei FC, Lin YT. Conventional versus endoscopic free gracilis muscle harvest. *Plast Reconstr Surg.* 2000;105(1):89–93.
22. Hasen KV, Gallegos ML, Dumanian GA. Extended approach to the vascular pedicle of the gracilis muscle flap: anatomical and clinical study. *Plast Reconstr Surg.* 2003;111(7):2203–2208.
23. Alkon JD, Smith A, Losee JE, et al. Management of complex groin wounds: preferred use of the rectus femoris muscle flap. *Plast Reconstr Surg.* 2005;115(3):776–783; discussion 784–785.
24. Hsu H, Chien SH, Wang CH, et al. Expanding the applications of the pedicled anterolateral thigh and vastus lateralis myocutaneous flaps. *Ann Plast Surg.* 2012;69(6):643–649.
25. Sbitany H, Koltz PF, Girotto JA, et al. Assessment of donor-site morbidity following rectus femoris harvest for infrainguinal reconstruction. *Plast Reconstr Surg.* 2010;126(3):933–940.
26. Kent KC, Bartek S, Kuntz KM, et al. Prospective study of wound complications in continuous infrainguinal incisions after lower limb arterial reconstruction: incidence, risk factors, and cost. *Surgery.* 1996;119(4):378–383.
27. Bandyk DF. Vascular surgical site infection: risk factors and preventive measures. *Semin Vasc Surg.* 2008;21(3):119–123.
28. Antonios VS, Noel AA, Steckelberg JM, et al. Prosthetic vascular graft infection: a risk factor analysis using a case-control study. *J Infect.* 2006;53(1):49–55.
29. Menzin J, Marton JP, Meyers JL, et al. Inpatient treatment patterns, outcomes, and costs of skin and skin structure infections because of Staphylococcus aureus. *Am J Infect Control.* 2010;38(1):44–49.
30. Calderon W, Chang N, Mathes SJ. Comparison of the effect of bacterial inoculation in musculocutaneous and fasciocutaneous flaps. *Plast Reconstr Surg.* 1986;77(5):785–794.

Visceral and Renal Artery Disease

26

Technical Aspects of Retrograde Open Mesenteric Stenting

Neel A. Mansukhani, MD and Andrew W. Hoel, MD

INTRODUCTION

Acute mesenteric ischemia (AMI) is an uncommon condition with significant associated morbidity and mortality. As such, a high index of suspicion coupled with prompt, accurate diagnosis is a critical first step in management of AMI. The subsequent comprehensive treatment of patients with suspected AMI is essential for optimal outcome. In this chapter, we will discuss retrograde open mesenteric stenting (ROMS) in the context of optimal management of AMI. Discussion will include diagnosis and initial management, the role of laparotomy in AMI, and revascularization options in the management of mesenteric ischemia. We focus on the role of ROMS in the management of AMI and detail the considerations and steps for this technique. We will end with a discussion of the postoperative care, follow-up, and published outcomes for ROMS.

DIAGNOSIS AND INITIAL MANAGEMENT OF ACUTE MESENTERIC ISCHEMIA

While treatment for chronic mesenteric ischemia (CMI) is associated with a 30-day mortality of 3%, mortality in AMI is markedly higher and has been reported from 14% to 75%. Presenting symptoms include abdominal pain in 96% and nausea in 56% of patients with AMI. One must have a high clinical suspicion for AMI in patients with a history of several comorbidities such as atrial fibrillation, diabetes, hypertension, hyperlipidemia, smoking, chronic obstructive pulmonary disease, a history of multiple peripheral vascular interventions, or a history of CMI.[1] Not surprisingly, patients presenting with AMI frequently describe symptoms consistent with CMI such as postprandial abdominal pain and weight loss.[2]

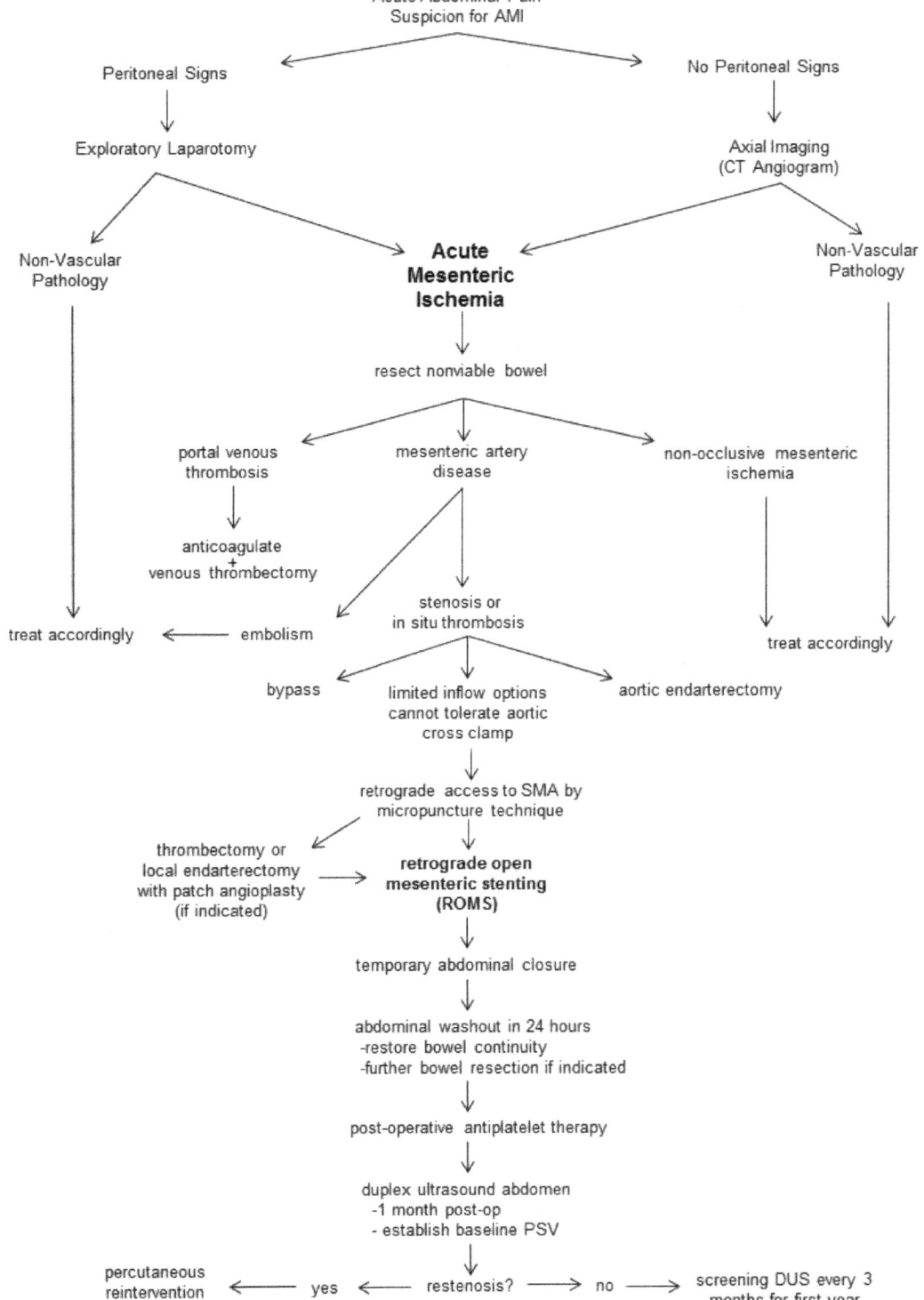

Figure 26-1. Treatment algorithm for patients with abdominal pain in which mesenteric ischemia is suspected. Adapted from Oldenberg et al.[3] and Falkensammer et al.[4]

In patients with suspected AMI, initial management should focus on accurate diagnosis, fluid resuscitation, and pain control. While patients with peritonitis and/or hemodynamic instability should proceed promptly to laparotomy with ongoing resuscitation, the majority of patients will undergo axial imaging (typically CT) as a key component of their initial work-up. Findings on CT will guide subsequent management. An algorithm for the evaluation of suspected AMI as well as the treatment is summarized in (Fig. 26-1). Beyond clear evidence of vascular occlusion, the findings on CT concerning for AMI include pneumatosis intestinalis, free fluid in the abdomen, and portal venous gas (Fig. 26-2). When an exploratory laparotomy is expedited without axial imaging, the first priority is establishing the diagnosis. Diagnosis of AMI is made or confirmed after visualization of ischemic bowel and/or signs of vascular compromise. This includes decreased or absent pulses in the case of mesenteric artery stenosis or thromboembolic occlusion and palpation/visualization of thrombus-laden mesenteric veins in the rare case of portal venous thrombosis. Angiography through femoral access can also be performed in this setting and is a useful adjunct in the diagnosis of AMI. After the diagnosis is made, it is important to decide on the optimal revascularization strategy. Although open surgical bypass is a reasonable, well-described strategy, ROMS is an appropriate alternative in many circumstances of AMI due to superior mesenteric artery (SMA) stenosis and/or in situ thrombosis. ROMS may even present a number of advantages when compared to surgical bypass. Patients may particularly benefit from ROMS when (1) inflow options are limited due to calcified or stenotic vessels; (2) conduit options are limited due to lack of available vein for a contaminated field; and (3) cardiac comorbidities preclude aortic cross clamp.

Outcomes for the treatment for AMI have recently been reported for various treatment modalities. In a high-volume tertiary referral center, postoperative mortality for AMI at 30 days and one year have been reported as low as 8% and 15%, respectively.[5] An independent and modifiable predictor of adverse outcome is prolonged symptom duration, with 30-day mortality as low as 14% for 12 hours or less time to intervention, and 75% for over 12-hour delay to intervention from time of symptom onset.[1] In a National Surgical Quality Improvement Program (NSQIP) series of 861 patients with AMI, bowel resection was reported as an independent predictor of 30-day postoperative

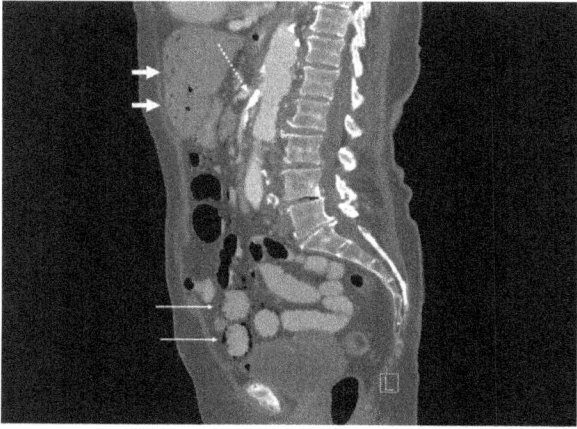

Figure 26-2. Representative sagittal image from a CTA on a patient that presented with suspected AMI. Note the pneumatosis intestinalis of small bowel in the pelvis (long arrows), portal-venous gas (short arrows), and the highly calcified proximal SMA (dashed arrow).

morbidity (56%) and mortality (27%)[6]; further suggesting that prolonged symptom duration is associated with worse outcome. Age is another factor associated with poor outcome. Age greater than 70 years is associated with 43% 30-day mortality, as compared to 23% 30-day mortality for age less than 70 years.[1]

LAPAROTOMY IN THE MANAGEMENT OF AMI

Exploratory laparotomy is warranted in the majority of patients presenting with AMI. In particular, patients with a concerning abdominal exam, laboratory abnormalities and characteristic findings on CT are more likely to need aggressive management. Furthermore, patients with AMI can present with an acute abdomen, particularly if they have prolonged symptoms before diagnosis. In these patients, mandatory laparotomy and visual inspection of the bowel are indicated. With findings of nonviable or ischemic bowel, temporary abdominal closure is often indicated even after definitive revascularization. This ensures that all nonviable bowel is removed and that intestinal continuity is safely restored in a subsequent procedure.

OPEN SURGICAL MESENTERIC REVASCULARIZATION

There are multiple options for open revascularization of the superior mesenteric artery applicable to both AMI and CMI. These options include autogenous vein graft or prosthetic bypass from a variety of inflow sites including antegrade bypass from the supraceliac aorta, retrograde bypass from the iliac arteries, or bypass from the renal or celiac arteries. In addition, local endarterectomy, and trans-aortic or "trapdoor" endarterectomy can also be performed if deemed suitable for these patients based on preoperative imaging.[2] In the treatment of CMI, a series of 80 patients had durable outcomes from aortic endarterectomy with a 3.7% rate of recurrent symptoms, compared to 10% symptomatic recurrence in patients who underwent open bypass procedure. Similar treatment in patients with AMI is associated with worse outcomes; in the same series, Mell et al. showed a 35% mortality for an aortic endarterectomy and a 28% mortality for bypass.[7] Although open surgical management remains common in the endovascular era, the significant associated morbidity and mortality with these procedures highlights an opportunity to pursue less invasive strategies for the management of AMI.

ENDOVASCULAR MANAGEMENT OF MESENTERIC ISCHEMIA

In the early 21st century, case series began showing promising results for endovascular treatment of CMI. In a 25-patient series of patients with CMI who underwent endovascular treatment for CMI, primary and primary-assisted patency at six months was 92%.[8] Another series of 59 patients with CMI showed a 96% procedural success rate. At an average of 39-month follow-up, 29% of patients had restenosis by angiography or duplex ultrasound (DUS) although only 17% of patients had recurrent symptoms.[9]

Mortality was compared for CMI and AMI over 18 years after intervention using the national inpatient sample; 6342 patients underwent percutaneous transluminal angioplasty and/or stenting (PTA/S), and 16,071 patients underwent open surgical bypass. In CMI, after PTA/S, mortality was 3.7% and 13% after bypass. In AMI, after PTA/S, mortality was 16% and 28% after bypass. Further analyzing the subset of patients with AMI, bowel resection after PTA/S was 3% and 7% for bypass, and mortality after bowel resection was 25% for patients treated with PTA/S, and 54% for patients after surgical bypass.[10]

In the largest series to date using an "endovascular first" treatment approach of AMI, there was a decreased mortality rate and decreased need for laparotomy. When treated endovascular, there was an 87% procedural success rate, with 69% of patients requiring exploratory laparotomy, 39% mortality, and an average of 52 cm of necrotic bowel. When treated with open surgical revascularization, 100% of patients were subject to exploratory laparotomy, with 50% mortality and an average of 160 cm of necrotic bowel. After initial endovascular treatment, patients were closely monitored and the decision to perform exploratory laparotomy was based on the presence of postoperative peritonitis or clinical deterioration. In the 13% of patients who failed endovascular treatment, mortality was 50%, equivalent to the mortality rate of open surgical revascularization.[11]

RETROGRADE OPEN MESENTERIC STENTING FOR ACUTE MESENTERIC ISCHEMIA—BACKGROUND

The endovascular-only treatment of AMI has the disadvantage of precluding visual inspection of the bowel in a patient presenting with acute signs of peritoneal irritation. The hybrid approach of ROMS was first described in 2004[12] and born out of necessity during intraoperative difficulties or failures of traditional open and endovascular treatment. When described in the early case series, surgeons had attempted open revascularization but were either limited by a patient who was too clinically unstable to tolerate an aortic cross clamp[13] or were unsuccessful due to a lack of antegrade or retrograde inflow secondary to severe calcification[14] or had failed initial revascularization using the endovascular first approach.[13,15] In one case report, the SMA ostium was covered during endovascular aneurysm repair (EVAR) rendering a traditional endovascular repair impossible. This was recognized intraoperatively during exploratory laparotomy and treated with ROMS.[16]

RETROGRADE OPEN MESENTERIC STENTING—TECHNIQUE

With either high suspicion or confirmed diagnosis of AMI, prompt surgical intervention is warranted. Here, we describe our favored technique for ROMS in a step-by-step fashion including the options and rationale for many of the steps. The use of a hybrid endovascular surgical suite provides optimal radiographic imaging; however, intervention can be performed with a mobile c-arm if necessary.

1. Position the patient supine with prep of the abdomen and bilateral groins. Prep of the left arm is occasionally helpful for retrograde brachial artery access. This possibility at the very least should be anticipated and the left arm placed on an arm board rather than tucked at the patient's side. The right arm should be tucked and it is generally most convenient to position the c-arm or fixed unit gantry on the patient's right side.
2. If the patient was brought to the operating room without CT angiography, diagnostic angiography can be performed at this time through femoral approach to image the

visceral arteries. However, with a high index of suspicion for AMI, direct evaluation of the abdominal viscera through laparotomy is the most efficient means for confirming the diagnosis.

3. Exploratory laparotomy is best performed through midline incision and should focus initially on inspection of the abdominal viscera and resection of gangrenous/perforated bowel with gastrointestinal staplers. Irrigation of any gross contamination can be performed at this time. Bowel anastomosis can be deferred until after revascularization.

4. Expose the superior mesenteric artery within the root of the small bowel mesentery distal to the middle colic artery by retracting the transverse colon cranially and the small bowel inferiorly and to the right. A diseased SMA can often be easily palpated in a thin patient. Incise the peritoneal lining over the SMA and isolate a segment of SMA proximally and distally and encircle with vessel loops. Side branches should also be controlled with vessel loops. The isolated SMA should be soft and of adequate caliber for sheath access. In addition, it is desirable to find an arterial segment that is relatively free of disease and as close to the origin of the middle colic artery as can easily be achieved.

5. Systemic heparin is typically administered at this point. We titrate the dose to achieve an activated clotting time greater than 275 seconds.

6. Retrograde access to the SMA is performed by micropuncture technique at a site of minimal disease with adequate caliber. We generally do not clamp the SMA or perform a surgical arteriotomy (i.e., with a knife) at this point until we have at the very least achieved wire access of the SMA—particularly if an endarterectomy appears likely based on preoperative imaging or the appearance of the vessel.

7. Occasionally thrombectomy is necessary, which can often also be judged by preoperative imaging or the appearance of the vessel. If this is the case, a longitudinal arteriotomy may be necessary with antegrade and retrograde Fogarty catheter thrombectomy. We generally use a 4-french Fogarty proximally and a 3-french Fogarty distally. After clot extraction, patch angioplasty can be performed before SMA stenting. While endarterecomy can be performed in conjunction with patch angioplasty, we do so cautiously and only if clearly necessary. This avoids the risk of passing a retrograde wire in a dissection plane at the proximal end of the endarterectomy.

8. Often a glide wire will easily cross a fresh in situ thrombosis at the origin of the SMA and the micropuncture sheath can be exchanged for a 25-cm, 6-Fr, or 7-Fr introducer sheath (Fig. 26-3). If the lesion is not easily traversed, a sheath is placed and a glide wire and catheter combination is used to traverse the lesion. In this case, it is often helpful to have femoral access so that aortography can be performed to establish a distal target. The use of a long, 25-cm sheath is preferable at this point because it avoids catheter and wire exchanges deep in the abdomen, which can be awkward, particularly in obese patients.

9. After traversing the lesion, a 5-Fr marker flush catheter is placed traversing the lesion. In a lateral projection, after removal of radiopaque retractors, simultaneous injection through the sheath and the flush catheter is performed allowing precise measurement of lesion length and vessel diameter.

10. A Rosen or other stiff wire is placed to the aorta traversing the lesion and the introducer sheath is advanced to the aorta. This occasionally requires predilation of the proximal SMA with a 3–4 mm × 4 cm angioplasty balloon.

11. Once the sheath is placed across the lesion, a properly sized balloon expandable stent or stent graft is placed in position, the sheath is withdrawn and the stent is deployed (Fig. 26-4). In general, we prefer the use of a stent graft in this situation for the potential

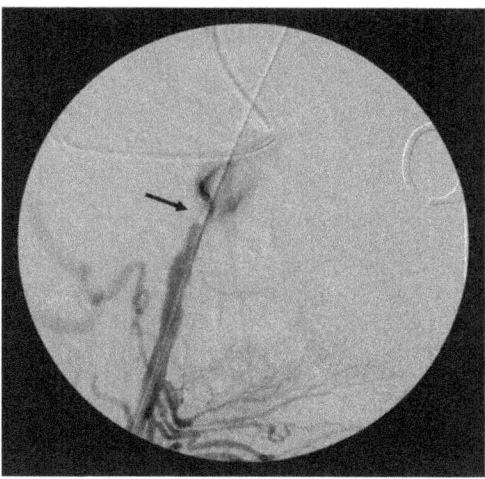

Figure 26-3. Retrograde angiography after wire access of the aorta from the SMA in the same patient seen in Figure 26-2. Black arrow denotes to proximal calcified high-grade stenosis of the proximal SMA.

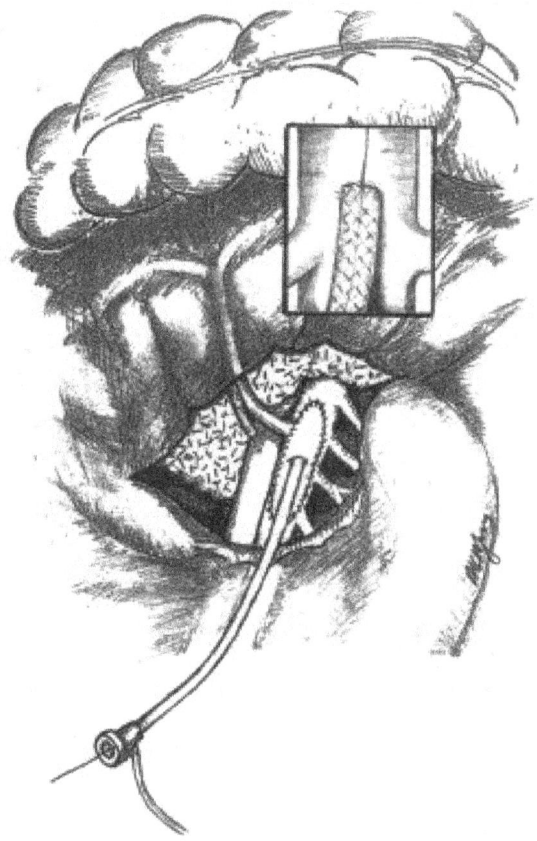

Figure 26-4. Line drawing of SMA exposure and access during ROMS demonstrating arterial access distal to the middle colic artery and placement of long introducer sheath. In this case, a longitudinal arteriotomy with patch angioplasty has been performed before sheath placement. From Wyers.[17] Used with permission.

to reduce rates of restenosis (see below). Postdilation and/or flare of the proximal portion of the stent can be performed at this time (Fig. 26-5). Completion angiography can then be performed through the sheath in both posterioanterior and lateral projection (Fig. 26-6). Manometry can be performed through the sheath or a catheter to confirm that there is no residual gradient.

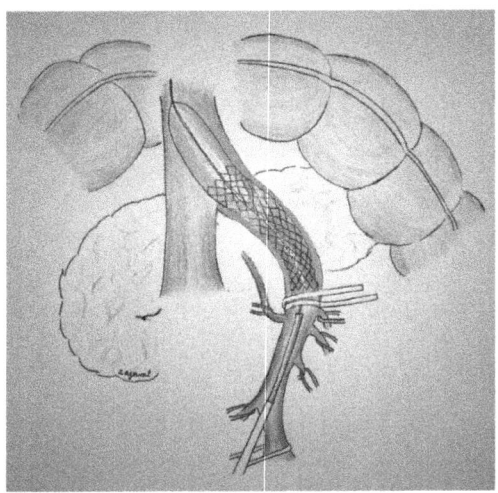 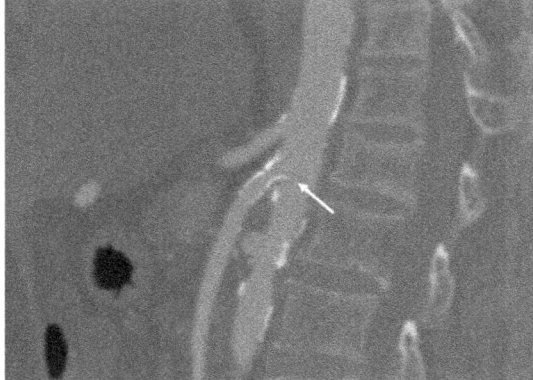

Figure 26-5. Proximal flare of the stent can be performed with a 2-mm oversized balloon, *A*. Follow-up CT angiography after SMA stent graft demonstrating a good proximal flare of the proximal portion of the stent, *B*, white arrow.

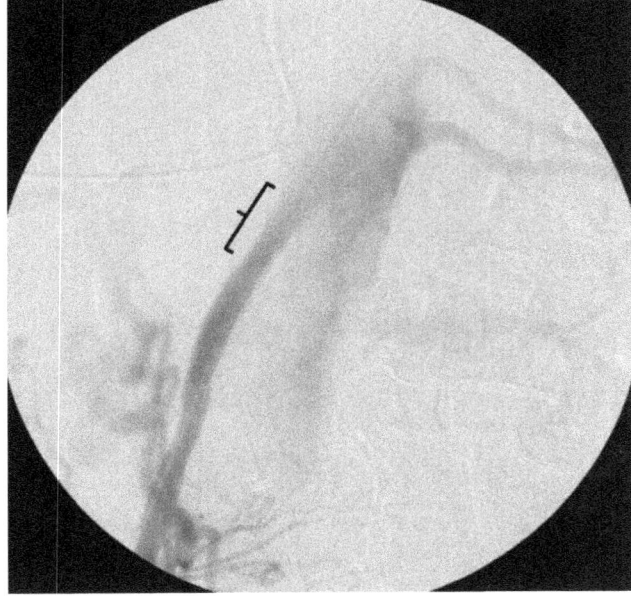

Figure 26-6. Retrograde completion angiography after stent graft to the proximal SMA (black bar) demonstrating brisk filling of the aorta and no visualized residual stenosis in the same patient from Figures 26-3 and 26-4. Manometry was performed through the sheath and demonstrated no pressure gradient.

12. Once satisfactory inflow has been achieved, wire and sheath can be removed and the SMA distal to the stent is controlled with concurrent control of branches and the distal outflow. If the SMA is not significantly diseased at the site of arteriotomy, it can be closed primarily in transverse fashion. However, if endarterectomy and/or patch angioplasty is necessary, it can be performed at this time. We typically use bovine pericardium or a vein patch for this portion of the procedure.

13. After the SMA is reperfused and hemostasis is confirmed, the peritoneum is closed over the mesentery and attention is returned to the abdominal viscera.

14. At this time, we typically perform temporary abdominal closure with planned washout in ~24 hours. Additional bowel resection or reanastomosis with restoration of gut continuity can be performed at reoperation.

POSTOPERATIVE CARE AND FOLLOW-UP

Patients should be started on antiplatelet therapy with aspirin immediately after the procedure if it was not initiated preoperatively. Clopidogrel should also be initiated as soon as possible and maintained for one month at minimum. After recovery we suggest follow-up imaging of the reconstruction. This can often be done with DUS, particularly in thin patients. We typically perform the first postoperative study at one month to establish a new baseline peak systolic velocity.

Surveillance

Endovascular treatment has been described as an option for bridge to definitive bypass as treatment of CMI in patients who are suboptimal for laparotomy and open revascularization due to poor nutritional status.[18] This is because of the high rates of restenosis observed following mesenteric stenting. ROMS is no different and close follow-up is warranted. We typically perform follow-up evaluation exclusively with clinical examination and duplex ultrasonography. The patient should undergo a mesenteric duplex at one month followed by every three months for the first year. As long as there is no evidence of early restenosis, we then expand the surveillance interval to six months after the first year postprocedure.

OUTCOME EVALUATION

Mortality

The first case series of ROMS showed low perioperative mortality of 16.7%.[13] Mortality at 20 months in this series was 66% and largely attributed to nonprocedure-related comorbidities, highlighting the poor overall medical conditions of patients with AMI. Table 26-1 lists all reported cases of ROMS since 2004. A total of 16 cases have been reported with generally low perioperative mortality that compares favorably to the overall mortality in the treatment of AMI (as noted above).

TABLE 26-1. CASE REPORTS AND CASE SERIES OF ROMS WITH ASSOCIATED OUTCOMES

Author	Year	Patients	Mortality Rate	Reintervention Rate	Outcomes
Milner et al.	2004	1	100%	—	Perioperative mortality due to multisystem organ failure
Wyers et al.	2007	6	Perioperative: 16% 20 months: 66%	16%	Perioperative: three required bowel resection, one perioperative death, five discharged home Follow-up: One alive and asymptomatic who required restent at 4.2 months One alive and asymptomatic One died of AML 20 months postop One died of presumed ruptured AAA one month post op One died of unknown cause 16 months post-op
Sonesson et al.	2008	6	33.30%	—	Two patients with atherosclerotic occlusion One patient with thrombotic occlusion with protein S deficiency who required extensive bowel resection (perioperative mortality) Three patients with acute SMA coverage during fenestrated graft placement, one with prolongued operation time, required bilateral fasciotomies for bilateral LE compartment syndrome, died perioperatively from MI
Do et al.[22]	2010	1	0%	100%	Asymptomatic one year post-op, required SMA restenting at nine months
Pisimisis et al.	2011	1	0%	—	Survived perioperative course, died at 11 months post-op secondary to advanced metastatic lung cancer
Sharafuddin et al.	2012	1	—	—	Series of 27 patients with attempted endovascular treatment of AMI. One treated with ROMS and considered failure of endovascular intervention. Outcome data not available

Secondary Interventions

The reintervention rate for endovascular treatment of CMI has been reported as high as 53%.[19] Primary patency for CMI status postendovascular treatment at one year is only 44%, with 100% primary-assisted patency.[20] Long-term complications and secondary interventions after ROMS for AMI likely roughly parallel those for other visceral stenting procedures. In the collected outcome data for ROMS since 2004, every patient requiring reintervention has been treated with percutaneous procedures. There is some data to suggest that the use of stent grafts in the visceral circulation is superior, particularly for complex and calcified lesions. The largest such report from Oderich et al. demonstrated a significantly lower rate of restenosis (92% vs. 53%, $P = .003$) and reintervention (91% vs. 56%, $P = .003$) as well as better patency at three years (92% vs. 52%, $P < .003$).[21]

SUMMARY

AMI is a condition with a variable presentation and a high morbidity and mortality. Therefore, the efficient and thorough evaluation and treatment of patients with suspected AMI is mandatory. The expanded use of endovascular procedures has the potential to improve patient outcomes compared to open surgical bypass in this patient population. Where an endovascular-only approach to AMI would incompletely treat irreversible visceral ischemia, ROMS allows less invasive treatment of arterial occlusion with concurrent direct evaluation and treatment of end-organ ischemia through laparotomy. As such, this technique is a useful adjunct for the treatment of AMI in this high-risk patient population.

REFERENCES

1. Kougias P, Lau D, El Sayed HF, et al. Determinants of mortality and treatment outcome following surgical interventions for acute mesenteric ischemia. *J Vasc Surg*. 2007;46:467–474.
2. Cho J-S, Carr JA, Jacobsen G, et al. Long-term outcome after mesenteric artery reconstruction: a 37-year experience. *J Vasc Surg*. 2002;35:453–460.
3. Oldenberg WA, Lau LL, Rodenberg TJ, et al. Acute mesenteric ischemia: a clinical review. *Arch Intern Med*. 2004;164:1054–1062.
4. Falkensammer J, Oldenburg WA. Surgical and medical management of mesenteric ischemia. *Curr Treat Options Cardiovasc Med*. 2006;8:137–143.
5. Ryer EJ, Kalra M, Oderich GS, et al. Revascularization for acute mesenteric ischemia. *J Vasc Surg*. 2012;55:1682–1689.
6. Gupta PK, Natarajan B, Gupta H, et al. Morbidity and mortality after bowel resection for acute mesenteric ischemia. *Surgery*. 2011;150:779–787.
7. Mell MW, Acher CW, Hoch JR, et al. Outcomes after endarterectomy for chronic mesenteric ischemia. *J Vasc Surg*. 2008;48:1132–1138.
8. Sharafuddin MJ, Olson CH, Sun S, et al. Endovascular treatment of celiac and mesenteric arteries stenoses: applications and results. *J Vasc Surg*. 2003;38:692–698.
9. Silva JA, White CJ, Collins TJ, et al. Endovascular therapy for chronic mesenteric ischemia. *J Am Coll Card*. 2006;47:944–950.
10. Schermerhorn ML, Giles KA, Hamdan AD, et al. Mesenteric revascularization: management and outcomes in the United States, 1988–2006. *J Vasc Surg*. 2009;50:341–349.
11. Arthurs ZM, Titus J, Bannazadeh M, et al. A comparison of endovascular revascularization with traditional therapy for the treatment of acute mesenteric ischemia. *J Vasc Surg*. 2011;53:698–705.
12. Milner R, Woo EY, Carpenter JP. Superior mesenteric artery angioplasty and stenting via a retrograde approach in a patient with bowel ischaemia: a case report. *J Vasc Endovasc Surg*. 2004;38:89–91.
13. Wyers MC, Powell RJ, Nolan BW, Cronenwett JL. Retrograde mesenteric stenting during laparotomy for acute occlusive mesenteric ischemia. *J Vasc Surg*. 2007;45:269–275.
14. Pisimisis GT, Oderich GS. Technique of hybrid retrograde superior mesenteric artery stent placement for acute-on-chronic mesenteric ischemia. *Ann Vasc Surg*. 2011;25:132.e7–132.e11.
15. Sharafuddin MJ, Nicholson RM, Kresowik TF, et al. Endovascular recanalization of total occlusions of the mesenteric and celiac arteries. *J Vasc Surg*. 2012;55:1674–1681.
16. Sonesson B, Hinchliffe RJ, Dias NV, et al. Hybrid recanalization of superior mesenteric artery occlusion in acute mesenteric ischemia. *J Endovasc Ther*. 2008;15:129–132.
17. Wyers MC. Acute mesenteric ischemia: diagnostic approach and surgical treatment. *Semin Vasc Surg*. 2010;23:9–20.
18. Biebl M, Oldenburg WA, Paz-Fumagalli R, et al. Endovascular treatment as a bridge to successful surgical revascularization for chronic mesenteric ischemia. *Am Surg*. 2004;70:994–998.

19. Brown DJ, Schermerhorn ML, Powell RJ, et al. Mesenteric stenting for chronic mesenteric ischemia. *J Vasc Surg*. 2005;42:268–274.

20. Schoch DM, LeSar CJ, Joels CS, et al. Management of chronic mesenteric vascular insufficiency: an endovascular approach. *J Am Coll Surg*. 2011;212:668–675.

21. Oderich GS, Erdoes LS, LeSar C, et al. Comparison of covered stents versus bare metal stents for treatment of chronic atherosclerotic mesenteric arterial disease. *J Vasc Surg*. 2013;58:1316–1324.

22. Do N, Wisniewski P, Sarmiento J, et al. Retrograde superior mesenteric artery stenting for acute mesenteric arterial thrombosis. *Vasc Endovascular Surg*. 2010;44:468–471.

27

Endovascular Approach to Gastroduodenal Artery Aneurysms

Monish Merchant, MD and Scott Resnick, MD

INTRODUCTION

Visceral artery aneurysms are a rare and potentially life-threatening disease entity with a reported prevalence of 0.1%–2%.[1] Modern high-resolution imaging has led to an increase in asymptomatic visceral aneurysm detection. Additionally, the advent of percutaneous biliary, hepatic, and renal interventions has resulted in a greater incidence of iatrogenic vessel injury and secondary pseudoaneurysms.

GDA aneurysms constitute approximately 1.5% of visceral artery aneurysms. Treatment of these aneurysms is directed toward an effort to prevent rupture. Regardless of size, if left untreated, there is approximately an overall 75% chance of rupture with a reported risk of mortality from 20% to 40%.[2-5]

Surgical and endovascular treatment of GDA aneurysms share the common goal of excluding an aneurysm from arterial circulation while preserving blood flow to distal organs. Endovascular management was initially introduced for patients at high surgical risk with significant comorbidities or aneurysms difficult to surgically access. Given the technical success, and the low procedural morbidity, endovascular exclusion has become the treatment of choice for most GDA aneurysms at many institutions.[2] Multiple endovascular treatment options exist and are dependent on aneurysm configuration, technical factors, individual patient, and operator preference.

ANATOMY

Normal

The GDA arises from the common hepatic artery through the celiac axis, which is the first wide ventral branch off the abdominal aorta arising just below the diaphragmatic hiatus at the level of the lower twelfth thoracic vertebrae. The celiac axis is generally oriented

281

caudad and forward, but can pass directly horizontal or even cranially. The common hepatic artery is one of three branch arteries off the celiac axis and is smaller than the splenic artery but larger than the left gastric artery. It is directed forward and toward the porta hepatis becoming the proper hepatic artery after the origin of the GDA.

The GDA is a short large branch oriented caudally, descending near the pylorus between the superior border of the duodenum and the neck of the pancreas; at the lower border of the duodenum the GDA bifurcates into its terminal branches the anterior-superior pancreaticoduodenal artery and the right gastroepiploic artery. The first branch of the GDA is the posterior-superior pancreaticoduodenal artery (retroduodenal artery) arising approximately 1–2 cm from its origin. A frequent branch off the posterior superior pancreaticoduodenal artery (50%) or proximal GDA (25%) is the supraduodenal artery of Wilke, which supplies both the anterior and posterior surfaces of the first part of the duodenum. Proximal to its division the GDA gives rise to two to three small branch arteries to the pylorus and pancreas.

Collateral Supply to GDA branches

Embolization of the GDA without significant clinical consequences is possible because of the rich collateral supply to the arteries originating from the GDA.

The anterior and posterior pancreaticoduodenal arteries give rise to the similarly named arcades, which are part of a rich vascular network supplying the head and uncinate process of the pancreas as well as the duodenal bulb. The arcades join behind the head of the pancreas forming a common trunk called the inferior pancreaticoduodenal artery that ends in an anastomosis with the superior mesenteric artery (SMA) or the first jejunal artery. The arcades also anastomose freely with the dorsal pancreatic artery, which frequently arises from the splenic artery.

A terminal branch from the GDA, the right gastroepiploic artery is the main artery to the stomach, following a winding course along the greater curvature of the stomach while giving rise to several ascending gastric branches that anastomose with descending branches from the right and left gastric arteries. Several omental branches also arise from the right gastroepiploic artery and form an anastomotic arcade with branches from the middle colic artery. Distally the right gastroepiploic artery ends in an anastomosis with the left gastroepiploic artery, which originates from the splenic artery.

Variant Anatomy

Identifying anatomic variations in the celiac axis, common hepatic artery, and GDA is important before intervention to avoid potential complications and aid in planning of the procedure. Song et al. evaluated 5002 patients for celiac axis and common hepatic artery variations. The common hepatic artery (CHA) was defined as an arterial trunk containing at least one segmental hepatic artery and the GDA. In patients with a definable CHA (98.7% of cases), the CHA originated from the celiac axis or its equivalent in 96.4% of cases. The most common variant in the origin of the CHA was from the SMA, which was found in 3% of the cases. In 0.16% of cases, the CHA originated from the left gastric artery. Although rare this variant is important to identify because the CHA has a transhepatic course with the segmental hepatic arteries arising proximally and then distally continuing as the GDA. The CHA was a direct branch of the aorta in 0.4% of the cases. In 1.1% of cases, the GDA originated separately without any hepatic arterial component. In the majority of these cases, the separate origin of the GDA was from the SMA.[6]

ETIOLOGY AND PATHOPHYSIOLOGY

GDA aneurysms are traditionally classified as either true aneurysms or pseudoaneurysms with different etiologies for each type.

In general, true aneurysms have all three layers of the arterial wall intact and are defined as localized dilation of an artery by more than 1.5 times the expected diameter. Unlike in aneurysms in the aortoiliac system, atherosclerosis seems to play a secondary role in true GDA aneurysms and does not always represent the first pathologic mechanism.[7] More commonly true aneurysms in the GDA are secondary to arterial wall degeneration, demonstrating a deficiency of the arterial media with loss or fragmentation of the elastic fibers and smooth muscle.

Flow-related true aneurysms in the GDA are secondary to absence/occlusion of the celiac axis or SMA. Decreased flow through the celiac axis can also be seen in median arcuate ligament syndrome. In these cases, the celiac to SMA or SMA to celiac collateral pathway results in increased blood flow in the GDA, as the pancreaticoduodenal arteries provide collateral supply to the branches of the stenotic, occluded, or absent artery. Aneurysmal dilation of the collateral vessels is thought to occur secondary to hemodynamic stress (high flow) and possibly turbulent flow (Figures 27-1 and 27-2).[8]

Congenital arterial wall defects can also lead to the formation of true aneurysms in the GDA. In one study, 18% of true GDA aneurysms were associated with other aneurysms in the arterial circulation, predominately in the mesenteric vessels.

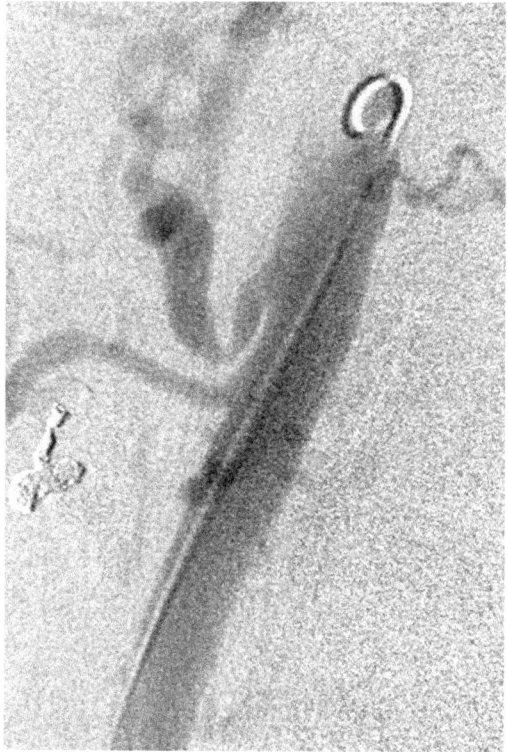

Figure 27-1. Lateral aortogram showing classic median arcuate ligament compression configuration of the celiac trunk with extrinsic downward displacement and compression with stenosis.

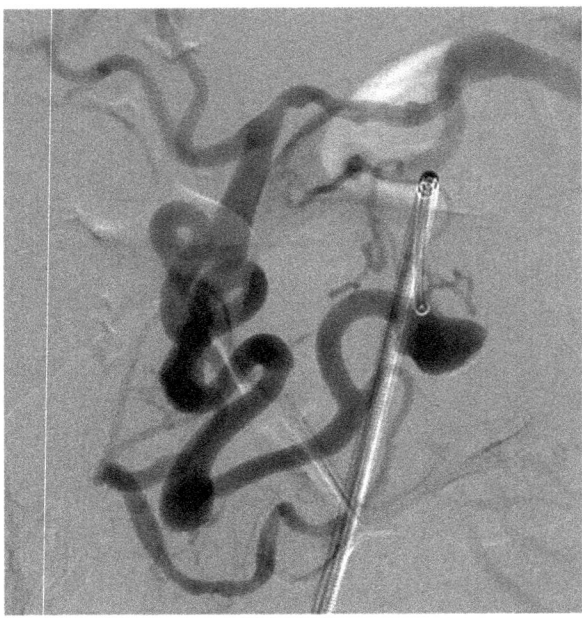

Figure 27-2. Selective SMA angiogram in setting of median arcuate ligament compression with markedly enlarged pancreaticoduodenal arcade and retrofill of celiac territory. Flow-related SMA branch vessel aneurysm is also seen.

Common congenital syndromes affecting the arterial wall include Marfan syndrome, Ehler–Danlos syndrome, hereditary hemorrhagic telangiectasia, Polyarteritis Nodosa, Kawasaki disease, and fibromuscular dysplasia.

The majority of GDA aneurysms are pseudoaneurysms,[9] defined by lack of a complete arterial wall and are effectively contained ruptures of the artery that is lined by adventitia or perivascular tissue. GDA pseudoaneurysms arise from a focal impairment in the integrity of the arterial wall leading to a contained hematoma followed by fibrosis and often by progressive enlargement. Insult to the arterial wall in the GDA is most commonly related to inflammation, infection, or trauma (accidental or iatrogenic).

The most common identified cause of GDA aneurysms is inflammation related to pancreatitis.[10] Activation and release of pancreatic enzymes causes rupture of the membrana elastica interna in the GDA, followed by thrombosis of the vasa vasorum causing necrosis and leading to a defect in the vessel wall (Figure 27-3). Inflammatory pseudoaneurysms may also form secondary to adjacent peptic ulcer disease, specifically ulceration along the posterior wall of the duodenum. GDA pseudoaneurysm from adjacent cholecystitis has also been described.[11]

Pseudoaneurysm formation in the GDA secondary to infection merits special consideration due to the proclivity to rapid expansion and rupture.[12] Vascular trauma with inoculation of bacteria into the vessel wall and septic emboli are the most common causes.[12] There is a limited role of endovascular therapy in these cases because of the potential for subsequent infection of therapy-related material.

Iatrogenic trauma to the GDA with focal wall disruption from surgical, endoscopic, and interventional radiologic procedures is known to result in pseudoaneurysm formation.

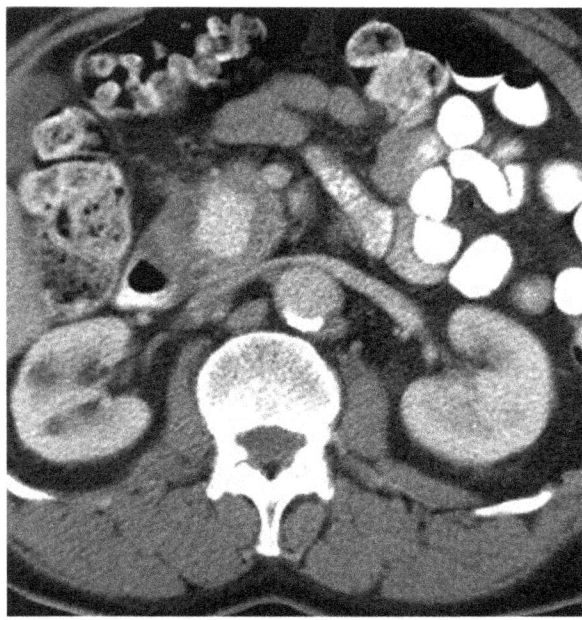

Figure 27-3. Large inflammation-surrounded GDA psuedoaneurysm in the setting of pancreatitis.

CLINICAL PRESENTATION

The clinical presentation of GDA aneurysms varies among patients with true aneurysms and pseudoaneurysms, with majority of the latter being ruptured at presentation. Rupture often presents with GI bleed, severe abdominal pain radiating to the back, and hemodynamic instability.[3,11] The mortality rate associated with rupture has been reported up to 40% and depends on the severity, rate of blood loss, and anatomical site of rupture.[3] Hemorrhage secondary to rupture can be contained in the retroperitoneum or may progress into the peritoneal cavity.[3] More commonly, there is extension of hemorrhage into the GI tract through the duodenum or stomach and less often through the biliary or pancreatic ductal system.[12] Bleeding into the pancreatic duct causing recurrent episodes of hemosuccus pancreatitis has been reported as well as bleeding into the common bile duct.[3,4]

In patients who have undergone recent percutaneous intervention of the GI system or with pancreatitis, any unusual signs or symptoms, especially those suggesting pseudoaneurysm, should be considered carefully given the potentially catastrophic consequences. There seems to be no correlation between size of the aneurysm or pseudoaneurysm and clinical presentation with risk of rupture.[2] This suggests that all GDA aneurysms, regardless of type or size, should be treated.

Moore et al. compiled a comprehensive search of true GDA aneurysms presented in the English literature from 1946 to 2001 and reported 35% were ruptured at patient presentation.[2] The majority of patients presented abdominal pain, which was slightly more common in ruptured aneurysms compared to unruptured aneurysms. Other presenting symptoms, likely related to compressive hematoma or external pressure by the aneurysm, include GI outlet obstruction, vomiting, jaundice, and diarrhea.[2,10] About 7% of GDA aneurysms were asymptomatic and discovered during diagnostic evaluation for other medical problems.[2]

Based on the rarity of GDA aneurysms and their deep-seated retroperitoneal location, it is unlikely they will be diagnosed by clinical examination and physical findings alone. Although larger aneurysms have been reported to present as a pulsatile abdominal mass or bruit.[2,10]

ENDOVASCULAR TREATMENT

Given the often difficult task of operatively identifying and isolating aneurysms of the peripancreatic arteries, endovascular techniques are being used increasingly for treatment, and in most centers are the first line of therapy.[2,10,13] Endovascular treatment provides an alternative to surgical repair with lower associated morbidity and mortality while reducing aneurysm-related symptoms with high technical success.[1,14]

Indications for Treatment

The indication for intervention is related to the high mortality risk associated with rupture of GDA aneurysms. Historical indications for treatment of visceral artery aneurysms include symptomatic aneurysms, documented evidence of growth, aneurysms in women of child-bearing age, and asymptomatic aneurysms over 2 cm in diameter. With the advent of endovascular options for management, the indications for treatment have broadened. Most authors advocate treatment of all GDA true and false aneurysms regardless of size. The natural history of untreated GDA aneurysms has not been well studied, but seems to be progression toward rupture.[3] There is no good predictive measure for potential rupture including size criteria. In a study of 48 true GDA aneurysms, all aneurysms less than 1 cm presented as a rupture.[2] The increased number of asymptomatic GDA aneurysms being identified, due to advanced imaging techniques, should be considered for aggressive endovascular treatment as the natural history is likely progression with eventual rupture in all cases.[3]

The majority of patients presenting with GDA aneurysms are candidates for endovascular treatment. Special consideration should be given to those with significant comorbidities (pancreatitis, abdominal sepsis, and hepatobiliary disease) that elevate the risk of major operative vascular repair, technically difficult surgical exposure potentially elevating the risk of iatrogenic injury, or congenitally abnormal and fragile arteries where surgical dehiscence is likely. Aneurysmal morphology favorable to endovascular treatment includes saccular aneurysms with a narrow neck and a single outflow artery. Patients are considered good candidates for endovascular treatment if the inflow and outflow GDA of the aneurysm can be accessed and occluded by a catheter-based system and organ perfusion can be maintained through collateral flow from the SMA and splenic artery.

Contraindications and Special Considerations

Contraindications to endovascular treatment are few and usually related to limited access to the GDA. Challenging local vascular anatomy related to tortuosity, narrowing, and/or sharp angulation can preclude access to the GDA, in which case alternative therapies should be pursued. Truly prohibitive anatomy is rarely encountered and often intervention is attempted even with severely narrowed or tortuous vessels. Sadek et al. described the "body floss" technique to treat a GDA aneurysm in a patient with a tortuous infrarenal aorta, precluding stable celiac catheter positioning from a femoral approach. They gained through-and-through access from the right brachial artery to the right femoral vein using a 0.018" wire to relieve the redundancy in the aorta allowing stable celiac catheter placement and successful exclusion of the GDA aneurysm.[11]

If direct access to the GDA from the celiac axis is not obtainable, then indirect access may be obtainable from the SMA or splenic artery through the pancreatico-duodenal arcades or left gastroepiploic artery. Another option is direct percutaneous puncture of the GDA aneurysm sac. Visualization and puncture of the aneurysm sac can be done using standard CT guidance, cone beam CT in the angio suite, or using ultrasound and/or fluoroscopic guidance. Using this technique, a percutaneous thrombin injection can be performed in GDA saccular true aneurysms or pseudoaneurysms with long narrow necks, similar to treatment of femoral artery pseudoaneurysms. Alternatively, the sac may be embolized with coils passed directly through the needle access. Nicholson et al. suggest that a percutaneous approach also be used in low flow pseudoaneurysms, which fill in the late venous phase on angiography or may not be seen at all.

If the celiac axis or SMA is not patent secondary to congenital absence, atherosclerotic disease, or median arcuate ligament syndrome, then treatment planning must include maintenance of GDA patency as this vessel serves as an important collateral pathway in this setting. Embolization of the GDA in these cases can cause gangrene of the gallbladder and stomach, splenic necrosis, or other disastrous complications.[3,8] Initial treatment options when GDA patency maintenance is required are endovascular stent placement or surgical bypass. However, if one of these cannot be performed, other options although not commonly employed include stent grafts, flow-directed stents, stent coiling for wide-necked aneurysms, or occlusion of the sac with onyx or glue while protecting artery by placing a balloon across the neck of the aneurysm.[13]

Although successful endovascular treatment of hemodynamically unstable patients has been described in the literature, some authors consider it a relative contraindication to endovascular treatment and advocate emergent open surgical repair. In these cases, treatment should be individualized to the patient and based on operator experience and comfort level.

TECHNIQUE

The end goal of endovascular treatment is to isolate the GDA aneurysm from the arterial supply, to avoid potential rupture or stop active hemorrhage. The success of endovascular treatment is dependent on high-quality preprocedural cross-sectional imaging, which allows evaluation of access vessel pathology, vessel tortuosity, suitability of a treatment strategy, and presence of aneurysms at other sites. Specific attention must be given to the patency of the celiac axis and SMA artery.

Access

Most GDA aneurysms that require treatment will be approached through common femoral artery puncture. Occasionally, an axillary, brachial, or radial artery approach is required for sharply angulated, stenosed, or tortious vessel. Usually a 5 or 6 Fr sheath is placed to secure access.

Visceral Angiography

It is essential that high-quality diagnostic angiographic images from the celiac axis and SMA be obtained to document adequate collateral flow and any anatomic variants to insure safe and successful treatment. Digital subtraction angiography, the preferred method of image acquisition for visceral angiography, is highly sensitive to motion artifact, which can cause significant image degradation during abdominal imaging. Bowel peristalsis and respiratory motion are the two common sources of motion during DSA.

Bowel peristalsis can be significantly decreased with the use of smooth muscle relaxants. Butylbromide (Buscopan) can be used with a recommended initial dose of 40 mg and should be increased by 20-mg increments when required. In some cases, complete bowel paralysis will require the addition of glucagon in 1 mg aliquots.

Respiratory motion is more difficult to control since very few patients are able to hold their breath without abdominal motion for more than 15 seconds. Motion is likely to be more pronounced if the patient is asked to take a deep breath in and hold it during acquisition of images; instead, it is the better to ask the patient to stop breathing at a comfortable position and to repeat similar breathing techniques on later imaging. Improvement in abdominal stillness can also be improved by pinching the patient's nose with a clip during breath holding. At our institution, we found that the best images were obtained during normal respiration with the use of masking techniques.

A wide variety of visceral selective catheters are available for celiac axis and SMA access. Catheter selection of the ostium, advancement into the vessel, and positional stability during manipulation all depend on the wall-seeking behavior of the catheter; it must be in contact with the vessel wall opposite the target branch orifice. The catheter selected should have no side holes, to avoid the formation of thrombi between the catheter tip and side holes. Either a 5 Fr or 4 Fr catheter can be used, with the 4 Fr systems generally having better tractability and the 5 Fr systems having better tip control. Occasionally larger catheter systems are useful when there is severe aortoiliac tortuosity.

Diagnostic angiograms are done by injecting 30–50 mL of iodinated contrast material at a rate of 5–6 mL/s. The arteriogram should be used to determine patency of the celiac axis and SMA as well as their branches. If there is a concern for median arcuate ligament syndrome, lateral projection arteriograms through the celiac axis in expiration and inspiration should be performed. Using the visceral angiogram, the remainder of the procedure can be planned with appropriate identification and selection of the GDA (Figure 27-4).

Super Selection of the GDA

Super selection of the GDA using a triaxial endovascular system with a 3 Fr microcathter is usually the method of choice. After super selection, diagnostic angiograms should be performed using pump injections with nondilute contrast material at flow rates of 3mL/s. Multiple projections may be needed for optimal visualization and proper identification of the aneurysm morphology, size, and location. If the aneurysm is located in the proximal GDA, additional angiograms from the common hepatic artery should be performed (Figure 27-5).

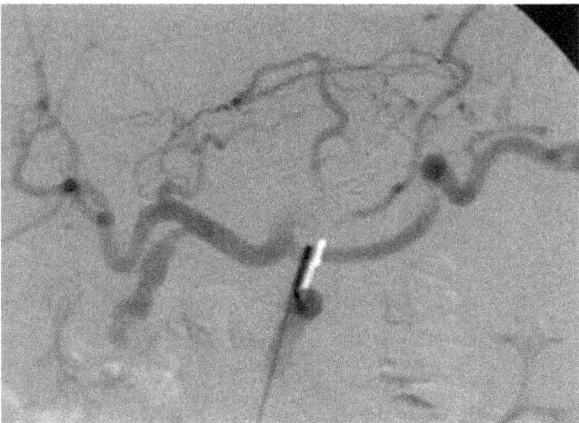

Figure 27-4. Celiac angiogram showing a fusiform aneurysm of the GDA arising from the common hepatic artery. Image courtesy of Dr. Mark Saker.

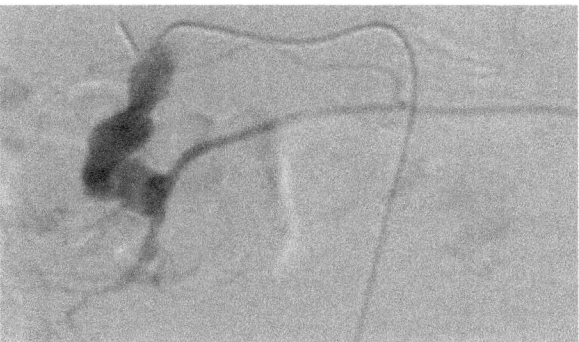

Figure 27-5. Selective GDA angiogram showing a fusiform aneurysm with outflow vessels, which should be embolized before embolizing the inflow artery. Image courtesy of Dr. Mark Saker.

EMBOLIZATION

Before embolization of the GDA, adequate patency of the celiac axis and SMA should be documented. The GDA can usually be sacrificed because of the rich collateral circulation to its branches. If only the inflow to the GDA is occluded, there is potential that there will be continued aneurysm perfusion with pressurization from retrograde flow through the collateral arteries. Therefore, treatment of GDA aneurysms involves embolization of the inflow artery and all outflow arteries. The outflow must be completely occluded first; this should be documented angiographically before occluding the feeding artery.

Careful evaluation and delayed angiography into the venous phase is necessary to identify and exclude all potential collateral outflow vasculature before proximal embolization is performed. In addition, low flow pseudoaneurysms may only be identified in later phase imaging (Figure 27-6). Special attention must be given to the smaller branches supplying the pylorus and duodenum as well as the supraduodenal artery of Wilke, because at times they can be difficult to identify angiographically.

During embolization, catheters should be flushed with nonheparinized saline and control angiograms should be obtained frequently. Positional stability of the

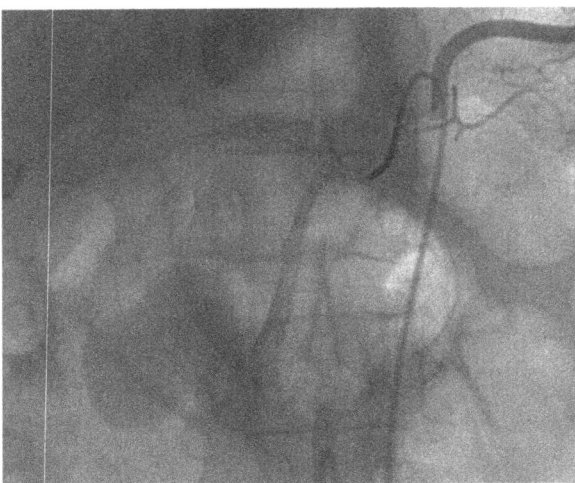

Figure 27-6. Late phase celiac angiogram with contrast opacified large low-flow GDA pseudoaneurysm to right of spine on AP image.

delivery catheter is very important, allowing precise delivery of embolic agents and minimizing the risk of nontarget embolization. Stability can often be improved with the use of specialized guiding sheaths and guide catheters.

Coil Embolization

Placement of vaso-occlusive coils on both sides of the GDA aneurysm is the most common endovascular technique used to exclude the defect from the arterial circulation. The GDA distal to the aneurysm must be accessible by a microcathter to employ this technique. Enriquez et al. found that there was a decreased rate of recannalization of the GDA after coil embolization to prevent hepaticoenteric flow when the most proximal coil was closer to the origin of the GDA. GDA diameter, length of the coil pack, and international normalization ratio did not show a statistically significant difference in rates of recannalization. Care must be taken that the proximal coil does not dislodge and embolize into the proper hepatic artery. With single vessel inflow and outflow anatomy, it is not necessary to embolize the aneurysm sac. In situations where multiple outflow vessels are identified, all of the outflow vessels should be individually embolized and coils should be placed bridging the aneurysm neck.[12,14,15]

Special consideration should be given to hemodynamically unstable patients where volume depletion causes reduced vessel size. Coil embolization in this setting can result in undersized coils with recanalization or coil migration when intravascular volume is restored. Coil over sizing is recommended in this situation.[16]

Pushable platinum coils are the most common type of coil used to achieve exclusion of the GDA aneurysm. In situations where pushable coils cannot be safely and easily used due to high risk of dislodgement and malpositioning, then using detachable coils may decrease procedural risk. Detachable coil systems permit controlled deployment and retrieval in cases of suboptimal positioning. They have shown to be equally as effective as pushable coils with decreased procedure times.[17] The drawbacks of using the detachable coils in the GDA are the difficulty of performing a controlled coiling when sharply angulated guiding catheters are used to select the celiac axis and technical success seems to be associated with operators' experience with the coils.

Amplatzer Vascular Plugs

In place of coils, Amplatzer Vascular Plugs (AVP) can be used to occlude the inflow and outflow arteries to a GDA aneurysm. The use of AVP compared to pushable coils has show a similar high technical success with low complication rates.[18] The ability to reposition and resheath the AVP before release allows for precise embolization. In most cases, a single plug is sufficient for complete vessel occlusion, decreasing procedural time, and reducing radiation exposure. Firm vessel attachment of the device can be obtained by selecting a size 30%–50% larger than the vessel diameter. The AVP 4 is the latest generation of plugs and is a double-cone-shaped nitol mesh mounted on a fixed-cone wire guide. The advantages of the AVP 4 compared to previous generations is that is can be deployed through a 4 Fr diagnostic catheter without the need for exchange of a vascular sheath or a guiding catheter.

In cases of smaller inflow and outflow arteries to the GDA aneurysm, the placement of a 4 Fr catheter for deployment of the AVP carries a high risk of spasm, dissection, and thrombosis; using pushable or detachable coil systems that are delivered through microcathters decreases this risk. Furthermore, tapered vessels may preclude adequate wall apposition of the AVP. Authors have described difficulty in advancing the AVP system in patients with a small angle (less than 20 degrees) between the aorta and celiac artery.[19]

Liquid Embolic Agents

Liquid embolic agents may play a role in the setting of distorted or tortuous anatomy of the GDA and in settings in which the outflow vessels from the aneurysm cannot be successfully catheterized, thus precluding coil placement. In such cases, liquid embolic agents such as N-butyl cyanoacrylate (glue) can be used to occlude the distal arteries. The rate of polymerization of NBCA can be altered, by changing the dilution ratio of ethiodized oil. Liquid embolic agents can also be beneficial in the setting of multiple outflow vessels or when there is persistent aneurysm flow despite coiling. Liquid agents have the potential for distal nontarget embolization if the injection rate is too rapid or polymerization time is prolonged.

ANEURYSM TREATMENT WHILE MAINTAINING PATENCY OF THE GDA

If the origin of either the celiac trunk or the SMA is occluded or stenosed, then treatment of a GDA aneurysm becomes much more complex. In this situation, it is essential to maintain patency of GDA because it serves as an important collateral pathway. Endovascular treatment options to maintain patency while still excluding the aneurysm include covered stent placement, primary coiling, and stent-assisted coiling of the aneurysm sac. Another option is to attempt revascularization of the celiac trunk or SMA with either transluminal endovascular intervention or open bypass before embolizing the GDA.

Covered stents offer the benefit of maintaining vessel patency and end organ perfusion, but certain anatomic considerations, such as vessel tortuosity, restrict their use. To place the stent, there must be sufficient vessel length on either side of the aneurysm to ensure a good seal. If the GDA is less than 6 mm in diameter, placement of a covered stent is not advised due to the increased risk of thrombosis in smaller vessels. Single vessel outflow anatomy is ideal for stent placement. If multiple outflow vessels are present, those vessels not bridged by the stent can continue to expose the aneurysm to systemic circulation and be a source of a type II endoleak. Caution should be taken when placing a covered stent to treat a GDA pseudoaneurysm because the disease process causing the defect (i.e., pancreatitis) is likely involving a greater length of the arterial wall than is apparent on angiography, leading to an increased risk of arterial rupture when a balloon expandable covered stent is placed. Stent grafts may not be appropriate if a pseudoaneurysm has ruptured into an adjacent vein, because of the possibility of AVM formation and continued aneurysm pressurization.

Although not regularly used, another option to maintain patency of the GDA is to pack coils into the aneurysm sac. The efficacy of this treatment is not well studied and we recommend this option only if a covered stent cannot be placed and open surgical repair is not an option. Primary coil embolization of pseudoaneurysms should not be done because the arterial wall lacks integrity and the coil pack may expand the sac, increasing the risk of rupture. If the aneurysm is wide-necked coiling of the aneurysm through the struts of a bare stent graft can be performed.

POST-THERAPY ANGIOGRAM

After the aneurysm has been excluded from the arterial circuation, selective angiograms through both the celiac trunk and SMA need to be performed (Figures 27-7 and 27-8). Again multiple projections and imaging in the venous phase should be obtained to evaluate for the possibility of addition vessels supplying the GDA aneurysm. If addition vessels are identified and cannot be accessed through an endovascular approach due to prior embolization, percutaneous thrombin injection is an option.

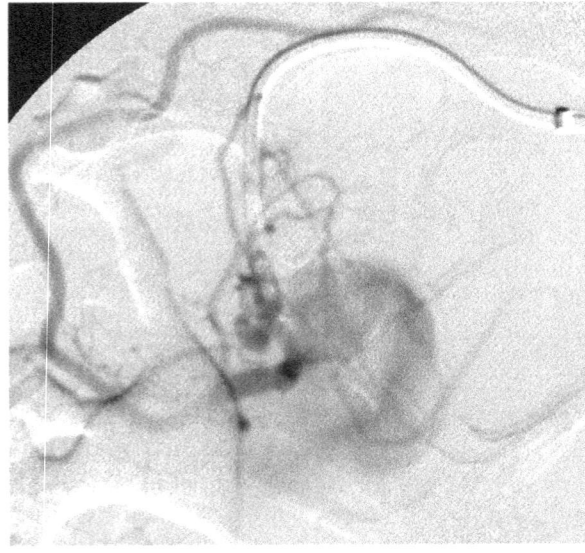

Figure 27-7. GDA angiogram with wide-neck low-flow pseudoaneurysm (same patient as Figure 27-6).

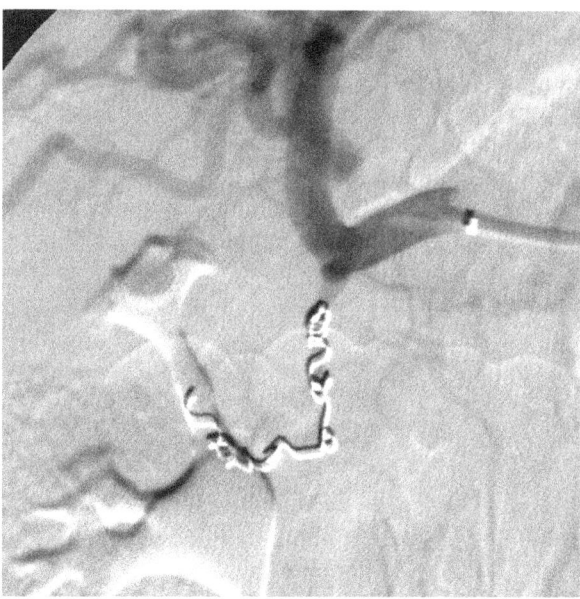

Figure 27-8. CHA angiogram with occluded GDA and absence of paeudoaneurysm filling following GDA coiled embolization (same patient as Figures 27-6 and 27-7).

FOLLOW-UP

Short- and long-term postprocedural follow-up imaging is important after endovascular GDA aneurysm repair, as recanalization requiring repeat intervention has been documented. Fankhauser et al. reviewed 185 minimally invasive visceral artery aneurysm repairs and showed 3% of treated aneurysms had persistent or recurrent flow on short-term repeat imaging. Follow-up imaging usually consists of CT angiography, MR angiography, duplex ultrasound, or a combination of these, to assess for sac flow, aneurysm size change, and adequacy of organ perfusion. Evaluation of postprocedural cross-sectional imaging at times may be difficult, secondary to metallic beam hardening artifact on CT and magnetic susceptibility artifact on MRI from the metallic embolic agents used to exclude the aneurysm. For this reason, if the aneurysm can be adequately evaluated by duplex ultrasound, it is the recommended modality. In instances where the aneurysm cannot be evaluated on cross-sectional imaging secondary to artifact and is not well visualized on duplex ultrasound, repeat angiogram may be necessary.

A specific follow-up imaging protocol after endovascular GDA aneurysm repair has not been validated; the timing to repeat imaging should take into account, the reason for intervention (bleeding/rupture versus enlargement), and the severity of the patient's illness. Patients who presented with hemorrhage and hemodynamic instability should be imaged sooner than nonbleeding aneurysms coiled due to size concerns. In acutely ill patients where residual contrast remains in the excluded portion of the artery on postprocedural angiogram, short-term (next day) follow-up with a noncontrast CT can be obtained to see if contrast is still present in the excluded portion of the vessel. If contrast is not evident on the next day CT, it can be assumed that the embolization was unsuccessful and there is continued systemic flow to the excluded segment.

At our institution, follow-up imaging in stable patients is obtained at one month, three months, and six months. If there is no evidence of aneurysm growth or continued perfusion, the follow-up interval is increased to annually. Although some authors have suggested that MRA is preferred over CT due to decreased artifact from the embolization material, we prefer the use CT for follow-up. CT follow-up is obtained with a triphasic protocol (noncontrast, early arterial phase, and portal venous phase). The initial noncontrast CT is done to visualize the extent of beam hardening artifact from the embolization material. The early arterial phase is used to visualize any continued perfusion to the excluded aneurysm and possible development of collateral vasculature. Finally, the portal venous phase is helpful to exclude late filling aneurysms with a type 2 endoleak-like configuration.

COMPLICATIONS

Although not common, complications related to endovascular repair of GDA aneurysms are usually related to nontarget embolization and catheter manipulation. Nontarget embolization can occur secondary to dislodgement of the coil or inappropriate deployment. There is potential for coil migration into the hepatic artery, which may cause acute liver enzyme derangement, but is not likely to cause long-term hepatic dysfunction if the portal vein is patent. Catheter manipulation in the celiac axis, SMA, or GDA can lead to dissection of the artery. GDA wire/catheter manipulation can cause intraprocedural aneurysm rupture. Other rare complications have been described in the literature, such as bile duct stricture 22 months after coil embolization of the GDA, presumably ischemia induced.[20] Also there are complications related to the access site such as psuedoaneurysm formation and access artery dissection.

SUMMARY

Although not extensively studied, recent literature suggests that the natural history of GDA aneurysms is progression to rupture. Due to this propensity, we recommend treating all GDA aneurysms regardless of size or type to prevent fatal complications related to rupture. The goal of both endovascular and surgical treatments is to isolate the aneurysm from the systemic circulation. Given the often difficult task to identify and isolate GDA aneurysms intraoperatively, endovascular repair is emerging as the treatment of choice for most patients. Endovascular repair has proven to be a viable treatment option with the benefit of low procedural morbidity and mortality. Also with the advent of smaller profile catheters and advancing endovascular techniques, the complication rates related to these procedures has been decreasing.[20]

REFERENCES

1. Huang YK, Hsieh HC, Tsai FC, et al. Visceral artery aneurysm: risk factor analysis and therapeutic opinion. *Eur J Vasc Endovasc Surg*. 2007;33(3):293–301.
2. Moore E, Matthews MR, Minion DJ, et al. Surgical management of peripancreatic arterial aneurysms. *J Vasc Surg*. 2004;40(2):247–253.

3. Habib N, Hassan S, Abdou R, et al. Gastroduodenal artery aneurysm, diagnosis, clinical presentation and management: a concise review. *Ann Surg Innov Res.* 2013;7(1):4.
4. Lykoudis PM, Stafyla VK, Koutoulidis V, et al. Stenting of a gastroduodenal artery aneurysm: report of a case. *Surg Today.* 2012;42(1):72–74.
5. Morita Y, Kawamura N, Saito H, et al. Diagnosis and embolotherapy of aneurysm of the gastroduodenal artery. *Rinsho Hoshasen.* 1988;33(5):555–561.
6. Song, SY, Chung JW, Yin YH, et al. Celiac axis and common hepatic artery variations in 5002 patients: systematic analysis with spiral CT and DSA. *Radiology.* 2010;255(1):278–288.
7. Pulli R, Dorigo W, Troisi N, et al. Surgical treatment of visceral artery aneurysms: a 25-year experience. *J Vasc Surg.* 2008;48(2):334–342.
8. Iyori K, Horigome M, Yumoto S, et al. Aneurysm of the gastroduodenal artery associated with absence of the celiac axis: report of a case. *Surg Today.* 2004;34(4):360–362.
9. Young R, Gagandeep S, Grant E, et al. Gastroduodenal artery pseudoaneurysm secondary to pancreatic head biopsy. *J Ultrasound Med.* 2004;23(7):997–1001.
10. Eckhauser FE, Stanley JC, Zelenock GB, et al. Gastroduodenal and pancreaticoduodenal artery aneurysms: a complication of pancreatitis causing spontaneous gastrointestinal hemorrhage. *Surgery.* 1980;88(3):335–344.
11. Sadek M, Rockman CB, Berland TL, et al. Coil embolization of a gastroduodenal artery pseudoaneurysm secondary to cholangitis: technical aspects and review of the literature. *Vasc Endovascular Surg.* 2012;46(7):550–554.
12. Chadha M, Ahuja C. Visceral artery aneurysms: diagnosis and percutaneous management. *Semin Intervent Radiol.* 2009;26(3):196–206.
13. Belli AM, Markose G, Morgan R. The role of interventional radiology in the management of abdominal visceral artery aneurysms. *Cardiovasc Intervent Radiol.* 2012;35(2):234–243.
14. Tulsyan N, Kashyap VS, Greenberg RK, et al. The endovascular management of visceral artery aneurysms and pseudoaneurysms. *J Vasc Surg.* 2007;45(2):276–283.
15. Nosher JL, Chung J, Brevetti LS, et al. Visceral and renal artery aneurysms: a pictorial essay on endovascular therapy. *Radiographics.* 2006;26(6):687–1704.
16. Mauro MA. *Image-guided Interventions.* Vol 2. 1st ed. Philadelphia, PA: Saunders/Elsevier-USA; 2008.
17. Dudeck O, Bulla K, Wieners G, et al. Embolization of the gastroduodenal artery before selective internal radiotherapy: a prospectively randomized trial comparing standard pushable coils with fibered interlock detachable coils. *Cardiovasc Intervent Radiol.* 2011;34(1):74–80.
18. Ng EH, Comin J, David E, et al. AMPLATZER Vascular Plug 4 for proximal splenic artery embolization in blunt trauma. *J Vasc Interv Radiol.* 2012;23(7):976–979.
19. Pech M, Mohnike K, Wieners G, et al. Advantages and disadvantages of the Amplatzer Vascular Plug IV in visceral embolization: report of 50 placements. *Cardiovasc Intervent Radiol.* 2011;34(5):1069–1073.
20. Fankhauser GT, Stone WM, Naidu SG, et al. The minimally invasive management of visceral artery aneurysms and pseudoaneurysms. *J Vasc Surg.* 2011;53(4):966–970.

28

Mesenteric Ischemia among Children and Young Adults: Etiology and Treatment

Erin C. Farlow, MD and Michael C. Dalsing, MD

MESENTERIC ISCHEMIA IN THE ADULT

Mesenteric ischemia is a disease process found rarely in patients less than 60 years of age because the etiology is generally the result of atherosclerotic occlusive disease. Chronic mesenteric ischemia can have various clinical presentations but involves a combination of the following signs and symptoms: slow weight loss, postprandial pain, emesis, diarrhea, and/or food fear over a period of weeks to months. Approximately 70% of chronic ischemia patients are women. Many of these patients also have a history of peripheral artery disease, stroke, or myocardial infarction. This type of ischemia is generally only seen when at least two of the three mesenteric vessels are stenotic or obstructed. When collateral arteries have been disrupted by prior intestinal resection, even one major mesenteric obstruction can cause symptoms. This slow onset of chronic mesenteric ischemia is distinctly different from acute mesenteric ischemia. However, acute mesenteric ischemia can result from a sudden occlusion of a preexisting chronic stenosis or a critical decrease in collateral flow in patients with chronic mesenteric ischemia. Alternatively, acute mesenteric ischemia can result from an acute embolus to or the sudden occlusion of a stenotic mesenteric artery in a patient without prior symptoms of chronic ischemia. Whatever the cause, the bowel is in eminent threat of loss with sudden onset severe abdominal pain with or without guarding. Mortality in patients with acute ischemia, in some studies, is in excess of 45%. Open surgical repair by thromboembolectomy or bypass has been the mainstay intervention but the recent use of endovascular stents in the treatment algorithm has reportedly decreased the perioperative morbidity and mortality.[1] Our aim as surgeons is to prevent this dire complication and to return the patient to a normal state of bowel perfusion and function.

MESENTERIC ISCHEMIA IN CHILDREN AND YOUNG ADULTS

Introduction

As is seen in the elderly with acute mesenteric ischemia, the most common presenting symptom is acute abdominal pain out of proportion to the physical examination. As the bowel ischemia becomes more profound, the patient may develop nausea, bowel emptying (vomiting and/or diarrhea), and occasionally hematochezia or melena. With progression, peritoneal signs develop and the physical examination becomes consistent with the pain expected on palpation. If bowel and potential liver ischemia progresses even further, approximately 50% of patients develop acidosis, acute renal insufficiency, and septic shock.[2] If the process is chronic in nature, the patient's symptoms often reflect the older patient with weight loss, food fear, and postprandial abdominal pain.

Mesenteric ischemia in patients under the age of 40 years is rare, and because of the lack of associated comorbidities, such as cardiac arrhythmia or associated peripheral and coronary artery disease, it is often not considered in the initial differential diagnosis. Therefore, the diagnosis is often made late in the clinical course. In a study by Ozturk et al., a group of 26 patients under the age of 40 years presented with acute mesenteric ischemia but only 6 of 26 (23%) had a preoperative diagnosis suggesting chronic mesenteric ischemia. The more common preoperative diagnoses included appendicitis, intussusception, and intra-abdominal abscess with the true cause of pain elucidated only during operative exploration.[2] Despite their otherwise often good general health, if the chronic disease progresses to acute ischemia or if acute ischemia is the initial presentation, these young patients can have a complication rate of 60% and mortality rates of 25%–30% due to the delay in diagnosis.

While occasionally caused by embolic or atherosclerotic occlusive diseases, the more common causes of mesenteric ischemia in the young can be broken into several groups including anatomic abnormalities, hypercoagulable states, inflammatory conditions, collagen vascular disorders, and environmental agents including smoking and cocaine use.[1–6]

Mesenteric ischemia in the youth is so rare that it presents in the literature as individual cases or small case series. Over a 16-year period, six patients under the age of 40 years were discovered who required revascularization for mesenteric ischemia at Indiana University Health (IUHealth). We did not consider cases such as bowel ischemia due to intrauterine pathology or those due to adhesion or torsion but only those associated with primary vascular occlusive disease. Review of these six cases in addition to a review of the literature form the basis of this report.

Illustrative Case Reports

Case 1. A 34-year-old woman presented with alcohol abuse, pancreatitis, and a 10-year history of postprandial pain and worsening weight loss. She had undergone cholecystectomy and had a previous celiac block in an attempt to alleviate the pain. Computerized tomographic angiography (CTA) scan performed as part of her subsequent evaluation demonstrated occlusion of the celiac and superior mesenteric arteries with extensive collaterals from the inferior mesenteric artery (IMA) (Fig. 28-1). Work-up was negative for elevation of inflammatory markers or evidence of a hypercoagulable state. She underwent a right iliac to distal superior mesenteric artery (SMA) bypass and left iliac to splenic artery bypass both with reversed saphenous vein graft. Postoperatively, she was given only aspirin without anticoagulation. Over the following year, she gained weight and experienced only minimal residual abdominal pain.

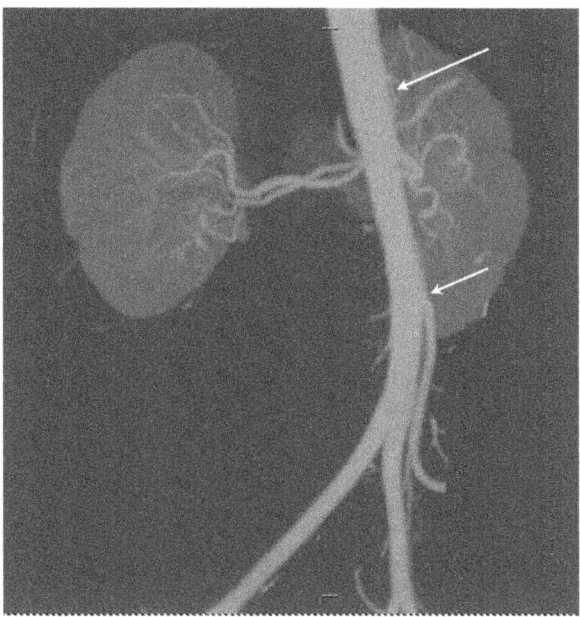

Figure 28-1. A three-dimensional CTA reconstruction of this patient demonstrating celiac and SMA occlusion (long arrow) with large IMA (short arrow) and collaterals.

Case 2. A 20-year-old African-American woman with a five-year history of Takayasu's arteritis presented with progressive worsening of abdominal pain and weight loss. She had known carotid, celiac, and SMA involvement. Repeat imaging demonstrated celiac artery stenosis of greater than 70% as well as greater than 50% stenosis of the SMA (Fig. 28-2). Despite the remission of her Takyasu's arteritis as indicated by a normal sedimentation rate, she continued to have pain suggestive of chronic mesenteric ischemia. The patient underwent a median arcuate ligament release and celiac and SMA bypass graft both with reverse saphenous vein originating from bilateral iliac arteries. Following this operative intervention, her symptoms improved dramatically. The patient remains on clopidogrel and low-dose steroids as adjusted by her rheumatologist.

Case 3. This 31-year-old woman had an extensive history of recurrent mesenteric ischemia. Unfortunately she had experienced a traumatic injury that led to back surgery that was complicated by a pulmonary embolism. Despite anticoagulation, she subsequently experienced an acute SMA embolus requiring emergent thromboembolectomy and patch angioplasty. Two years later, she developed stenosis of the SMA patch repair (Fig. 28-3), which responded to a 6 × 27 mm Express LD stent (Boston Scientific Corp.) placed at the SMA origin (Fig. 28-4). Postoperatively, she has been maintained on aspirin and warfarin to assist with stent patency thought to be required due to her recurrent episodes of embolism and thrombosis. Postoperatively, the patient remained pain free; however, the stent became occluded within one year as determined by CTA obtained during a brief hospitalization for an episode of self-limited abdominal pain. Shortly after her admission, her pain resolved and she tolerated a diet well. Given her asymptomatic nature, no further interventions were performed.

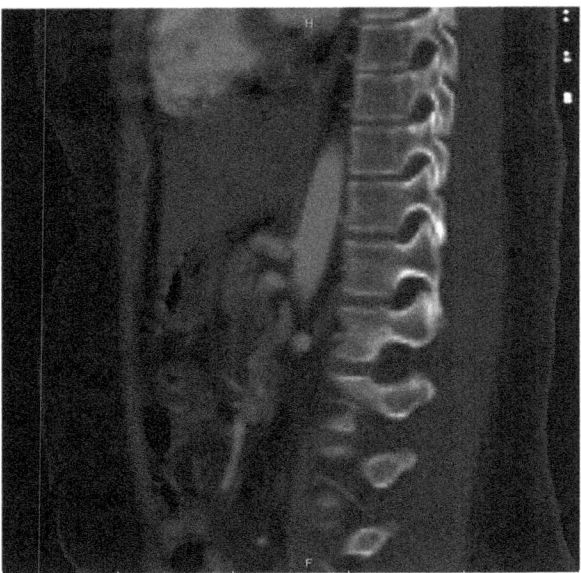

Figure 28-2. This CT angiogram sagittal view of the aorta demonstrates high-grade stenosis of the celiac and SMA in this patient with Takayasu's disease.

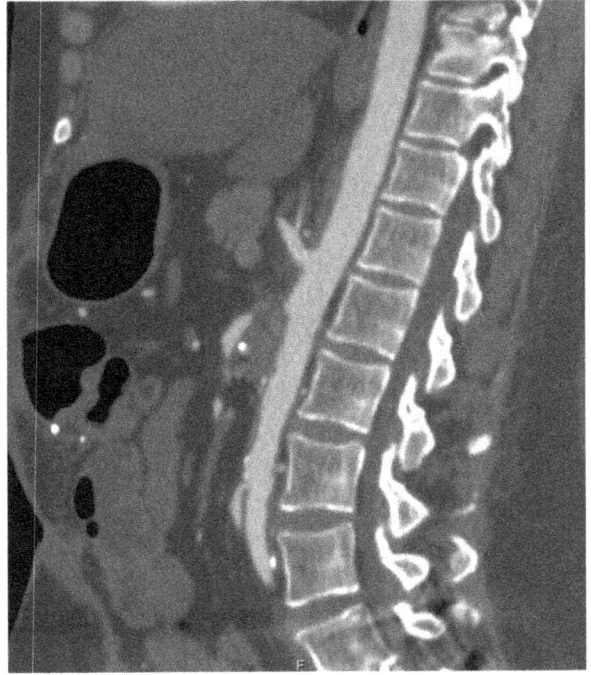

Figure 28-3. This CT angiogram sagittal view of the aorta shows stenosis of the SMA postpatch angioplasty with surrounding postsurgical soft tissue reaction.

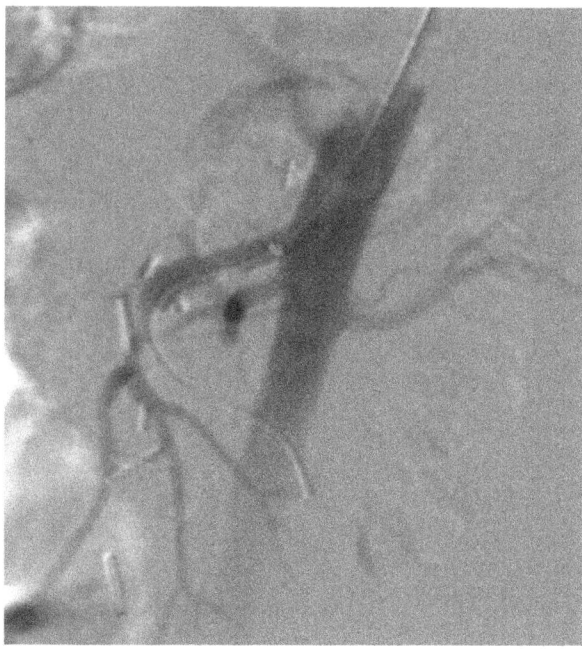

Figure 28-4. The patient with patch occlusion has a widely patent SMA following stent insertion as confirmed by this postoperative angiogram.

Case 4. A 37-year-old man with a history of afibrinogenemia (requiring multiple cryoprecipitate infusions), psoriasis, polyarteritis nodosum, a 36 pack a year smoking history, and a history of stroke presented with intermittent abdominal pain. On computerized tomography (CT) imaging, the patient was found to have splenic and hepatic infarcts. Laboratory results included protein C deficiency of 43% (normal 70%–180%), a fibrinogen level near zero, and antithrombin III level of 20 (normal 22–31). Antinuclear antibody (ANA) and erythrocyte sedimentation rate (ESR) were normal. CTA showed an occlusion of the celiac axis and a 95% stenosis of the SMA. Multiple renal arteries also demonstrated greater than 50% stenosis. He underwent an aorta to SMA and an aorta to IMA bypass both with polytetrafluoroethylene (PTFE) grafts. The patient could not be anticoagulated because of recurrent gastrointestinal bleeding episodes. At two years, the IMA bypass was occluded, but the SMA bypass remained patent without symptom recurrence.[5]

Case 5. A 33-year-old man with a history of hypertension and a 20-pack-year smoking history presented with recurrent episodes of abdominal pain. Ten days after his initial presentation, he developed rebound abdominal tenderness and was found to have necrosis of the stomach, small bowel, and colon without pulsatile flow in the SMA. After transfer to our facility for further management, CTA demonstrated no direct flow to the celiac, SMA or IMA. He underwent bypass with reversed saphenous vein graft from the right common iliac to SMA and from the left common iliac to the IMA. While the patient had a prolonged recovery with development of an enterocutaneous fistula and the need for additional bowel resection, he was eventually anticoagulated with enoxaparin and transitioned to warfarin as an outpatient. In follow-up 1.5 years later, the patient was gaining weight well and was without abdominal pain.[5]

Case 6. A 30-year-old woman with a history of Takayasu's arteritis and hypertension presented with a four-month history of abdominal pain and a 50-pound weight loss. Endoscopy showed a lesser curve ulcer, and magnetic resonance angiography (MRA) suggested stenosis of all major mesenteric arteries. She deteriorated after undergoing an angiogram that confirmed the MRA findings but which also demonstrated portal venous air and bowel pneumatosis. She underwent emergent right common iliac-to-SMA bypass graft with reversed saphenous vein along with bowel resection. She had an ESR of 33 (normal <20), but all other coagulation and inflammatory serum studies obtained were normal. She was discharged home with aspirin alone. She had a patent bypass without symptom recurrence at two years.[5]

Etiologies Associated with Mesenteric Ischemia in the Child and Young Adult

Congenital Aortic Anomalies

Coarctation or aortic dysplasia most frequently occurs at the aortic arch; however, 0.5%–2% of cases occur in the descending or abdominal aorta. This may be caused by unequal fusion or obliteration of one of the primordial aortic buds. While the cause of a mid-aortic coarctation is not fully understood, there has been some association with rubella and an increased incidence of associated neurofibromatosis.[4] Approximately one-fifth of patients with coarctation or hypoplastic aorta have concurrent renal artery and mesenteric artery stenosis.[7]

Aortic duplication, partial or complete, is very rare and is associated with mesenteric ischemia in 22% of patients so affected. This pathology is postulated to occur secondary to malfusion of the dorsal and ventral aorta during the fourth to seventh weeks of gestation. If the ventral aorta does not appropriately fuse and regress into the splanchnic vessels, this can lead not only to mesenteric ischemia but also to hypertension secondary to renal artery stenosis with commonly associated claudication or even more severe lower extremity ischemia.[7]

A 25-year retrospective review conducted at the University of Michigan by Upchurch and colleagues found 17 patients from age 2 to 17 who presented with critical stenosis of the celiac or SMA. Fifteen of the 17 were caused by abnormal fusion of the visceral vessels to the aorta with 14 having aortic coarctation. All 15 of these patients also had renal artery stenosis with associated renovascular hypertension. Of the 10 that required operative intervention, only two patients complained of symptoms of intestinal ischemia.[4]

Treatment for these rare conditions is highly individualized. Factors to consider include the age and size of the patient, the length of stenosis or occlusion, the clinical consequences of the pathology, and the potential need for additional surgery in the future. The aortic coarctation must be addressed; depending on the length of stenosis and the specific location, patients may benefit from aortoplasty with prosthetic patch or thoracoabdominal aortic bypass.[4,8] Depending on the age of the child, aortic bypass can be challenging to plan appropriately. With the growth that will occur before adulthood, the graft selected must be of adequate diameter and have adequate redundancy to allow for vertical growth without physiologic graft stenosis. From the visceral standpoint, if the length of stenosis or occlusion is short, the child may adequately be treated with celiac or SMA reimplantation. If the length of stenosis is longer and the patient is young, the diameter of the saphenous vein will likely be inadequate to act as an arterial conduit and is more likely to become aneurysmal. In that scenario, the best graft may be an internal iliac artery. If the patient is fully grown and the saphenous vein is of adequate caliber, this would be an adequate conduit with good length for multiple visceral bypasses. Other occasionally performed procedures include intimectomy and/or reimplantation of the celiac artery at the SMA origin.[4]

Given the rarity of these anatomic anomalies, long-term benefit of endovascular repair is unknown. Angioplasty has been performed with restenosis seen at a rate of 25% at one year. Early restenosis can be decreased with insertion of stents, but this increases the need for reintervention from 10% to up to 20% even over short follow-up periods. Open bypass or angioplasty remains the most reliable reconstruction at the present time.[7]

Median Arcuate Ligament Syndrome

Median arcuate ligament syndrome (MALS) is observed in patients with diaphragmatic compression of the celiac artery and reportedly can cause abdominal pain, nausea, vomiting, and other symptoms of chronic ischemia. It most frequently presents in women during the third to fifth decade of life and is a diagnosis of exclusion. Celiac artery angulation and compression with poststenotic dilatation seen on CTA and ultrasound may be visualized with respiratory variation causing worsening of the symptoms. Acute ischemia is rarely seen in these patients, except in the setting of a concomitant hypercoagulable state with acute celiac thrombosis or in patients with concomitant SMA or IMA stenosis. Meta-analysis by Jiminez and colleagues evaluated treatment algorithms for MALS. Until recently, open surgical release of the diaphragm causing celiac compression with celiac ganglion resection and frequently celiac artery bypass, depending on the appearance of the artery after release of the extrinsic compression, was the standard treatment. More recent studies suggest laparoscopic release with possible follow-up angioplasty/stenting of the celiac artery is a viable option. In one report of laparoscopic repair, patients report an immediate improvement in symptoms in 85% of cases as compared with 78% in the open group. Complications associated with laparoscopic release are rare and include celiac artery, aortic and gastric artery bleeding, pneumothorax, and/or phrenic nerve injury as well as a 9% incidence of conversion to an open repair. Stroke, bypass graft thrombosis, gastroesophageal reflux, pancreatitis, splenic infarction, and pancreatitis were seen following the open bypass. No perioperative mortality was seen in either group, and the treatments were considered equivalent with late recurrence of symptoms of 6.8% and 5.7% in the open and laparoscopic groups, respectively.[9] This is contrary to previously suggested recurrence rates of 22% in patients undergoing open release and bypass compared to 44% in open release alone cases.[9,10] While the majority of patients do not require additional procedures after laparoscopic release, 14% underwent angioplasty with or without stenting or open angioplasty or bypass in an effort to further improve symptoms. Case reports suggest that the need for arterial reconstruction can be limited to the select patients with chronic symptoms due to irreversible intimal and medial hyperplasia or intrinsic stenosis caused by the chronic external compressive trauma.[9]

Valvular Heart Disease

While valvular and other heart disease is a more common problem in elderly patients, embolic occlusion of the visceral vessels is occasionally seen in patients with congenital valvular abnormalities or infectious endocarditis.[2] The clinical presentation in these patients is as acute mesenteric ischemia rather than a history of chronic weight loss or food fear. Embolectomy should be performed expeditiously with postoperative anticoagulation.

Additionally, congenital or infectious valve abnormalities should be addressed to prevent further embolism.

Hypercoagulable State

Thrombophilia can be caused by a variety of genetic variations in components of the coagulation cascade. While abnormalities including elevated Factor VIII, protein C deficiency, protein S deficiency, and Factor V Leiden mutation may increase the risk for arterial thrombosis, thrombus in an otherwise nonatherosclerotic aorta or mesenteric vessel is rare given the high flow state.[11] Other factors that can worsen preexistent hypercoagulable states includes pregnancy, oral contraceptive use, smoking, and polycythemia vera. These patients generally present in extremis with acute mesenteric ischemia and should be placed on immediate anticoagulation to prevent extension of the thrombus. Following embolectomy, thrombolysis, or bypass and bowel resection as necessary, these patients should be continued on life-long anticoagulation. A complete hypercoagulable work-up should be undertaken in the postoperative period.

Patients with thrombophilia including Factor V Leiden, protein C and S deficiency, prothrombin gene mutation, anti-thrombin III deficiency, and methylene-tetrahydrofolate reductase gene mutation are more likely to experience mesenteric vein or portal vein thrombosis than arterial thrombosis. Thrombosis of the superior mesenteric vein or portal vein accounts for 5%–15% of all clinical mesenteric ischemia. Treatment of patients with mesenteric venous thrombosis is generally nonoperative in nature with immediate anticoagulation involving initially low-molecular-weight heparin followed by a vitamin K antagonist, antibiotics, bowel rest, and supportive fluid resuscitation. With this treatment, between 40% and 80% of patients demonstrate at least partial recanalization of the portal vein and rapid clearly of the distal vein thrombosis, which allows bowel survival. Patients with poor recanalization develop an increased risk of GI bleed from thin walled varices as well as ascites. While there are centers that have undertaken portal vein thrombolysis, this is not recommended by most reporting physicians. Since the use of anticoagulation for this pathology, mortality has decreased significantly from 80%–100% to 35% or less.[12]

Vasculitides

Systemic vasculitis, while more frequently affecting the lungs and renal vasculature, does occasionally have GI pathology leading to mesenteric ischemia. The most common vasculitides that cause GI pathology are polyarteritis nodosa (PAN), systemic lupus erythematosus (SLE), and Henoch–Schonlein purpura. However, taken together, these vasculitides are responsible for less than 5% of mesenteric ischemia cases observed.[13] Case reports also describe bowel infarction associated with giant cell arteritis, Churg–Strauss disease, rheumatoid vasculitis, Kawasaki disease, and Takayasu's arteritis. When patients have nonspecific complaints and signs often associated with inflammatory diseases such as a recent viral prodrome, myalgias, arthralgias, kidney disease, or in patients of a young age without other definable cause of intestinal ischemia, vasculitis should be more highly considered. In 85% of cases, mesenteric vasculitis most commonly affects the SMA with ileum and jejunal involvement.

In medium and small vessel vasculitis, skip lesions within multiple vessels are seen and the chronicity of lesions is quite variable.[3] PAN mesenteric ischemia presents with an acute surgical abdomen 31% of the time compared with only 11% of the time in SLE.[3] When SLE is in remission, the incidence of mesenteric ischemia decreases to <1%.

In large vessel vasculitis, the presentation is similar to that seen with small and medium vessel conditions, but in the quiescent state, the patient's stenosis may be permanent causing persistence of symptoms. Takayasu's arteritis is more common in Asian women up to 40 years old. It presents as a granulomatous inflammation with atrophy of the media and intimal hyperplasia.[14]

Patients should undergo immunologic work-up including titers for perinuclear antineutrophil cytoplasmic, anti-beta-2 glycoprotein I, antinuclear, anti-DNA, and anti-smooth muscle and anticardiolipin antibody evaluation. Depending on preoperative clinical systemic inflammatory signs or pathologic signs at operation, diagnosis and work-up may occur preoperatively or postoperatively. When the bowel is ischemic without necrosis, the treatment of choice is initially supportive. The algorithm used by Rits and associates in a case series for initial medical treatment in otherwise stable patients includes 40 mg prednisone daily for four to six weeks, and aspirin followed by a slow taper over months if symptom free. If the symptoms recur or persist, then operative intervention is undertaken. With this algorithm, 7 of 15 patients in their group were in remission at the time of surgical intervention.[13] Additional immunomodulators including cyclophosphamide to induce quiescence may be beneficial.[3] Ideally, these patients do not undergo revascularization or stenting in the acute period since during that time they have a higher risk of graft failure and thrombosis. When revascularization is undertaken, the goal is to avoid the inflamed fields for both inflow and outflow anastomoses, which means normal arteries must house the bypass anastomotic sites. In addition to mesenteric reconstruction, these patients often require concurrent renal revascularization.[13] Whether or not stenting and angioplasty is appropriate in the setting of acute inflammation is unproven since only case reports with short-term follow-up are available for review. However, some case reports demonstrate technical success in this disease setting at least initially. Whether restenosis rates will be worse than the 22%–44% demonstrated in atherosclerotic disease is yet to be determined.[14]

Thromboangiitis Obliterans

Thromboangiitis obliterans, also known as Buerger's disease, is seen predominantly in heavy smokers between 20 and 40 years of age with a male predominance. It affects the small and medium vessels of the extremities and is a nonatherosclerotic inflammatory disease. Generally, it presents as painful ischemia to the digits of the hand or foot. Advanced disease will often show corkscrew collateral vessels on extremity angiography. Mesenteric vessel involvement, although very rare, can occur at any point in the patient's disease process; however, it is most often seen years after initial extremity symptoms. Patients with mesenteric ischemic often present with symptoms of chronic ischemia with significant weight loss, but they occasionally become acutely ill. Angiographic corkscrew collaterals may be apparent, although they are less prominent than is seen in the extremities.[6] While the diagnosis is clinical in nature in general, when biopsy is performed, the pathologic specimen will demonstrate acute inflammation of the entire vessel wall with cellular thrombus, perivascular fibrosis, and recanalization in the chronic state. The small bowel is affected more frequently than the colon. Depending on the degree of vessel involvement, treatment options may be limited. Smoking cessation is heavily encouraged and mandatory for effective treatment of these patients. Some may benefit from a lumbar sympathectomy or prostaglandin treatment for symptomatic relief, but more severe disease may require bowel resection. Given the involvement of small vessels in this disease process, patients rarely benefit from operative revascularization. The mortality for this disease process is approximately 30%.[6,15]

Cocaine Use

Cocaine is a stimulant that prevents the reuptake of norepinephrine. This leads to sympathetic stimulation including tachycardia and hypertension along with peripheral and regional vascular constriction. While myocardial infarction is a commonly recognized complication of cocaine use, mesenteric ischemia is seen infrequently and is caused by vasospasm of the smaller branches of the mesenteric vessels leading to nonocclusive mesenteric ischemia. Pathologic specimens from these patients may show anything from no detectable thromboembolic or atherosclerotic disease of the mesenteric vessels with bowel necrosis to larger mesenteric vessel intimal injury with platelet aggregation. The latter is often reported in the coronary vasculature with cocaine-induced myocardial ischemia.[16] The vasoconstrictive effect of cocaine on these vascular beds is found to be amplified with the addition of tobacco use. Treatment is often initially supportive with fluid hydration and antibiotics. Due to the occasional large vessel involvement, CTA is beneficial to determine a treatment plan. If immediate exploratory intervention is undertaken, intraoperative evaluation to confirm large vessel patency is prudent. Intra-arterial agents including papaverine, glucagon, phenoxybenzamine, and isoproterenol may also be utilized to promote vasodilation and improved blood flow in the setting of ischemic but not necrotic bowel.[17] If the bowel is necrotic, segmental resection should be performed after adequate resuscitation. Vascular bypass or stenting is only occasionally undertaken, and in a review of the literature, only 2 of 15 patients required a bypass.[16]

Fibromuscular Dysplasia

Fibromuscular dysplasia (FMD) in the pediatric population accounts for 70% of patients with renovascular hypertension. It is nonatherosclerotic, noninflammatory disease characterized by intimal and media fibroplasia/hyperplasia causing arterial stenosis. Medial fibroplasia accounts for the majority of patients treated. It is more predominant in younger and middle aged women. FMD affects renal arteries in 60%–75%, carotids in 25%–30%, and other arteries in up to 30% of cases. Twenty-five percent have multiple vascular beds involved. Angiographic examination can demonstrate a string of beads appearance.[18] Patients may present with postprandial pain, nausea, and vomiting in the setting of hypertension. If FMD is suspected, the exam should include an evaluation for abdominal bruits. Further work-up with mesenteric duplex and CTA are appropriate. While angioplasty and stenting have been attempted in this disease process, it seems that aorto-mesenteric bypass is a more reliable treatment option.[19]

Specifics of Operative Interventions

SMA Reimplantation

In many cases, the cause of mesenteric ischemia is limited to ostial lesions with SMA or celiac stenosis from congenital abnormalities or prior vasculitis. Especially concerning in children and young adults is the longevity of any repair. If anatomically possible, SMA reimplantation into the infrarenal aorta should be considered.[20] This prevents the need for suprarenal cross-clamping with potential renal ischemia, avoids the harvest of autogenous bypass conduit, and prevents the danger of infection or future size discrepancy in patients who undergo prosthetic bypass.

Bypass Grafts

When bypass grafting must be performed, the site of origin can be the supra or infrarenal aorta or the iliac arteries. The choice of conduit is important. In childhood, the internal iliac artery is preferred if adequate length can be obtained since the saphenous vein is very thin walled and, therefore, more prone to aneurysmal degeneration. Once a patient is grown, the saphenous may act as the best conduit in terms of easy of harvest and adequate length for even bifurcated grafts or C-loop alignment as the anatomy may require.

Prosthetic Bypass Graft Conduit

In a review by Davenport and colleagues of 156 adult patients with chronic mesenteric ischemia, vein revascularization was used in 28% and a prosthetic bypass graft in 72%. They found no difference in postoperative complications or hospital length of stay (11 vs. 15 days) between the vein and nonvein conduits. Even when patients who also required a bowel resection were removed from the analysis, the mortality was actually higher in the vein bypass group but not statistically so; 13.5% versus 4.5% (p=0.121). Early graft failure occurred in 4 of 44 (9.1%) vein grafts compared to 4 of 112 of the nonvein grafts (3.6%).[21] With the retrospective nature of this study, one must consider a possible patient selection bias before applying the data broadly, but it does suggest that prosthetic bypass material can be a viable substitute when optimal vein conduit is not available. Certainly, caution must still be used if the patient is not fully grown or if there is any concern that bowel integrity has been compromised.

Open Verses Endovascular Repair

While the data cannot be fully translated from the generally older population with chronic mesenteric ischemia to the youthful population, a review by Oderich and colleagues evaluated the outcomes of endovascular and open repairs. Their review found that in the open group, bypasses were performed with polyester grafts in 45%, PTFE in 18%, and vein in 34% of cases. In the endovascular repair, 70% underwent angioplasty with stenting and 73% had single vessel intervention. They found that perioperative mortality was greater in the open group compared with the endovascular group (7% vs. 3%), but that primary patency was much greater at one year in the open group (89% vs. 74%).[22] Given the small number of young patients reported, determination of mortality data is difficult. It does appear that the use of stents or angioplasty in youths varies widely based on surgeon preference.

Stents

The introduction of stents into the treatment algorithm for mesenteric ischemia must be undertaken cautiously. Stents are generally limited to short length disease and have generally been bare metal to prevent the coverage of early branch points. A report by Malgor et al. reviewed mesenteric stents placed in 101 patients over a 10-year period. SMA stenting compared to SMA and celiac or celiac-alone stenting showed no difference in morbidity, mortality, or recurrence of symptoms. Celiac artery stenting alone, however, was associated with a higher risk of recurrence. Freedom from restenosis at three years was between 34% and 47% in the three groups evaluated. Twenty-three of 101 patients developed recurrent symptoms and 24 were asymptomatic. Independent predictors of restensoses were prior mesenteric intervention and small SMA diameter. By three years of follow-up, 33% of the patients required reintervention for stent stenosis or occlusion.[23] Given the frequency of reintervention over a relatively short period of time, the use of stents in the younger population may be questionable.

Surgical Complications

Depending on the etiology and eventual surgical approach used to treat the problem, complications vary widely. Rits and colleagues showed that with open revascularization in 15 vasculitis patients, there was one gastrointestinal hemorrhage, an ileus requiring reexploration, and a superior mesenteric vein thrombosis, but no 30-day mortality.[13] Additional complications seen in the broader patient population reported by Ozturk et al. were as high as 61.5% and included wound infections, intra-abdominal abscesses, pneumonias, sepsis, and bowel anastomotic leaks. Patients had increased morbidity and mortality associated with the extent of ischemia, the extent of resection, acidosis, acute renal failure, respiratory failure, and the need for second-look operations.[2]

Acute mesenteric ischemia perioperative mortality remains significant despite aggressive care. Patients who require bowel resection associated with acute mesenteric ischemia have a 30-day postoperative morbidity of 56.6% and a postoperative mortality of 27.9%.[23] Depending on the disease process, mortality can range from 0% to 90%.[3,5,13,24]

Long-term complications associated with open operative intervention include the possibility for the patient to outgrow the visceral or aortic graft placed and depends on the age of the patient and the size of the graft at the time of implantation. This must be considered at the time of initial operation and redundancy of graft length should be allowed for if the patient still has a significant growth potential. Additionally, the diameter of synthetic grafts used should be carefully selected to avoid the need for a repeat operation due to limited flow. Better growth and remodeling as the patient matures may be achieved with the use of an autogenous graft, including harvest of the internal iliac artery for shorter graft segments.

Postoperative Care

Medications

Given the wide range of etiologies causing mesenteric ischemia symptoms in these children and young adults, the need for antiplatelet and anticoagulant therapy must be considered on an individual basis. In patients with vasculitis, adequate immunosuppression and antiplatelet agents are adequate. However, in patients with an acute occlusion, a hypercoagulable state must be considered. If elucidated, patients will require lifelong anticoagulant with heparin, low-molecular-weight heparin, or oral anticoagulants. Additional options include direct factor Xa inhibitors, which are becoming more readily available; however, dosing and indications are not yet available for the pediatric population.

Smoking Cessation

While smoking is associated with atherosclerotic disease in coronary, peripheral, and mesenteric vascular disease, it is critically important in patients with Buerger's disease and has been found to compound the effect of cocaine on mesenteric vasoconstriction. Outside of these considerations, chronic smoking may decrease the longevity of the bypass graft or other intervention used to treat the patient. Overall, it should be heavily discouraged with cessation counseling offered for best results.

Postoperative Follow-up

Given the young age of these patients, special attention should be paid to the detrimental effect of radiation from recurrent CT angiograms with the possibility of hematologic and other malignancies. It has been our routine to follow patients with symptomatic improvement at one month postoperative with a physical examination that includes the patient weight as well as a mesenteric duplex to evaluate graft or stent patency. This is repeated every six months thereafter. Provided the bypass or endovascular repair shows no progression of disease after one to two years of follow-up, the frequency of graft surveillance may be decreased to yearly. With the rigidity of stent materials, flow velocities as determined by duplex imaging are frequently elevated even immediately following intervention, and, therefore, baseline and sequential velocity measurements are particularly important in these patients. A significant increase over baseline velocities would lead to more aggressive imaging. CT angiogram or conventional angiographic evaluation may become necessary if the patient is developing recurrent symptoms or if duplex ultrasound evaluation is inadequate or demonstrates progressive disease.

CONCLUSIONS

To diagnose mesenteric ischemia in the young population, clinicians must have a high index of suspicion and complete a thorough initial history and physical examination. The etiologies are broad including hypercoagulable states, anatomic anomalies including mid-aortic coarctation, vasculitides, and environmental factors, but the presentation is rather standard and indicative of mesenteric ischemia. However, since mesenteric ischemia in the child and young adult is so rare, it is often not considered in the initial diagnostic algorithm and, therefore, there may be a significant delay in diagnosis. Because of this reality, outcomes vary widely and are most influenced by recognizing the disorder before overt bowel ischemia. If discovered before bowel ischemia, the mortality can be minimal with early intervention. But, with the onset of acute mesenteric ischemia, survival is often poor and so the overall mortality of all patients treated varies from 0% to 90%. In the setting of acute mesenteric ischemia, the initial treatment is unchanged from acute mesenteric ischemia in adults and consists of fluid resuscitation, broad spectrum antibiotics, bowel rest, and imaging often with CT angiogram. If vascular compromise is found, anticoagulation becomes an integral component of initial management to prevent thrombus propagation. Additional work-up varies based on initial clinical symptoms but may include a hypercoagulable panel and an inflammatory markers panel when the patient is otherwise stabilized. The overall goals of management should be to remove frankly necrotic bowel, reperfuse ischemic bowel, limit resection length when possible to prevent short-gut syndrome, and treat the underlying etiology when determined. Medications including immunosuppressants, anticoagulants, and antiplatelet agents should be considered for particular disease states. Depending on the etiology, recurrence of vascular occlusive disease or embolic states may remain high and lifelong, which means that follow-up is necessary to assure preservation of perfusion to the remaining intestine.

REFERENCES

1. White CJ. Chronic mesenteric ischemia: diagnosis and management. *Progress Cardiovasc Dis.* 2011;54(1): 36–40.
2. Ozturk G, Aydinli B, Atamanalp SS, et al. Acute mesenteric ischemia in young adults. *Wien Med Wochenschr.* 2012;162(15–16):349–353.
3. Passam FH, Diamantis ID, Perisinaki G, et al. Intestinal ischemia as the first manifestation of vasculitis. *Semin Arthritis Rheum.* 2004;34(1):431–441.
4. Upchurch GR, Jr., Henke PK, Eagleton MJ, et al. Pediatric splanchnic arterial occlusive disease: clinical relevance and operative treatment. *J Vasc Surg.* 2002;35(5):860–867.
5. Sanders BM, Dalsing MC. Mesenteric ischemia affects young adults with predisposition. *Ann Vasc Surg.* 2003;17(3):270–276.
6. Cho YP, Kwon YM, Kwon TW, Kim GE. Mesenteric Buerger's disease. *Ann Vasc Surg.* 2003;17(2):221–223.
7. Ma H, Kandil A, Haqqani OP, et al. Endovascular treatment of stenoses in a pediatric patient with incomplete aortic duplication, mesenteric ischemia, and renovascular hypertension. *J Vasc Surg.* 2013;57(1):214–217.
8. Lillehei CW, Shamberger RC. Staged reconstruction for middle aortic syndrome. *J Pediatr Surg.* 2001;36(8):1252–1254.
9. Jiminez JC, Harlander-Locke M, Dutson EP. Open and laparoscopic treatment of median arcuate ligament syndrome. *J Vasc Surg.* 2012;56:869–873.
10. Reily LM, Ammar AD, Stoney RJ, Ehrenfeld WK. Late results following operative repair for celiac artery compression syndrome. *J Vasc Surg.* 1985;2:79–91.
11. Bosma J, Rijbroek A, Rauwerda JA. A rare case of thromboembolism in a 21-year old female with elevated factor VIII. *Eur J Endovasc Surg.* 2007;34:592–594.
12. Bonariol L, Virgilio C, Tiso E, et al. Spontaneous superior mesenteric vein thrombosis (SMVT) in primary protein S deficiency. A case report and review of the literature. *Chirurgia Italiana.* 2000;51(2):183–190.
13. Rits Y, Oderich GS, Bower TC, et al. Interventions for mesenteric vasculitis. *J Vasc Surg.* 2010;51(2): 392–400.
14. Lima LT, Christopoulos GB, Braga VM, et al. Treatment of mesenteric angina in patients with Takayasu's arteritis. *Rev Bras Reumatol.* 2011;51(2):188–195.
15. Lee KS, Paik CN, Chung WC, et al. Colon ischemia associated with Buerger's disease: case report and review of the literature. *Gut Liver.* 2010;4(2):287–291.
16. Myers SI, Clagett GP, Valentine RJ, et al. Chronic intestinal ischemia caused by intravenous cocaine use: report of two cases and review of the literature. *J Vasc Surg.* 1996;23(4):724–729.
17. Hon DC, Salloum LJ, Hardy HW, Barone JE. Crack-induced enteric ischemia. *N J Med.* 1990;87(12):1001–1002.
18. Sugiura T, Imoto K, Uchida K, et al. Fibromuscular dysplasia associated with simultaneous spontaneous dissection of four peripheral arteries in a 30-year-old man. *Ann Vasc Surg.* 2011;25(6):838.e9–11.
19. Patel NC, Palmer WC, Gill KRS, Wallace MB. A case of mesenteric ischemia secondary to fibromuscular dysplasia (FMD) with a positive outcome after intervention. *J Interv Gastroenterol.* 2012;2-4:199–201.
20. Meacham PW, Dean RH. Chronic mesenteric ischemia in childhood and adolescence. *J Vasc Surg.* 1985;2:878–885.
21. Davenport DL, Shivazad A, Endean ED. Short-term outcomes for open revascularization of chronic mesenteric ischemia. *Ann Vasc Surg.* 2012;26:447–453.
22. Oderich GS, Malgor RD, Ricotta JJ, 2nd. Open and endovascular revascularization for chronic mesenteric ischemia: tabular review of the literature. *Ann Vasc Surg.* 2009;23(5):700–712.
23. Malgor RD, Oderich GS, McKusick MA, et al. Results of single- and two-vessel mesenteric artery stents for chronic mesenteric ischemia. *Ann Vasc Surg.* 2010;24(8):1094–1101.
24. Gupta PK, Natarajan B, Gupta H. Morbidity and mortality after bowel resection for acute mesenteric ischemia. *Surgery.* 2011;140:779–787.

29

Radiofrequency Renal Sympathetic Denervation

Heather L. Gill, MD, MPH and Nicholas J. Morrissey, MD

BACKGROUND

The incidence and prevalence of hypertension is growing at an alarming rate. Currently in the developed world, 65% of adults over the age of 60 are classified as hypertensive. In the United States, 75 million adults are affected, with over 1 billion people affected worldwide. Hypertension is estimated to be responsible for approximately 7 million deaths annually.[1] In recent years, there has also been a spike in the proportion of patients with refractory or resistant hypertension.[2] Refractory hypertension is defined as blood pressure (BP) that remains above target levels despite the concurrent use of three or more antihypertensive drugs of different classes including a diuretic, at their maximum highest tolerated levels.[3] It is estimated that 25%–35% of adults never reach their target BP goals. In the United States, this figure may be as high as 50%. In the past decade, the percentage of patients on at least three medications with uncontrolled hypertension has risen from 15.9% to 28.8%.[2] This leads to increased risks and complications.

Failure to meet BP targets is most commonly caused by noncompliance with lifestyle and medications.[4] Other rarer causes of refractory hypertension include renal artery stenosis, obstructive sleep apnea, chronic renal failure, aortic coarctation, hyperaldosteronism, and pheochromocytoma. An in-depth work up of these possible inciting factors must be completed on all patients who present with refractory hypertension before other therapies are considered.[5]

PATHOPHYSIOLOGY

An in-depth discussion of the pathophysiology of the mechanism of sympathetic activity on hypertension is beyond the scope of this chapter; however, a brief overview will be presented here. Sympathetic nerves enter the kidneys through the adventitia of the renal arteries. Sympathetic stimulation at the renal level increases renin secretion through β1 adrenergic receptors. It also increases the overall Remin Angiotensin Aldosterone System activity.

Finally, it increases tubular sodium and water reabsorption through α2 adrenergic receptors. This then induces renal artery vasoconstriction with a resultant decrease in renal blood flow and glomerular filtration rate.[6,7] These factors combine to cause increases in BP. These factors also lead the afferent nerves to travel back to the hypothalamus signaling decreased renal perfusion and renal ischemia, which leads to increased sympathetic stimulation.

HISTORICAL BACKGROUND

Sympathetic denervation has been known as a treatment for hypertension for the better part of the past century. In the late 1930s–1950s, surgical sympathectomy was used to treat severe hypertension. It was done as thoracic, abdominal, or pelvic surgery to achieve a radical sympathetic block. It was shown to be successful in decreasing BP, preserving end organ function, and decreasing mortality. However, it was also associated with significant morbidity in the form of orthostatic hypotension, orthostatic bradycardia, excessive sweating, palpitations, breathlessness, bowel dysfunction, and sexual dysfunction.[8] From 1938 to 1947, a large trial followed 1733 patients. A total of 1266 patients underwent splanchnicectomy or surgical resection of the splanchnic nerves innervating both kidneys, and 467 were treated medically. The five-year mortality in the surgical group was 19% compared to 54% in the medical group. This survival advantage was shown to persist up to 10 years after the surgery.[9] With the advent of effective pharmacologic therapy to treat hypertension, however, the surgical treatment fell out of favor. With the advancement in endovascular therapies and the possibilities for localized renal sympathetic denervation, this treatment has begun to be reinvestigated.

CATHETER-BASED RENAL SYMPATHETIC DENERVATION

Catheter-based sympathetic denervation is a localized minimally invasive endoluminal technique allowing for complete sympathetic denervation of the kidneys with minimal systemic side effects. There are three main methods currently in practice or under investigation. These are radiofrequency ablation (RFA), ultrasound (US) ablation, and direct pharmacologic ablation.[7] Given the large potential population demand, this is an area of intense research and development. There are anecdotal online reports suggesting that there may be upwards of 40 renal denervation devices in development. From a business standpoint, the global market for renal denervation is expected to reach 560 million dollars by 2015.[10]

RADIOFREQUENCY RENAL SYMPATHETIC DENERVATION

The first and most studied methods of catheter-directed renal sympathetic denervation is that of RFA. This can theoretically be done using a standard electrophysiology catheter, but there are currently many specialized systems under investigation. These include but are not limited to the Symplicity Renal Denervation catheter (Medtronic Inc. Minneapolis, Minnesota), the EnligHTN RFA Catheter (St. Jude Medical Inc., St. Paul, Minnesota), the Vessix V2 RFA catheter (Vessix Vascular Inc. Laguna Hills, California), the OneShot RFA catheter (Covidien Inc., Mansfield, Massachusetts), the ThermoCool cryoablative catheter

(Biosene Webster Inc., Diamond Bar, California), and the Chilli II irrigative RFA catheter (Boston Scientific Inc., San Jose, California). There are currently four devices approved for general use in Europe, one in Canada, and none in the United States.[8] Treatment techniques vary according to the system used. Generalities are access to the renal arteries in a standard angiographic fashion, short duration RFA followed by wire, catheter, and sheath removal according to standard angiographic practices. In general, anatomic limitations are that the renal arteries must be larger than 3 mm for some devices and 4 mm for others. There must also be a treatment length of >20 mm. Most devices can be used from either brachial or femoral access. Some patients report an intense visceral abdominal pain during the procedure and this is often managed through pain control without any negative side effects.[6,7]

What follows is a brief description of the main catheters currently under investigation.

Symplicity Renal Denervation System

The most studied catheter at this point in time is the Symplicity Renal Denervation system from Medtronic. The Symplicity catheter is a single-use disposable catheter with a single platinum electrode that delivers low-level RFA to the renal artery. It is compatible with a 6 French sheath. The catheter tip is deflectable and is controlled at the handle to assist with placement within the artery. It is also torqueable to allow for several points of contact to be able to treat different areas of the artery. An integrated extension cable connects the catheter to the simplicity generator. A series of 2-minute ablations is performed along the endoluminal surface of the entire renal artery. Potential drawbacks to this system are the increased procedural time, 40 minutes in early studies, which has decreased with experience.

EnligHTN RFA Catheter

The EnligHTN RFA catheter is a single-use multielectrode RFA catheter from St. Jude Medical. It is placed through an 8 French guiding catheter and then delivers four sequential ablations in 90-second intervals. This theoretically allows for less manipulation and shorter total procedure time.

Vessix V2 RFA Catheter

The Vessix V2 catheter from Vessix Vascular is a low pressure balloon catheter with RF probes mounted on the exterior. The catheter is advanced into the renal artery over a guidewire. Once in place, the balloon is insufflated to low atmospheric pressures (3 mm Hg) and is activated to provide low-power RF energy over the entire course of the artery for 30 seconds. This has the theoretical advantage of being over the wire and thus simple to use as well as occluding blood flow allowing for more directed energy as well as one-shot treatment. Variable sizes can accommodate renal arteries as small as 3 mm.

OneShot RFA Catheter

The OneShot RFA system from Covidien is compatible with a 7 French sheath. It is a balloon catheter that goes over a 0.014 guidewire. RF energy is delivered through a spiral electrode surrounded by irrigation holes to allow for cooling to nontreated areas. This allows for a single treatment per artery with theoretically more consistent and reliable treatment patterns.

ULTRASONIC ABLATIVE RENAL SYMPATHETIC DENERVATION

Ultrasonic ablation while less studied is another emerging catheter-directed renal sympathetic denervation technique. The two systems currently under investigation are the Paradise catheter system (ReCor Medical Inc. Ronkonkoma, New York) and the Therapeutic intravascular US system (TIVUS; Cardisonic Ltd, Tel Aviv, Israel).

PARADISE System

The PARADISE system is a 6 French compatible balloon catheter with a central core US. It has a self-centering transducer to ensure the greatest accuracy with the least amount of adverse tissue loss. The US core causes frictional heating of the tissues while the balloon cools the endoluminal surface.

TIVUS

The TIVUS system is a 6 French compatible catheter that tracks over a 0.014 guidewire. The US probe does not touch the surface and leads to remote ablation without damaging the endoluminal surface. It is self-regulating and thus monitors local temperatures to prevent overheating.

TISSUE-DIRECTED PHARMACOLOGIC ABLATION

While less studied than the other two, tissue-directed pharmacologic ablation are in the preclinical stages of investigation. Bullfrog microinfusion catheters consist of a balloon that as it inflates a small needle becomes unsheathed, which then punctures the arterial wall. This allows for direct administration of pharmacologic agents such as vincristine into the adventitial space. This has been successful in swine models but is yet to be explored in humans.[11]

EVIDENCE

To date, the literature on this subject consists of many small case series with two large trails. There are many trials actively recruiting patients and the results of these are expected to change the field over the next five years.

In 2009, Krum et al. published a proof of concept series of 45 patients who underwent renal sympathetic denervation using the Symplicity system. All patients were on at least three antihypertensive medications with systolic BP above 160. At one month, there was a mean decrease in systolic and diastolic BPs of 14 mm Hg and 10 mm Hg, respectively. At one year, the decreased were 27 mm Hg and 17 mm Hg, respectively. There were no adverse events.[12] This trial showed that RSD was safe; however, it was criticized for the small number of patients, the lack of a control group, and questions regarding the inclusion and exclusion criteria. This led to the Symplicity HTN 1 trial that took the same cohort but increased the number of patients and increased the follow-up. This trial consisted of 153 nonrandomized patients that were on a mean of five antihypertensive medications with mean office BP readings of $176 \pm 17 / 98 \pm 15$ mm Hg. The mean estimated glomerular filtration rate was 83 ± 20. The median procedure time was 38 minutes. A total of 149/153 (97%) patients had no complications. Of those that sustained complications (three pseudoaneurysms and one renal artery dissection stented at completion of procedure), none went on to have repeated intervention or long-term complications. The mean decrease in BP was 20/10, 24/11, 25/11, 23/11, 26/14, and 32/14 at 1, 3, 6, 12, 18, and 24 months, respectively, thus showing a sustained decrease over time. At one year, 69% of patients were classified as responders (>10 mm Hg drop in BP). At two years, 82% had responded. At two years, all patients had stable renal function and there were no documented cases of renal artery stenosis.[13] While the results of this trial were encouraging, there still lacked a control group.

The next important trial was the Symplicity HTN 2 trial. This was a prospective randomized controlled trial involving 106 patients on at least three antihypertensive medications with an office SBP > 160 mm Hg in nondiabetic patients or >150 mm Hg in diabetic patients. The primary end point was change in office sitting BP at 6 months. Fifty-two patients were randomized to the RSD group and 54 patients to the control group. There were no catheter-related morbidity or mortality. At six months, the treatment arm had a mean decrease in BP of 32/12 mm Hg, whereas the control group had no change in their BP. This was statistically significant. As well at six months, 84% of patients in the treatment group were considered responders, while 35% of those in the control group had decreases of 10 mm Hg. This difference was also significant. At one year, there was a sustained decrease in the BP (–28/–10 mm Hg) with no change in renal function. Control patients were allowed to crossover to the treatment group at six months if they so desired. For those that crossed over, they had a decrease in BP six months later of –24/8 mm Hg.[14] Again the results seem very encouraging; however, there has been criticism over the lack of blinding and the fact that the end point was a single office BP measurement.

ONGOING TRIALS

Symplicity HTN 3

Began recruiting patients in September 2011. Designed as a multicenter prospective single-blinded randomized controlled trial to look at safety and efficacy. They have a target goal of 500 patients at 87 centers in the United States. Primary end points are a change in 24-hour average ambulatory BP at six months and adverse events at one month.

Arsenal

Open label trial in Europe/Australia of the EnligHTN system. Began recruiting in 2011 with planned completion in 2013. Interim results showed a one-month mean decrease in BP of 28/10 mm Hg with over 78% of patients responding. There were four hematomas, three vasovagal episodes with sheath pull, and two procedural bradycardic episodes.

Reduce HTN

European and Australian trial for the Vessix V2 system that began recruitment in February 2012. Estimated completion in 2014 with a total of 64 patients. Primary outcome is safety with a secondary outcome of six-month change in office and 24-hour ambulatory BP measurements. Interim results show a mean decrease in BP of –30/11 mm Hg.

Rapid

Open label trial in Europe and New Zealand studying the OneShot catheter. Began recruitment in May 2012 with completion expected in 2013 with a total of 40 patients. Primary end point is safety and BP change at six months.

Swan HT

Study looking at the ThermoCool catheter. Recruiting all patients with BP > 140/90 mm Hg. Began recruitment in 2011 with expected end date of 2016 with 800 patients.

Save

Study looking at ThermoCool and Chilli 2 catheter systems. Began recruitment in May 2012 and plans completion in December 2019 with a goal of 500 patients. Primary end point is change in office BP at six months. Secondary end points are 48 months outcomes for BP, renal artery blood flow and dimensions, renal function, and difference in number of antihypertensive medications.

Ralise

Trial looking at PARADISE US ablation system. Safety trial of 20 patients with secondary end point of change in ambulatory BP and number of antihypertensive medications. Midterm data on 15 patients shows a three-month decrease in BP of 32/16 mm Hg.

LIMITATIONS

While the early results from trials do appear to be encouraging, there are still some major limitations. The first being anatomical considerations. Most of the catheter systems in use today require the renal artery to be at least 4 mm in diameter and to have a working length of at least 20 mm. Secondly, some procedures have been limited by pain. Some patients experience a deep visceral pain with the procedure that has been reported to be a cause for termination of the procedure. Thirdly while there are small reports showing no change in renal function over time, animal models have shown that with endoluminal ablation the renal arteries can become fragile and thus prone to stenosis and aneurysm. In the short term, this has not been a problem in humans; however, long-term data is lacking.

CONCLUSION

For the better part of 80 years, it has been known that sympathetic denervation leads to reductions in BP and the associated morbidities. In recent years, however, the advent of minimally invasive catheter-directed treatment modalities have permitted the development of local renal sympathetic denervation. This has allowed for the benefits of sympathetic denervation without the major adverse systemic effects. The early evidence shows that for patients with resistant hypertension, renal sympathetic denervation appears to be a viable option for BP control. Although the studies have been small, the effects have been impressive enough to generate tremendous enthusiasm among those who treat hypertension. Thus far, the impact on the renal arteries appears to be insignificant, thus emphasizing the safety of the procedure. At the same time, the impact on BP is significant and thus far appears durable. The enthusiasm for the procedure is reflected in the number of devices being developed and studied for safety and efficacy. In the near future, the results of current studies will determine the role of renal sympathetic denervation in the treatment of resistant hypertension. In addition, the role of this technology in hypertension treatment could increase if the safety and long-term benefits compare favorably to the best current medical regimens. We should look forward with enthusiasm to the results of ongoing trials.

REFERENCES

1. Go AS, Mozaffarian D, Roger VL, et al. Executive summary: heart disease and stroke statistics—2013 update: a report from the American Heart Association. *Circulation.* 2013;127(1):143–152.
2. Egan BM, Zhao Y, Axon RN, et al. Uncontrolled and apparent treatment resistant hypertension in the United States, 1988 to 2008. *Circulation.* 2011;124(9):1046–1058.
3. Calhoun DA, Jones D, Textor S, et al. Resistant hypertension: diagnosis, evaluation, and treatment: a scientific statement from the American Heart Association Professional Education Committee of the Council for High Blood Pressure Research. *Circulation.* 2008;117(25):e510–e526.
4. De Souza WA, Sabha M, de Faveri Favero F, et al. Intensive monitoring of adherence to treatment helps to identify "true" resistant hypertension. *J Clin Hypertens.* 2009;11(4):183–191.
5. Chiong JR, Aronow WS, Khan IA, et al. Secondary hypertension: current diagnosis and treatment. *Int J Cardiol.* 2008;124(1):6–21.
6. Polimeni A, Curcio A, Indolfi C. Renal sympathetic denervation for treating resistant hypertension. *Circulation.* 2013;77(4):857–863.
7. Bunte MC, Infante de Oliveira E, Shishehbor MH. Endovascular treatment of resistant and uncontrolled hypertension: therapies on the horizon. *JACC Cardiovasc Interv.* 2013;6(1):1–9.
8. Froeschl M, Hadziomerovic A, Ruzicka M. Renal sympathetic denervation for resistant hypertension. *Can J Card.* 2013;29(5):636–638.
9. Smithwick RH, Thompson JE. Splanchnicectomy for essential hypertension: results in 1,266 cases. *JAMA.* 1953;152(16):1501–1504.
10. Renal Denervation Devices Market (Symplicity, EnligHTN, OneShot, V2, Paradise, TIVUS, Bullfrog, Surround Sound, Micro-Infusion, Ultrasound and Radiofrequency)— Global Industry Analysis, Size, Share, Growth, and Forecast, 2012–2021. http://www.transparencymarketresearch.com/renal-denervation-devices-market.html. February 2013.
11. Stefanadis C, Toutouzas K, Synetos A, et al. Chemical denervation of the renal artery by vincristine in swine. A new catheter based technique. *Int J Cardiol.* 2012. doi:10.1016/j.ijcard.2012.01.002.
12. Krum H, Schlaich M, Whitbourn R, et al. Catheter-based renal sympathetic denervation for resistant hypertension: a multicentre safety and proof-of-principle cohort study. *Lancet.* 2009;373:1275–1281.
13. Symplicity HTN-1 Investigators. Catheter-based renal sympathetic denervation for resistant hypertension: durability of blood pressure reduction out to 24 months. *Hypertension.* 2011;57:911–917.
14. Esler MD, Krum H, Schlaich M, et al. Renal sympathetic denervation for treatment of drug-resistant hypertension: one-year results from the Symplicity HTN-2 randomized, controlled trial. *Circulation.* 2012;126:2976–2982.

30

Renal Artery Reconstruction Techniques for Aneurysms and Occlusive Disease: Approach and Conduits

Dhiraj M. Shah, MD; R. Clement Darling III, MD; and Philip S.K. Paty, MD

Renal artery occlusive disease and aneurysmal disease have been successfully treated surgically over the years. However, with the recent paradigm shift to endovascular techniques for repair of renal artery disease, the incidence of surgical renal artery reconstruction has lessened. Still, surgical armamentarium is necessary, even today, for renal artery reconstructions for cases that are not amenable to endovascular repair, concomitant aortic surgery, and renal artery disease and also for those who have failed endovascular treatment of both occlusive and aneurysmal diseases. In this chapter, we delineate our experience of surgical repair of renal artery disease, both occlusive and aneurysmal, its approach and technical aspects, and best conduit for repair. To date, our experience with more than 1000 renal artery reconstructions for occlusive disease and 48 patients with repair of renal artery aneurysm comprise this text.

OCCLUSIVE DISEASE

Atherosclerotic renal vascular occlusive disease management has changed. The typical indication of hypertension for symptomatic disease has extended itself to repair of renal artery disease with greater than 70% stenosis in asymptomatic patients. Proponents of this concept suggest that over 44% of the renal artery with stenosis greater than 75% went on to occlude.[1] Although the true incidence of renal artery stenosis from atherosclerotic disease is small (0.1% of the population), it increases to 4% of all hypertensive patients: 10%–20% in patients with concomitant hypertension, coronary artery disease, and about 50% of patients with peripheral vascular disease. Typical indications for treatment of renal artery stenosis is renovascular hypertension, but no more than 60%–70% of patients with hypertension improve after renal artery revascularization and only 5%–30% of patients are actually cured.[2] However, the results are still better than those for best medical treatment in many small and randomized controlled trials. Poor patient selection and inadequate work-up will produce inferior results. However, it is difficult to sort out and pick out the winners.[3] The only variable that seems to be important is the degree of hypertension and the status of the kidney. Severe hypertensive patients with diastolic >110 torr and normal kidney size with severe renal artery stenosis have the best chance of improvement after renal artery revascularization.

The next indication is ischemic nephropathy. The goal of any treatment is to prevent disease progression and save the kidney. However, in general, creatinine improves in about 25% of the patients, stabilizes in about 50% of the patients, and is worse in another 25% of the patients. Best result from most of this disease is obtained with severe declining renal function. Patients with flush pulmonary edema are another group who present with bilateral renal artery stenosis, ischemic kidney, hypertension, and heart failure. The success for renal artery revascularization in these patients can reduce the need for further hospitalization in 70% of the patients. Proponents of asymptomatic renal artery stenosis treatment suggest that the kidney will continue to get worse. However, that thought is not borne out by data although most of these are treated by endovascular treatment. Occasionally, surgical treatment is done in concomitant renal artery stenosis over 75%.

SURGICAL THERAPY

Bypass for renal artery stenosis can be divided into anatomic and extra-anatomic. Anatomic bypasses arise from the aorta or from aortic bypass grafts but also include thromboendartectomy and renal artery reimplantation. These reconstructions have both high flow and excellent patency, and our preferred therapy. Extra-anatomic bypasses are hepatorenal, splenorenal, and rarely iliorenal or mesorenal revascularizations. These are secondary procedures reserved for challenging anatomy and patients with significant comorbidities. Ultimately, there is nephrectomy that still has a limited role even today for hypertension.

Anatomic Bypass

Aortorenal Bypass as Adjunct to Aortic Reconstruction

The most common aortorenal bypass is as part of aortobifemoral bypass or repair of an abdominal aortic aneurysm. Addition of left renal artery reconstruction to aortic surgery through a left retroperitoneal approach has not increased the incidence of adverse outcomes in our hands (morbidity 4%).[4] However, significantly higher morbidity occurs when bilateral renal artery reconstructions are performed (10%). The aorta is exposed by a left flank incision. Division of the lumbar branch of the left renal vein is required as is division

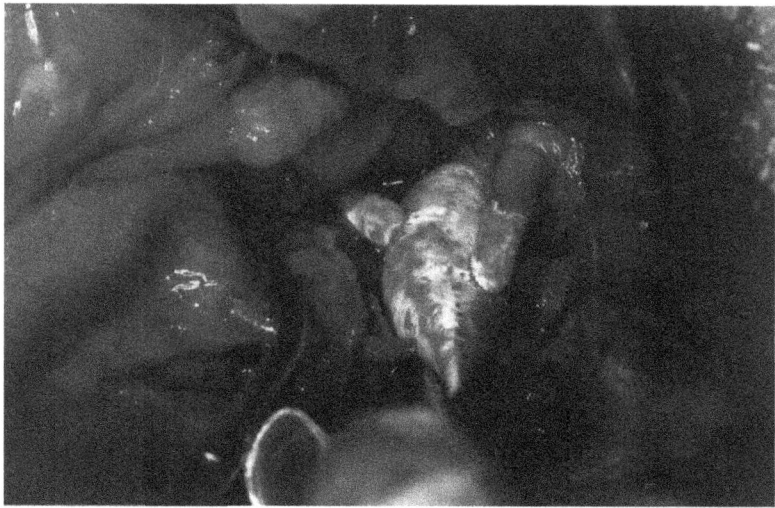

Figure 30-1. Renal artery bypass with aortic reconstruction. From Byrne and Darling.[6] Used with permission.

of the left crus of the diaphragm to facilitate exposure of the left renal artery. The right renal artery can also be exposed in its proximal 1–2 cm from this approach, although it is difficult before division of the aorta. Limbs of 6 mm expanded polytetrafluoroethylene (ePTFE) are sewn onto the aortic graft before suprarenal or infrarenal aortic clamping (Fig. 30-1).[5] The patient is given a bolus of 30 IU per kilogram body weight of heparin. We do not routinely flush the kidney with cold saline or ice pack the kidney to prolong warm ischemia time during revascularization. After clamping the aorta proximally and transecting it, the right renal artery can be accessed more readily if needed. The renal artery or arteries are clamped before aortic clamping. The proximal aorta-graft anastomosis is completed and suture line tested. The ePTFE graft limb is now sewn end-to-end onto the appropriate renal artery. The clamp is then repositioned below the origin of the renal artery bypass graft and the renal artery is perfused. Intraoperative continuous wave Doppler is used to confirm blood flow. The distal aortic, iliac, or femoral anastomoses are then completed.

Primary Aortorenal Bypass

The infrarenal aorta is commonly used as inflow (Fig. 30-2). Reversed greater saphenous vein or 6 mm ePTFE is used as the conduit. This is usually sewn in an end-to-side fashion onto the aorta. Occasionally, the suprarenal aorta may be used as the inflow source, which makes the bypass more anatomic but translates into a more difficult exposure. This is not commonly used for bilateral primary renal artery bypasses. A laparotomy incision is made. The supraceliac aorta is exposed for inflow through either a medial visceral rotation or traversing the lesser sac and a bifurcated graft can be used for reconstruction of both renal arteries. Alternatively, if the infrarenal aorta is of good quality, an infrarenal aorta to renal artery bypass can be performed through either a bilateral subcostal incision, a transverse abdominal incision, or a conventional laparotomy exposure. The posterior peritoneum overlying the aorta is incised and the ligament of Treitz is divided to allow reflection of the duodenum downward and to the right. The incision in the peritoneum is then continued

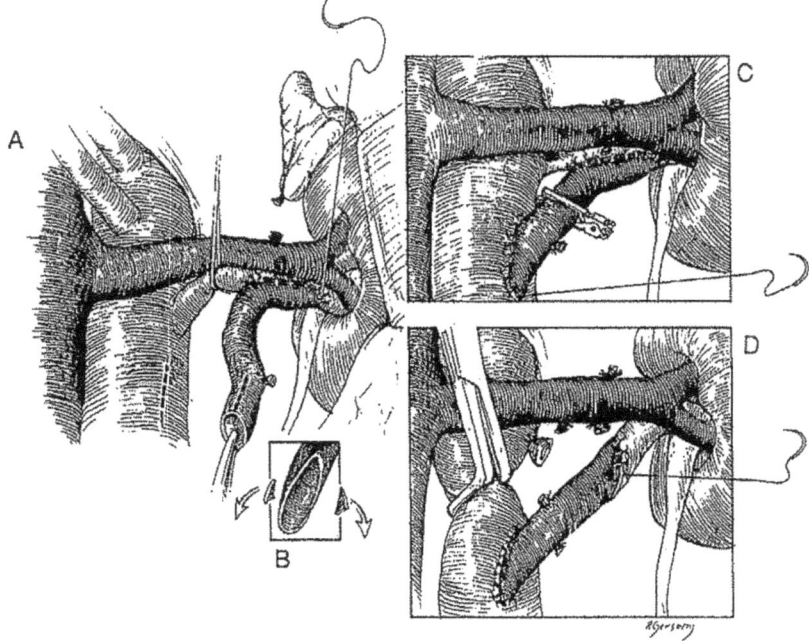

Figure 30-2. Aortorenal bypass grafting with end-to-side and end-to-end anastomoses. An end-to-end anastomosis between the graft and the native renal artery is generally preferred. From Benjamin and Dean.[7] Used with permission.

along the inferior border of the pancreas to the patient's left. By entering an avascular plane at the inferior border of the pancreas, the left renal hilum can be exposed. The left renal artery lies deep to the vein. It is necessary to divide the lumbar branch of the left renal vein to safely retract the vein and allow exposure of the left renal artery. Division of the supra-renal and gonadal veins may also be required. Exposure of the origin of the right renal artery will require division of two to three lumbar veins and retraction of the left renal vein superiorly while the inferior vena cava (IVC) is retracted to the patient's right. To approach the *distal right renal artery*, the hepatic flexure of the ascending colon is taken down and the right colon retracted inferiorly. Next, the duodenum is reflected medially to expose the IVC and right renal vein. The right renal artery is usually inferior to the renal vein. The right renal vein is carefully mobilized and retracted superiorly to expose the artery.

Transaortic Thromboendarterectomy

We perform this through a retroperitoneal incision through the 10th intercostal space, dividing the lumbar branch of the left renal vein and the left crus of diaphragm to facili-tate exposure. The left kidney is mobilized and reflected anteriorly. The aorta is clamped above the celiac axis and below the renal arteries. Clamps are placed on both renal arteries and the mesenteric vessels. A "trapdoor" incision is made in the aorta along the postero-lateral portion of the aorta and the aorta is endarterectomized to include the renal artery origins. Endarterectomy requires an "eversion" technique to ensure an adequate end point (Fig. 30-3). Others use a transperitoneal approach. In this case, a medial visceral rotation must be performed to allow exposure to the visceral artery origins before proceeding

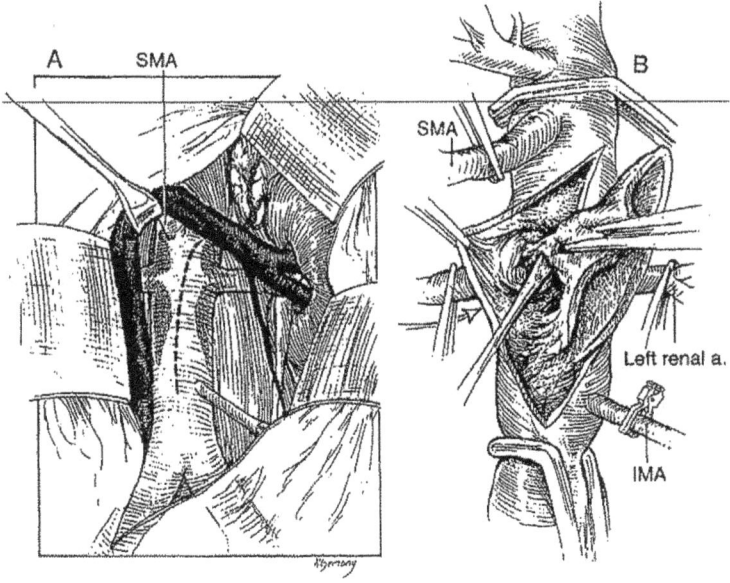

Figure 30-3. Transperitoneal approach for a longitudinal transaortic endarterectomy. *A*, Dashed line shows the location of the aortotomy. *B*, The plaque is transected proximally and distally, and the renal arteries are everted to remove the atherosclerotic plaque from each renal ostium. The aortotomy is closed with a running 4-0 or 5-0 monofilament polypropylene suture. IMA, inferior mesenteric artery; SMA, superior mesenteric artery. From Benjamin and Dean.[7] Used with permission.

to endarterectomy. An alternative to a conventional trapdoor incision is a transverse aortotomy carried across the origins of both renal vessels and which, in theory, allows more distal endarterectomy of both renal arteries.

Renal Artery Reimplantation

Occasionally, with sufficient dissection and mobilization of the renal arteries, there may be redundancy to allow division of the renal artery distal to the stenosis, leaving enough length for reimplantation of the renal artery directly into the infrarenal aorta.

Ex vivo Reconstruction

This is usually required when previous renal artery stents or bypasses have failed or when the distal renal branches are severely diseased. It is rarely used in our practice. The warm ischemia time of a kidney undergoing in situ revascularization is 30 minutes. With ex vivo reconstruction and cooling of the kidney to a core temperature of 10–15°C, the operating time can be prolonged to two to three hours. A standard flank nephrectomy incision is made. Gerota's fascia is divided and a nephrectomy performed with a cuff of IVC. The kidney is perfused with chilled preservation solution. Reversed saphenous vein is used. After completion of the arteriovenous anastomoses, the kidney is returned to its fossa and the renal vein is reanastomosed first and then the vein graft to aorta anastomosis is completed.

Extra-Anatomic Bypass

Splenorenal Bypass

Splenorenal bypass is performed in select cases. It is important to confirm the presence of an undiseased celiac axis before surgery by mesenteric angiography with both an anteroposterior and a lateral contrast injection. We usually employ a left subcostal incision; however, a laparotomy incision can also be used. The colon is identified and the splenic flexure is mobilized to reveal the tail of pancreas. The pancreas is reflected superiorly by mobilizing its inferior border. A retropancreatic plane is developed and the splenic artery is mobilized as far distally as the splenic hilum. The left renal artery lies above and behind the left renal vein. The renal artery is carefully separated from the vein. The splenic artery is mobilized and divided as far distally as possible. The renal artery is also divided and spatulated. It is then sewn end-to-end with the left renal artery. After completion of the anastomosis, it is important to ensure no kinking of an excessively redundant splenic artery. Intraoperative continuous wave Doppler interrogation will confirm normal flow to the left kidney.

Hepatorenal Bypass

This technique is performed through a right subcostal incision or a midline laparotomy approach. Again, a patent, nondiseased celiac axis is a prerequisite. The lesser omentum is incised to expose the hepatic artery proximal and distal to the gastroduodenal artery. Then the duodenum is mobilized and retracted medially to identify the IVC. The right renal vein is located. The right renal artery crosses the right crus of the diaphragm and psoas muscle behind the IVC and the right renal vein. It is carefully separated from the renal vein. Reversed greater saphenous vein is used as the conduit. The proximal anastomosis is created end-to-side on the hepatic artery. The vein graft is laid anterior to the IVC and sutured end-to-end with the transected right renal artery.

Iliorenal Bypass

Iliorenal bypass is a rarely performed operation although it has seen resurgence with recent "debranching" procedures that accompany endovascular treatment of thoracoabdominal aortic aneurysms. It requires a relatively "disease-free" common iliac artery. Classically, a midline abdominal incision is made. The right or left colon is reflected medially to expose the ipsilateral renal and common iliac arteries. Either a reversed saphenous vein graft or a synthetic graft can be used. The inflow requires an end-to-side technique onto the common iliac artery while employing an end-to-end anastomosis on the recipient renal artery. Alternatively, a right or left retroperitoneal incision can be made to access the appropriate renal artery for unilateral reconstruction.

Mesorenal Bypass

This is often described but rarely performed as evidenced by the paucity of reports in the literature. The superior mesenteric artery (SMA) is exposed either by a retroperitoneal approach or by a medial visceral rotation. Conventional wisdom is that manipulation of this vessel should be reserved only for hypertrophic SMAs to reduce the risk of "steal" and subsequent bowel ischemia. Recent reports dispute this. In our experience, a reversed vein graft is sutured end-to-side onto the proximal SMA and end-to-end to the renal artery. Published outcomes are reasonable.

NEPHRECTOMY

For atrophic kidneys (less than 8 cm in length), renal revascularization is pointless as there is little or no chance of better blood pressure control or resurrection of renal function. Nephrectomy is therefore reserved for patients with renovascular hypertension in whom the kidney has no excretory function (less than 10% on radionuclide renography) and an occluded artery. In this situation, sacrifice of the kidney will not affect renal function while potentially curing or improving hypertension. Historically, it only resolved hypertension in little over one-third of patients while halving renal excretory function in all. Nephrectomy is still occasionally employed, usually for atrophic, nonfunctioning kidneys that are felt to be driving high blood pressure.

CONCLUSIONS

Atherosclerosis of the renal artery is a difficult subject. Technical success and clinical benefit do not necessarily go hand in hand. The conclusive role of intervention has still to be determined. Patency rates are high for all surgical reconstructions but renal artery stenting has demonstrable advantages over simple balloon angioplasty. Although renal artery reconstruction has been practiced for decades, it is only now that its role and indications are becoming established with well-designed randomized control trials. In the next decade or two, the role of revascularization should be further objectively elucidated.[8]

SURGICAL TREATMENT OF RENAL ARTERY ANEURYSM

Aneurysms of the renal artery are no longer considered rare although the exact incidence is difficult to determine; estimates from angiographic studies for aneurysmal disease range from 0.7% to 0.9%. Autopsy studies have shown an incidence of 0.01%; however, aneurysms may be small or intraparenchymal and thus overlooked. The incidence rises to 2.5% when evaluation is performed for hypertension and to 9.2% in patients with fibromuscular disease of the renal artery. With the advent of more sensitive diagnostic imaging, these aneurysms have been identified with increasing frequency. Despite numerous reports, controversy still exists regarding the significance of renal artery aneurysms, in particular for small (<2.5 cm) aneurysms in asymptomatic patients.[9] Older reports suggest that these aneurysms, if asymptomatic, should be managed with observation. However, renal aneurysms may eventually lead to rupture, renovascular hypertension, renal infarction from embolization, thrombosis, or arteriovenous fistula formation. At our institution, we have adopted an aggressive approach in the management of renal artery aneurysms, providing that they could be repaired electively with minimal morbidity and mortality.[10]

To date, 48 renal artery aneurysms were repaired at our institution. The records of all patients operated on for renal artery aneurysm at the Albany Medical Center Hospital were reviewed. All patients were offered surgical repair. Three patients refused surgery. Diagnosis was established on the basis of angiography and CAT scan of the abdomen (Fig. 30-4). The remaining patients underwent extraparenchymal renal artery aneurysm repair in vivo. Variables examined in this group of patients included age, sex, hypertensive status, renal function, the presence or

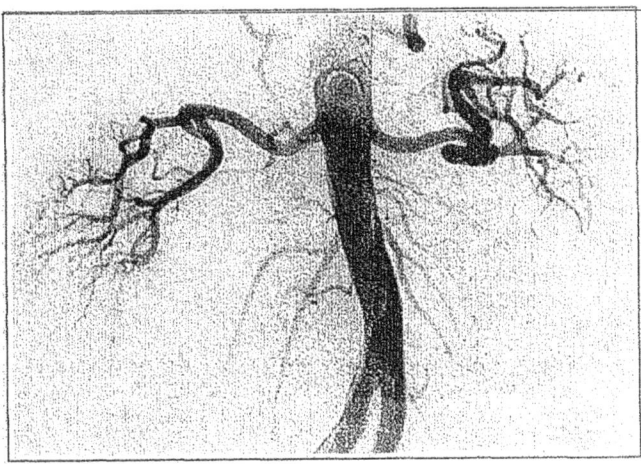

Figure 30-4. Angiogram demonstrating a typical saccular extraparenchymal left renal artery aneurysm at a primary bifurcation. Aneurysm diameter is 1.5 cm. From Kreienberg et al.[10] Used with permission.

absence of pain and associated vascular disease (aneurysm or occlusive disease), and type of renal aneurysm repaired. Two of these patients had small (<2 cm) aneurysms and were asymptomatic, the patient who refused had an aneurysm related to renal artery dissection and eventually expired from rupture of thoracic aortic dissection.

Sixteen patients had left-sided aneurysms and 20 were on the right with five patients having bilateral aneurysms. Twenty-eight of the aneurysms were saccular and the other 13 were fusiform. The aneurysms had mean size of 2.4 cm (range 1.5–4.0) and occurred in either the main renal artery (16 patients), at the hilar bifurcation (24 patients), or at a secondary bifurcation (one patient).

Clinical presentation of these aneurysms varied. Fourteen patients were asymptomatic and the aneurysms were identified in the work-up of other problems. Four presented with pain related to the aneurysm. Twelve patients had an associated abdominal aortic aneurysm and in four patients the renal aneurysm was diagnosed on the preoperative angiogram for occlusive disease. In two patients, the renal aneurysm was associated with neurofibromatosis. Preoperative laboratory evaluation revealed that all patients in this series had normal renal function by blood urea nitrogen and serum creatinine values. Five patients had renal vein renin sampling in the course of evaluation. These patients were hypertensive and the renin levels were found to lateralize to the affected side.

All surgical repairs were performed through a retroperitoneal approach. The procedures performed included arterioplasties, 6 mm PTFE bypasses based on aortic replacement grafts, and renal artery was reimplanted into the aortic replacement graft. Two aortic-based 6-mm PTFE bypasses were used and one patient underwent a saphenous vein interposition graft after bifurcation plasty of the branch renal arteries. Following these procedures, no patient had deterioration of renal function. Ten patients with preoperative hypertension, saccular type primary bifurcation aneurysms who underwent arterioplasty, are now normotensive and require no antihypertensive medications (Figs. 30-5–30-7). There were no operative mortalities. The mean follow-up for these patients is 1.5 years and duplex ultrasound revealed all reconstructed arteries to be patent.

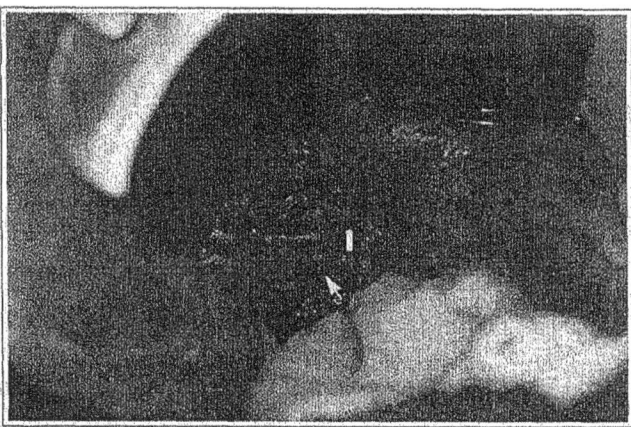

Figure 30-5. Intraoperative photograph demonstrating retroperitoneal exposure of a right renal artery aneurysm. From Kreienberg et al.[10] Used with permission.

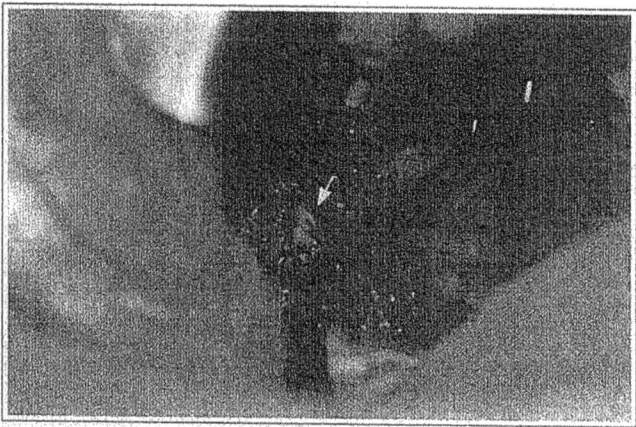

Figure 30-6. Intraoperative photograph demonstrating redundant renal artery aneurysm sac after partial excision of aneurysm. From Kreienberg et al.[10] Used with permission.

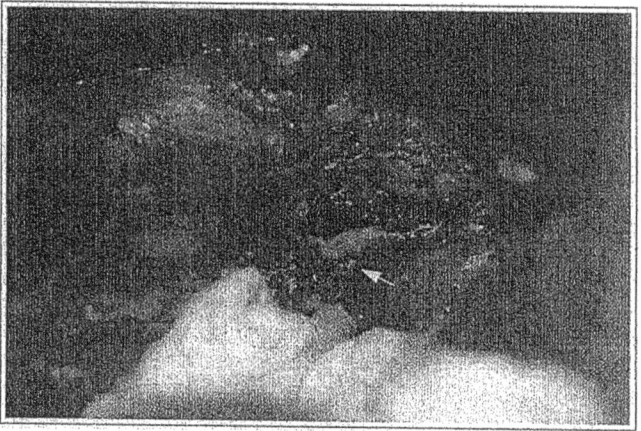

Figure 30-7. Intraoperative photograph demonstrating completed arterioplasty of renal artery after excision of renal artery aneurysm. From Kreienberg et al.[10] Used with permission.

CONCLUSION

The clinical importance of extra-parenchymal renal artery aneurysms lies in establishing the morbidity attributable to intact aneurysms including the development of hypertension, loss of renal function, or rupture.[11] The vast majority of these lesions, however, are asymptomatic. Previous studies have mandated that the indication for repair of these aneurysms should include symptomatic patients with suspected aneurysmal expansion, aneurysms associated with functionally important renal artery stenoses, aneurysms that harbor thrombus particularly when embolization is present, and operation for all women of childbearing age because of the increased risk rupture. These recommendations have been reiterated in the literature more recently. However, controversy still exists as to the significance of small asymptomatic aneurysms.

The concern regarding rupture of small asymptomatic aneurysms has motivated surgeons to carry out early repair. However, the true risk of rupture of renal artery aneurysm may have been overestimated. Early reports noted rupture rates up to 24% and were more likely to develop in patients with aneurysm >2 cm. Tham et al. followed 69 patients for a mean duration of 4.3 years without development of any symptoms or rupture.[12] However, in this study, 54 of the 69 patients had aneurysms less than 1 cm. Hageman et al. reported on 29 patients with saccular aneurysms.[13] Nineteen of 29 patients with aneurysm <2 cm were followed for eight years with no ruptures occurring. In this study, patients were followed with serial angiography in 50% of cases. These studies demonstrate that these aneurysms when small can be safely followed. However, all these patients will require follow-up and either CAT scans or angiography in the process. Thus, if surgical repair can be performed safely with minimal morbidity, then the follow-up can be obviated.

Repair of these extra-parenchymal aneurysms carries very little risk. Hageman reported zero mortality and no worsening of renal function in his series.[13] Similarly, Lumsden et al. reported only one death in his series 10 repairs and this was a myocardial infarction in a patient who had undergone concomitant suprarenal aortic aneurysm repair.[14] The other nine patients all had no change in renal function and recovered uneventfully. These results are similar to that presented in our series of 19 patients. There were no deaths and no patient suffered worsening of renal function. Therefore, it may be reasonable in good risk patients with extra-parenchymal aneurysms to offer surgical repair as it carries minimal risk, avoids the small but present risk of rupture, and obviates the need for continued imaging by CAT scan or angiography.

REFERENCES

1. Edwards MS, Corriere MA. Contemporary management of atherosclerotic renovascular disease. *J Vasc Surg*. 2009;50(5):1197–1210.
2. Fenstad ER, Kane GC. Update on the management of atherosclerotic renal artery disease. *Minerva Cardioangiol*. 2009;57(1):95–101.
3. Textor SC. Atherosclerotic renal artery stenosis: overtreated but underrated? *J Am Soc Nephrol*. 2008;19(4):656–659.
4. Darling RC, III., Kreienberg PB, Chang BB, et al. Outcome of renal artery reconstruction: analysis of 687 procedures. *Ann Surg*. 1999;230(4):524–532.

5. Darling RC, III., Kreienberg PB, Shah DM, et al. Aortic reconstruction and concomitant renal artery revascularization using the retroperitoneal approach: techniques and results. *Semin Vasc Surg.* 1996;9(3):231–235.

6. Byrne J, Darling RC III. Atherosclerotic renovascular disease. In: Cameron JL, Cameron AM, editors. *Current Surgical Therapy, Tenth Edition.* Philadelphia: Elsevier; 2011. pp. 822–829.

7. Benjamin ME, Dean RH. Techniques in renal artery reconstruction: part I. *Ann Vasc Surg.* 1996;10:306.

8. Mehta M, Darling RC III, Roddy SP, et al. Outcome of concomitant renal artery reconstructions in patients with aortic aneurysm and occlusive disease. *Vascular.* 2004;12(6):1–6.

9. Cinat M, Yoon P, Wilson SE. Management of renal artery aneurysms. *Semin Vasc Surg.* 1996;9:236–244.

10. Kreienberg PB, Darling RC III, Chang BB, et al. Surgical management of extraparenchymal renal artery aneurysms. *Vasc Surg.* 1998;32(6):587–593.

11. Stanley JC, Rhodes EL, Gewertz BL, et al. Renal artery aneurysms: significance of macroaneurysms exclusive of dissections and fibrodysplastic mural dilations. *Arch Surg.* 1975;110:1327–1333.

12. Tham G, Ekelund L, Herrlin K, et al. Renal artery aneurysms: natural history and prognosis. *Ann Surg.* 1983;197:348–352.

13. Hageman JH, Smith RF, Szilagyi E, Elliot JP. Aneurysms of the renal artery: problems of prognosis and surgical management. *Surgery.* 1978;84:563–572.

14. Lumsden AB, Salam TA, Walton KJ. Renal artery aneurysm: a report of 28 cases. *Cardiovasc Surg.* 1996;4:185–189.

Upper Extremity Diseases

31

Axillosubclavian Arterial Injuries: Endovascular versus Open

Aaron C. Baker MD, MS and W. Darrin Clouse, MD

INTRODUCTION TO AXILLOSUBCLAVIAN ARTERIAL INJURY

Injuries to blood vessels in the thoracic inlet continue to present significant challenges to trauma and vascular surgeons. As with other vascular injuries, there is a severity spectrum depending on mechanism, anatomic location, temporal circumstances, and concomitant injuries. How to manage each particular incident can be quite different and may depend on the experience and expertise of the trauma team caring for the patient. Not only can life-threatening hemorrhage occur, but also ischemia leading to ischemic neuropathy/plexopathy, compartment syndromes, and muscular contracture. Associated injuries to the thorax, as well as brachial plexus, bony shoulder girdle, and soft tissues frequently contribute to dysfunction. Ultimately, in some instances, amputation may be the result in both the acute or chronic setting after injury.

Today, advancements in modern imaging technologies, experience in critical care, acceptance of damage control principles, and the revolution in endovascular therapies have provided a more contemporary perspective on upper extremity junctional zone injuries. In both civilian and military settings, the experiences and principles of the past, along with appreciation for these advancements, have provided a platform of reevaluation in recognition, diagnosis, and management.

This chapter serves to review current paradigms in diagnosis and treatment of subclavian and axillary artery injuries. Use of modern endovascular techniques is becoming more realistic in many acute trauma settings, and, similar to other vascular injury territories such as with blunt aortic injury, shows significant promise. Effort to better understand benefits, drawbacks, and selection for endovascular treatment is engaging and continues. We further aim to describe how specific injury features speak to advantages and disadvantages of both open and endovascular management.

GENERAL COMMENTS

Reports from both civilian and military settings have shown the distribution and outcomes of major vascular injuries going as far back as the Civil War. Most reports detail all sustained vascular injuries or combined extremity vascular injuries. While some focus on details of vascular injuries to the upper extremity, more directed and specific outcomes of upper extremity vascular injuries, particularly axillosubclavian injuries, in most series can be difficult to discern since many trauma patients are lost to follow-up or die from more serious concomitant injuries. Nevertheless, some patterns regarding axillosubclavian vascular injury can be seen across these available studies, and several general comments pertaining to axillosubclavian vascular injury can be made.

- Upper extremity vascular trauma is less common than that in the lower extremity in both military and civilian environments.
- Penetrating mechanism is more common than blunt force, especially in the military setting.
- In civilian reports, blunt mechanism has an overall higher morbidity and mortality compared to penetrating injury.
- Mortality related to axillosubclavian arterial injury after either endovascular or open intervention is 10%–20% and usually due to associated injury.
- The axillary and subclavian arteries in the junctional zone are the most infrequently injured vessels of the upper extremity.
- Primary repair, patch angioplasty, and autologous vein grafting are common techniques used to repair traumatic subclavian and axillary injuries in the arm. However, prosthetic grafts in this location are not unreasonable due to size match, and the usual critical condition in many of these patients.

While hemorrhage and critical ischemia are the key, hard determinants indicating need for intervention and repair, a deeper understanding of the presentation and diagnostic nuances of this arterial segment is essential. This allows one to optimize management decisions, including situations when nonoperative, endovascular, or open operative management can be applied.

Unstable patients should be taken to the operating room. Stable patients may undergo further diagnostic imaging to better prepare for treatment. Preoperative evaluation should include chest X-ray. This can reveal fractured ribs and clavicles, hemopneumothoraces, missle fragments, and may provide information about the mediastinum. Bilateral arm blood pressures using continuous wave Doppler (i.e., measurement of an injured extremity index) is a quick and easy extension of the physical exam, which allows more objective diagnosis of an inflow or arterial injury. In a hemodynamically stable patient, computed tomography-angiography (Fig. 31-1) has proven itself and offers the opportunity for determining the location and nature of vessel injury, defines other concomitant injuries, and allows optimization of either open or endovascular operative planning. Duplex ultrasound can be used to quickly evaluate the axillary artery, but is limited in evaluation of the subclavian artery due to the depth and bony features of the thoracic inlet. Standard intra-arterial arteriography remains useful and may provide either catheter-based endovascular repair or control. Duplex is mostly relegated to assessment and indirect measures of reduced flow in this anatomic location with injury definition difficult.

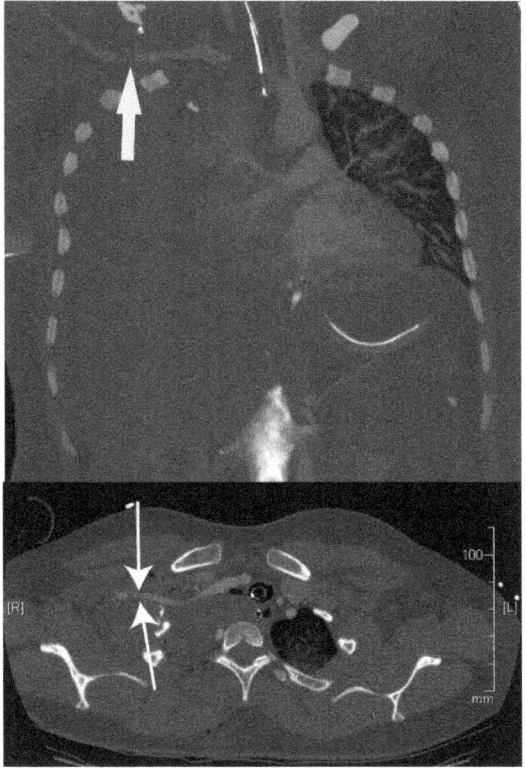

Figure 31-1. CT angiogram showing a partially transected axillary artery after gunshot wound.

GENERAL OPEN OPERATIVE STRATEGY IN THE MODERN AGE

Traditionally, the open operative strategy for complex extremity vascular injury was guided by the dictum "life over limb." Experience in the wars in Afghanistan and Iraq with damage control resuscitation and damage control surgical strategies has shown that in many instances, even with a significantly mangled extremity, it is now possible to save both life and limb acutely. Understanding of damage control adjuncts such as temporary vascular shunts and a methodical evaluation of axillosubclavian injuries can assist in minimizing morbidity and mortality while attempting to maximize functional outcomes in these formidable scenarios.

Most subclavian and axillary artery injuries are accompanied by major associated injuries. This is not surprising as these arteries are protected by muscle mass and the bony shoulder girdle. Thoracic wall and intracavitary injury, which may include pulmonary, cardiac, mediastinal vascular trauma, along with rib, clavicle, and soft tissue destruction, are commonplace. As the brachial plexus is intimately located with these arteries, blunt traction and tear, or direct penetrating division of plexus components may occur and commonly the degree of neurologic injury best defines outcome for these patients. When faced with arterial injury in conjunction with these major concomitant injuries, several broad concepts should be reviewed. In axillary artery injuries, in particular, humeral fractures should be brought to

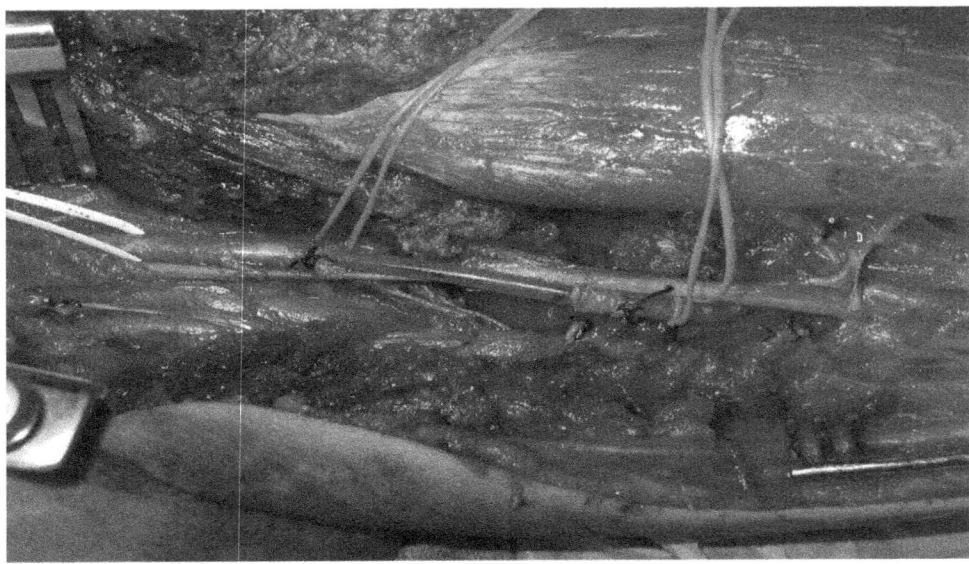

Figure 31-2. Temporary shunt placement in the distal axillary/proximal brachial artery.

length with either permanent or temporary fixation before definitive vascular repair. Temporary vascular shunts may be considered to expeditiously restore perfusion when other injuries require life-saving attention, or the patient's condition requires abbreviated maneuvers (Fig. 31-2). This now proven strategy allows for expedited perfusion to the extremity, a more thoughtful and complete assessment in urgent fashion, and an easier platform for definitive arterial and/or venous reconstruction.

Debridement of all clearly devitalized tissue should be performed. When extensive, primary amputation may occasionally need to be considered, particularly with scapulothoracic dissociation. Generally, we pursue anatomic reconstruction. In our experience, it is very rare that bypass grafting in these injuries requires planes away from the anatomic neurovascular bundle. Consideration must be given to primary repair of concomitant nerve/plexus injuries versus tagging the nerve ends for delayed neurorrhaphy once the wound has been stabilized.

This arterial injury pattern often requires that the surgeon be able to apply a diverse armamentarium of techniques. Efficient application requires adequate foresight of potential intraoperative and postoperative issues during the diagnostic and assessment stage. Failure to correctly prepare can prolong operative time and inadvertently result in suboptimal outcomes.

A FURTHER WORD ON TEMPORARY VASCULAR SHUNTS IN AXILLOSUBCLAVIAN ARTERIAL INJURY

Temporary intravascular shunts can allow for rapid restoration of distal limb perfusion when immediate vascular reconstruction is not possible (Fig. 31-2). This may be due to delays involving orthopedic fixation, wound debridement and definition, vein harvest, lack of clinical expertise at the initial treating facility, or addressing more life-threatening injuries. The use of intravascular shunting has been specifically applied within the military setting as a method to stabilize and temporize peripheral vascular injuries, avoid vascular reconstructions in austere, forward environments with limited resources and time, and allow for restitution and preservation of extremity perfusion during transport to definitive care. Furthermore, shunting has been used during mass casualty events and during damage control in those with significantly adverse physiology or concomitant bony injuries. As such, robust, systematic evaluations of use during Operation Iraqi Freedom (OIF) and Operation Enduring Freedom (OEF) have been performed, which demonstrate vascular shunts are safe and effective in preventing limb loss.[1-3] Additional case series have also been performed within the civilian population. These series report similar results and considerations regarding the use of shunts. Controversies regarding the use and theoretic benefit of venous shunts and therapeutic, or pharmacologic, shunting remain to be further studied and defined, along with the proper posture of shunting during transport in civilian settings.

Collectively, these experiences have defined the feasibility and usefulness of temporary shunting in the upper extremities, particularly proximally in the arm. Certainly, there appears to be no harm in early reperfusion using shunts. The potential drawbacks of unrecognized vessel injury by shunts, or the necessity for more extensive repairs owing to shunts and securing mechanisms seem negligible overall. Even when faced with primary upper extremity vascular injury at the time of definitive management, initial shunt use can be quite effective in providing time for operative planning, orthopedic lengthening/fixation, and autologous vein harvest. This simple strategy allows for earlier flow restoration and time to better define the vascular injury and may create a more precise final revascularization with improved neuromuscular outcome. Although dedicated assessment of temporary intravascular shunt use in axillary and subclavian artery injury is less common than more distally in the arm, success in utilization has been appreciated. Thus, selective use based on factors of time and degree of ischemia, patient stability, and associated issues make temporary intravascular shunting a viable option for these injuries.

CONSIDERATIONS IN OPEN MANAGEMENT OF SUBCLAVIAN ARTERY INJURIES

The relatively short length of the subclavian vessels along with the bony structure and musculature that surrounds them makes injury to these proximal most upper extremity vessels rare. However, subclavian vascular injury should be considered based on pattern of penetration or when the bony structures of the thoracic outlet such as the first rib or clavicle are fractured. While injury to the subclavian is more common in penetrating trauma, reports from military and civilian settings show subclavian artery injuries in general are a rather infrequent arterial injury.[4-10] Subclavian artery injury may not present with critical ischemia given the robust collateral circulation around the shoulder. Absence of distal pulses in an upper extremity, reduction in the injured extremity index (<0.9; compared to uninjured arm), or the presence of hemodynamic collapse with apparent mechanism should be considered highly suspicious for subclavian artery injury. In fact, many patients with subclavian artery injury will present in shock. Hemopneumothorax is common. More subtle physical signs can include significant supraclavicular and low cervical swelling or tracheal compression from an expanding hematoma. Immediate control may require manual pressure or Foley catheter tamponade. Concomitant injuries to the cervical, thoracic spine may be present and upper brachial plexus injuries along with associated venous injury will be common, and meticulous assessment for these injuries should be performed during the initial evaluation.

The proximal portion of the right subclavian artery can be exposed through a median sternotomy. This may require a clavicular extension with or without clavicular resection (Fig. 31-3). The origin of the left subclavian artery is in a more posterior location on the aortic arch and is classically exposed through a left

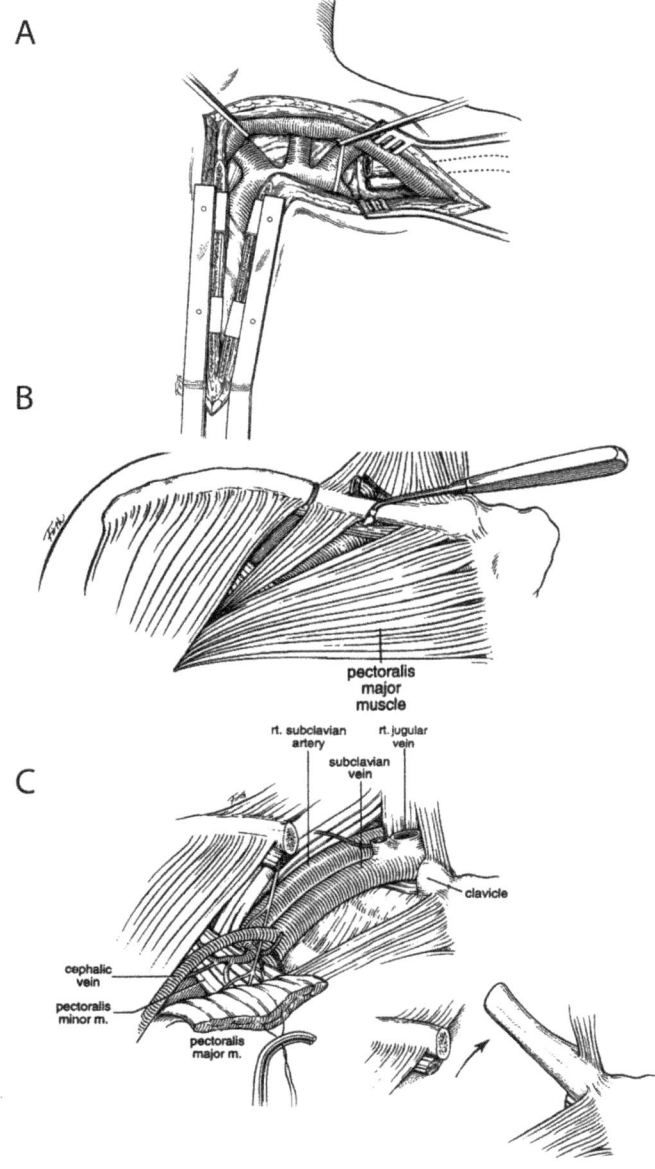

Figure 31-3. *A,* Clavicular extension of median sternotomy allows exposure of left subclavian artery. *B* and *C,* Resection of the medial half of the clavicle can be used to aid in exposing the subclavian and axillary vessels. Reprinted with permission from Demetriades et al.[12]

anterolateral thoracotomy, usually in the 4th interspace. Occasionally, particularly in thin patients, the proximal left subclavian can be controlled through a median sternotomy with a supraclavicular or cervical extension. Combining this with the anterolateral thoracotomy provides the "trapdoor" configuration exposing the proximal left subclavian artery. With the clavicular extension, the entire left subclavian artery can be exposed.

When the goal is to expose the mid-portion of the subclavian artery, a combined supraclavicular/infraclavicular two-incision technique has been described, but in the authors' experience, a single-incision approach with subperiosteal clavicular resection with or without simultaneous reconstruction of the clavicle seems most expeditious and flexible. The distal subclavian artery and proximal axillary artery is also potentially treatable from a two-incision approach, but injury management may require a lateral clavicular resection, again with or without bony replacement, and the author's preference is again a single-incision approach. The extent of proximal exposure necessary in subclavian artery injury is predicated on injury mechanism, injury location, patient stability, and surgeon experience. As will be discussed later, the advent of endovascular control techniques, using balloon occlusion, may provide inflow control and the ability to perform directed subclavian exposure through clavicular incision in situations when open control may have dictated more proximal exposure.

Dissection in the area of the subclavian artery and vein should be performed with care given the abundance of adjacent nerve structures at risk for inadvertent injury. Aside from the brachial plexus and vagus nerve, the phrenic nerve sits on the anterior scalene muscle and should be identified and avoided (Fig. 31-4). The

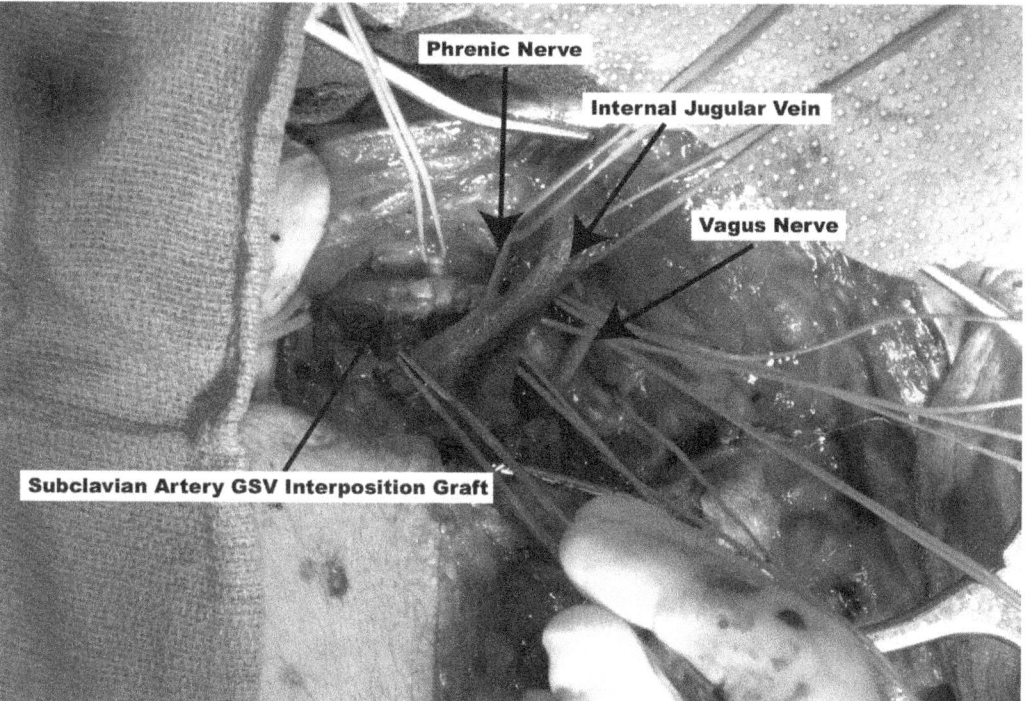

Figure 31-4. Right subclavian artery repair using greater saphenous vein interposition graft and pledgets in a 30-year-old man with penetrating injuries to the central chest. The complexity of the anatomy in the area of the subclavian artery and vein necessitates meticulous dissection during operative exposure.

abundance of collaterals around the shoulder and neck may allow for ligation of the subclavian artery in emergency situations with maintenance of upper extremity viability. Temporary shunting, however, may be considered and in the author's opinion provides a better alternative to ligation in most circumstances. Tension-free repair of the subclavian artery cannot be overemphasized as the vessel is relatively thin, nonmuscular, and delicate. Due to this, primary repair and patch angioplasty is challenging. If these are entertained, use of pledgets is recommended. Prosthetic material can be used as an interposition graft for these larger, more proximal great vessel and upper extremity reconstructions. Autologous conduit such as saphenous vein, paneled saphenous vein, internal jugular vein, or even femoral vein can be entertained depending on size and length considerations (Fig. 31-5). The choice is dependent on patient condition and associated soft tissue injury. In more extensive injuries, ligation and revascularization using bypass with inflow based more proximally such as from ascending aorta, the innominate artery, or carotid systems may also be an option.

CONSIDERATIONS IN OPEN MANAGEMENT AXILLARY ARTERY INJURIES

Axillary artery injuries are more common than subclavian artery injuries because they lack the protection of the structures of the thoracic outlet. This more superficial course leads to the axillary artery accounting for 2%–3% of arterial injury.[4-11] Similar to the subclavian, penetrating trauma is the most common mechanism of axillary artery injury. However, in contrast to isolated subclavian artery injuries in which the patient will present in shock, isolated injuries to the axillary artery rarely present with hemodynamic collapse. More common hallmarks include absent distal pulses or reduced injured extremity index (<0.9), pulsatile bleeding, and/or an expanding hematoma. The rich collateral network may preclude the development of critical ischemia, and an axillary artery injury may not be readily recognized without the aid of the continuous wave Doppler and measurement of the injured extremity index. CTA or arteriography is useful diagnostic tools in certain situations including those in which an endovascular therapy is being considered. However, with good physical examination, continuous wave Doppler use, and other noninvasive imaging modalities, most axillary artery injuries can be diagnosed without arteriography. Duplex ultrasonography is more useful distally in the axillary artery, but may still be limited. Anterior dislocation of the humeral head or fractures of the humerus can result in axillary artery injury and concomitant injuries to the nearby nerves of the brachial plexus and axillary vein are common.

Sterile preparation of the ipsilateral neck, chest, supraclavicular fossa, and the circumferential arm will be essential to obtain proximal control. Attempting to obtain proximal control within an area of a hematoma should be approached with caution to decrease excessive blood loss and damage to adjacent nerve structures.

An infraclavicular incision made two fingerbreadths below and parallel to the clavicle will allow for access to the proximal axillary artery. The clavipectoral fascia is next divided through the superior aspect of this incision opening a space, which allows visualization of the proximal axillary artery. Identification and division of the pectoralis minor muscle through this exposure is frequently necessary to show the entire axillary artery. Exposure of the subclavian artery as discussed previously may also be required for more proximal axillary artery injuries. This two-incision

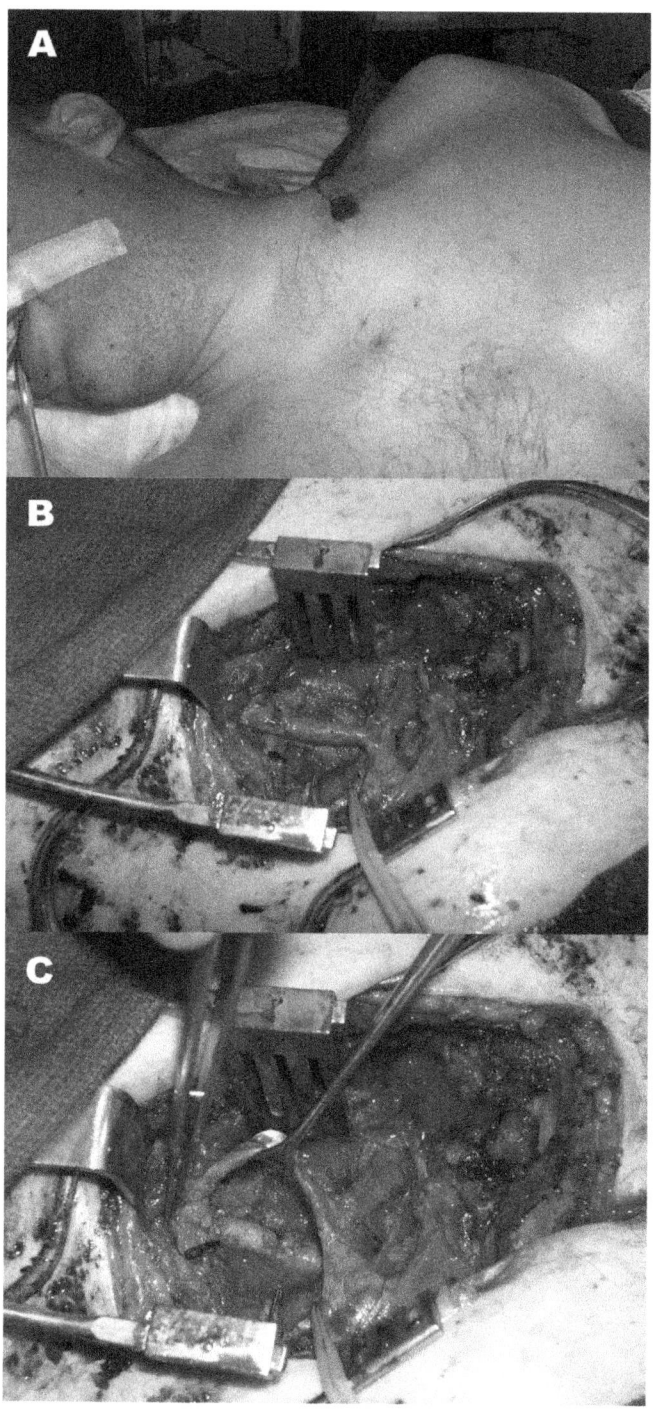

Figure 31-5. *A*, A gunshot wound to zone 1 of the neck is shown. *B* and *C*, A supraclavicular incision was performed, and a subclavian artery and vein injury were identified. A partial subperiosteal clavicular resection was used for exposure. A subclavian artery Great Saphenous Vein (GSV) interposition graft was performed as well as a subclavian vein to internal jugular GSV bypass.

supraclavicular and infraclavicular exposure can be helpful in approaching these injuries, but injuries to the distal subclavian/proximal axillary artery may require clavicular resection for adequate visualization. Precise arterial clamping is essential given the proximity to the axillary vein and brachial plexus.

A primary end-to-end repair of the axillary artery can be performed with ligation and division of side branches as needed to mobilize the artery and allow for a tension-free anastomosis. However, most axillary artery injuries require more complex reconstruction, usually consisting of an interposition graft. Similar to subclavian artery management, autologous vein from various locations used either as a simple interposition or paneled graft provides a reasonable conduit particularly in the setting of a significant soft tissue injury. Prosthetic graft is a rational alternative should size mismatch exist or patient's injuries preclude vein harvest. As noted, some have suggested that the rich collateral supply of the upper extremity will allow for ligation of the axillary artery, but recent experiences with temporary intravascular shunting may allow for perfusion with patient stabilization and return at a future time point for definitive repair. Maintenance of flow in and repair of the axial vessel of the upper extremity is especially important in the setting of soft tissue wounds where an otherwise robust collateral circulation may have been interrupted.

A BRIEF COMMENT ON VENOUS INJURY

Axillosubclavian venous injury can have dire consequences. In a study by Demetriades et al. looking at penetrating injuries to the subclavian and axillary vessels, venous injury had a significantly higher mortality than arterial injury.[12] Ligation of the named veins of the upper extremity can be performed in austere conditions or when another life-threatening injury takes precedence with relatively low morbidity; however, the optimal management of upper extremity venous injury remains controversial. Extremity venous repair gained popularity during the Vietnam War with Rich reporting 377 venous injuries, in which 124 (32.9%) were repaired. Lateral suture was the most common repair performed (n = 106) followed by end-to-end anastomosis (n = 10), vein interposition graft (n = 5), and vein patch graft (n = 3).[13]

In further experience in Iraq and Afghanistan, Gifford and colleagues, in 2009, identified venous repair as independently protective against amputation (RR = 0.2; 95% CI [0.04–0.99], P = .05) during evaluation of 125 extremity vascular injuries, of which 35 were in the upper extremity.[14] This has led to the authors' relatively aggressive stance to repair upper extremity veins, particularly in the proximal arm where the larger veins represent watershed areas of venous drainage. Upper extremity vein repair should also be considered in instances where this is a multimechanistic injury resulting in major soft tissue defects likely to compromise venous return through an otherwise robust collateral network. In these instances, it is the authors' observation that maintenance or reestablishment of the main axial venous outflow is important in quality limb salvage (Fig. 31-5).

As such, the most difficult injuries in the axillosubclavian segment in which to perform venous reconstruction are those likely to benefit. Primary lateral venorrhaphy, patch angioplasty, or debridement and primary anastomosis are legitimate techniques. Use of panel grafts for size match is useful, but time consuming. When the saphenous vein is of reasonable size, the authors have used simple interposition vein grafting, widely spatulating for anastomotic creation, accepting up to a 50% vessel size reduction. Our observation has been that venous repair helps with immediate extremity venous decompression and reduces venous hemorrhage in massive injuries. Rich and colleagues have suggested that roughly half of venous repairs will thrombose in the near term. Yet, after thrombus maturation and remodeling, half of these will recanalize.[13] The degree of meaningful venous return remains to be defined.

ENDOVASCULAR MANAGEMENT OF AXILLOSUBCLAVIAN ARTERIAL INJURY

Use of endovascular technologies in diagnosis and management of injury to the subclavian and axillary arteries continues to evolve. Indeed, this approach has now become commonplace in both civilian and combat settings.[15–18] Specific application of catheter-based treatments in proximal upper extremity and junctional zone injuries may offer advantages both in acute vessel injury and in less urgent or delayed traumatic sequelae such as arteriovenous fistula and pseudoaneurysm (Fig. 31-6). In particular, endovascular techniques avoid emergent operative dissection near the brachial plexus and venous structures and may provide earlier hemorrhage control by balloon occlusion techniques. Furthermore, it allows the surgical team to address other life-threating injuries and avoid the morbidity of a median sternotomy, thoracotomy, or junctional zone open exposure. Endovascular repair has been suggested to decrease operative time, blood loss, fluid requirements, and possibly length of stay.[17]

Use of covered stents is becoming a feasible definitive management alternative for these injuries in both penetrating and blunt trauma.[17,19–23] Even when hard signs of vascular injury and hemodynamic instability are present, patients now may be considered for emergent endovascular repair in the operating room. When, either for anatomic reasons or inability to gain wire access across the injury, open repair is deemed necessary, balloon control proximal to the injury is quite useful and facilitates repair, and may allow for selective reduction in degree of open exposure required for repair. These types of endovascular maneuvers require timely endovascular capability and personnel expertise within a highly functional care system. Fixed hybrid operating room technology with state-of-the-art imaging has made this possibility realistic. In those hemodynamically stable, or with soft signs of vascular injury, the use of noninvasive anatomic imaging, particularly CTA in the axillosubclavian segment, allows for injury diagnosis, definition, and more complete endovascular treatment planning (Fig. 31-1).

Control and definitive endovascular management of axillosubclavian arterial injuries may require antegrade femoral access, retrograde ipsilateral brachial access, or both. Passing the wire under fluoroscopic guidance across vessel disruption may be challenging, particularly in complete transection. Secondary to the shorter distance from the access site to the injury, many consider the retrograde brachial approach preferred owing to improved pushability and steerability. Directional catheters, balloon centering guidance, and wire snare capture from combined antegrade-retrograde access "rendezvous" are described techniques used to facilitate wire access (Fig. 31-7).[15,17,18] Both self-expanding and balloon expandable covered stents have been reported effective in managing axillosubclavian injuries (Fig. 31-8). Bare metal stents have been used for treatment of small dissections or intimal flaps.

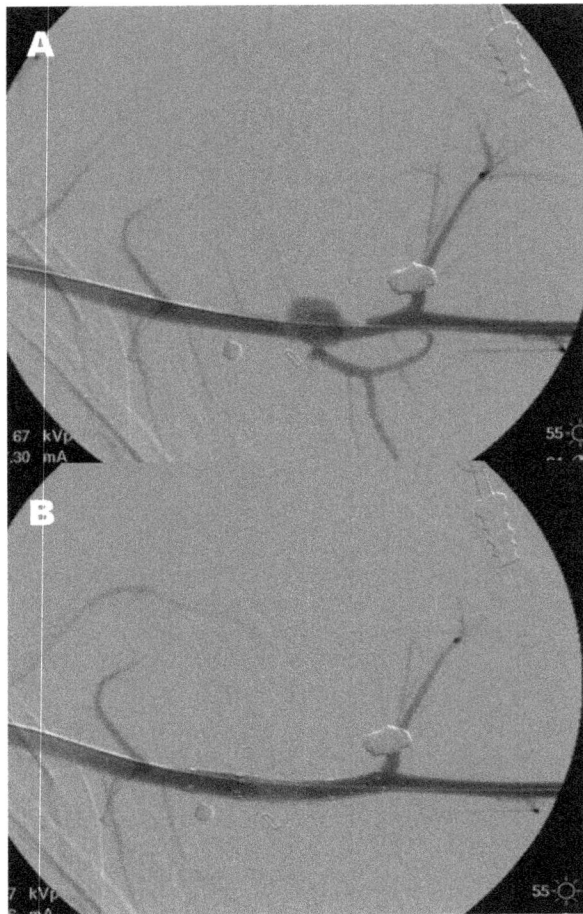

Figure 31-6. *A*, A large 6-cm pseudoaneurysm of the axillary brachial junction was identified. *B*, A retrograde left brachial artery endovascular approach allowed for deployment of covered stents. This repair remains patent at six years follow-up.

We generally begin with femoral access for arteriography and inflow occlusion if necessary. We then attempt wire crossing and use brachial access adjunctively and promptly if antegrade passage is difficult. Our preference is use of self-expanding stent grafts due to angulation and potential motion translation from the arm in areas constrained by the clavicle and first rib. These are oversized to 15%–25% of the treatment vessel. Understanding of the contralateral vertebral artery is necessary with selective coverage of the ipsilateral vertebral, and only entertained if the contralateral is continuous and not hypoplastic or atretic. Postdeployment balloon angioplasty within the covered stent should usually be avoided to prevent injury tearing and enlargement, thus increasing the risk of repair failure. Occasionally, gentle angioplasty is needed to provide adequate stent graft expansion.

Reports describing use of endovascular repair in subclavian and axillary artery injury began to appear more than a decade ago. In a multiinstitutional communication on the use of the self-expanding Wallgraft endoprosthesis (Boston Scientific, Natick, MA) for the treatment of 18 subclavian arterial injuries, White and colleagues showed the

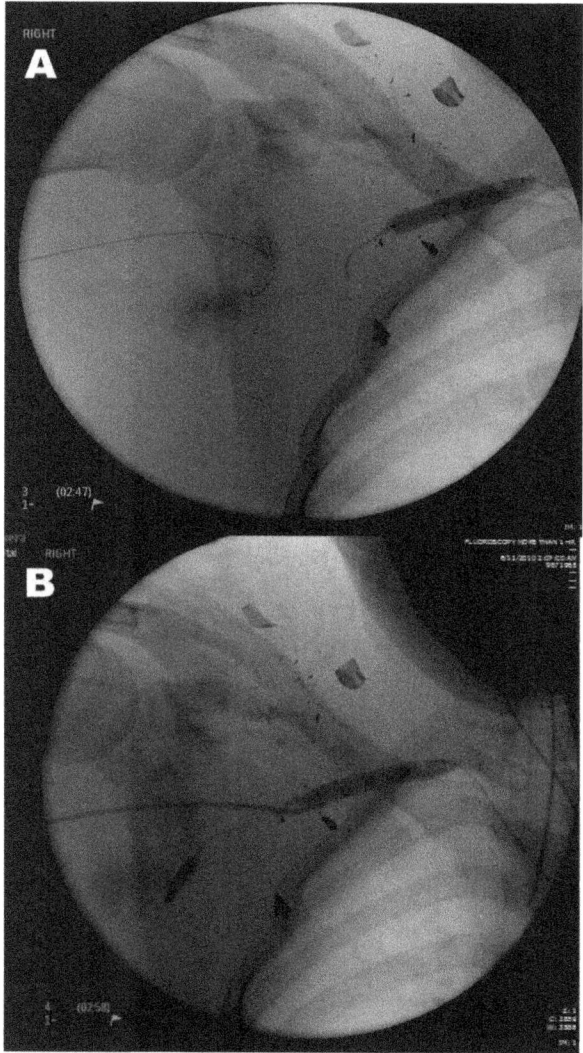

Figure 31-7. *A*, Arterial transection with proximal balloon occlusion utilization through femoral access and "rendezvous" access through brachial site to traverse lesion. *B*, Successful traverse of lesion following "rendezvous" technique. Reprinted with permission from DuBose et al.[15]

endoprosthesis achieved full exclusion in 90% of injuries.[21] Freedom from open revision was achieved in 100% of subclavian injuries at one year without procedure-related mortality. The most common postprocedure complication involved stenosis or occlusion.

du Toit and colleagues reported 57 patients with penetrating subclavian artery injury that underwent stent graft treatment during a ten-year period.[20] One patient in this series died due to other injuries, and three (5%) developed early, nonlimb threatening stent graft occlusion. Complete follow-up data was available for 16 patients at a mean of 61 months (range 8–104 months), which showed that five patients had arm claudication and >50% in-stent stenosis on arteriogram. These patients were successfully treated with balloon angioplasty. Three additional asymptomatic patients in the

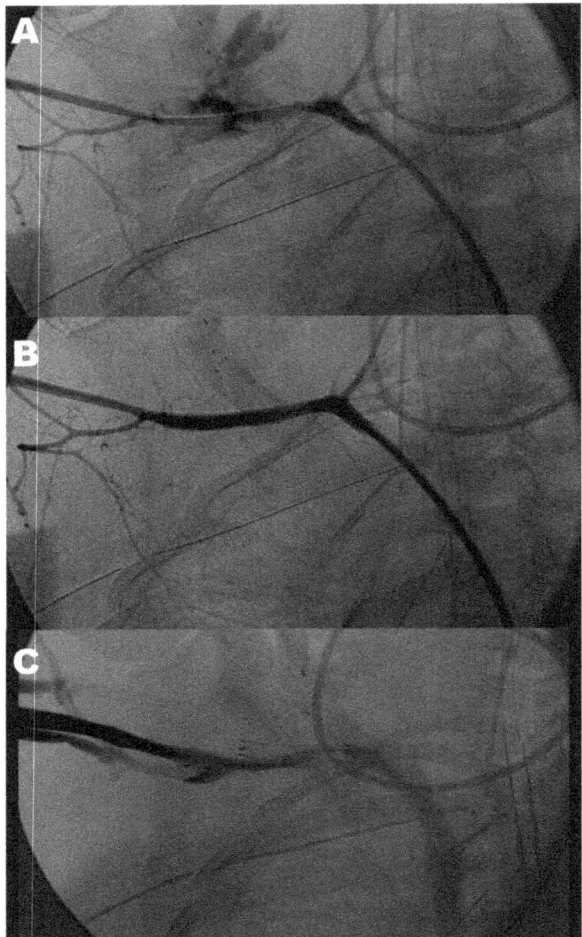

Figure 31-8. *A,* Partial transection of axillary artery after gunshot wound. *B,* Endograft exclusion of injured axillary artery. *C,* Assessment of axillary and subclavian vein after endograft deployment. Images of *A* and *B* reprinted with permission from DuBose et al.[15]

follow-up cohort had stent occlusion, but did not require reintervention. Hershberger et al. reviewed 195 studies on endovascular treatment of injury to the aortic arch and supra-aortic arteries between 1995 and 2007.[24] When endovascular treatment of subclavian (*n* = 91) and axillary (*n* = 12) artery injuries were assessed, technical success rates were 96.7% and 100%; peri-procedural morbidity 12.1% and 8.3%; and mortality 3% and 0%, respectively. Complications included access site pseudoaneurysm, in-stent stenosis with arm claudication, stent fracture, and thrombosis.

Recently, collective reviews of the available low-level literature on endovascular management of axillosubclavian injury have become available.[15,18] These have included reports of small clinical series and the now available few institutional reports comparing open versus endovascular management. Even in the face of significant lead-time and selection biases, these have iterated the need to acutely convert to open repair when attempting endovascular management is quite low (5% or less) and technical success is 93%–100%. Later reintervention is estimated to be necessary in some 4%–8%.

The majority of these can be managed with catheter-based therapies with reported indications including in-stent stenosis, thrombosis, and endoleak. No clear mortality benefit of endovascular treatment over open repair is currently appreciated.[18] The risk of stroke is less than 2% regardless of open or endovascular treatment selection. Arm amputation, excluding the decision for primary amputation and those for major brachial plexus injury, occurs in some 1.5%. Primary patency of axillary and subclavian artery stent grafts is projected to be nearly 95% at one year and approximately 75% at five years.[15–18]

In our own literature review of 37 reports published between 1994 and 2011, a total of 186 patients with axillosubclavian arterial injuries managed with endovascular repair were identified. The majority of injuries were caused by a penetrating mechanism and were pseudoaneurysms (Figs. 31-9 and 31-10). In comparison to most of the reports on open axillosubclavian injury where the injury is managed acutely, endovascular management has been used to address injuries presenting both acutely and delayed (Fig. 31-11). No patients in this review died directly from their arterial injury. Postprocedure follow-up was variable and ranged between 1 and 104 months. While

Mechanisms of Axillosubclavian Artery Injuries Treated with Endovascular Repair

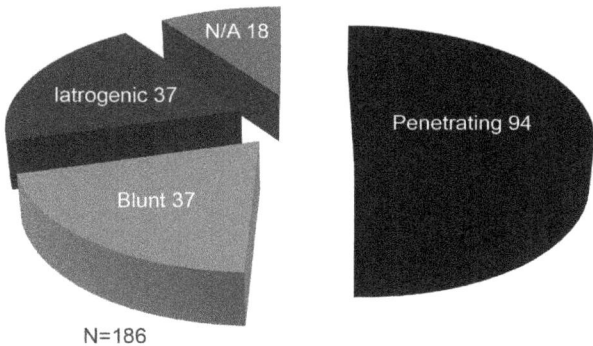

Figure 31-9. Distribution of mechanism of axillosubclavian injuries treated with endovascular repair in cumulative review of case reports in 186 patients. References available upon request.

Types of Axillosubclavian Artery Injuries Treated with Endovascular Repair

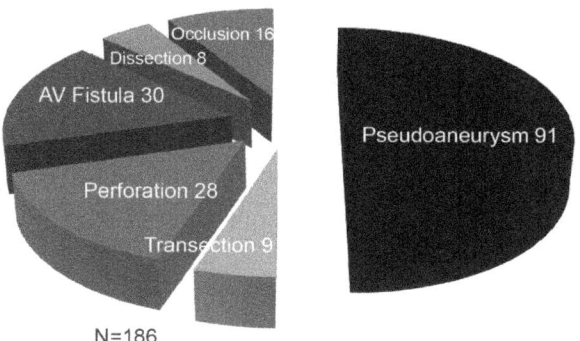

Figure 31-10. Distribution of type of axillosubclavian injuries treated with endovascular repair in cumulative review of case reports in 186 patients. References available upon request.

Time to Endovascular Interventions in Axillosubclavian Injuries

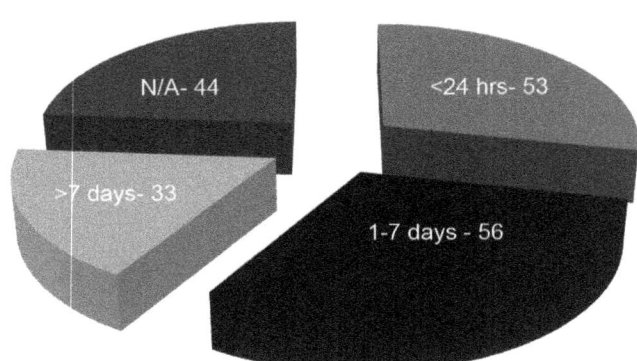

N=186

Figure 31-11. Time to endovascular treatment of axillosubclavian injuries in cumulative review of case reports in 186 patients. References available upon request.

TABLE 31-1. COMPLICATIONS IN ENDOVASCULAR TREATMENT OF AXILLOSUBCLAVIAN INJURIES

Complication	*N = 186*	Percent
No reported complications	157	84.4
Stent fracture, occlusion, or stenosis requiring reintervention	13	6.9
Endoleak requiring reintervention	1	0.5
Asymptomatic occlusion or stenosis >50% not requiring reintervention	7	3.7
Access site complication	3	1.6
Conversion to open	5	2.6

stent patency data for 70 patients was unavailable, 97 patients had 100% patency in follow-up and three patients had patency between 80% and 99%. This data should be approached with some healthy skepticism, however, as the length of follow-up is quite broad. A total of five (2.6%) patients were reported as being converted to open. A complete list of complications for these patient reports is shown in Table 31-1.

Although graft infection is a legitimate concern, there is no indication that this poses undue risk in this anatomic position. In fact, the authors are not aware of a report or experienced any upper extremity stent graft–related infectious complications in grafts placed in Iraq, Afghanistan, or in civilian trauma practice in the United States. Thus, despite concern regarding durability of endovascular stent graft use in trauma patients, results are encouraging for this anatomic location.

Certain limitations to the endovascular approach must be recognized. As noted, the personnel, facilities, and trauma system must provide for rapid diagnostic and multimodality treatment capability. Hybrid operating rooms, born out of the transformation in disease-related vascular and endovascular surgery, truly provide state-of-the-art treatment arenas for trauma. They provide a singular setting in which to have the full spectrum of therapeutic options in vascular injury and perform other treatment maneuvers such as thoracotomy, laparotomy, orthopedic stabilization, and other procedures. While these facilities are now quite apparent in many high-level trauma centers, access to fluoroscopy and device inventory still remains a limiting factor in many locations.

Concomitant axillosubclavian venous injury is difficult to treat by endovascular modalities, and while venography at the time of arterial treatment seems prudent, use of stent grafts or remote occlusion techniques in these veins is less defined, and ongoing venous hemorrhage is a concern. Similarly, visualization, assessment, and some understanding of brachial plexus integrity are appreciated with open exposures. With endovascular repair, this is functionally assessed in a delayed fashion and may lead to arterial reconstruction in some in whom amputation is realized. Finally, injury anatomy may limit endovascular application. While open revascularization constructs are not constrained by this per se, designed stent grafts allowing for proximal traumatic reconstruction of the innominate bifurcation and/or vertebral artery preservation are not available.

COMPLICATIONS AFTER REPAIR OF AXILLOSUBCLAVIAN ARTERIAL INJURY

Complications after axillosubclavian arterial injury and repair include reperfusion injury, graft stenosis and thrombosis, anastomotic hemorrhage, infection, and pseudoaneurysm formation. Stroke, as noted, occurs rarely, and other systemic complications are patient specific. With endovascular repair, access site complications such as hemorrhage and hematoma, pseudoaneurysm, neurologic compromise, and arteriovenous fistula are possible as with any endovascular intervention. The risk of any one or combination of these varies based on type and severity of injury and has not been well defined in the literature. Most of the series on upper extremity vascular injury focus more on mortality and successful limb salvage than specific rates of repair-related complications. However, these are important to keep in mind when one cares for a patient with this injury pattern. The authors' own experience reported in an analysis of combat upper extremity vascular injuries from OIF involving 45 patients showed early complications after open repair were significant and involved infection (4.7%), thrombosis (9.3%), anastomotic hemorrhage (2.3%), and early amputation (9.3%).[5] Upper extremity fasciotomy performance requires clinical judgment. This can be quite challenging and must be considered in a spectrum of ischemic duration (four to six hours upper limits), degree of ischemia based on collateralization, as well as venous injury and the burden of musculoskeletal injury and wounds. Late ongoing surveillance of vascular repair in subclavian and axillary arterial injuries, with modalities such as duplex ultrasound or CTA, is recommended to reduce the risk of late repair–specific complications. This is obviously challenging in trauma patients. The lack of such surveillance data in both open and endovascular repair is truly a limiting factor in honing contemporary approach.

There is some indication that functional ability is the harbinger of true outcome, as opposed to arterial related problems. Brown et al. did a retrospective review of 71 patients who underwent open operative management after upper extremity arterial injury.[25] The limb salvage rate was 94% and follow-up after injury was 6.3 months (range 0–33 months). Patients who sustained blunt injury were more likely to have severe disability than patients with a penetrating injury. Patients with concomitant orthopedic injury were as likely to have a full functional recovery as those without an orthopedic injury. The importance of associated nerve injury was highlighted as patients who had either a concomitant nerve injury or combined nerve and orthopedic injuries were less likely to regain function. Additionally, patients who had delayed repair of nerve injuries were more likely to have severe disability or amputation in follow-up. These authors found that injuries deemed severe enough to require fasciotomy did not have a significant functional recovery and were left with the most severe disability. Thus, while restoration of arterial perfusion, by either open or catheter-based methods, is quite feasible, nerve and soft tissue disruption remain formidable and are true determinants of functional outcome. Clearly, in addition to repair specific information, more high-quality data are needed to provide a better understanding of how treatment strategies for injuries to the blood vessels in the upper extremity junctional zone affect patient's lives and function.

OPEN OR ENDO? A FINAL WORD ON THE EVOLUTION

Mortality for axillosubclavian arterial injury is 10%–20% with associated limb loss less than 2% in more recent reports. Currently, there is no indication either open or endovascular repair confers an improved survival advantage when compared. Use of endovascular technology to repair subclavian and axillary arterial injury is now highly visible and has been shown feasible and safe. Its application has now been extended to unstable patients owing to hybrid operating rooms and technical expertise. At best, it is definitive management. Within the available literature, and in our experience, this is being born out in those able to be treated with stent grafting. At worst, it might be a bridge to either earlier inflow control or a delayed more controlled revascularization in a stabilized, nonhemorrhaging patient.

Open repair remains a life-saving definitive reconstruction with rare need for reintervention. It takes longer, leads to more blood loss and fluid requirement, carries wound/incision morbidity, and likely longer length of stay. Open repair is not as anatomically constrained as endovascular repair providing for the breadth of anatomic needs. Today's environment mandates the vascular surgeon have expertise in both endovascular and open repair, allowing for direct, individualized treatment in each situation.

REFERENCES

1. Chambers LW, Green DJ, Sample K, et al. Tactical surgical intervention with temporary shunting of peripheral vascular trauma sustained during Operation Iraqi Freedom: one unit's experience. *J Trauma*. 2006;61:824–830.
2. Rasmussen TE, Clouse WD, Jenkins DH, et al. The use of temporary vascular shunts as a damage control adjunct in the management of wartime vascular injury. *J Trauma*. 2006;61: 8–12; discussion 12–15.
3. Taller J, Kamdar JP, Greene JA, et al. Temporary vascular shunts as initial treatment of proximal extremity vascular injuries during combat operations: the new standard of care at Echelon II facilities? *J Trauma*. 2008;65:595–603.
4. Clouse WD, Rasmussen TE, Peck MA, et al. In-theater management of vascular injury: 2 years of the Balad Vascular Registry. *J Am Coll Surg*. 2007;204:625–632.

5. Clouse WD, Rasmussen TE, Perlstein J, et al. Upper extremity vascular injury: a current in-theater wartime report from Operation Iraqi Freedom. *Ann Vasc Surg*. 2006;20:429–434.
6. Debakey ME, Simeone FA. Battle injuries of the arteries in World War II: an analysis of 2,471 cases. *Ann Surg*. 1946;123:534–579.
7. Graham JM, Feliciano DV, Mattox KL, et al. Management of subclavian vascular injuries. *J Trauma*. 1980;20:537–544.
8. Hughes CW. Arterial repair during the Korean war. *Ann Surg*. 1958;147:555–561.
9. Lin PH, Koffron AJ, Guske PJ, et al. Penetrating injuries of the subclavian artery. *Am J Surg*. 2003;185:580–584.
10. Rich NM, Baugh JH, Hughes CW. Acute arterial injuries in Vietnam: 1,000 cases. *J Trauma*. 1970;10:359–369.
11. Graham JM, Mattox KL, Feliciano DV, DeBakey ME. Vascular injuries of the axilla. *Ann Surg*. 1982;195:232–238.
12. Demetriades D, Chahwan S, Gomez H, et al. Penetrating injuries to the subclavian and axillary vessels. *J Am Coll Surg*. 1999;188:290–295.
13. Rich NM, Hughes CW, Baugh JH. Management of venous injuries. *Ann Surg*. 1970; 171:724–730.
14. Gifford SM, Aidinian G, Clouse WD, et al. Effect of temporary shunting on extremity vascular injury: an outcome analysis from the Global War on Terror vascular injury initiative. *J Vasc Surg*. 2009;50:549–555; discussion 555–546.
15. DuBose JJ, Rajani R, Gilani R, et al. Endovascular management of axillo-subclavian arterial injury: a review of published experience. *Injury*. 2012;43:1785–1792.
16. Fox CJ, Patel B, Clouse WD. Update on wartime vascular injury. *Perspect Vasc Surg Endovasc Ther*. 2011;23(1):13–25.
17. Shalhub S, Starnes BW, Hatsukami TS, et al. Repair of blunt thoracic outlet arterial injuries: an evolution from open to endovascular approach. *J Trauma*. 2011;71:E114–E121.
18. Sinha S, Patterson BO, Ma J, et al. Systematic review and meta-analysis of open surgical and endovascular management of thoracic outlet vascular injuries. *J Vasc Surg*. 2013;57:547–567 e548.
19. Carrick MM, Morrison CA, Pham HQ, et al. Modern management of traumatic subclavian artery injuries: a single institution's experience in the evolution of endovascular repair. *Am J Surg*. 2010;199:28–34.
20. du Toit DF, Lambrechts AV, Stark H, Warren BL. Long-term results of stent graft treatment of subclavian artery injuries: management of choice for stable patients? *J Vasc Surg*. 2008;47:739–743.
21. White R, Krajcer Z, Johnson M, et al. Results of a multicenter trial for the treatment of traumatic vascular injury with a covered stent. *J Trauma*. 2006;60:1189–1195; discussion 1195–1186.
22. Xenos ES, Freeman M, Stevens S, et al. Covered stents for injuries of subclavian and axillary arteries. *J Vasc Surg*. 2003;38:451–454.
23. Danetz JS, Cassano AD, Stoner MC, et al. Feasibility of endovascular repair in penetrating axillosubclavian injuries: a retrospective review. *J Vasc Surg*. 2005;41:246–254.
24. Hershberger RC, Aulivola B, Murphy M, Luchette FA. Endovascular grafts for treatment of traumatic injury to the aortic arch and great vessels. *J Trauma*. 2009;67:660–671.
25. Brown KR, Jean-Claude J, Seabrook GR, et al. Determinates of functional disability after complex upper extremity trauma. *Ann Vasc Surg*. 2001;15:43–48.

32

Uncommon Upper Extremity Arterial Disorders

Thom W. Rooke, MD and Cindy Felty MSN, RN, CNP

Aren't all upper extremity arterial disorders uncommon?

Hardly. Upper extremity arterial disorders, while less prevalent overall than those of the lower extremity, are routinely encountered in clinical practice. The causes of upper extremity arterial disorders include both common and uncommon etiologies. For purposes of further examination, arterial disorders can be discussed in terms of three broad categories: those that occur *extrinsic* to the arterial wall, those that directly *involve* the arterial wall, and those that occur *within* the lumen of the artery. Disorders affecting the arterial wall can be further divided into *structural* versus *vasomotor* abnormalities.

DISORDERS OCCURRING OUTSIDE THE ARTERIAL WALL

Some of the most common disorders affecting the upper extremity arteries originate outside of the vessels. For example, positional compression at the thoracic outlet is so common that it can almost be considered a variant of normal.[1] It is only in a small minority of patients (particularly those with cervical ribs, fibrous bands, or other structural abnormalities) that the degree of positional obstruction is severe enough to produce symptoms consistent with the "thoracic outlet syndrome." In its usual mild form, this entity is seen far too frequently to be considered an "uncommon arterial disorder." However, unusual causes of thoracic outlet syndrome do occur and may prove difficult to diagnose and/or treat (Fig. 32-1).

Under certain conditions, the upper extremity arteries can be impinged or compressed even when the arm or shoulder is in a neutral position. Classic causes include tumors of the shoulder and lung (such as Pancoast tumors),[2] hematomas that may result from blunt or penetrating trauma, iatrogenic causes, and so on, and even the over exuberant use of tourniquets.[3,4]

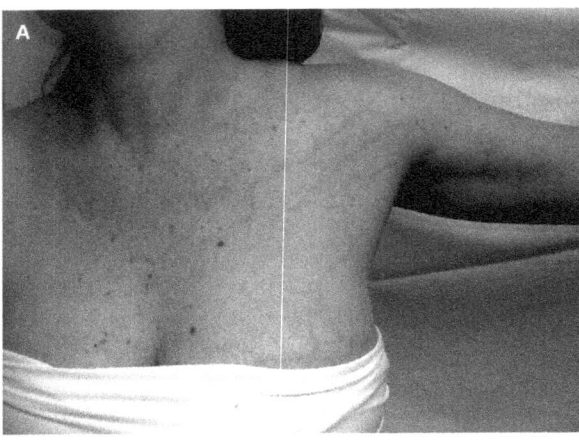
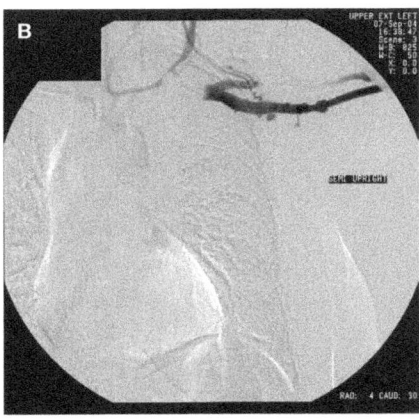
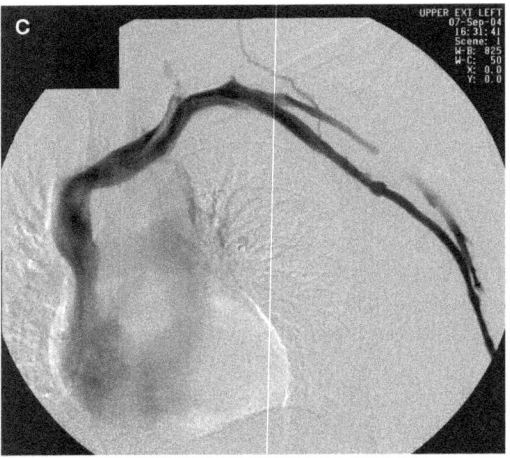
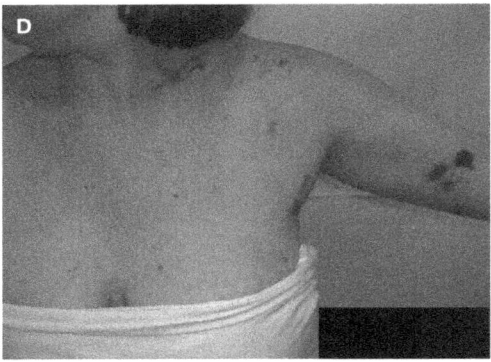

Figure 32-1. *A,* A 45-year-old woman reached for a cup of coffee and experienced a "snapping" sensation in her left shoulder accompanied by severe pain. Examination an hour later revealed a prominent superficial venous pattern consistent with acute collateral vein enlargement secondary to deep venous obstruction. *B,* The patient was taken for urgent venography. The observed axillary vein obstruction was thought to represent acute DVT. *C,* With abduction of the arm, the obstruction disappeared. The cause was subsequently determined to be extrinsic compression of the subclavian-axillary vein by a fractured and displaced first rib. *D,* The patient underwent immediate first rib resection. During the immediate postoperative recovery period, her prominent superficial venous pattern resolved, indicating restoration of deep venous flow.

Extrinsic arterial disorders include more than the various "things that cause compression of an otherwise normal artery." For example, arteriovenous (AV) malformations and AV shunts interfere with arterial perfusion by stealing flow from otherwise normal arteries. Malformations, fistulas, and shunts may be associated with mass effect, tenderness, pain, problems related to high arterial flow, and an assortment of pathological manifestations that are completely independent of any ischemic problems that may also be associated with arterial "steal."

DISORDERS OCCURRING IN THE ARTERIAL WALL

Structural Disorders

The most common structural abnormality of the upper extremity arterial wall (or for that matter almost any arterial bed) is *atherosclerosis*. Atherosclerotic plaques tend to occur most commonly in proximal arteries (subclavian, innominate, and axillary arteries) and less commonly in distal ones (radial and ulnar); this "proximal versus distal" pattern is typical for most arterial distributions.

Other less common noninflammatory, nonatherosclerotic disorders can affect the upper limb and produce obstructive narrowing in the arteries. Among the unusual disorders is *fibromuscular dysplasia* (FMD). Although this entity seems to be most common in renal and carotid vessels, it can affect almost any artery in the body including those of the upper extremity.[5] The exact incidence of FMD is unknown; national registries are currently under way, which may help to better define the incidence/prevalence of FMD throughout the body.[6]

Disorders involving abnormal vascular proteins, fibrins, or other connective tissues can rarely affect the vessels of the upper extremity along with others throughout the body. The best example of this type (although not necessarily the most common condition producing these changes) is Ehlers–Danlos syndrome. Many similar, and far rarer, abnormalities, diseases, or syndromes have been described but are beyond the scope of this chapter.

A variety of inflammatory conditions can also affect the arteries of the upper extremities. Among the best known examples of these are the giant cell arteritides. Giant cell (or temporal) arteritis typically affects those 50 years or older, while Takayasu arteritis is seen almost exclusively in those less than 50 years.[7] These well-described vasculitides frequently affect the upper extremity vessels, producing long, tapered hour-glass lesions and/or complete occlusions (Fig. 32-2). Treatment classically involves immunosuppression with corticosteroids, but more recent studies suggest an increasing role for nonsteroid and/or novel immunosuppressive agents.[8–10]

An assortment of unusual vasculitides can affect the smaller vessels of the upper extremity. These include such diverse disorders as livedo vasculitis,[11] cutaneous polyarteritis nodosa,[12] Behcet's syndrome,[13] Wegener's granulomatosis,[14] and a host of others. Most of these are vascular inflammatory conditions of uncertain etiology, often associated with markers of inflammation such as a high sedimentation rate. Treatment with steroids, immunosuppressive agents, and/or anti-inflammatory drugs may be useful, but the response to treatment is often variable and unpredictable. Thromboangiitis obliterans (Buerger's disease) is a special case of arterial inflammatory disease.[15] This condition, which almost always involves the upper extremities, is clearly "inflammatory" (based on histology), although the erythrocyte sedimentation rate is typically low (often less than five). Treatment hinges almost entirely on successfully removing the toxin (acquired through smoking or use of tobacco products); if the patient abstains from tobacco, substantial improvement typically follows without any other treatment. In contrast, if the patient continues to use tobacco, there is essentially no therapy that is effective.

Several noninflammatory "vasculopathies" also affect the upper extremity arteries. Of these, the connective tissue diseases—particularly scleroderma—are most prevalent.

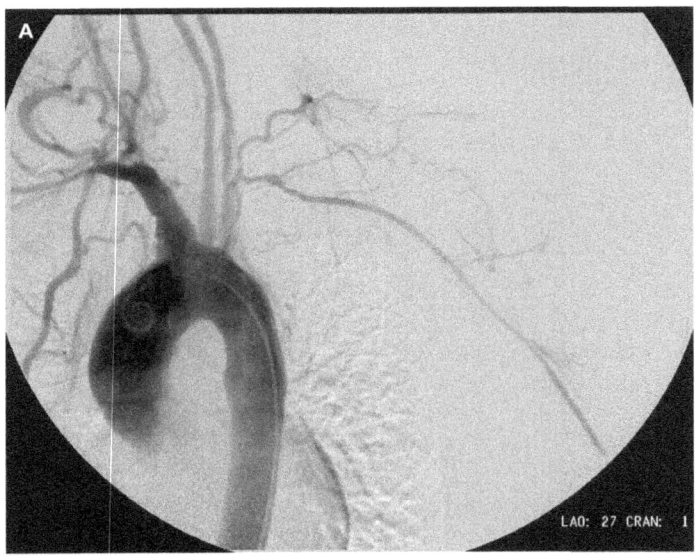

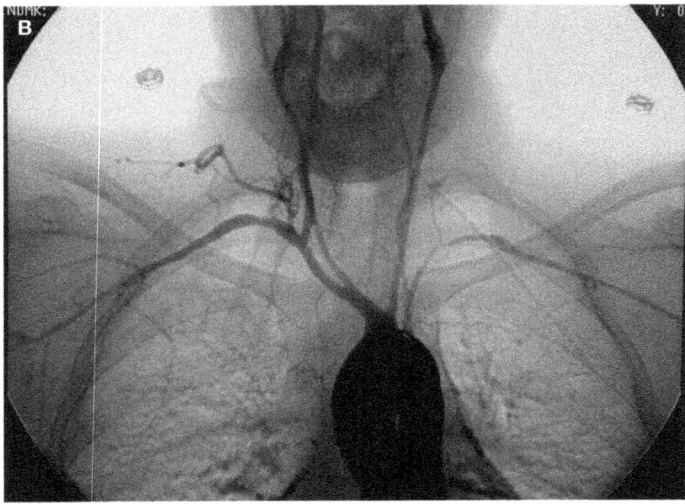

Figure 32-2. *A,* A 37-year-old female with Takayasu arteritis. Note the long, tapered narrowing in the brachial-axillary artery. *B,* A 72-year-old female with giant cell arteritis. Tapered narrowings are noted in the right sub-clavian (arrow) and left subclavian (circle) arteries.

Scleroderma (and the "CREST" syndrome) are less common but by no means rare causes of upper extremity (and in particular digital) ischemia. Because there is no way to treat scleroderma effectively, its arterial manifestations are likewise extremely difficult to treat. Medical therapy is often ineffective, and there is no reliable surgical treatment. In our experience, the use of upper extremity pneumatic pumps to force blood antegrade through the narrowed/obstructed arteries is one of the few therapeutic modalities that can be effective.[16]

Repetitive motion, vibration, repeated low-level trauma, and other mechanical forces can disrupt or damage arteries; this often occurs chronically and may not be immediately attributed to "trauma." Disease of this type involving the distal ulnar artery ("hook of the hamate") is well recognized.[17] As a result of low-grade trauma (and possibly concomitant genetic factors?), the ulnar artery undergoes changes that lead to redundant elongation, occlusion, aneurysm formation, thrombosis, distal embolization, and other problems. Surgical approaches may prove useful in correcting this relatively uncommon problem.

As noted above, the plethora of problems that can affect upper extremity arteries often lead to stenosis or occlusion, but the artery may react in other ways. Aneurysm formation is one of them. Upper extremity aneurysms, like aneurysms elsewhere, may be either saccular or fusiform in shape depending on their location and etiology. In addition, long segments of upper extremity artery may occasionally undergo aneurysmal dilatation producing a condition often referred to as "arteriomegaly." Aneurysms, perhaps more than any other arterial disorder, require the attention of a surgeon as opposed to an internist. Along with aneurysms, *dissections* can and do affect the arteries of the upper extremity and may lead to catastrophic consequences including diffuse regions of infarction. Like aneurysms, the causes of dissections are too numerous to cover in this setting.

Although extremely rare, blood vessels (including arteries) can undergo malignant transformation and give rise to angiosarcomas or similar tumors.[18] These malignancies are among the most aggressive and difficult to treat, and limb loss or death is a common outcome. With the exception of Kaposi sarcoma, these cancers—thankfully—tend to be extremely rare (Fig. 32-3).

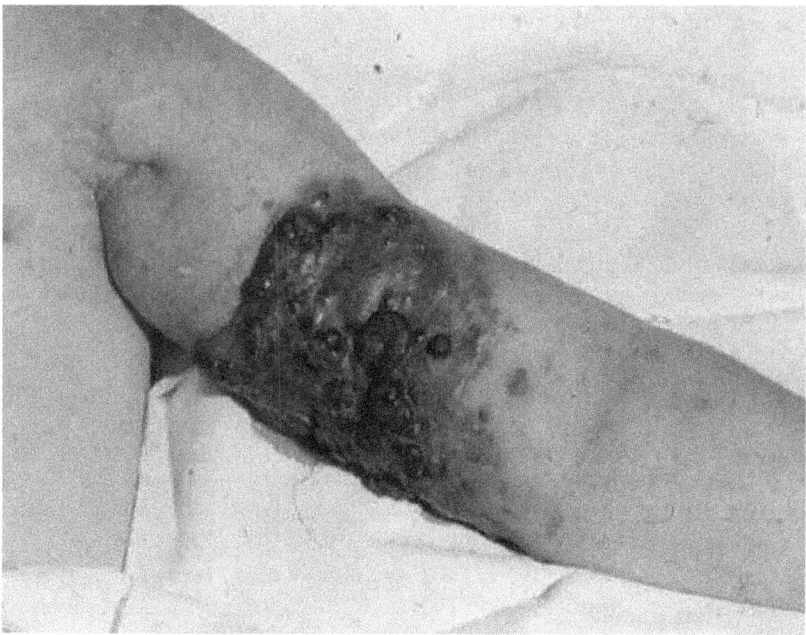

Figure 32-3. Angiosarcoma affecting the upper extremity.

VASOMOTOR DISORDERS

Vasomotor abnormalities (i.e., Raynaud's phenomenon) are extremely common and typically do not constitute an "unusual" disorder of the upper extremity. Indeed, episodic low cutaneous blood flow of the type seen with primary Raynaud's is so common (particularly in women) that it clearly constitutes a variant of normal. In many cases, an otherwise mild tendency toward vasoconstriction crosses the line into vasospasm because of secondary factors such as hypothyroidism, beta-blocker use, smoking/tobacco, and many others. Some patients are unusually sensitive to ergo-containing compounds; in the past, ergotamine toxicity has occasionally led to severe cases of vasospasm resulting in digital tissue damage and infarction.[19]

Most upper extremity vasospastic disorders can be treated conservatively by (1) elimination of any underlying vasoconstrictive factors, (2) avoidance of cold, (3) use of warm clothing, and (4) vasodilator agents (if necessary). Sympathetic nerve interruption (i.e., sympathetic nerve blocks or surgical sympathectomies) may occasionally be useful.[20] When all else fails, physical relocation to a warmer climate often produces substantial relief.

DISORDERS OCCURRING WITHIN THE ARTERIAL LUMEN

In many cases, the cause of an arterial problem can be found within the lumen of the artery. Examples include emboli, thrombosis in situ, hyperviscosity, and other common or not-so-common problems. *Emboli* are probably the most common intraluminal problems, and whether or not to classify a particular embolus as "unusual" depends on its etiology. Emboli derived from atrial fibrillation, atherosclerotic plaques, or cardiac valvular disease *are not* very unusual, while emboli coming from, for example, traumatically released bone marrow (i.e., "fat emboli") *are* unusual.

Unusual conditions leading to *intraluminal thrombosis* include cryoglobulinemia and other abnormalities of circulating proteins.[21] In cryoglobulinemia, the offending protein undergoes changes that lead to clotting when the temperature falls below a certain threshold (as may be found in the distal extremities, which are typically cooler than core body temperature). This can lead to significant perfusion abnormalities, particularly in the small vessels, and may cause infarction of the extremity. Various forms of thrombophilia can produce similar results. Among the most devastating of these are those caused by *disseminated intravascular coagulation* (DIC)–type phenomenon.[22] Certain infectious processes and tumors/malignancies can lead to DIC-mediated activation of the clotting system with horrendous peripheral arterial consequences in the upper extremities. The most devastating of these is "purpura fulminans," which involves aggressive small vessel thrombosis in the extremities and may predispose to limb loss.[23]

The special role of trauma as a cause of upper extremity limb problems deserves a final mention. Trauma is capable of producing problems that are extrinsic to the artery or may involve the structure of the wall and/or trigger vasoconstriction or may lead to intraluminal clotting. The unique ability of trauma to affect arteries in so many ways is not simply academic; when trauma has resulted in a disruption of arterial flow, it is critical to think about each of these components (extrinsic, wall, intraluminal) and make certain that each has been properly addressed and treated as appropriate.

Indeed, it is entirely possible that a particular episode of upper extremity trauma (seen with a motor vehicle accident, fall, etc.) could require surgery to minimize or alleviate extrinsic compressive factors (like hematoma or compartment syndrome), treatment of a disrupted arterial wall, and subsequent anticoagulation to address trauma-related intravascular clotting. In addition, trauma can induce vasospasm that may further complicate an injury and require specific medical therapy.

REFERENCES

1. Sanders RJ, Hammond SL. Management of cervical ribs and anomalous first ribs causing neurogenic thoracic outlet syndrome. *J VascSurg*. 2002;36:51–56.
2. Detterbeck FC. Changes in the treatment of Pancoast tumors. *Ann Thorac Surg*. 2003;75:1990–1997. The Society of Thoracic Surgeons, Elsevier.
3. Burnand KM, Lagocki S, Lahiri RP, et al. Persistent subclavian artery stenosis following surgical repair of non-union of a fractured clavicle. *Grand Rounds*. 2010;10:55-58. http://www.grandrounds-e-med.com/articles/gr100012.pdf.
4. Machleder HI, Sweeney JP, Barker WF. The pulseless arm after brachial artery catheterization. *Lancet*. 1972;1:407–409.
5. Gray GH, Young JR, Olin JW. Miscellaneous arterial diseases. In: Young JR, Olin JW, Bartholomew J, eds. *Peripheral Vascular Diseases*. 2nd ed. St. Louis: Mosby-Yearbook; 1996:425–440.
6. Olin JW, Froehlich J, Gu X, et al. The United States Registry for fibromuscular dysplasia: results in the first 447 patients. *Circulation*. June 26, 2012;125(25):3182–3190.
7. Hellman DB. Giant cell arteritis, polymyalgia rheumatic, and Takayasu's arteritis. In: Firestein GS, Budd RC, Harris ED, Jr., et al, eds. *Kelly's Textbook of Rheumatology*. 8th ed. Philadelphia, PA: Saunders Elsevier; 2008:chap 81.
8. Hoffman GS, Cid MC, Heiklmann DB, et al. A multicenter randomized double blind placebo-controlled trial of adjuvant methotrexate treatment for giant cell arteritis. *Arthritis Rheum*. 2002;46:1309–1318.
9. Martinez-Taboada VM, Rodrigues-Valverde V, Carreno L, et al. A double-blind placebo controlled trial of etanercept in patients with giant cell arteritis and corticosteroid side effects. *Ann Rheum Dis*. 2007;67:625–630.
10. Seitz M, Reichenbach S, Borel HM, et al. Rapid induction of remission in large vessel vasculitis by IL-6 blockade. *Swiss Med Weekly*. 2011;141:E1–E4.
11. Papi M, Didona B, De Pità O, et al. Livedo vasculopathy vs. small vessel cutaneous vasculitis. *Arch Dermatol*. 1998;134:447–452.
12. Morgan AJ, Schwartz RA. Cutaneous polyarteritis nodosa: a comprehensive review. *Int J Dermatol*. 2010;49:750–756.
13. Hatemi G, Silman A, Bang D, et al. Management of Behcet disease: a systematic literature review for the European League against Rheumatism evidence-based recommendations for the management of Behcet disease. *Ann Rheum Dis*. 2009;68:1528–1534.
14. Ramsey MK, Owens D. Wegener's granulomatosis: a review of the clinical implications, diagnosis, and treatment. *LabMedicine* 2006;37(2):114–116.
15. Olin JW. Thromboangiitis obliterans (Buerger's disease). *N Engl J Med*. 2000;864(12):864–869.
16. Pfizenmaier DH, Kavros SJ, Liedl DA, Cooper LT. Use of intermittent pneumatic compression for treatment of upper extremity vascular ulcers. *Angiology*. 2005;56(4):417–422.
17. Mehlhoff TL, Wood MB. Ulnar artery thrombosis and the role of interposition vein grafting: patency with microsurgical technique. *J Hand Surg*. 1991;16A:274–278.
18. Koch M, Nielsen GP, Yoon SS. Malignant tumors of blood vessels: angiosarcomas, hemangioendotheliomas, and hemangiopericytomas. *J Surg Onc*. 2008;97:321–329.

19. Garcia GD, Goff JM, Hadro NC, et al. Chronic ergot toxicity: a rare cause of lower extremity ischemia. *J Vasc Surg*. 2000;31:1245–1247.
20. Lowell RC, Gloviczki P, Cherry KJ, et al. Cervicothoracic sympathectomy for Raynaud's syndrome. *Int Angiol*. Jun, 1993;12(2):168–172.
21. Ferri C. Review: mixed cryoglobulinemia. *Orphanet J Rare Dis*. 2008;3:25. doi:10.1186/1750-1172-3-25.
22. Bick RL. Disseminated intravascular coagulation: A review of etiology, pathophysiology, diagnosis, and management: guidelines for care. *Clin Appl Thomb Hemost*. Jan, 2002;8(1):1–31.
23. Chalmers E, Cooper P, Forman K, et al. Purpura fulminans: recognition, diagnosis, and management. *Arch Dis Child*. 2011.doi:10.1136/adc.2010.199919.

33

Hand Ischemia after Radial Artery Cannulation: When Is Operation Indicated?

R. James Valentine, MD

The superficial location of the radial artery at the wrist makes it a convenient site for direct cannulation. Placement of indwelling radial artery catheters for continuous blood pressure monitoring and blood sampling has become routine in the operating room and intensive care units, and past estimates suggest that more than 8 million arterial catheters are placed perioperatively in the United States each year.[1] The radial artery has also gained popularity as a favored access site for percutaneous coronary angiography, using 5 Fr or 6 Fr sheaths. Fortunately, these procedures are associated with extremely low complication rates, owing to the paired blood supply of the forearm and hand. Although radial artery flow reduction or thrombosis occurs in up to one-third of patients after decannulation,[2,3] very few develop clinical hand or digital ischemia. However, sporadic cases of hand or finger gangrene after radial artery cannulation have been reported, and the incidence is expected to rise as transradial coronary interventions continue to increase. The purpose of this chapter is to discuss the etiology, risk factors, and treatment of hand ischemia after radial artery cannulation.

ANATOMY

The radial and ulnar arteries represent the paired blood supply to the forearm and hand. The radial artery usually branches from the brachial artery bifurcation at the level of the radial tuberosity, but a higher origin is found in up to 9% of subjects.[4] In the forearm, the radial artery lies beneath the brachioradialis muscle and becomes superficial at the wrist, where it lies between the tendons of the brachioradialis and flexor carpi radialis. The ulnar artery runs under the flexor digitorum superficialis and emerges on the radial side of the flexor carpi ulnaris tendon at the wrist.

The arterial supply in the hand is variable. Most commonly, the forearm arteries terminate in superficial and deep palmar arteries that connect the two circulations. Although much attention has been focused on which of the two arteries represents the "dominant" artery of the hand, the crucial anatomy relates to the status of the palmar arches. The superficial palmar arch is largely supplied by the ulnar artery, while the deep palmar arch is largely supplied by the radial artery. The dominant blood supply to the digital arteries of the thumb and index fingers is from the deep arch, while the superficial arch is the dominant supply to the other fingers (Fig. 33-1). The arches are sometimes incomplete, but one of the two arches is patent in most individuals. However, the anatomy of the palmar arches is highly variable and there are numerous

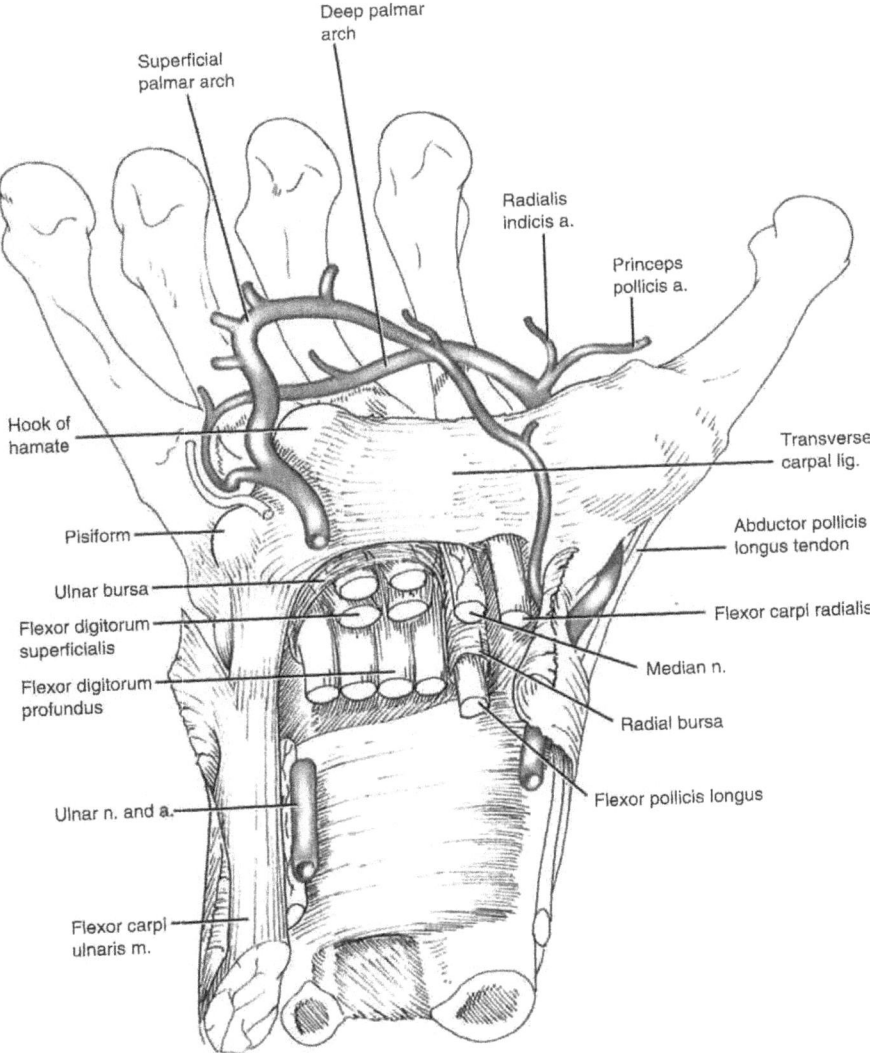

Figure 33-1. Arterial anatomy of the hand. The ulnar artery is the dominant supply of the superficial palmar arch, and the radial artery is the dominant supply to the deep arch. Note that the arterial supply of the thumb and index fingers is derived principally from the deep palmar arch. From Wind and Valentine.[5]

patterns reported within "complete" palmar circulations. In a detailed anatomic study using stereotactic angiography in 220 cadaver hands, Ikeda et al.[6] found incomplete deep arches in 23% and incomplete superficial arches in 3.6% of specimens. The authors subdivided complete deep arches into four subtypes and complete superficial arches into eight subtypes. In contrast, in a study of 45 fresh limbs from cadavers, Gellman et al.[7] found incomplete superficial palmar arches in 15.5% of specimens. However, there was no specimen is which both arches were incomplete in either study.

ISCHEMIC COMPLICATIONS OF RADIAL ARTERY CANNULATION

Thrombosis is a common sequela of radial artery cannulation, but clinical hand ischemia is very rare. In prospective studies, radial artery flow reduction or thrombosis has been documented in 25%–33% of patients after radial artery cannulation for hemodynamic monitoring, but hand ischemia has been estimated to occur in about .09%.[8,9] Radial artery occlusion represents the most common complication of transradial cardiac catheterization, with a published incidence of 2%–18%.[10] Fortunately, hand ischemia after transradial cardiac catheterization has only rarely been reported. Considering the huge number of arterial cannulas placed and the increasing use of transradial cardiac catheterization, one might expect a large number of reported cases of hand ischemia in the literature. However, published experience has generally been limited to sporadic cases. Our five-year experience with eight patients who developed hand ischemia after radial artery cannulation for monitoring represents one of the largest series.[11]

Although thrombotic occlusion of the radial artery rarely leads to hand ischemia, the presence of thrombus appears to be a prerequisite for hand ischemia. In patients with indwelling arterial catheters for hemodynamic monitoring, the incidence of radial artery thrombosis appears to relate to the degree with which the catheter fills the arterial lumen.[8] A number of technical risk factors for radial artery thrombosis have been proposed, including larger size catheters (>20-guage catheters), use of polypropylene (versus Teflon) catheters, multiple puncture attempts, female gender (due to smaller artery size), and infiltration of local anesthetics around the artery.[8,9] Risk factors associated with radial artery thrombosis after cardiac catheterization include prolonged high-pressure compression, repeat entry, and larger sheath size.[8]

It is not clear why a small subset of patients with radial artery thrombosis progress to hand ischemia. The most common explanation is embolization from a radial artery thrombus, as suggested by Lee and colleagues.[12] This is corroborated by the tendency for occlusion of the digital arteries supplied by the radial side of the palmar arch (Fig. 33-2). Catheter flushing, external catheter thrombus, and air embolus have all been proposed as contributing factors.[9] A number of patient-specific risk factors for hand ischemia have been proposed (Table 33-1), but none is uniformly present in all cases.

SHOULD A MODIFIED ALLEN TEST BE PERFORMED PRIOR TO CANNULATION?

The anatomic variation of the superficial and deep palmar arches has been well documented.[6,7,9] Although preoperative evaluation of adequate collateral blood supply is necessary before radial artery harvest, it remains controversial whether documentation is

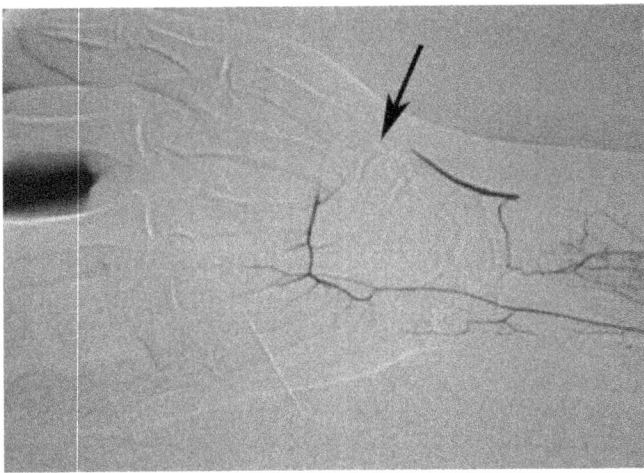

Figure 33-2. Arteriogram of a patient who developed severe finger and hand ischemia after radial artery cannulation. Note the absence of flow in the deep palmar artery and severe spasm of the ulnar artery and residual palmar segment. From Valentine et al.[11] By permission of the *Journal of the American College of Surgeons*.

TABLE 33-1. RISK FACTORS FOR ISCHEMIC COMPLICATIONS OF RADIAL ARTERY BLOOD PRESSURE MONITORING

Patient-Specific Risk Factors

    Prior arterial injury

    Female gender

    High-dose vasopressors

    Profound circulatory failure

    Malignancy

    Heparin-induced thrombocytopenia

    Disseminated intravascular coagulation

    Hypercoagulable states

Catheter-Related Risk Factors

    Cannulation >7 days

    Increased number of attempts

    Catheter type (Teflon vs. polypropylene)

    Length (shorter = more risk)

    Catheter diameter >20 gauge

necessary before radial artery cannulation. Much of the controversy surrounds the modified Allen test, which has been shown to be a poor predictor of hand ischemia after radial artery cannulation. Radial artery cannulation has been performed without ischemic complications in patients with abnormal Allen test results.[13–15] Furthermore, hand ischemia has been reported after radial artery cannulation in patients with normal Allen tests.[16,17] In their evaluation of 93 hands, Jarvis et al. compared the modified Allen test with Doppler ultrasound and calculated a diagnostic accuracy rate of 80%, sensitivity of 76%, and specificity of 82%.[18] Addition of adjuncts such as pulse oximetry, plethysmography, or reactive hyperemia has not been shown to improve the overall accuracy.[9] Although the Allen test is generally considered important in selection of patients for radial artery harvest, the preponderance of the literature suggests that it is not necessary before routine radial artery cannulation. Some cardiologists feel that it is not necessary to assess the palmar blood supply prior to transradial cardiac catheterization.[19]

DIAGNOSIS

As noted above, the vast majority of patients with cannulation-induced radial artery thrombosis are asymptomatic. However, a small subset will develop hand ischemia, and early recognition is the most important factor in reducing permanent injury. The following are typical presentations: darkening of the skin ranging from a dusky appearance to mottling and cyanosis, pain and weakness in the fingers and hand, delayed capillary refill, and an absent radial pulse. Doppler signals are typically absent in the ipsilateral radial artery, palmar arches, and affected digital arteries. Ischemia may involve only the first three fingers or the entire hand, depending on the degree of involvement.

UT SOUTHWESTERN EXPERIENCE

We previously reported eight patients who developed radial artery–induced thrombosis and hand ischemia at our institution between 1999 and 2004.[11] The mean age of the cohort was 63 ± 10 years, and four were women. All patients underwent radial artery cannulation in the operating room for arterial monitoring using 20-gauge, one-inch polyurethane devices that were placed percutaneously over a standard 22-gauge needle with a .018 wire guide. Catheters remained in place from six hours to 14 days before vascular consultation. All patients had grade IIb ischemia involving the first three fingers ($n = 4$) or the entire hand ($n = 4$), and most had several of the risk factors shown in Table 33-1. Noninvasive tests confirmed that Doppler signals were absent in the ipsilateral palmar arches and radial arteries of all eight patients. Ulnar signals were absent distal to the mid-forearm in the four patients with hand ischemia; Doppler signals were monophasic in the ulnar arteries of the other four patients with finger ischemia. Two of the four patients with hand ischemia underwent catheter arteriograms, which showed occlusion of the radial artery and severely reduced flow in the palmar arteries believed to be the consequence of vasospasm.

Radial artery revascularization was attempted in five patients. Three underwent thrombectomy and patch angioplasty ($n = 3$) while two had vein interposition bypass ($n = 2$). Two patch angioplasty repairs thrombosed but the other three repairs remained patent for 30–59 months. However, the type of repair had no effect on ultimate outcome: regardless of the repair patency, four patients who survived to discharge developed finger gangrene, two of whom required finger amputation. This is most likely due to embolic occlusion of the digital arteries, which is not correctable by restoration of flow in the palmar arch.

Three patients in our series did not undergo operative repair. Treatment was aimed at the underlying pathology, including anticoagulation and administration of intra-arterial vasodilators. Although use of lytic agents was considered, all patients had a contraindication. One patient had complete reversal of ischemia, while two others developed digital gangrene or permanent neurologic sequela.

Our small experience underscores the fact that hand ischemia after radial artery cannulation for hemodynamic monitoring is very rare, but associated with a high risk of tissue loss or amputation. We have not encountered any patients who developed hand ischemia after transradial coronary catheterization. In patients with hand ischemia, our study suggests that operative repair offered no advantage over medical therapy in prevention of digital gangrene. Based on this experience, we hypothesized that digital gangrene resulted from distal embolization from the site of initial arterial thrombosis and was not remediated by radial artery revascularization.

TREATMENT

Once recognized, treatment of hand ischemia should consist of increasing blood flow, treating vasospasm, and preventing extension of thrombus. First, the patient's hemodynamic status should be optimized, correcting volume deficits and weaning intravenous inotropic agents as possible. Unless there are clear contraindications, the patient should be systemically anticoagulated with intravenous heparin. If the radial artery cannula is still present, it should be removed. Some authors have reported success in reversing ischemic symptoms with aspiration of thrombus at the catheter tip or intra-arterial administration of vasodilators. Administration of intra-arterial vasodilators appears to be particularly helpful to treat arterial spasm associated with transradial catheterization; treatment with a "cocktail" of nitroglycerine and calcium channel blockers has been immediate and effective.[3,10] However, catheter removal is recommended in patients with hand ischemia after radial artery cannulation for monitoring to be certain that it is not contributing to flow reduction. Intra-arterial lytic therapy should be considered, but most if not all patients will have contraindications—as was the case in our series. Catheter-based arteriography will help to define the location and degree of arterial occlusion, and the catheter can be used for intra-arterial injections. We have successfully treated three patients with intra-arterial infusion of tolazoline or papaverine through catheters placed in the distal brachial artery (unpublished data).

The decision for surgical exploration should be individualized. Ischemia limited to one to three digits is usually due to embolization; affected patients are unlikely to benefit from operative intervention. Similarly, patients with symptomatic hand ischemia associated with residual Doppler signals in the palmar arch will benefit from medical therapy including administration of vasodilators. However, patients with ischemia of the entire hand associated with absent arterial flow merit prompt operative thrombectomy and radial artery revascularization. Our experience suggests that replacement of the injured radial artery segment with autologous vein interposition graft is a better option than simple patch angioplasty in these circumstances. We routinely inject vasodilators into the radial artery at the time of thrombectomy. In rare cases, more distal revascularization into the hand and digits may be required. Lee et al. described direct reconstruction of the common digital arteries of the index and middle fingers using a vein graft from the palmar arch.[20] Despite restoration of flow into the palmar arch, amputation of the distal digits is often required.

SUMMARY AND CONCLUSIONS

Although thrombosis is a common sequela of radial artery catheterization, hand ischemia is very rare. A number of patient-specific and catheter-related risk factors for ischemia have been proposed. Embolization is the most likely explanation why some patients with radial artery thrombosis progress to gangrene; operative repair of the radial artery does not appear to offer any advantage over medical therapy in prevention of digital gangrene. Although theoretically useful, the use of lytic agents is often contraindicated in affected patients. Systemic anticoagulation and administration of intra-arterial vasodilators represent the cornerstones of treatment; operative thrombectomy and radial artery revascularization are indicated in patients with ischemia of the entire hand.

REFERENCES

1. Gardner RM. Direct arterial pressure monitoring. *Curr Anaesth Crit Care*. 1990;1:239–246.
2. Sfeir R, Khoury S, Khoury Gh, et al. Ischaemia of the hand after radial artery monitoring. *Cardiovasc Surg*. 1996;4:456–458.
3. Shroff A, Siddiqui S, Burg A. Identification and management of complications of transradial procedures. *Curr Cardiol Rep*. 2013;15:350.
4. Uglietta JP, Kadir S. Arterigraphic study of variant arterial anatomy of the upper extremities. *Cardiovasc Intervent Radiol*. 1989;12:145–148.
5. Wind GG, Valentine RJ. *Anatomic Exposures in Vascular Surgery*. 3rd ed. Philadelphia, PA: Wolters Kluwer/Lippincott Williams & Wilkins, 2013, p. 227.
6. Ikeda A, Ugawa A, Kazihara Y, Hamada N. Arterial patterns in the hand based on a three-dimensional analysis of 220 cadaver hands. *J Hand Surg*. 1988;13A:501–509.
7. Gellman H, Botte MJ, Shankwiler J, Gelberman RH. Arterial patterns of the deep and superficial palmar arches. *Clin Ortho Rel Res*. 2001;383:41–46.
8. Scheer BV, Perel A, Pfeiffer UJ. Clinical review: complications and risk factors of peripheral arterial catheters used for haemodynamic monitoring in anaesthesia and intensive care medicine. *Crit Care*. 2002;6:198–204.
9. Brzezinski M, Luisetti T, London MJ. Radial artery cannulation: a comprehensive review of recent anatomic and physiologic investigations. *Anesth Analg*. 2009;109:1763–1781.
10. Kanei Y, Kwan T, Nakra NC, et al. Transradial cardiac catheterization: a review of access site complications. *Cath Cardiovasc Interv*. 2011;78:840–846.
11. Valentine RJ, Modrall JG, Clagett GP. Hand ischemia after radial artery cannulation. *J Am Coll Surg*. 2005;201:18–22.
12. Lee KL, Miller JG, Laitung G. Hand ischemia following radial artery cannulation. *J Hand Surg*. (Brit) 1995;20B:493–495.
13. Slogoff S, Keats AS, Arlund C. On the safety of radial artery cannulation. *Anesthesiology*. 1983;59:42–47.
14. Abu-Omar Y, Mussa S, Anastasiadis K, et al. Duplex ultrasonography predicts safety of radial artery harvest in the presence of an abnormal Allen test. *Ann Thorac Surg*. 2004;77:116–119.
15. Barbeau GR, Arsenault F, Dugas L, et al. Evaluation of ulnopalmar arterial arches with pulse oximetry and plethysmography: comparison with the Allen's test in 1010 patients. *Am Heart J*. 2004;147:489–493.
16. Arthurs GJ. Case report: digital ischemia following radial artery cannulation. *Anaesth Intensive Care*. 1978;6:54–55.
17. Mangar D, Laborde RS, Vu DN. Delayed ischemia of the hand necessitating amputation after radial artery cannulation. *Can J Anaesth*. 1993;40:247–250.

18. Jarvis MA, Jarvis CL, Jones PR, Spyt TJ. Reliability of Allen's test in selection of patients for radial artery harvest. *Ann Thorac Surg.* 2000;70:362–365.
19. Ghuran AV, Dixon G, Holmberg S, et al. Transradial coronary intervention without pre-screening for a dual palmar blood supply. *Int J Cardiol.* 2007;121:320–322.
20. Lee MK, Lee O, Kong MH, et al. Surgical treatment of digital ischemia occurred after radial artery cannulation. *J Korean Med.* 2001;16:375–377.

34

Treatment Strategies for Access-Related Hand Ischemia

Thomas S. Huber, MD, PhD and Salvatore T. Scali, MD

INTRODUCTION

Access-related hand ischemia (ARHI), commonly known as "steal syndrome," is one of the most challenging clinical problems for the access surgeon. The construction of an anastomosis between an artery and a vein (i.e., arteriovenous fistula) results in a predictable decrease in the perfusion pressure distal to the anastomosis that can lead to ischemia if the compensatory mechanisms are inadequate. Several clinical predictors have been identified, but their collective positive predictive value is not sufficient to identify scenarios when the hemodialysis access should not be attempted. The diagnosis of ARHI is largely a clinical one that can be corroborated in equivocal cases with noninvasive vascular laboratory studies. The treatment goals are to reverse the hand ischemia and to preserve the access with the paramount concern to avoid any long-term hand disability. There are a variety of remedial treatment strategies and they should be viewed as complementary with the choice contingent upon the responsible underlying mechanism, the severity of the symptoms, the patient comorbidities, and the utility (or potential utility) of the access itself. The distal revascularization and interval ligation (DRIL) procedure is our preferred treatment because it reverses the ischemic symptoms and salvages the access in approximately 90% of the cases. The chapter will review the management of ARHI including the pathophysiology, clinical presentation, and treatment options along with an update of our recent DRIL experience and our current treatment algorithm.

PATHOPHYSIOLOGY AND RISK FACTORS

The construction of an anastomosis between an artery and a vein creates a high flow, low resistance circuit with the blood preferentially directed toward the venous outflow as a result of the pressure gradients (Fig. 34-1). The blood flow in the axial artery immediately

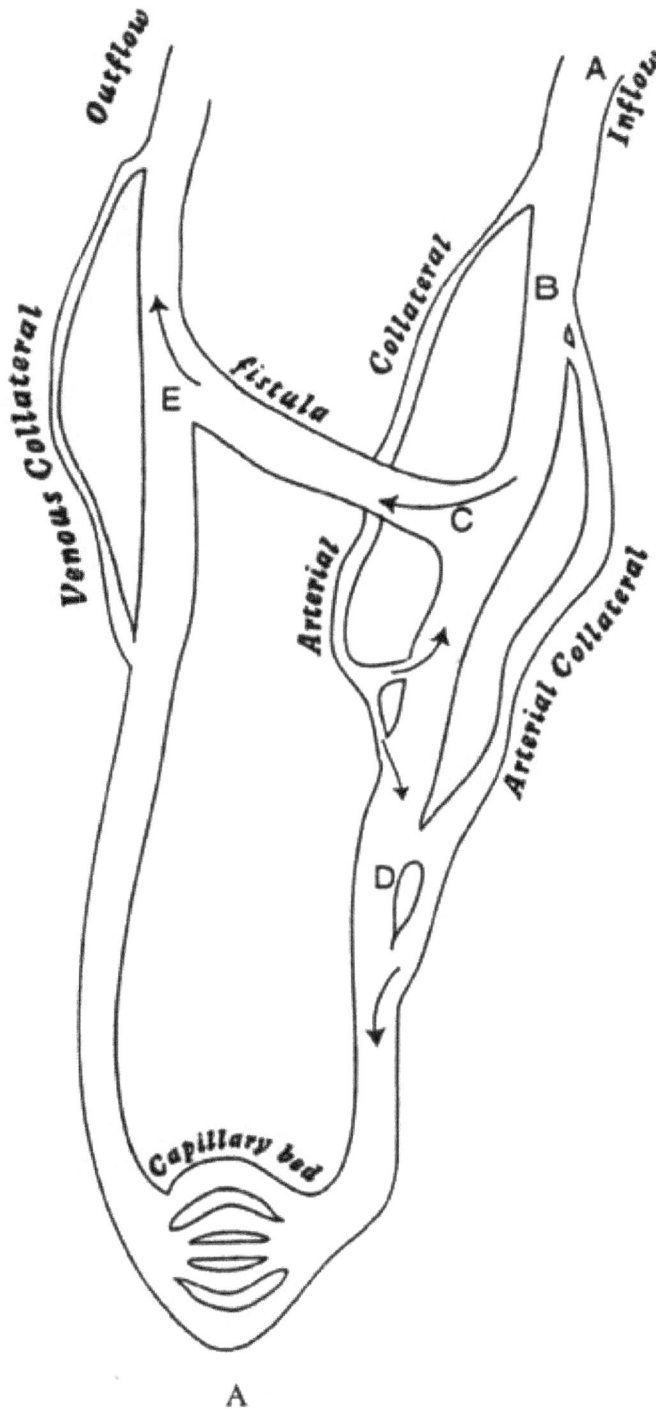

Figure 34-1. A representative diagram of an autogenous arteriovenous hemodialysis access is shown. Note the retrograde blood flow through the anastomosis from the arterial segment immediately distal to the anastomosis. The perfusion of the tissues distal to the anastomosis is supplied predominantly by the arterial collaterals. Reproduced with permission from Wixon et al.[1] Figure used in *Contemporary Vascular Surgery* 2011. Used with permission.

distal to the anastomosis can be retrograde, antegrade, or "to and fro" depending on these gradients and the timing of the cardiac cycle. Perfusion of the tissue distal to the access is typically augmented through vasodilation of the inflow arteries, collateral recruitment, and an increase in the cardiac output. Papasavas et al.[2] reported that the construction of an arteriovenous access results in a decrease in the ipsilateral digital pressures in approximately 80% of patients. This "physiologic steal" is usually well tolerated, but can become clinically significant when the compensatory mechanisms are inadequate. The presence of significant occlusive disease within the inflow (e.g., subclavian) or outflow (e.g., ulnar) arteries can further exacerbate the hemodynamic changes resulting from the access, potentially leading to ischemia. Specifically, the increased blood flow in the extremity resulting from the access can cause an energy loss and pressure decrease in a "subcritical" proximal lesion similar to the response of an aortoiliac lesion to a vasodilator. Occlusive disease in the forearm or hand, commonly seen in the diabetic population, can further exacerbate the drop in arterial pressure from the access alone.

ARHI occurs in up to 20% of brachial artery–based access procedures with roughly half (i.e., 10% of all brachial artery–based procedures) classified severe (grade 1, mild; grade 2, moderate; grade 3, severe)[3] and meriting some type of remedial treatment. ARHI can occur after distal radial artery–based procedures, but the incidence is significantly less (2%) than the brachial artery–based procedures and treatment is rarely required. The underlying hemodynamic changes with radial artery–based accesses are similar to those outlined above (i.e., decreased arterial pressure distal to the anastomosis). ARHI can also occur after radial artery–based procedures as a result of retrograde flow through the palmar arch and this is potentially reversible by occluding the distal radial artery with a suture or coil.

A variety of clinical factors have been identified as *preoperative* predictors of ARHI. These include age, female gender, diabetes, coronary artery disease, hypertension, tobacco abuse, peripheral vascular arterial occlusive disease, brachial artery–based accesses, previous episodes of ARHI, large conduits, and multiple prior access procedures. Indeed, it has been our anecdotal impression that patients who develop ARHI are at extremely high risk for recurrence with each subsequent access attempt, thereby emphasizing the limitations of ligating an access on one extremity with the intention of simply placing a new access on the contralateral side. This list of clinical predictors is very extensive and encompasses a large percentage of patients with end-stage renal disease. Unfortunately, there are no predictive models that are sufficiently accurate to preclude constructing an access in an "at-risk" patient. Similar to the clinical predictors, preoperative finger pressure or digital brachial indices (DBIs) measured in the vascular laboratory have also been inconclusive. They can be used in concert with the clinical predictors, but the absolute threshold values are unclear (i.e., DBI <0.45, 0.6, 1.0).

CLINICAL PRESENTATION AND DIAGNOSIS

Patients with ARHI can present with the typical features of either acute or chronic extremity ischemia. In our own DRIL experience, the presentation was trimodal with a third of the patients presenting within seven days of the index procedure, a third within 7–30 days and the final third presenting after 30 days.[4] The signs and symptoms associated with acute ARHI include the classic "6 P's"—pain, paresthesia, paralysis, pulselessness, poikilothermia, and pallor. Similar to acute lower extremity ischemia, a motor deficit is particularly worrisome and merits emergent treatment. Chronic ARHI can present with either rest pain or tissue loss. Notably, this can manifest months to years after the index procedure, particularly in diabetic patients with advanced forearm vascular disease.

The diagnosis of ARHI is predominantly a clinical one based on the history and physical examination with imaging (both noninvasive and invasive) reserved for equivocal cases. The differential diagnosis of hand complaints after an access procedure includes diabetic peripheral neuropathy and carpal tunnel syndrome, but ARHI should be considered first and foremost. It is important to ask patients about their dialysis session since the associated hypotension and hypovolemic can often precipitate hand complaints in patients that are otherwise asymptomatic. The physical exam may occasionally confound the diagnosis in the presence of a palpable pulse. Although it may seem contradictory to have a palpable pulse and an "ischemic" hand, all postoperative symptoms must be attributed to ischemia until proven otherwise. It has been our anecdotal impression that the threshold for ischemic symptoms in the upper extremity may be different than for the lower extremity with symptoms developing at a much higher absolute pressure in the upper extremity. Access-related neuropathy can lead to pain, weakness, and paralysis of the muscles in the hand and forearm without significant tissue necrosis. In the most extreme scenario, patients can develop ischemic monomelic neuropathy, characterized by intense, neuropathic pain that occurs in the early postoperative period. This rare entity is seen almost exclusively in older, diabetic patients with peripheral vascular disease. Nerve conduction studies in this setting demonstrate axonal loss and reduced sensory and motor nerve conduction velocities. The selective involvement of the nerves likely results from their greater metabolic requirements and tenuous blood supply (relative to the muscle tissue). Urgent, definitive treatment to reduce the underlying ischemia is mandatory to present long-term disability.

Noninvasive vascular laboratory studies can help corroborate the diagnosis for patients with equivocal symptoms. The diagnosis of ARHI may be excluded if the pressure measurements and the corresponding Doppler waveforms are completely normal (i.e., symmetric wrist/digital pressures, triphasic radial/ulnar waveforms, and normal finger PPGs). However, this scenario is quite rare with the more common one being a patient with equivocal symptoms, diminished wrist/DBIs, and monophasic Doppler waveforms at the wrist. Not surprisingly, compression of the access usually results in the normalization of the wrist pressures and waveforms. We have taken an aggressive approach in these equivocal cases, assuming that all of the hand complaints were due to ARHI and have treated them accordingly. Catheter-based arteriography has been used as a diagnostic study, but it is important to remember that ARHI is a hemodynamic problem and arteriography is largely an anatomic study albeit an important part of the treatment algorithm to rule out any significant inflow lesions.

INDICATIONS AND TREATMENT STRATEGIES FOR ARHI

The treatment goals for patients with ARHI are to reverse the hand ischemia and salvage the access although the paramount concern is to prevent any long-term hand disability. The natural history of ARHI is poorly documented, although all patients with moderate to severe ischemia (i.e., grades 2 and 3) likely merit intervention. It has been our anecdotal impression that patients with mild symptoms (i.e., grade 1) may improve over time although they merit close observation. Papasavas et al.[2] reported no additional decreases in the digital pressures after a month postoperatively despite the significant early drop noted above. In contradistinction, it has been our impression that patients with moderate symptoms rarely improve.

There are a variety of different treatment options for patients with ARHI (Table 34-1). Although we favor the DRIL procedure (Fig. 34-2), the various treatments should be viewed as complementary since they may afford advantages in specific cases. It is important to remember that the ultimate goal of the remedial procedures is to correct the adverse hemodynamic changes resulting from the access. Zanow et al.[6] constructed a pulsatile flow circuit of an upper extremity arteriovenous access, complete with collateral channels, to examine these changes. Not surprisingly, they found a decrease in the flow through the access (i.e., "flow-limiting" strategy) improved the distal perfusion. Siting the arteriovenous anastomosis more proximally on the arterial tree (i.e., proximalization of the arterial inflow [PAI], Fig. 34-3) also improved the distal perfusion while ligating the axial artery immediately distal to the anastomosis in an attempt to limit the retrograde perfusion had little effect. Both the DRIL and PAI resulted in a dramatic improvement in the distal perfusion with the PAI having the greatest benefit. Interestingly, the ligation component of the DRIL only increased distal flow 10% and the overall benefit of the DRIL was reduced at higher access flow rates. Illig et al.[7] measured arterial pressures and flow rates in nine patients undergoing the DRIL procedure. They reported that there was a "pressure sink" in the brachial artery with a mean pressure of 102 ± 17 mm Hg in the proximal brachial artery that decreased to 47 ± 38 mm Hg at the anastomosis and that the flow in the brachial artery distal to the anastomosis was retrograde when the fistula was open. Following the DRIL procedure, the pressure gradient in the brachial artery was essentially unchanged. However, the pressure in the brachial artery bypass and the brachial artery distal to the ligation were 104 ± 27 mm Hg (i.e., systemic pressure) and that these values did not change with compression of the access. Reifsnyder and Arnaoutakis[8] also measured the inflow arterial pressures in a small group of patients ($N = 9$) with ARHI and found that the axillary pressures were higher than the proximal brachial pressures (153 vs. 116 mm Hg). These data suggest that the pressure drop resulting from the arteriovenous fistula may start more proximal on the arterial tree than previously suspected.

Several investigators have attempted to classify ARHI into "high flow" or "low flow" although the absolute threshold for differentiating these states and their clinical significance remain unresolved. Clearly, the flow rates in the access contribute to the hemodynamic changes although it is unclear whether they are independent of the other factors involved in the adaptive (or maladaptive) responses.

TABLE 34-1. TREATMENT OPTIONS FOR ACCESS-RELATED HAND ISCHEMIA

Access ligation

Correction of arterial inflow stenosis/occlusion

Flow-limiting procedures (i.e., banding, outflow reduction, anastomosis reduction)

Proximalization of arterial anastomosis (PAI)

Revision using distal inflow (RUDI)

Distal revascularization and interval ligation (DRIL)

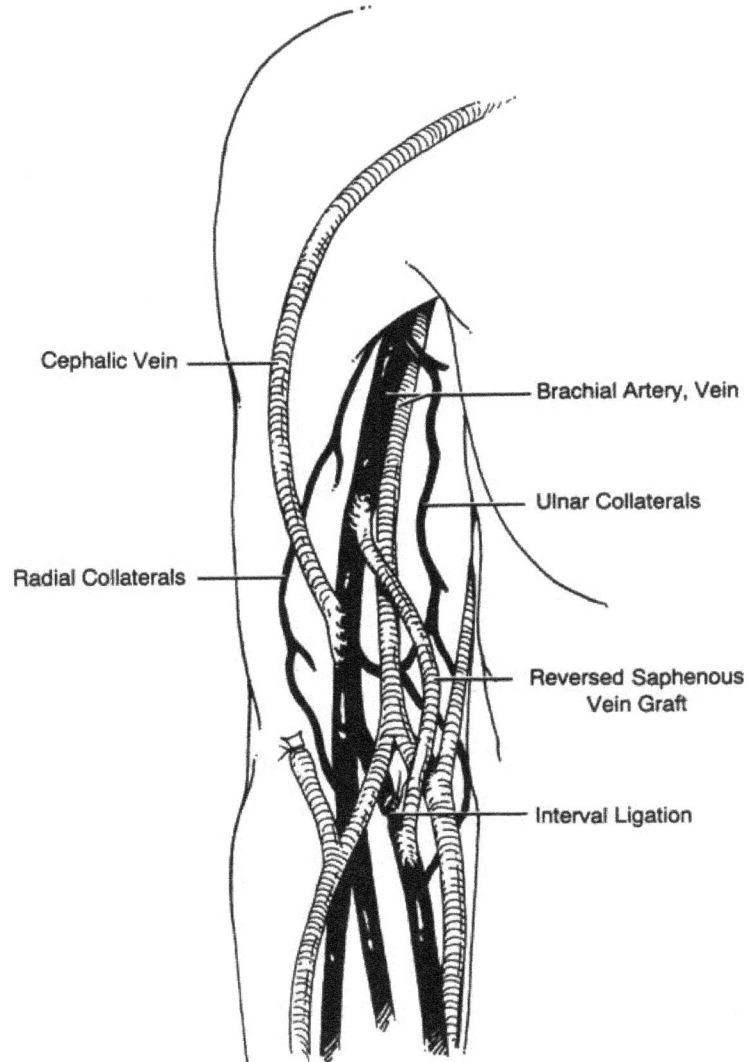

Figure 34-2. A diagram of a distal revascularization and interval ligation (DRIL) procedure is shown for a patient with an autogenous brachial-cephalic access. Note the brachial–ulnar saphenous vein graft and the ligature on the proximal ulnar artery. Reproduced with permission from Berman et al.[5] Figure used in *Contemporary Vascular Surgery* 2011. Used with permission.

Ligation

Ligating the access eliminates the arteriovenous access and reverses the hemodynamic changes. It should eliminate the ischemic symptoms provided that it is performed in a timely fashion. However, it has been our experience that a small percentage of patients will have some residual paresthesia, presumably from an ischemic neuropathy. The obvious disadvantage of ligation is the loss of the access, a major concern for patients with limited options. However, it is a reasonable approach for patients with acute ARHI after a prosthetic access given its limited patency. Notably, Scheltinga et al.[9] reported that prosthetic

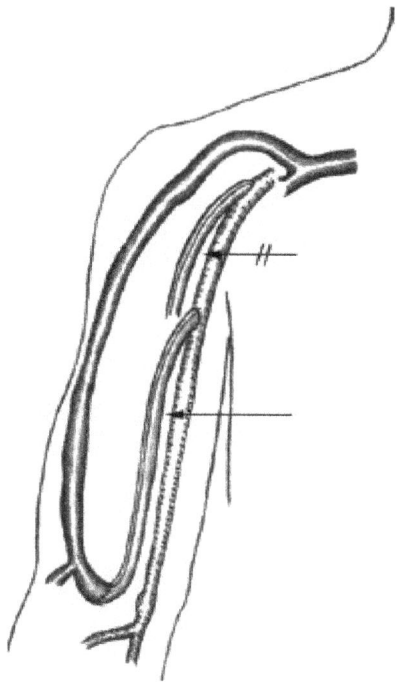

Figure 34-3. Proximalization of the arterial inflow (PAI) is shown for a brachial-cephalic autogenous access. Note that the autogenous access has been dissembled and an interposition graft (4- or 5-mm PTFE) inserted between the more proximal brachial artery and the proximal segment of the original autogenous access. Reproduced with permission from Zanow et al.[14] Figure used in *Contemporary Vascular Surgery* 2011. Used with permission.

accesses were more often associated with acute symptoms (<24 hours) while autogenous accesses were associated with chronic symptoms (>1 months) in their systematic review of the literature. Ligation may also be an appropriate treatment option for patients with severe comorbidities that preclude a more significant operation, those with limited conduit that preclude a DRIL, and those with persistent ischemic symptoms that have failed another remedial procedure (e.g., prior DRIL or banding).

Correction of Arterial Inflow Stenosis

A stenosis in the inflow vessels proximal to the arteriovenous access may contribute to the development of ARHI. Ideally, these should be identified and corrected before the index access procedure. The incidence of inflow lesions as a contributing factor has been somewhat variable in the literature, occurring less than 10% of the time in our own experience. This variability is likely due to differences in the preoperative evaluation. In our own practice, we obtain upper extremity arterial pressure measurements and Doppler waveforms in the noninvasive vascular laboratory as part of our preoperative algorithm and our criteria for a suitable inflow artery include an adequate diameter (i.e., brachial artery ≥3 mm and radial artery ≥2 mm) and the absence of a hemodynamically significant inflow lesion based on the pressures and waveforms. Regardless, a catheter-based arteriogram should be performed as part of the diagnostic and treatment algorithm for all patients with ARHI to exclude a proximal lesion.

Flow-Limiting Procedures

There are a variety of "flow-limiting strategies" designed to improve distal perfusion while maintaining the access. These approaches are based on the hemodynamic principle that increased resistance in the access will increase distal perfusion through a decrease in the relative resistance through the peripheral arterial bed. These various approaches include arterial inflow reduction, anastomotic narrowing, and venous outflow reduction. The most popular technique is "banding" or narrowing a proximal segment of the vein used for the access. Notably, these techniques have been around for long period of time, but remain somewhat controversial. Gupta et al.[10] recently reported their experience with a variety of remedial therapies for ARHI and concluded that "banding" had a low success rate and a high likelihood of reintervention. The fundamental problem with all of these strategies is finding the tenuous balance between the relative resistance that achieves adequate distal perfusion, yet maintains access patency and facilitates effective dialysis. Furthermore, the biologic behavior and the associated hemodynamics of the access may change over time (e.g., inflow artery dilation and outflow vein dilation) and, therefore, the assumptions and modifications made intraoperatively may not be sustained. Notably, the flow through a *large* arteriovenous access is independent of the extent of the communication between the vessels once the anastomosis exceeds 75% of the arterial diameter. This hemodynamic principle underscores the futility of trying to reduce the size of the anastomosis since reducing the anastomotic length of a 3-mm brachial artery to less than 2.25 mm (i.e., <75% diameter) would likely result in early thrombosis.

Part of the recent enthusiasm for these flow-limiting approaches has been predicated upon the use of objective measurements to quantify distal perfusion and access flow. Zanow et al.[11] reported a series of 95 patients with "high flow" accesses (autogenous >800 mL/min, prosthetic >1200 mL/min) that underwent flow-directed narrowing of their access using a combination of a plication suture and a prosthetic cuff (Fig. 34-4). Long-term relief of symptoms was achieved in 86% of the patients. They used target flow rates of 400 mL/min for the autogenous accesses and 600 mL/min for the prosthetic ones although they stated in the discussion of their manuscript that a target of 750 mL/min may be more appropriate for the prosthetic accesses. Scheltinga et al.[12] performed a systematic review of "banding" as a "flow reduction" procedure and reported that the success rate was <50% if performed without the guidance of flow measurements or digital pressures. However, they concluded it was very effective when flow rate was monitored and concluded that it was the procedure of choice for "high flow" accesses (i.e., >1.2 mL/min). Thermann et al.[13] reported that flow-directed banding was effective in the setting of mild, short-duration skin lesions, but ineffective for longer-term lesions and those with more extensive tissue loss. They concluded that more complex surgical solutions may be required in the setting of these more chronic, extensive lesions.

Miller et al.[14] have described a minimally invasive variant coined the MILLER banding procedure (Minimally Invasive Limited Ligation Endoluminal-Assisted Revision) and have reported fairly impressive results. The technique involves narrowing the access over an angioplasty balloon using a suture. They reported successful relief of symptoms in 109/114 (96%) patients with ARHI with a six-month patency rate of 75%. Shemesh et al.[15] described a novel "banding" variant in which the restrictive band is place in the midportion of the access between the "arterial" and "venous" cannulation sites. This creates a pressure gradient between the "arterial" and "venous" sites that maintains adequate access flow and effective dialysis, a scenario that the

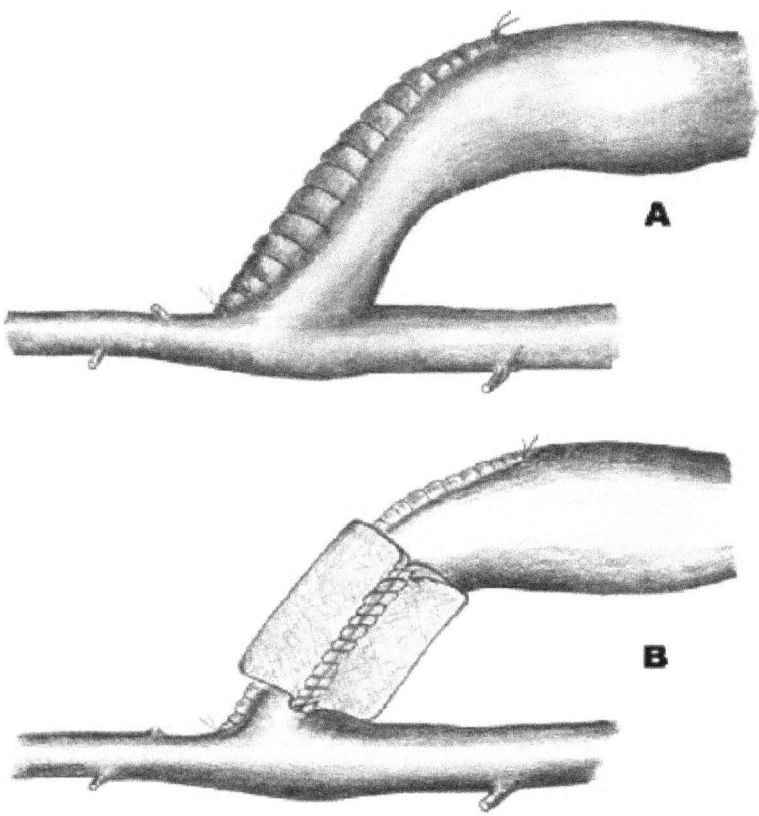

Figure 34-4. The technique described by Zanow et al.[9] to narrow the proximal autogenous access is illustrated. *A,* A continuous suture is used to plicate and narrow the proximal portion of the access. *B,* A ePTFE "cuff" is placed around the access at the proximal portion of the suture line to prevent further access dilation. Reproduced with permission from Zanow et al.[9] Figure used in *Contemporary Vascular Surgery* 2011. Used with permission.

authors claim is effective for ARHI and "low-flow" states. Other investigators have suggested that ligation (or embolization) of accessory veins or side branches can reduce the flow through the access and the ischemic symptoms.

Proximalization of Arterial Inflow

Resiting the access anastomosis more proximal on the arterial tree (e.g., resiting from brachial artery at antecubital to brachial artery near the axilla) may improve the perfusion to the hand. Theoretically, this is based on the larger caliber of the proximal vessel, the smaller concomitant pressure drop from the arteriovenous access, and the more extensive collateral network. In reality, the technique may represent a variant of the flow-limiting approaches given the described approach of using a 4- or 5-mm expanded polytetrafluoroethylene (ePTFE) interposition graft. Notably, Zanow et al.[16] reported that the PAI procedure was associated with the resolution of symptoms in 84% of their cases (*N* = 30) and that the patency rates were excellent. They concluded that it was a good alternative to the DRIL procedure and recommend its use for ARHI resulting from lower flow states (i.e., autogenous access <800 mL/min and prosthetic access <1000 mL/min). Thermann and Wollert[17] reported complete resolution of symptoms in 65% of their cases encompassing both radial (N = 5) and brachial artery–based access procedures (N = 18). They reported that the procedure was associated with increased radial artery flow and decreased access flow, but concluded that it was not effective for patients with severe tissue loss. Jennings et al.[18] have reported using the PAI approach "prophylactically" with good results in small group of patients (N = 4) deemed high risk for ARHI.

The PAI technique is appealing since it does not require ligating an axial artery and the hemodynamic models suggest that it is comparable to the DRIL. Furthermore, it may be suitable for patients that do not have adequate autogenous conduit for a DRIL procedure. However, the published experience is fairly limited, and it requires converting an autogenous access to a composite prosthetic/autogenous access and, thereby, increases the infectious and thrombotic complications with the latter particularly worrisome given the small caliber of the graft (i.e., 4- or 5-mm ePTFE).

Revision Using Distal Inflow

The revision using distal inflow (RUDI) involves resiting the arteriovenous anastomosis further distal on the arterial tree by disconnecting the original anastomosis and interposing a vein bypass graft (Fig. 34-5). This essentially converts a brachial artery–based access to a radial artery–based access. Notably, either the proximal (i.e., antecubital) or distal (i.e., wrist) radial artery may be used as the inflow source for the access. As noted above, the incidence of ARHI is dramatically lower for distal radial artery–based access procedures when compared to the brachial artery–based procedures and is also likely lower for proximal radial artery–based procedures. Although this seems somewhat counterintuitive given the close proximity of the brachial artery and the proximal portion of the radial artery (and the potential for retrograde flow from both the radial and ulnar arteries through the fistula), the limited clinical experience seems to support the RUDI. Notably, Callaghan et al.[20] reported that the RUDI relieved the precipitating ischemic symptoms and was associated

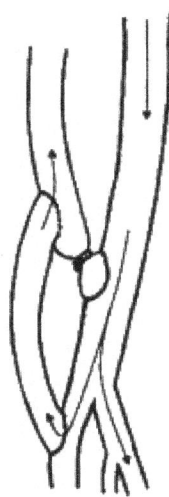

Figure 34-5. Revision using distal inflow is illustrated. Note that the brachial artery anastomosis to the brachial-cephalic access was ligated. An interposition graft was constructed using saphenous vein from the radial artery to the proximal aspect of original access. Reproduced with permission from Scali and Huber.[19] Figure used in *Contemporary Vascular Surgery* 2011. Used with permission.

with favorable hemodynamic changes although it was associated with a high access failure rate. Further justification for the RUDI is provided by the lower incidence of ARHI for the de novo proximal radial artery–based procedures when compared to the brachial artery–based ones. Both Whittaker[21] and Gupta et al.[10] have reported a 2% incidence of ARHI with the de novo proximal radial artery–based procedures. Indeed, Gupta et al.[10] report that they have changed their clinical practice, incorporating more proximal radial artery–based procedures. One potential advantage to the RUDI is that it maintains perfusion through the axial artery. Paradoxically, the major disadvantage is that it converts a brachial artery–based access to a radial artery–based one. This is potentially problematic, despite the favorable reports above, given the smaller caliber of the radial artery and the high prevalence of occlusive disease in the forearm vessels that can limit their ability to vasodilate and increase flow in a response to the access. Indeed, the presence of significant forearm arterial occlusive disease is likely one of the explanations for the inferior success rates for distal radial-cephalic autogenous accesses that are particularly poor in the elderly, diabetics, and women.

DISTAL REVASCULARIZATION WITH INTERVAL LIGATION AND THE UNIVERSITY OF FLORIDA EXPERIENCE

The DRIL procedure likely represents the best option for most patients with ARHI. However, it is worth emphasizing that Schanzer et al.[22] first described the procedure in 1988 and the overall published experience is relatively limited given the overwhelming number of patients on hemodialysis. The hemodynamic basis for the technique is the low resistance arterial bypass that overcomes the high resistance collateral circulation and the ligation that prevents retrograde flow from the distal vessels through the fistula. Interestingly, these components that afford the hemodynamic advantage (i.e., arterial bypass and ligation) have been cited as limitations. Concerns have been raised that the DRIL creates a scenario in which perfusion of the hand is dependent on the bypass and that graft thrombosis could be catastrophic. However, this logic is partly flawed because it is the collateral network (i.e., profunda brachial) rather than antegrade flow past the anastomosis that is responsible for the distal perfusion in the absence of the brachial bypass that comprises the DRIL.

We have recently updated our DRIL experience that now encompasses a total of 134 procedures in 126 patients.[4] The majority of the patients were female (59%) and diabetic (69%) while 13% had ≥2 prior access attempts and 15% had a prior episode of ARHI (Table 34-2). All of the access procedures were based on the brachial artery and the overwhelming majority was autogenous (Table 34-3). Motor dysfunction was the leading presenting symptom, but many of the patients had multiple complaints (i.e., paresthesia and motor dysfunction) (Fig. 34-6). The average time from index access creation to DRIL was 82 ± 153 days, but there was trimodal distribution of symptoms as noted above (i.e., <7, 7–30, >30 days) (Fig. 34-7). Saphenous vein was used for the bypass conduit in 75% of the cases with arm vein used in 18%. The average postoperative length of stay was 4.2 ± 4.8 days, the 30-day mortality rate was 2%, and the overall postoperative complication rate was 27% with wound complications accounting for the leading cause (Table 34-4). The DRIL resulted in significant increases in the wrist/brachial (WBI) and digital/brachial (DBI) indices WBI, 0.31 ± 0.25 ($P = .02$); DBI, 0.25 ± 0.29 ($P = .03$) (Fig. 34-8). The presenting symptoms resolved in 82% of patients (Fig. 34-9), and 85% continued to use the index hemodialysis access at last follow-up.

TABLE 34-2. PATIENT DEMOGRAPHICS AND COMORBIDITIES

Demographics	$n = 126$
Age, mean (SD), years	57 (12)
Gender (% female)	59
Comorbidities	
Hypertension	95%
Diabetes	69%
Dyslipidemia	55%
Coronary artery disease	49%
Smoking	46%
Congestive heart failure	21%
Prior hand ischemia	15%
Prior access attempts (≥2)	13%

Abbreviation: SD, Standard deviation.

Source: Reproduced with permission from Scali et al.[3]

TABLE 34-3. BREAKDOWN OF ACCESS CONFIGURATIONS

Access Configurations	$n = 126$
Autogenous brachial-cephalic upper arm direct access	46%
Autogenous brachial-basilic upper arm transposition	36%
Autogenous/cadaveric brachial-axillary indirect femoral vein	16%
Prosthetic brachial-axillary access	2%

Source: Reproduced with permission from Scali et al.[3]

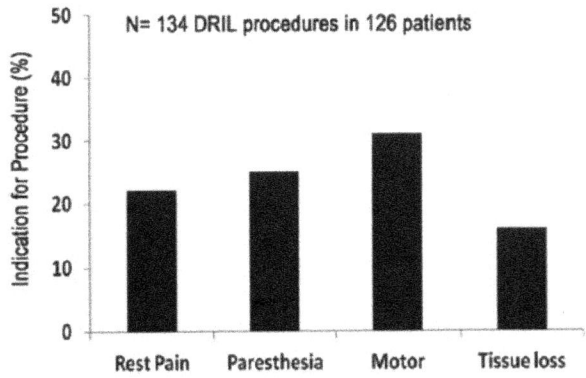

Figure 34-6. The predominant indication for the DRIL procedure in the University of Florida experience is shown. Reproduced with permission from Scali et al.[3]

The cumulative loss of primary and primary-assisted patency for the DRIL bypass (± standard error of the mean) were 5 ± 2% and 4 ± 2% at one year and 22 ± 5% and 18 ± 5% at five years, respectively (Fig. 34-10). Several univariate predictors of primary patency failure were identified with ≥2 prior access procedures having the greatest hazard ration (HR 4.1 (1.6–10.4)) (Table 34-5). The brachial-brachial bypass occluded

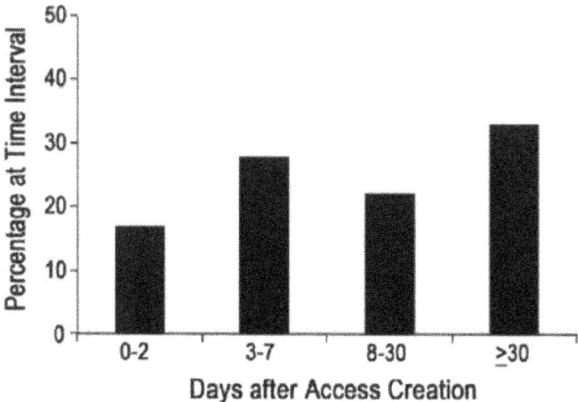

Figure 34-7. The timing of the DRIL procedure relative to the index access procedure that causes the ARHI in the University of Florida experience is shown. Reproduced with permission from Scali et al.[3]

TABLE 34-4. POSTOPERATIVE MORBIDITY AND MORTALITY

Morbidity	27%
Wound	19%
Peripheral nerve	3%
Cardiac	2%
Gastrointestinal	2%
Cerebrovascular	1%
Thirty-day mortality	2%

Source: Reproduced with permission from Scali et al.[3]

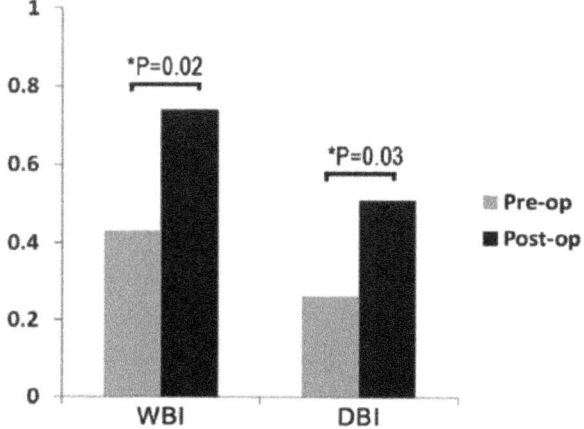

Figure 34-8. The mean preoperative (pre-op) and postoperative (post-op) wrist/brachial (WBI) and digital/brachial (DBI) indices in the University of Florida experience are shown. Significant increases ($P < .05$) were noted for both indices after the DRIL procedure. Reproduced with permission from Scali et al.[3]

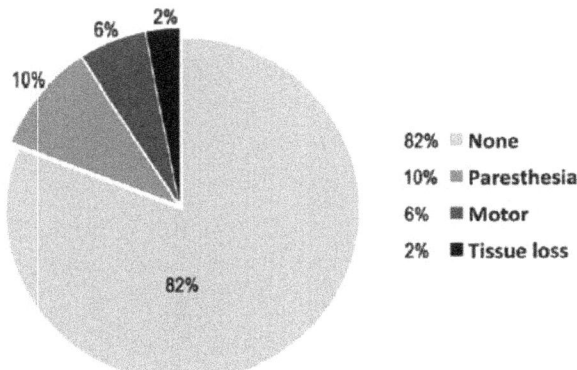

Figure 34-9. The proportions of patients with symptom relief and residual symptoms after the DRIL in the University of Florida experience are shown. Reproduced with permission from Scali et al.[3]

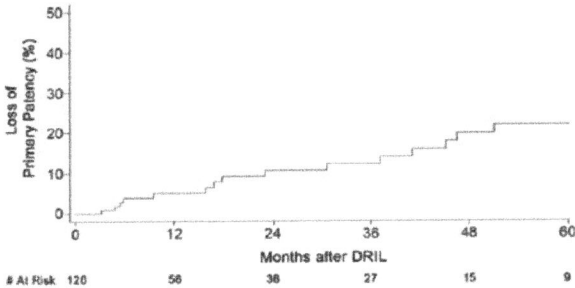

Figure 34-10. The cumulative incidence of the loss of primary patency after the DRIL procedure along the number of patients at risk in the University of Florida experience is shown. Note that the standard errors are <10% throughout. Reproduced with permission from Scali et al.[3]

TABLE 34-5. UNIVARIATE PREDICTORS OF LOSS OF PRIMARY PATENCY

Predictor[a]	HR	CI	P-value
≥2 prior access creations	4.1	1.6–10.4	.004
Nonautogenous brachial-cephalic/brachial-basilic access[b]	3.4	1.4–8.3	.009
Complication from DRIL	3.3	1.2–8.9	.02
Autogenous vein conduit	0.2	0.06–0.58	.004
Autogenous brachial-cephalic upper arm direct access	0.2	0.04–0.8	.02

Abbreviations: CI, confidence interval; HR, hazard ratio.

[a]Cumulative incidence regression was used to determine univariate associations between patient covariates and DRIL bypass primary patency. Cumulative incidence regression was used due to the competing risk of patient mortality.

[b]Nonautogenous brachial-cephalic/brachial-basilic access includes configurations of autogenous indirect femoral vein translocation brachial-axillary access, cadaveric femoral artery/vein brachial-axillary access, and prosthetic brachial-axillary access.

Source: Reproduced with permission from Scali et al.[3]

in 11 patients with three being asymptomatic and eight undergoing a second DRIL procedure. One patient with a failed DRIL procedure had persistent hand dysfunction that predated the original DRIL: no amputations resulted from the DRIL thromboses. All-cause mortality was 28 ± 5% at one year and 79 ± 6% at five years (Fig. 34-11).

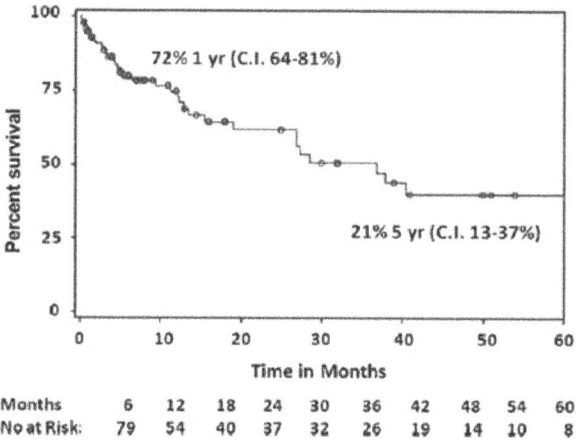

Figure 34-11. The Kaplan–Meier curves for patient survival along with the number of patients at risk in the University of Florida experience are shown. Note that the standard errors are <10% throughout. Reproduced with permission from Scali et al.[3]

TABLE 34-6. MULTIVARIATE PREDICTORS OF ALL-CAUSE MORTALITY

Predictor[a]	HR	CI	P-value
Age >40 years	8.3	2.5–33.3	.0004
Grade 3 ischemia	2.6	1.5–4.6	.0008
Complication from DRIL	2.4	1.3–4.5	.004
Smoking history (past/current)	2.2	1.3–4	.007
No prior access procedures	0.5	0.3–0.9	.02

Abbreviations: CI, confidence interval; HR, hazard ratio.

[a]Cox proportional hazard regression analysis.

Source: Reproduced with permission from Scali et al.[3]

Multivariate analysis identified age >40 years, Grade 3 ischemia, any complication after DRIL, and smoking history as predictors of mortality after the DRIL (Table 34-6). The model predicted better survival if the patients had no prior permanent access attempts before the index access creation for which the DRIL operation was performed.

Our DRIL experience (in terms of access patency, relief of symptoms, and bypass patency) has been corroborated by other, large experiences in the literature. Aimaq et al.[23] published their DRIL experience (N = 81) and reported a 17% complication rate and five-year access and bypass survival rates of 56% and 97%, respectively. Notably, the symptomatic outcomes varied with the presenting complaints; 82% and 90% of those with rest pain and tissue loss, respectively, had relief, but only 56% of those with neuropathy were symptom-free. Similarly, Anaya-Ayala et al.[24] reported that the DRIL procedure (N = 33) was associated with relief of the presenting symptoms in 77% of their cases with one-year secondary patency rates for both the access and bypass of 94%. Notably, failure of a DRIL bypass in their series resulted in gangrene of the hand requiring a transmetacarpal amputation. Gupta et al.[10] echoed our enthusiastic support for the procedure in their recent publication concluding that the "DRIL is particularly effective".

RATIONAL APPROACH TO THE MANAGEMENT OF ARHI

Our general approach to ARHI is outlined in Fig. 34-12. However, we readily concede that the clinical decisions can be difficult in terms of recommending treatment for patients with equivocal symptoms and selecting the optimal approach. Furthermore, our approach continues to evolve based on the published literature and our own experience. The clinical decisions are contingent upon several factors, somewhat independent of the advantages and disadvantages of the remedial treatments outlined above. These include the underlying cause of the ischemia (e.g., potential inflow lesion), the utility (or potential utility of the access), future access options, patient comorbidities, and available conduit.

The initial decision point in our algorithm is to determine whether the patient is sufficiently healthy to withstand the proposed treatment. Clearly, there are different risks involved with the various options ranging from percutaneous catheter-based procedures to the DRIL with its obligatory vein harvest and brachial bypass. This balance between the risks and benefits of the treatment must be assessed at each step of the algorithm with simple ligation being the fall back or bailout procedure. Admittedly, the assessment of the risks and benefits of the various remedial procedures are impacted by the time course of the presenting symptoms, in that patients with acute symptoms have already undergone an operation and therefore were

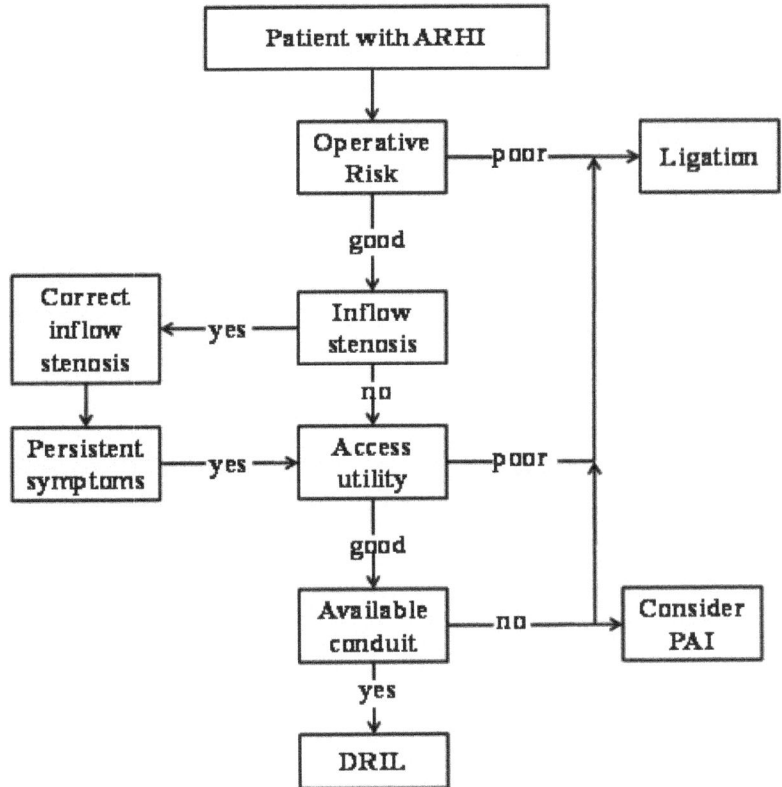

Figure 34-12. Our current treatment algorithm for patients with ARHI is illustrated. A full description of the flow diagram is described in the text. Reproduced with permission from Scali and Huber.[19] Figure used in *Contemporary Vascular Surgery* 2011. Used with permission.

deemed sufficiently healthy to undergo the index access procedure. In practice, it is unusual to deem a patient a prohibitive risk to undergo a remedial procedure.

The next step in the algorithm is to determine whether there is a potential inflow lesion. As mentioned above, the incidence of a significant inflow lesion in our experience is quite low, but this has not been the experience of others. An arteriogram (either catheter-based or CTA) should be obtained to rule out a proximal lesion. It is our preference to perform a catheter-based arteriogram in our hybrid operating room and correct any significant lesions at the same time. These lesions usually occur at the origin of the subclavian artery and are amenable to angioplasty in combination with stenting. In the absence of a significant inflow lesion, we proceed down the outlined algorithm, but it is worth emphasizing that it is important to work through the various steps and potential outcomes before embarking on a specific treatment. Notably, we obtain a catheter-based arteriogram at the time of our DRIL procedures, but it would be unusual for us to correct the lesion and abort the DRIL hoping that correcting the inflow lesion would be sufficient to relieve the presenting symptoms.

An important consideration in the treatment algorithm is the utility or potential utility of the access. Admittedly, this concern is somewhat irrelevant for patients with a functional autogenous access and chronic hand ischemia. However, it is very pertinent for patients with acute symptoms and either a prosthetic or autogenous access and for those with chronic symptoms and a prosthetic access. The treatment choice represents a balance between the likelihood (and potential duration) of the access being functional and the added morbidity associated with the remedial procedure. In our own DRIL experience, the successful autogenous access maturation rate for procedures performed emergently was comparable to our larger cohort of access procedures. However, the autogenous access maturation rates reported from the Dialysis Access Consortium, a randomized controlled NIH-funded trial, were a sobering 38%.[25] We have generally ligated the access for patients with acute hand ischemia secondary to a prosthetic access in the absence of a contributory inflow lesion. We have performed a few DRIL procedures for patients with chronic ischemic symptoms and a prosthetic access. However, these were very select patients with limited options and a prosthetic access that had worked or was expected to work for some time.

The final decision in our treatment algorithm is the status of the conduit and the feasibility of its use in the brachiobrachial bypass that comprises the DRIL. Similar to lower extremity bypasses, the greater saphenous vein is our preferred conduit and we have used >3 mm as our diameter criteria for a suitable vein. We have been reluctant to harvest the saphenous vein below the knee in patients with significant peripheral vascular disease. In patients that do not have suitable saphenous vein, we have used the cephalic or basilic vein in select cases, attempting to balance the benefit of preserving the current access against the loss of a future access option. We recommend against the use of prosthetic and cryopreserved cadaveric vein conduits. For patients that lack a suitable autogenous conduit for a DRIL, PAI with a small caliber PTFE graft may be a reasonable alternative to ligation. However, our experience has been fairly limited and we would echo the report cited above that it is probably not effective for patients with severe tissue loss.[17] Unlike the description of Zanow et al.[16] that reported using a 4- or 5-mm graft, we have used a 4–7 tapered graft or a 6-mm straight ePTFE graft.

We have had limited experience with the various flow-limiting procedures and the RUDI, and, therefore, they have not played a major role in our treatment algorithm. Our enthusiasm for the flow-limiting approaches is tempered by the inconsistent reports in the literature and the requisite, tenuous balance between adequate distal perfusion and sufficient access flow to sustain effective dialysis. However, the various flow-limiting strategies may be effective for patients that have very high flow rates, particularly those with cardiac dysfunction. The RUDI has a tremendous amount of theoretical appeal, particularly in patients with limited conduit in which a DRIL procedure may not be feasible. Although the published results are very limited, the consistent observation that the de novo proximal radial artery–based access procedures have a lower incidence of ARHI than brachial artery–based procedures is compelling. Our enthusiasm for the RUDI has been tempered by our large diabetic population and relatively poor experience with radial-cephalic autogenous accesses in this cohort. In contrast, we have had an excellent experience with the DRIL procedure and this success has both reinforced our approach and diminished our enthusiasm for the other alternatives.

It is worth emphasizing that the management or treatment of ARHI really begins during the preoperative evaluation. The likelihood of hand ischemia should be determined with each access procedure based on the clinical predictors outlined above and all preventative strategies to reduce the incidence should be implemented. All potential inflow arterial stenoses should be identified and corrected. The operative procedure should be selected or designed to minimize the risk of ischemia in patients deemed "at risk." This potentially includes using a small diameter conduit (e.g., 3-mm cephalic vein vs. 6-mm basilic vein) where applicable and/or siting the arterial anastomosis at a location less likely to lead to hand ischemia. As noted above, the incidence of ARHI appears to decrease as the anastomosis is sited either further distal (i.e., proximal radial artery and distal radial artery) or proximal (i.e., proximal brachial artery) from the brachial artery at the antecubital fossa. For example, we would construct an upper arm loop using the proximal brachial artery near the axilla in high-risk patients that require a prosthetic brachial-axillary access rather than using the brachial artery at the antecubital fossa.

A remedial plan should be generated in the operating room at the time of the index procedure to address any potential hand ischemia. Occasionally, we will obtain a saphenous vein survey during the preoperative workup to identify all potential conduits for a DRIL. In the most extreme circumstances, we have performed a preemptive DRIL procedure at the time of the index access although these have been reserved for patients with significant ipsilateral tissue loss or prior ARHI.

ADDITIONAL CONSIDERATIONS

DRIL Failure

Despite our enthusiasm for the DRIL procedures, we have had a few cases in which the procedure was ineffective in terms of relieving the initial symptoms. In these instances, it has been difficult to determine whether the persistent symptoms were a result of the initial ischemic nerve injury or frank ongoing ischemic complaints. Our generic approach in these settings is to obtain upper extremity arterial pressures and Doppler waveforms along with a graft scan of the brachial artery bypass that comprises the DRIL procedure. We have a low threshold for obtaining a catheter-based arteriogram since it can help identify potential problems in the arterial inflow, bypass conduit, and forearm outflow. Remedial treatment is often dictated by abnormalities on the arteriogram. In the absence of an identifiable problem, the remedial options include ligation and some type of flow-limiting strategy as outlined above. Unfortunately, PAI and RUDI are not practical options after a DRIL procedure.

ARHI After Radial Artery–Based Procedures

Hand or digital ischemia can occur after distal radial artery–based procedures. The underlying hemodynamic changes are similar to those outlined for the brachial artery–based procedures and result in a pressure drop distal to the anastomosis. This is not usually a problem given the dual nature of the circulation to the hand and the dominance of the ulnar artery in the majority of individuals. However, it can become problematic in patients with significant forearm or hand arterial occlusive disease and for those individuals with a dominant radial artery. The dominant artery to the hand should be identified preoperatively with an Allen's test and this is included among the noninvasive studies performed in the vascular laboratory in our algorithm. Access procedures should generally not be performed using the dominant artery to the hand, either the radial or the ulnar, despite the favorable report by Bourquelot et al.[26] due to the risk of hand ischemia associated with the functional access and the potential for the artery to thrombose when/if the access fails. Hand ischemia can also occur after radial artery–based procedures as a result of retrograde flow from the ulnar artery and palmar arch.

The treatment options for patients with hand ischemia secondary to a radial artery–based access are theoretically similar to those outlined above for the brachial artery–based procedures with the exceptions of the DRIL and RUDI. However, ligation remains the most common definitive treatment. Any hemodynamically significant inflow lesions can be corrected, particularly those in the dominant ulnar artery. The radial artery distal to the fistula can be interrupted using either ligatures or coils for individuals with significant retrograde flow through the palmar arch. Notably, Chemla et al.[27] documented hemodynamic improvement in terms of hand perfusion after balloon occlusion of the distal radial artery.

REFERENCES

1. Wixon CL, Hughes JD, Mills JL. Understanding strategies for the treatment of ischemic steal syndrome after hemodialysis access. *J Am Coll Surg*. 2000;191:301–310.
2. Papasavas PK, Reifsnyder T, Birdas TJ, et al. Prediction of arteriovenous access steal syndrome utilizing digital pressure measurements. *Vasc Endovascular Surg*. May, 2003;37(3):179–184.
3. Sidawy AN, Gray R, Besarab A, et al. Recommended standards for reports dealing with arteriovenous hemodialysis accesses. *J Vasc Surg*. Mar, 2002;35(3):603–610.
4. Scali ST, Chang CK, Raghinaru D, et al. Prediction of graft patency and mortality after distal revascularization and interval ligation for hemodialysis access-related hand ischemia. *J Vasc Surg*. Feb, 2013;(2):451–458.
5. Berman SS, Gentile AT, Glickman MH, et al. Distal revascularization-interval ligation for limb salvage and maintenance of dialysis access in ischemic steal syndrome. *J Vasc Surg*. 1997;26:393–404.
6. Zanow J, Krueger U, Reddemann P, Scholz H. Experimental study of hemodynamics in procedures to treat access-related ischemia. *J Vasc Surg*. Dec, 2008;48(6):1559–1565.
7. Illig KA, Surowiec S, Shortell CK, et al. Hemodynamics of distal revascularization-interval ligation. *Ann Vasc Surg*. Mar, 2005;19(2):199–207.

8. Reifsnyder T, Arnaoutakis GJ. Arterial pressure gradient of upper extremity arteriovenous access steal syndrome: treatment implications. *Vasc Endovascular Surg*. Nov, 2010;44(8):650–653.

9. Scheltinga MR, van HF, Bruijninckx CM. Time of onset in haemodialysis access-induced distal ischaemia (HAIDI) is related to the access type. *Nephrol Dial Transplant*. Apr 29, 2009;24:3198–3204.

10. Gupta N, Yuo TH, Konig G, et al. Treatment strategies of arterial steal after arteriovenous access. *J Vasc Surg*. Jan 26, 2011;54:162–167.

11. Zanow J, Petzold K, Petzold M, et al. Flow reduction in high-flow arteriovenous access using intraoperative flow monitoring. *J Vasc Surg*. Dec, 2006;44(6):1273–1278.

12. Scheltinga MR, van HF, Bruyninckx CM. Surgical banding for refractory hemodialysis access-induced distal ischemia (HAIDI). *J Vasc Access*. Jan, 2009;10(1):43–49.

13. Thermann F, Ukkat J, Wollert U, et al. Dialysis shunt-associated steal syndrome (DASS) following brachial accesses: the value of fistula banding under blood flow control. *Langenbecks Arch Surg*. Nov, 2007;392(6):731–737.

14. Miller GA, Goel N, Friedman A, et al. The MILLER banding procedure is an effective method for treating dialysis-associated steal syndrome. *Kidney Int*. Feb, 2010;77(4):359–366.

15. Shemesh D, Goldin I, Olsha O. Banding between dialysis puncture sites to treat severe ischemic steal syndrome in low flow autogenous arteriovenous access. *J Vasc Surg*. Aug, 2010;52(2):495–498.

16. Zanow J, Kruger U, Scholz H. Proximalization of the arterial inflow: a new technique to treat access-related ischemia. *J Vasc Surg*. Jun, 2006;43(6):1216–1221.

17. Thermann F, Wollert U. Proximalization of the Arterial Inflow: new Treatment of Choice in Patients with Advanced Dialysis Shunt-Associated Steal Syndrome?. *Ann Vasc Surg*. Oct 28, 2009;23:485–490.

18. Jennings WC, Brown RE, Ruiz C. Primary arteriovenous fistula inflow proximalization for patients at high risk for dialysis access-associated ischemic steal syndrome. *J Vasc Surg*. Mar 30, 2011;54:554–558.

19. Scali ST, Huber TS. Treatment strategies for access-related hand ischemia. *Semin Vasc Surg* 2011;24:128–136.

20. Callaghan CJ, Mallik M, Sivaprakasam R, et al. Treatment of dialysis access-associated steal syndrome with the "revision using distal inflow" technique. *J Vasc Access*. Jan, 2011;12(1):52–56.

21. Whittaker L, Bakran A. Prevention better than cure. Avoiding steal syndrome with proximal radial or ulnar arteriovenous fistulae. *J Vasc Access*. Mar 31, 2011;12:318–320; BADFD2EF–44D1.

22. Schanzer H, Schwartz M, Harrington E, Haimov M. Treatment of ischemia due to "steal" by arteriovenous fistula with distal artery ligation and revascularization. *J Vasc Surg*. Jun, 1988;7(6):770–773.

23. Aimaq R, Katz SG. Using distal revascularization with interval ligation as the primary treatment of hand ischemia after dialysis access creation. *J Vasc Surg*. Apr, 2013;57:1073–1078; discussion.

24. Anaya-Ayala JE, Pettigrew CD, Ismail N, et al. Management of dialysis access-associated +ACI-steal+ACI-syndrome with DRIL procedure: challenges and clinical outcomes. *J Vasc Access*. Jul, 2012;(3):299–304.

25. Dember LM, Beck GJ, Allon M, et al. Effect of clopidogrel on early failure of arteriovenous fistulas for hemodialysis: a randomized controlled trial. *JAMA*. May 14, 2008;299(18):2164–2171.

26. Bourquelot P, Van-Laere O, Baaklini G, et al. Placement of wrist ulnar-basilic autogenous arteriovenous access for hemodialysis in adults and children using microsurgery. *J Vasc Surg*. May, 2011;53(5):1298–1302.

27. Chemla E, Raynaud A, Carreres T, et al. Preoperative assessment of the efficacy of distal radial artery ligation in treatment of steal syndrome complicating access for hemodialysis. *Ann Vasc Surg*. Nov, 1999;13(6):618–621.

35

Hand Ischemia

Jason M. Souza, MD and Gregory A. Dumanian, MD

Hand ischemia is rendered difficult by what it is not: It is not pure vascular surgery, it is not pure hand surgery, and it is not common. The anatomy is relatively unfamiliar and the physiology of hand blood flow is generally misunderstood. The disease entities causing hand ischemia are in some instances unique to the hand in comparison to the rest of the body. The surgical adjuncts of microscopes and tourniquets are not used in most vascular surgery practices. Finally, the postoperative splints, rehabilitation protocols, nerve issues, and prostheses in cases of failed salvage are all the domain of hand surgery rather than vascular surgery. The goal of this chapter is to provide a framework with which to approach a patient with hand ischemia.

HAND BLOOD FLOW ANATOMY AND PHYSIOLOGY

The parallel blood supply to the hand from the radial and ulnar arteries has been extensively studied in the dissection laboratory. In their landmark 1961 study, Coleman and Anson demonstrated an anatomic connection between the radial and ulnar arteries in 80% of hands.[1] A "complete palmar arch" was defined to be present when the superficial palmar arch was contiguous with, or "completed" by, a branch from the deep palmar arch, the radial artery itself, or a persistent median artery. It stands to reason that for hands with an "incomplete arch," damage to the radial artery at the wrist should theoretically cause decreased blood flow to the thumb, while an ulnar artery injury would yield only ulnar-sided ischemia. Based on their anatomic dissections, Coleman and Anson also identified the ulnar artery as the dominant hand vessel, given that it was found to be the larger artery and the principal supplier to the superficial palmar arch.

However, blood flow physiology is significantly different from blood vessel anatomy. Differences between radial and ulnar artery contributions to hand blood flow were garnered from observations of World War II soldiers undergoing arterial ligations in the forearm. Surprisingly, soldiers with radial artery ligations had five times the rate of hand tissue loss than did soldiers who underwent ligation for ulnar artery trauma. The physiologic basis for this observation was later revealed with the use of pulse volume recording (PVR). In an effort to better appreciate the relative importance of radial artery perfusion before harvest for coronary artery bypass grafting, PVR was used to quantify the flow to the thumb, index, and small fingers during sequential compression of the radial or ulnar artery.[2] Manual compression of the radial artery at the wrist caused the loss of pulsatile flow seen on PVRs of the thumb and fifth fingers in approximately 20% of hands, while compression of the ulnar artery caused similar flat line PVR tracings in only 4% of hands (Figs. 35-1 and 35-2). These findings suggested that the radial artery served as the dominant source of blood flow to the hand five times as often as the ulnar artery.

In addition to challenging the concept of ulnar artery dominance, these PVR studies also refuted the traditional teaching that the hand is composed of two potentially

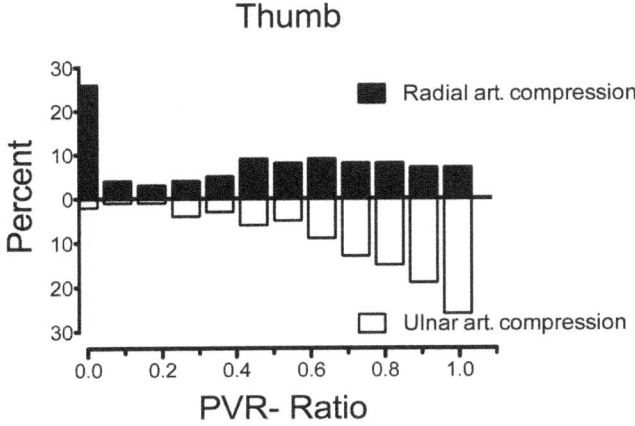

Figure 35-1. Percent reduction in surface area under PVR tracing for thumb with either radial or ulnar artery compression at the wrist. 294 hands. Twenty-five percent of thumbs lose pulsatile flow with compression of the radial artery at the wrist, while 3% of thumbs lose pulsatile flow with ulnar artery compression. A PVR tracing = 1 shows no change in blood flow with compression of the artery, while a PVR tracing = 0 shows a complete loss of pulsatile flow.

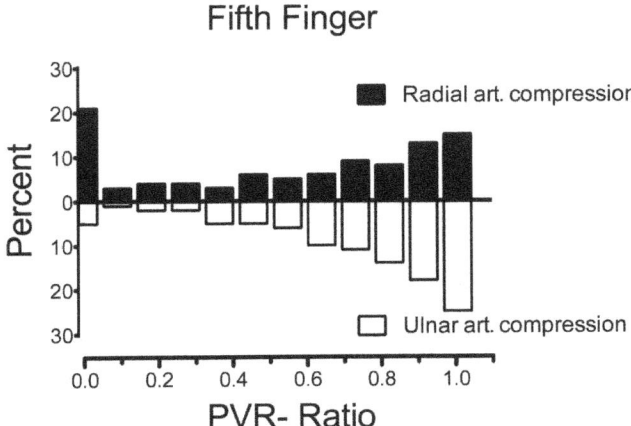

Figure 35-2. Percent reduction in surface area under PVR tracing for fifth finger with either radial or ulnar artery compression at the wrist. 578 hands. Twenty-one percent of fifth fingers lose pulsatile flow with compression of the radial artery at the wrist, while 5% of fifth fingers lose pulsatile flow with ulnar artery compression. A PVR tracing = 1 shows no change in blood flow with compression of the artery, while a PVR tracing = 0 shows a complete loss of pulsatile flow.

separate vascular beds. Based on Coleman and Anson's anatomical study, the 20% of hands that lack a patent palmar arch should act as two independently perfused vascular beds, with the radial and ulnar arteries serving as end arteries. However, it was observed that hands that lose pulsatile blood flow to the thumb with radial artery compression at the wrist also demonstrate loss of pulsatile blood flow to the fifth finger 70% of the time. In only 1% of all tested hands was blood flow maintained in the small finger when radial artery compression caused a loss of pulsatile blood flow in the thumb (Fig. 35-3). Based on these PVR studies, the hand most frequently acts as a single vascular bed supplied by two different arteries. As a result, a pressure drop in one vessel affects the entire hand, rather than causing an isolated radial or ulnar-sided perfusion defect. Clearly, anatomy does not always correlate with physiology. In the overwhelming majority of hands, the radial and ulnar digits act more similarly than dissimilarly

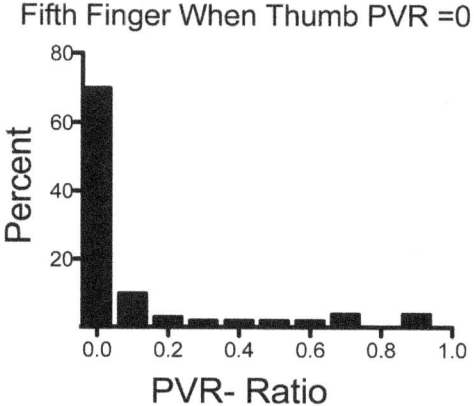

Figure 35-3. Percent reduction in fifth finger PVR tracings in the 86 hands that lost thumb blood flow with radial artery compression at the wrist. Seventy percent of fifth fingers also lost pulsatile flow, demonstrating that the fifth finger and the thumb act similarly. On the right, 4% of these 84 hands maintained normal blood flow to the fifth finger despite losing pulsatile flow to the thumb with radial artery compression. This minority of tests hands have two distinct vascular beds.

in response to changes in perfusion pressure. Images of ischemic hands demonstrate digits affected simultaneously on the radial and ulnar sides of the hand (Figs. 35-4 and 35-5). This single vascular bed concept is critical when bypass grafting of the hand is considered. Rather than needing to revascularize multiple arteries, increased inflow to the hand *at one site* will usually improve blood flow throughout the hand.

VASCULAR PHYSICAL EXAMINATION

Palpation of the brachial and radial artery pulses is mandatory in the initial evaluation of blood flow in the hand. The radial artery pulse can also be palpated in the anatomic snuffbox on the dorsal radial aspect of the hand. The ulnar artery is typically difficult to palpate, due to the stout flexor carpi ulnaris tendon overlying the vessel. A handheld Doppler is a useful adjunct to assess blood flow in distal hand vessels that are too small to be palpated. Just as in the lower extremities, the pitch and character of the Doppler tone provides information about the quality of flow.

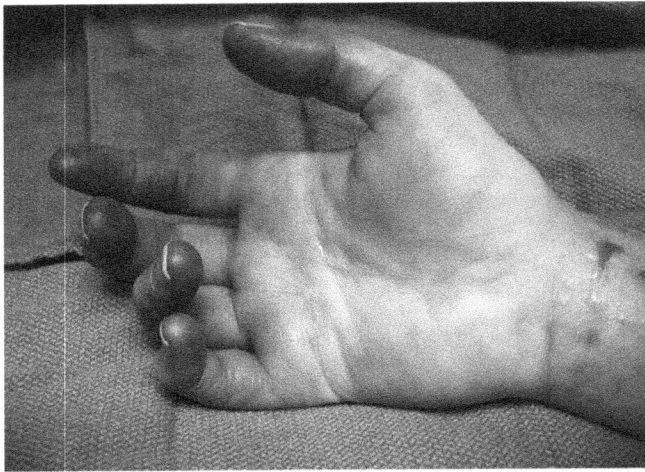

Figure 35-4. Global hand ischemia in a critically ill patient on vasopressors.

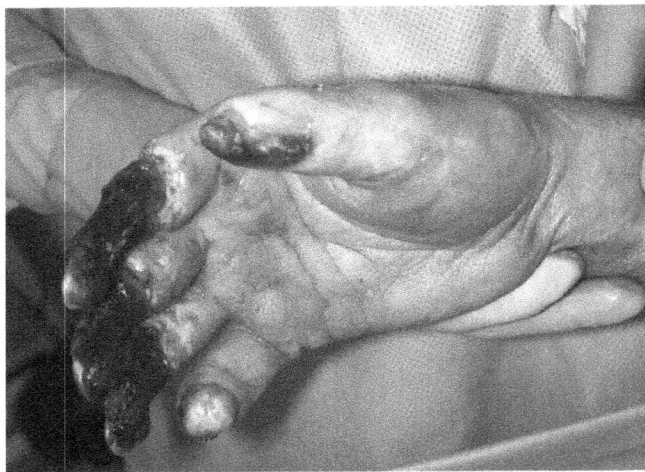

Figure 35-5. Multiple necrotic digits demonstrating the hand acting as a single vascular bed.

To better evaluate the relative contributions of the radial and ulnar arteries to hand blood flow, Allen, a medical student, devised the Allen's test. To perform the test, the hand is first exsanguinated of blood with making of a fist, followed by rapid opening and closing of the hand with the examiner occluding the radial and ulnar arteries at the wrist. With the arteries still compressed, the subject opens the fingers, but in a relaxed and normal cascade so as not to artificially cause blanching of the skin. The examiner then releases either the radial or the ulnar artery, to assess the reperfusion of the hand from that vessel. The fingers should appear pink within five seconds. Digits that remain pale demonstrate either a lack of patency of the released artery at the wrist or inadequate hand perfusion through the unimpeded vessel. The Allen's test is especially important for testing the patency of the ulnar artery before arterial catheter placement, as thrombosis or injury to the radial artery can lead to ischemic complications in patients with insufficient ulnar flow. Infrequently, the hand does not blanch despite compression of both the radial and ulnar arteries during exsanguination. In this case, the presence of a persistent median artery should be considered. A persistent median artery is an embryologic remnant that runs within the carpal tunnel and usually undergoes apoptosis during upper limb development. However, a well-performed cadaveric study demonstrated the presence of this anatomic variant in 15.5% of specimens.[3]

In addition to the pulse exam and Allen's test, evaluation of the soft tissues of the hand can provide valuable insight into the nature, pattern, and chronicity of an ischemic problem. An isolated area of ecchymosis or eschar formation is suggestive of an embolus or distal thrombus, while diffuse, distal tip changes are consistent with generalized hypo-perfusion due to systemic hypotension or thrombosis of a proximal vessel. Absence of hair growth or clubbing of the fingernail may imply chronic ischemia.

DIAGNOSTIC TESTING

In addition to a thorough history and physical exam, noninvasive vascular tests and imaging serve as important adjuncts to the initial vascular assessment of patients with hand ischemia. Segmental arterial pressure measurements, like those frequently performed for evaluation of lower extremity vascular disease, provide valuable information about the level and degree of upper extremity ischemia. Standardized as a digital brachial index (DBI), a ratio of 0.7 is considered indicative of adequate perfusion. PVRs, which quantitatively assess the volume of inflow and outflow to the digits, are also helpful in characterizing the pattern of ischemia.

In terms of imaging modalities, color duplex imaging offers a noninvasive evaluation of vessel flow and is frequently used to visualize upper extremity masses that may impinge on vascular structures. Additional noninvasive imaging modalities include the computed tomography angiogram (CTA) and the magnetic resonance angiography (MRA), although both require intravenous contrast to produce images of sufficient clarity. CTA has found widespread application in the trauma setting, where images can rapidly be obtained without the need for intra-arterial catheterization.[4] While MRA is commonly used to identify vascular lesions in the lower extremity, the image resolution provided by current MRA technology precludes visualization of the fine vessels of the hand and is thus not useful for assessment of chronic hand ischemia.

Despite the convenience of these noninvasive modalities, the intricate detail and real-time sequential images provided by contrast arteriography make this the gold standard for visualizing the vasculature of the upper extremity. Close collaboration between vascular and hand surgeons increases the range of interventions that can be applied to the evaluation and management of upper extremity ischemia. Vascular surgeons can offer proximal bypass grafts or provide techniques of angioplasty or intra-arterial thrombolysis to improve patency before distal reconstruction or in cases where distal reconstruction is not feasible (Fig. 35-6A–D).

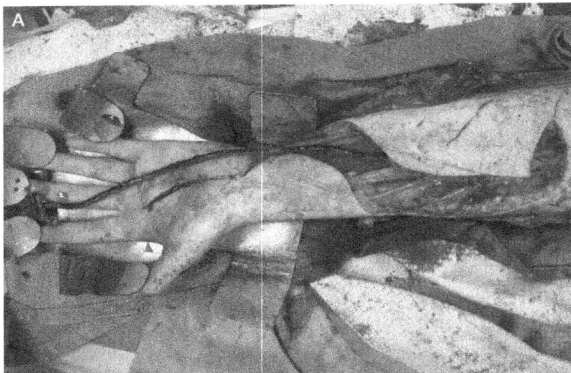
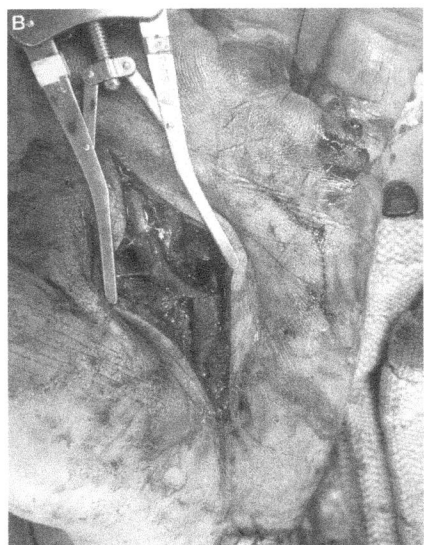
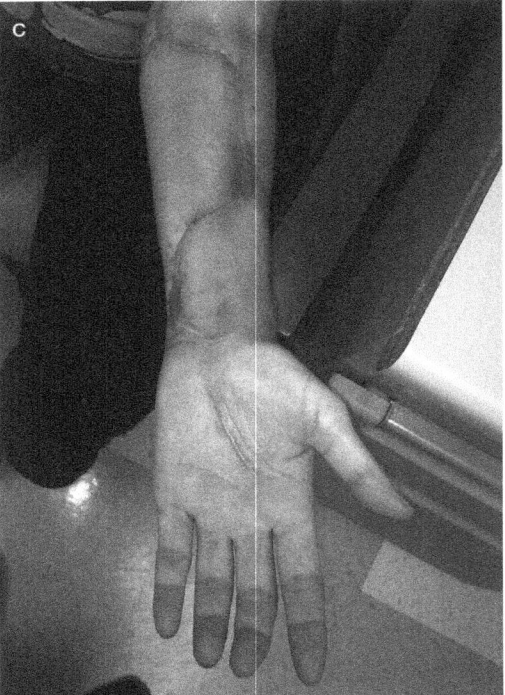
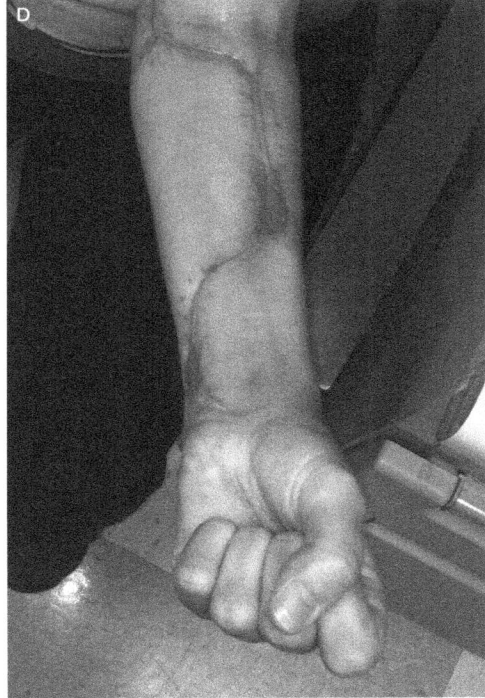

Figure 35-6. *A*, Non-reversed saphenous vein graft bypass from the brachial artery to the superficial palmar arch for management of ischemia of the left hand complicated by ulnar and radial artery injury after attempted distal thrombectomy. *B*, Distal anastomosis performed end-to-side into the superficial palmar arch. The saphenous vein graft and proximal anastomosis performed by the vascular surgery service. The distal anastomosis and tunneling of the graft through the wrist after endoscopic carpal tunnel release performed by the plastic surgery service. *C*, The patient is asymptomatic and demonstrates full extension six months after the procedure. *D*, Full flexion.

ACUTE HAND ISCHEMIA

A thorough history and physical examination must be obtained upon the presentation of an individual with a cool, mottled, and painful hand. Patient age, handedness, smoking history, occupation, heart history, trauma, athletic history, recent upper extremity surgery or catheter placement, and history of a hypercoagulable state must be obtained. The presence or absence of a sinus rhythm, evidence of endocarditis and septic emboli, pulses at the level of the humerus and wrist, an Allen's test, and the presence of Doppler signals in the palm and fingers are mandatory. This initial history and exam seeks to identify the etiology of the ischemia as embolic, thrombotic, or due to a systemic low-flow state. This preliminary evaluation will often also provide information about the level and degree of the ischemia. Hand ischemia in the setting of penetrating trauma presents less of a diagnostic challenge, but does require a determination as to the degree of ischemia that warrants revascularization. Critical hand ischemia, defined by inadequate capillary refill, inaudible palmar or digital Doppler signals, or DBI less than 0.7, should be addressed surgically. Revascularization for noncritical ischemia is more controversial, but may be pursued with the aims of preventing future critical ischemia or the development of subclinical ischemic symptoms, such as cold intolerance or numbness.

The management of patients with acute hand ischemia due to nontraumatic causes is rendered more difficult by several factors. First, due to its relative rarity, many cases present late, with tissue loss that is unrecoverable. The "acute" presentation of digital ischemia from emboli due to aneurysmal disease is often actually attributable to the accumulation of multiple sequential distal vessel occlusions that occur over a prolonged period of time in subacute fashion. This is the pathophysiology that underlies both subclavian artery and ulnar artery aneurysmal disease. "Acute" emboli are typically difficult to retrieve with a Fogarty catheter due to their multiple, small, and distal nature. In these cases, definitive management usually consists of therapeutic thrombolysis, systemic anticoagulation, and pain control. Any patient presumed to have hand ischemia from an embolic source should undergo an echocardiogram to look for mural thrombi or valvular disease (Figs. 35-7 and 35-8). Chest imaging should also be entertained to assess for a subclavian aneurysm from shoulder hypermobility or artery impingement from thoracic outlet syndrome.[5] Along with these other tests, an arteriogram that includes the take-off of the subclavian artery from the aorta is typically required to complete the work-up of a proximal source of emboli to the arm and hand.

Acute ischemia due to radial arterial injury following arterial catheterization should be treated with immediate catheter removal. If this does not improve the hand, then an immediate exploration is required to repair the injured radial artery. In the case of radial artery thrombosis, the thrombus may be sufficiently proximal to be managed through direct thrombectomy. The location of the radial artery thrombus can frequently be identified with the aid of a pencil Doppler alone. In this rare case, the pattern of ischemic skin changes typically involves all digits, as suggested by the blood flow studies previously discussed. Catheter-related radial artery trauma can also lead to ischemia due to distal microemboli. These can present as isolated skin changes involving the thumb or radial digits (Fig. 35-9). As in the case of aneurysmal disease, catheter-assisted embolectomy is generally not practical due to the small caliber of the involved vessels. In these instances, intra-arterial infusions of thrombolytic agents are often helpful. To minimize systemic side effects, an intra-arterial injection of tissue plasminogen activator (tPA) at 10% of the systemic dose is administered

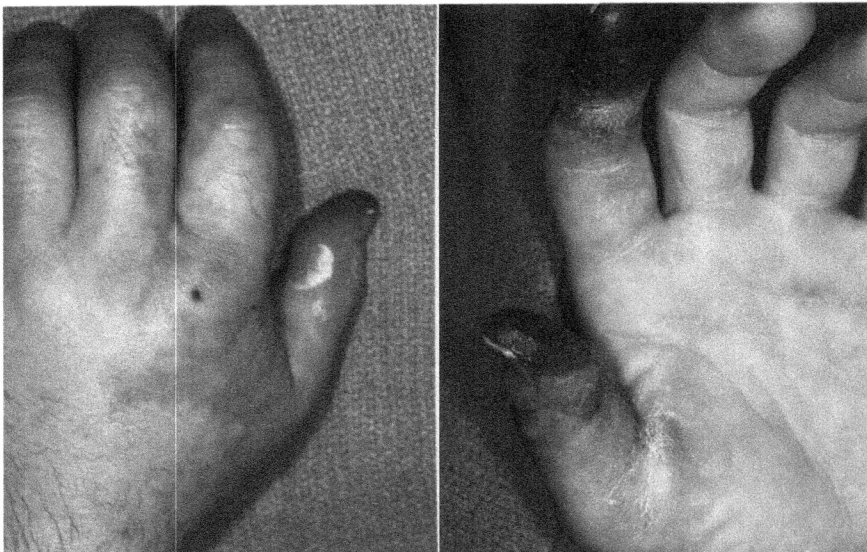

Figure 35-7. Volar and dorsal views of a patient with acute hand ischemia, presenting one full week after the beginning of severe pain. He was treated for thumb and index finger paronychias initially.

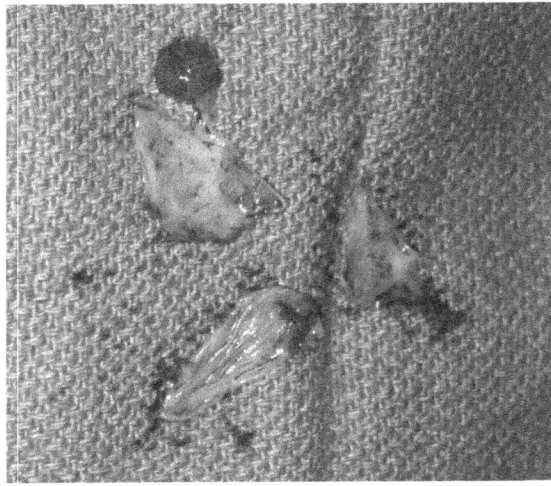

Figure 35-8. Nonseptic degenerative lesion excised from his aortic leaflets at the time of aortic valve replacement.

through the radial artery after inflation of an upper forearm tourniquet for 30 minutes (Fig. 35-10A, B). By minimizing the total volume of the injected vascular bed, the tourniquet allows the tPA therapy to be effective while avoiding dosages that could cause systemic fibrinolysis. Alternatively, the tPA can be administered over time using a super-selective catheter threaded from the groin. A prophylactic carpal tunnel release and intrinsic muscle fasciotomies should be performed in hands that have had a prolonged ischemic event.

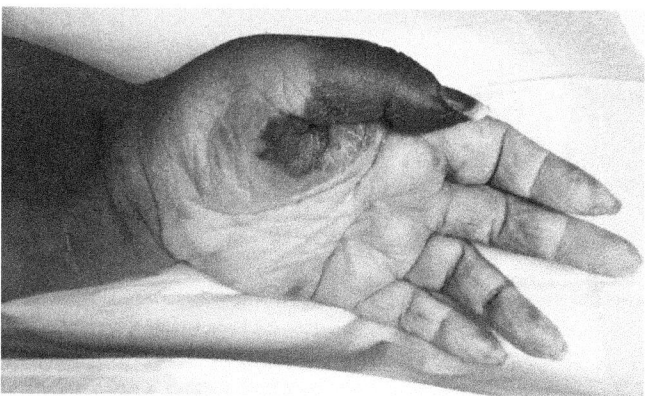

Figure 35-9. Isolated thumb ischemia after attempted radial arterial line placement.

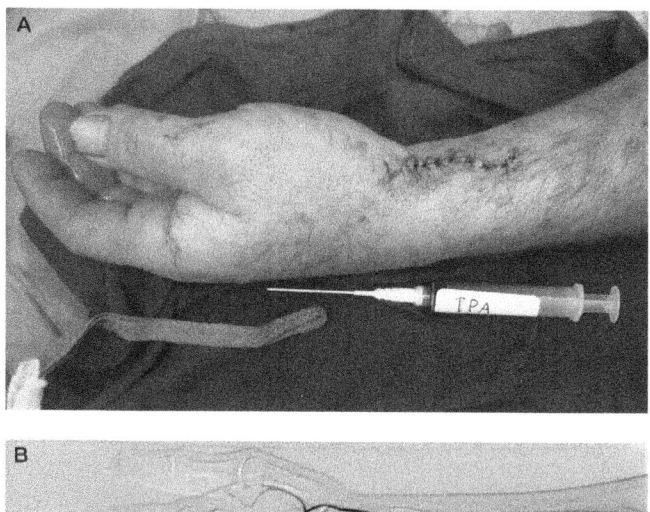

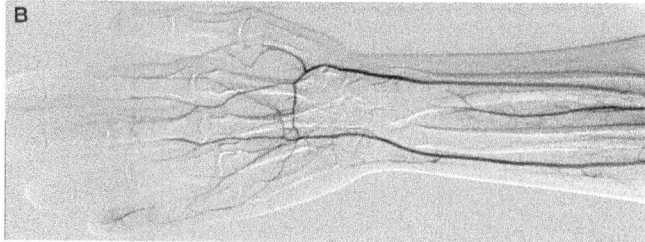

Figure 35-10. Hand ischemia due to radial artery placement with distal emboli. *A,* Successful treatment with radial artery repair, carpal tunnel release, and infusion of tPA under tourniquet. *B,* Pre-treatment arteriogram of above patient demonstrating distal occlusions of multiple digital arteries and illustrating need for thrombolysis.

Vasopressor-associated hand hypo-perfusion and ischemia occurs in critically ill patients in ICU settings. Other than removal of any arterial blood pressure catheters in line with the extremity, surgical treatment of the hand ischemia is typically not feasible in these patients. When possible, therapeutic anticoagulation should be considered. Conservative management of the ischemic digits is typically in order. Aggressive attempts at amputation tend to suffer from marginal ischemia and necrosis along the suture lines and should be avoided. Fortunately, the degree of tissue loss tends to be *less* marked than would otherwise be expected based on the patient's initial presentation. Long-term finger motion and function tends to be poor.

Supracondylar fractures, most commonly seen in children, represent an additional cause of acute limb ischemia. The associated distal limb ischemia is either due to an intimal stretch injury at the time of the bony injury or due to compression of the artery following reduction of the fracture. Supracondylar fractures complicated by limb ischemia must be taken urgently to the operating room. Following bony reduction by the orthopedic service, the hand is evaluated for a palpable pulse at the wrist and capillary refill in the hand. Controversy exists regarding the degree of distal perfusion that is considered adequate after fracture reduction. We feel a palpable pulse at the wrist should be restored before leaving the operating room, to not only prevent ischemic compromise but also ensure normal growth of the maturing arm. If distal perfusion is deemed to be inadequate, the brachial artery is explored. If the artery is found to be within the fracture line, the fixation must be removed and the artery restored to its normal position. If the artery is not found to be impinged by the fracture, and pulsatile flow is absent after adventitial stripping, then an intimal injury must be suspected. Excision of the damaged artery and repair possibly with a vein graft is necessary to reestablish a pulse at the wrist. This often requires microsurgery and consideration of a postrevascularization fasciotomy.

CHRONIC HAND ISCHEMIA

Patients with chronic hand ischemia present with painful digital ulcers, cold intolerance, or numbness. In the absence of obvious ischemic lesions, patients with chronic hand ischemia report a history of numbness or cold intolerance that is most notable when stressed or in a cold environment. These symptoms are suggestive of impaired peripheral tissue perfusion that is often unmasked in the setting of increased demand. Alternatively, patients with chronic hand ischemia may present with the "acute" appearance of ischemic skin changes. As previously discussed, this presentation of "acute" on chronic hand ischemia can be understood as a recent embolic episode that acts upon a partially occluded vascular tree to push the compromised hand into the ischemic zone. The main etiologies for chronic hand ischemia can generally be divided into recurrent embolization, small vessel thrombosis, and vasospastic disease.

Embolic sources of chronic hand ischemia can frequently be traced to the ulnar and subclavian arteries. The ulnar artery is the most common site of arterial aneurysms in the upper extremity. Color duplex imaging can be used to identify the aneurysm, but must be accompanied by an arteriogram to investigate for downstream emboli. Given the possibility of a subclavian artery aneurysm, any arteriogram should begin at the aortic arch to rule out emboli coming from a subclavian ostial lesion. When present, an ulnar or subclavian aneurysm causes chronic hand ischemia through a process of repeated distal embolization. Anticoagulation is the first-line treatment of emboli-induced ischemia, followed by the prevention of further embolic events. Subclavian artery injury from atherosclerosis, excess mobility, or brachial plexus compression can be addressed through a combination of endovascular techniques, brachial plexus decompression, and subclavian artery resection and replacement. These entities are beyond the scope of this chapter.

Ulnar artery aneurysms should be addressed through exploration, with subsequent ligation of the artery or bypass reconstruction. If possible, bypass reconstruction is preferred. Historically, vein grafts have served as the staple conduits for distal bypass, but arterial conduits have gained increasing popularity due to improved handling characteristics, better size and taper, and the suggestion of improved patency rates.[6] However, the increased morbidity and complexity of harvesting an arterial conduit may offset these advantages. As with much of hand surgery, the use of a tourniquet allows the microvascular reconstruction to be performed in a bloodless surgical field.[7] Adventitiectomies of the superficial palmar arch and common digital vessels, much like those performed for patients with scleroderma, serve as useful adjuncts to ulnar artery replacement. To achieve this, extensile palmar incisions are often required in addition to the ulnar artery exposure.

Just as ulnar artery aneurysms can cause downstream emboli to the ulnar digits, so too can ulnar artery thrombosis. In so-called "hypothenar hammer syndrome," the ulnar side of the hand is used to strike objects during manual labor, traumatizing the ulnar artery against the hook of the hamate. Patients present with a constellation of symptoms that varies based on the degree of collateral flow through the radial artery and the presence or absence of embolic phenomena. Contrast angiography demonstrates a cork-screw appearance of the ulnar artery. In less severe cases, patients can be managed with behavioral modification, smoking cessation, or vasodilator therapy. However, presented with ischemic symptoms and a DBI less than 0.7, surgical management is indicated. Catheter-based thrombolysis is usually ineffective due to the chronic nature of the disease process. Just as with ulnar artery aneurysms, excision and ligation of the diseased arterial segment will prevent new emboli from occurring. However, to prevent cold intolerance and optimize hand function, bypass reconstruction of the residual ulnar artery is preferred.

A third group of patients present with chronic, intermittent digital ischemia attributable to vasospastic disease. In these cases, the digital vessels undergo inappropriate vasoconstriction in response to cold, stress, or a variety of other stimuli. When these vasospastic symptoms occur in the absence of an underlying systemic or occlusive disorder, the ischemia that results is reversible and unlikely to cause ulcerations or digit-threatening ischemia. These patients have primary vasospastic disease, or Raynaud's *disease*, which is associated with a relatively benign prognosis. First-line therapies emphasize behavioral modification, in particular cold avoidance, smoking cessation, and discontinuation of medications with vasoactive side effects. Calcium channel blockers, angiotensin-converting enzyme inhibitors and angiotensin receptor blockers, endothelin receptor antagonists, phosphodiesterase inhibitors, and antiplatelet therapy serve as the cornerstone for medical therapy. However, the myriad of pharmacologic therapies being applied underscores the lack of a single definitive medical therapy. Initially injected into the hand for treatment of hyperhidrosis, botulinum toxin A has proven useful as a low-morbidity intervention for those cases refractory to behavioral or conventional medical therapy.[8,9] Treatment with 50–100 units of agent divided into 15–20 subdermal injections has been shown to help a percentage of patients in terms of wound healing, pain, and digital blood flow. It is unclear how often these agents need to be reinjected. It is also unclear if patients with intrinsic vascular abnormalities or a vaso-occlusive component of their disease will do as well as patients with ischemia purely due to vasospasm.

Chronic hand ischemia due to secondary vasospastic disease, or Raynaud's *phenomenon*, occurs in the setting of an underlying collagen vascular or occlusive disease. Most cases are due to scleroderma, which causes chronic hand ischemia through a combination of thrombotic and vasospastic mechanisms. Classically, the arterial pathology in a scleroderma hand exhibits a combination of diffuse intimal hyperplasia and adventitial fibrosis. While the proximal radial and ulnar arteries tend to be relatively unaffected, as one moves distally from the wrist, the vessels of the hand begin to develop a constricting fibrosis that causes them to appear small on an arteriogram (Fig. 35-11). The superficial palmar arch is often thrombosed, although the deep arch is often patent. Additional thromboses tend to occur at the level of proximal interphalangeal (PIP) joint. Similar to Raynaud's *disease*, initial management emphasizes behavioral and pharmacologic therapies. Likewise, more recent studies have demonstrated a benefit to botulinum injection in these patients. A recent review of botulinum toxin for management of Raynaud's *phenomenon* pooled data from five studies performed between 2004 and 2010.[10] Overall, all reports demonstrated an improvement in pain symptoms, but a cohesive interpretation of these findings is precluded by the use of varied botulinum doses and distribution of injection as well as the inclusion of patients with a number of different collagen vascular diseases. Thus, while initial reports have been encouraging, botulinum therapy has not yet supplanted digital sympathectomy as the gold standard therapy for medically refractory disease.

Surgical treatment of chronic hand ischemia due to scleroderma is reserved for cases that have failed medical therapy. These patients generally present as worsening digital ulcerations or an increased frequency of vasospastic episodes.[7] Frequently, these scleroderma-associated ischemic symptoms exist in conjunction with challenging joint contractures, calcinosis, and a contracted soft tissue envelope. Thus, it is imperative that the goals of surgical therapy be clearly defined in terms of realistic pain,

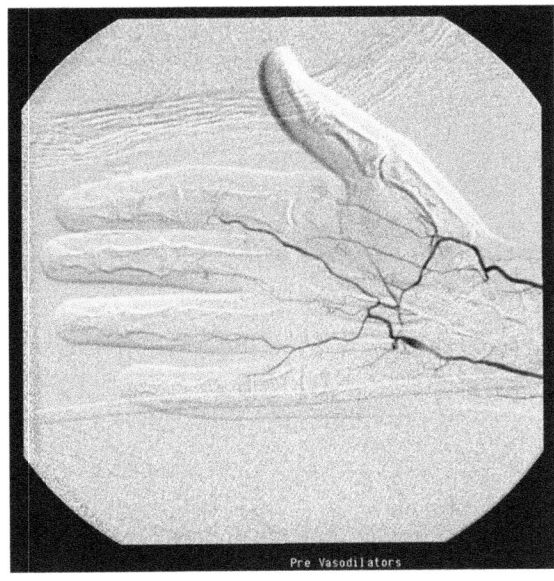

Figure 35-11. Arteriogram of a patient with digital ulcerations due to scleroderma and a proximal compression of the ulnar artery in Guyon's canal.

aesthetic, and functional outcomes. In the case of tissue necrosis involving a significant proportion of the distal finger, the patient may be better served with distal amputation than a complex attempt to restore perfusion to the compromised tissue. Overall, surgical treatment of the scleroderma hand aims to address the increased sympathetic tone and adventitial fibrosis through digital sympathectomy or improve distal flow through microscope-assisted bypass grafting of occluded vessel segments. Digital sympathectomy is a bit of a misnomer, because the procedure is more directed at periadventitial stripping of fibrotic tissue than it is a sympathectomy. The digital arteries are innervated through sympathetic fibers that leave the common digital nerves at right angles over a 2–3-cm area proximal to the PIP joints. In a classic digital sympathectomy, Bruner incisions are used to expose both the radial and ulnar digital arteries from the palmar arch to the PIP joint (Fig. 35-12A, B). Microscope-assisted adventitial stripping relieves the circumferential constriction and alleviates sympathetically mediated vasoconstriction, leaving the vessels in a relatively dilated state. Adventitial

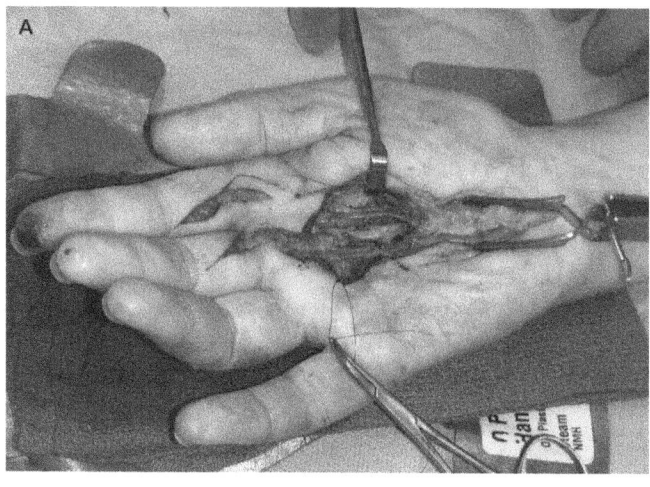

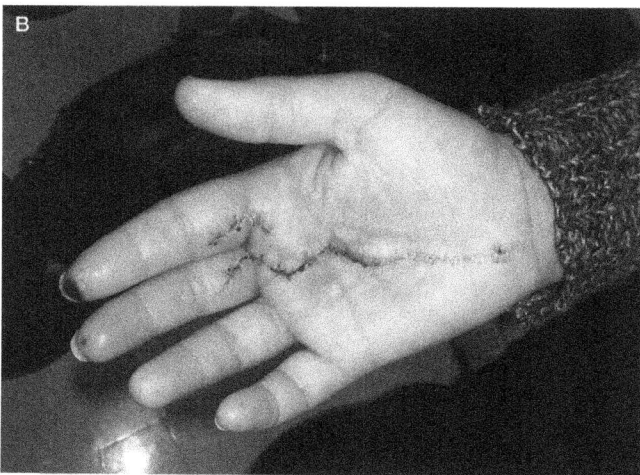

Figure 35-12. Intraoperative, *A*, and postoperative, *B*, views of digital sympathectomy/radical adventiectomy for the arteriogram seen in Figure 35-11.

stripping for a length of 2 cm proximal to the PIP joint is usually sufficient to divide the sympathetic innervation to the fingertip. However, there is some rationale for continuing the adventitiectomy along the common digital arteries as they run proximally to the superficial palmar arch. Some advocate even more proximal dissection, with the goal of dividing the superficial palmar fascial bands, which may be an additional source of ulnar artery compression. Regardless of the extent of dissection, it is imperative not to damage any connections between the deep and superficial palmar arches, as these collaterals may be serving as the principal source of inflow to the digits. Two helpful procedural adjuncts are a brachial plexus nerve block, which improves blood flow in the postoperative period, and intraoperative use of topical papaverine to ameliorate any arterial spasm induced by vessel manipulation during the procedure.

In cases in which digital sympathetectomy yields inadequate improvement in flow, bypass grafting may be indicated. Bypass grafts have typically been considered surgical challenges, with diagrams demonstrating multiple arterial microanastomoses with reimplantation of each of the common digital arteries end-to-side off of the bypass graft.[11] The need for bypass grafting in addition to, or in place of digital sympathectomy, can sometimes be predicted based on the preoperative angiogram and the response to a diagnostic bupivacaine block. A critical issue in deciding between a long vessel adventitiectomy and a distal hand bypass is the presence or absence of "in-line" flow. Vessels of narrow caliber but with evidence of continuous flow through the superficial palmar arch would be treated with digital sympathectomy, while digits supplied through collateral flow from the deep palmar arch would be potential candidates for a hand bypass procedure. Bypasses are done in a unique manner for hand ischemia in comparison to other types of vascular surgeries.[12,13] First, a tourniquet provides a bloodless surgical field and prevents clot formation while inflated, but necessitates that the procedure be performed within the customary two-hour window. Second, the superficial palmar arch or a single common digital artery can provide improved perfusion throughout the hand while serving as the sole source of outflow for the bypass graft (Figs. 35-13 and 35-14). As previously discussed, the hand acts as a single vascular bed, thus one vessel can revascularize the entire hand. This decreases

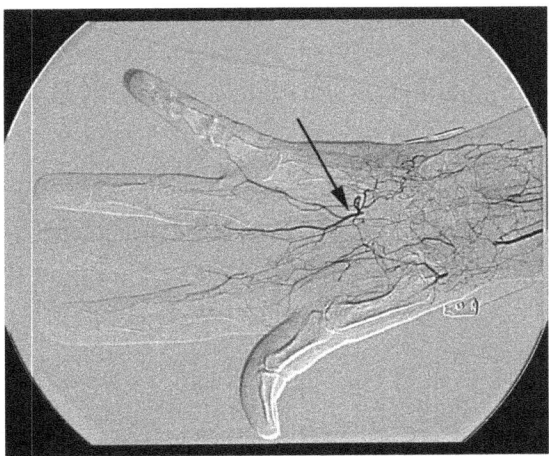

Figure 35-13. Arteriogram of a patient with scleroderma with large area necrosis middle finger and small tip necrosis index finger. She has a radial artery pulse at the wrist. The arrow demonstrates a patent superficial arch.

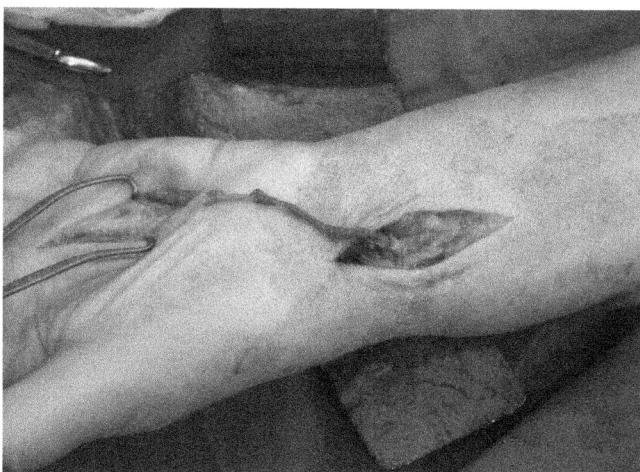

Figure 35-14. Bypass from the radial artery through the carpal canal end-to-end to the superficial palmar arch using the thoracodorsal artery for conduit.

operative times and allows the procedure to be done within one tourniquet run. Third, the tunneling of the graft within the tight confines of the skin of the hand can be difficult. An alternative technique is to perform the proximal anastomosis of a reversed lesser saphenous vein graft to either the radial or ulnar artery, and to tunnel the graft through the carpal canal that has been enlarged with the aid of an endoscopic carpal tunnel release. The palmar tissue bridge that is preserved by this technique serves to protect the graft and is less prone to kinking than a subcutaneous tunnel. The graft is allowed to fill with blood while still under the tourniquet to ensure proper length of the construct. The distal anastomosis is done to a vessel selected with the help of a preoperative arteriogram, either end-to-end or end-to-side, depending on whether or not there is a proximal occlusion present. Once the tourniquet is deflated, the newly revascularized hand frequently exhibits a reperfusion-associated coagulopathy that does require additional time to achieve adequate hemostasis.

AMPUTATIONS

Despite improved therapies and techniques aimed at limb salvage, amputation remains an important component of the care of the ischemic hand patient. The primary goal of surgery is a mobile, pain-free digit. Digital length is secondary. An intact, stiff finger plagued by pain from persistent ischemia often represents a worse outcome than a shortened digit with well-healed amputation incisions and good soft tissue coverage of the transected digital nerves. When necessary, digital amputations can be performed as an office procedure under local anesthesia and without requiring discontinuation of anticoagulation therapy. Fish-mouth incisions with dog-ears taken out in the mid-lateral lines tend to do well. The skin edges tend to be prone to necrosis due to suture compression. As a result, there should be absolutely no tension on the skin flaps, which requires the bone to be resected more proximally than initially thought necessary. The bone end should be contoured so as not to look bulbous. In general, the amputations across the midportion of the middle phalanx have unreliable healing for a patient with a necrotic digital tip, and the PIP joint does not tend to maintain its motion. Conversely, amputations across the proximal phalanx tend to heal completely, and metacarpophalangeal movement tends to be maintained. Nerves found on either side of the tendon sheath should be placed on traction and divided as proximally as possible to decrease the chance of a symptomatic neuroma found under the skin. Similarly, traction should be placed on both flexor tendons before a proximal division to decrease the chance of an infected tendon end festering in the mid-palm. The flexor tendons specifically should *not* be sewn to the extensor tendon mechanism for added bone coverage. The profundus tendon placed and fixed on unusual tension in that manner is a cause of "quadrigia" and decreased motion of adjacent fingers. Digital prostheses are available for the patient with amputations. While not improving function, custom-made digits made out of latex materials can assist patients in camouflaging the sequelae of their vascular injuries.

POSTOPERATIVE CARE

Digital tip ulcers are treated with gentle wound care, very conservative removal of necrotic tissue, and a topical antimicrobial with a silver containing compound. If bypass surgery is performed, prevention of occlusion of the graft from wrist flexion or pressure on the graft can be achieved with a volar well padded splint placed in the operating room with the metacarpophalangeal joints extended and the PIP joints flexed slightly. Splints helps to immobilize the soft tissues to achieve early postoperative healing and they also help with postoperative pain. Patency of the bypass graft is followed in the postoperative period with an arterial saturation monitor placed on a finger. Early digit motion and nighttime splints in full extension help to prevent PIP flexion contractures that develop in these sympathectomy patients prone to develop thick scar. If a bypass graft is done, a well-padded wrist splint with the fingers free worn for three to four weeks will help to prevent occlusion of the graft from wrist flexion or direct compression.

CONCLUSIONS

The complete treatment of a patient with hand ischemia requires a working knowledge of vascular surgery, hand surgery, and reconstructive microsurgery. Lasting improvements in hand function are achievable using the principles presented in this chapter.

REFERENCES

1. Coleman SS, Anson BJ. Arterial patterns in the hand based upon a study of 650 specimens. *Surg Gyncol Obstet*. 1961;113:409.
2. Dumanian GA, Segalman K, Beuhner JW, et al. Analysis of digital pulse-volume recordings with radial and ulnar artery compression. *Plast Reconstr Surg*. 1998;102:1993–1998.
3. Gellman H, Botte MJ, Shankwiler J, Gelberman RH. Arterial patterns of the deep and superficial palmar arches. *Clin Orthop Relat Res*. 2001;383:41–46.
4. Anderson SW, Foster BR, Soto JA. Upper extremity CT angiography in penetrating trauma: use of 64-section multidetector CT. *Radiology*. 2008;249:1064–1073.

5. Durham JR, Yao JST, Pearce WH, et al. Arterial injuries in the thoracic outlet syndrome. *J Vasc Surg*. 1995;21:57.

6. Masden DL, Seruya M, Higgins JP. A systematic review of the outcomes of distal upper extremity bypass surgery with arterial and venous conduits. *J Hand Surg*. 2012; 37A:2362–2367.

7. Dumanian GA, Chen A. Microsurgery in a bloodless field. *Microsurgery*. 2000;20:221–4.

8. Van Beek AL, Lim PK, Gear AJ, Pritzker MR. Management of vasospastic disorders with botulinum toxin A. *Plast Reconstr Surg*. 2007;119:217.

9. Fregene A, Ditmars D, Siddiqui A. Botulium toxin type A: A treatment option for digital ischemia in patients with Raynaud's phenomenon. *J Hand Surg*. 2009;34A:446–452.

10. Iorio ML, Masden DL, Higgins JP. Botulinum toxin A treatment of Raynaud's phenomenon: A review. *Semin Arthritis Rheum*. 2012;41:599–603.

11. Wilgis EF. Evaluation and treatment of chronic digital ischemia. *Ann Surg*. 1981;193:693-698.

12. Jones NF. Ischemia of the hand in systemic disease. The potential role of microsurgical revascularization and digital sympathectomy. *Clin Plast Surg*. 1989;16:547–556.

13. Kryger ZB, Rawlani V, Dumanian GA. Treatment of chronic digital ischemia with direct microsurgical revascularization. *J Hand Surg*. 2007;32A:1466–1470.

Complex Arterial and Venous Diseases

36

Endovascular Treatment of the Aorta in Marfan Syndrome Patients

Alyson L. Waterman, MD, MPH and Adam W. Beck, MD

The vascular manifestations of Marfan syndrome, specifically dissection, aneurysm and rupture, are the largest cause of morbidity and mortality for affected individuals. Bentall's method of replacement of the ascending aorta was initially described in 1968, and is now commonly used to prophylactically treat aortic root dilation in Marfan patients.[1] This preventative intervention revolutionized the care of these patients and greatly improved their life expectancy.[2] However, despite improved survival following ascending aortic repair, Marfan patients continue to experience degeneration of the remainder of their aorta throughout their lives, often requiring multiple remedial aortic interventions or treatment of other aortic segments.

Reoperative surgery in these patients is known to have a higher risk of morbidity and mortality than the initial treatment. In their study including 675 Marfan patients undergoing aortic root replacement, Gott et al. reported that 14% of patients had a history of previous aortic surgery.[3] Those patients who had a history of previous aortic operation had a 60-day mortality that was fivefold higher than those who had not. Gott's study also showed that subsequent dissection or rupture of the residual aorta was the leading cause of late death (defined as greater than 30 days). Other authors have also reported that reoperation rates for Marfan patients are as high as 27%,[4] with a mortality rate of reoperation up to 31%.[5]

As Marfan patients who have been treated with standard open operations advance in age and experience progression of their aortic pathology, options for safe open interventions diminish. The advent of endovascular therapies has provided an attractive alternative for treatment of patients who are high risk for open operation, but these interventions have not been widely accepted in connective tissue disorder (CTD) patients due to concerns about durability. In the 2008 Expert Consensus Document on the Treatment of Descending Thoracic Aortic Disease Using Endovascular Stent Grafts, The Society of Thoracic Surgeons Endovascular Surgery Task Force stated that "stent grafting in patients with Marfan syndrome or any other know connective tissue disorder is not recommended [as] there is limited information regarding the impact of persistent radial forces of a stent graft in the abnormal and weak aorta."[6] Despite these concerns, multiple case reports and series in the literature demonstrate that practitioners are using these techniques in Marfan patients with mixed results (Table 36-1).[7–18] The patients who have been offered endovascular options in these series are generally those felt to be at high medical or surgical risk for open repair due to previous operations or comorbid conditions.

At the University of Florida we frequently treat patients with Marfan syndrome, and we have recently published our experience with endovascular treatment of the aorta in Marfan patients, detailing our short- and mid-term outcomes.[16] With respect to endovascular intervention, in order to categorize our results, we placed patients into three groups: (1) those deemed on follow-up to have successful therapy (Fig. 36-1A–C), (2) those with primary treatment failure (Fig. 36-2A, B), or (3) those with secondary treatment failure (Fig. 36-3A–C). Successful therapy was defined as complete clinical and radiographic exclusion of the target pathology or thrombosis of the false lumen in the stented aorta with no subsequent interventions required during follow-up. Primary treatment failure was defined as a type I endoleak around the endograft, persistent false lumen flow in the stented aorta leading to aneurysmal degeneration, and/or need for subsequent operative interventions (open or endovascular) to address the original presenting aortic pathology. Secondary treatment failure was defined as initially successful treatment of the target aortic pathology with aortic degeneration at a site proximal or distal to the stent requiring further intervention that was unrelated to the original presentation or endovascular procedure performed.

In our series, 16 Marfan patients underwent 19 aortic endovascular procedures over a 10-year period for varying indications. Six patients were deemed to have successful therapy, seven had primary treatment failure, and two had secondary treatment failure (one patient was lost to follow-up). When examining our results by indication, it was notable that all but one of the primary treatment failures were in patients with chronic dissection. Below, we report our results in combination with those of the existing literature, sorted by indication.

ACUTE DISSECTION WITH MALPERFUSION

While type A dissection remains a surgical emergency only treatable by open aortic repair, acute type B dissection is generally treated conservatively unless the presentation is complicated by things such as concomitant rupture, acute false lumen aneurysm, or distal malperfusion. In our series, two patients with known Marfan syndrome presented with acute dissection of the descending thoracic aorta with malperfusion. Both patients were effectively treated in the acute setting with placement of an endograft, with one having a successful result in follow-up to date. The other patient was considered a secondary treatment failure due to persistent false lumen flow in the more distal aorta leading to aneurysmal degeneration. A second endograft was placed in this patient, which led to successful false lumen thrombosis, and the patient now has a stable repair without further intervention.

Zaman et al. reported similar success in a patient who presented with acute dissection and lower extremity paralysis due to malperfusion.[7] After endograft placement, successful thrombosis of the false lumen occurred with improved distal perfusion and resolution of the paralysis. Geisbusch et al. similarly reported a patient with acute

TABLE 36-1. SUMMARY OF PUBLISHED DATA ON ENDOVASCULAR THERAPY FOR MARFAN SYNDROME BY INDICATION

	N	Prior Procedures	Technical Success Yes	PTF	STF	Subsequent Procedures	Mortality	Follow-up Length (mos)
Eid-Lidt et al. (2013)	10							60
CTBAD/aneurysm	10	1 (n = 5)	6	4	–	3	2	
Gelpi et al. (2013)	1							12
CTBAD/aneurysm	1	3	1	–	–	0	0	
Waterman et al. (2012)	16							13.7
CTBAD/aneurysm[a]	11	1–5	6	7	2	8	4	
Acute dissection	2		3	6	1			
Pseudoaneurysm	2		1	1	1			
Anastomotic disruption	1		1					
Geisbusch et al. (2008)	6							31
CTBAD	5	1–3 (n = 4)	3	2	1	2	0	
Acute dissection	1		3	2	1			
Marcheix et al. (2008)	15							25
CTBAD	15	1 (n = 11)	3	10	2	8	3	
Baril et al. (2006)	6	1 (n = 4), 2 (n = 2)	3	1	?	4	0	29
Aneurysm	3		2	1	1			
Pseudoaneurysm	3		1	1	1			
Botta et al. (2006)	1							12
CTBAD/aneurysm	1	2	1	–	–	0	0	

(Continued)

TABLE 36-1. (Continued)

	N	Prior Procedures	Technical Success			Subsequent Procedures	Mortality	Follow-up Length (mos)
			Yes	PTF	STF			
Dong Xu et al. (2005)	2	0	2	–	–	0	0	12–16
CTBAD/aneurysm	2							
Ince et al. (2005)	6	1 (n = 5)	2	4	–	2	1	12–74
CTBAD/aneurysm	6							
Fleck et al. (2003)	1	4	1	–	–	0	0	36
Pseudoaneurysm	1							
Roux et al. (2002)	1	2	1	–	–	0	0	n/a
Pseudoaneurysm (Asc)	1							
Zaman et al. (2002)	1	n/a	1	–	–	0	0	12
Acute dissection	1							
Total number of patients	66							

Abbreviations: CTBAD, chronic type B aortic dissection; n/a: not available; PTF, primary treatment failure; STF, secondary treatment failure.
[a]One patient lost to follow-up.

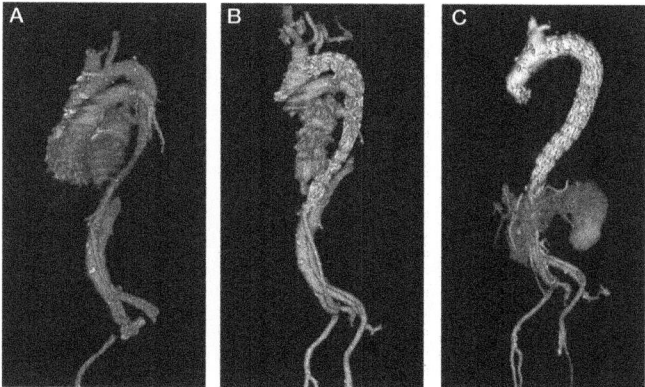

Figure 36-1. Successful treatment with a TEVAR after prior ascending/arch/valve conduit. These figures show the initial 3D reconstruction (*A*) with favorable aortic remodeling throughout the thoracic aorta at 3 months (*B*) and 4 years (*C*).

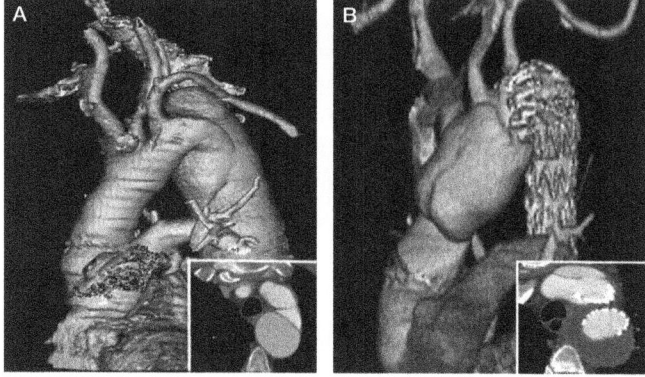

Figure 36-2. Primary treatment failure in a patient with a prior ascending valve conduit. The pre-op scan is shown (*A*) as is the retrograde dissection after TEVAR with aneurysmal degeneration of the transverse aorta (*B*). This patient required an open arch reconstruction.

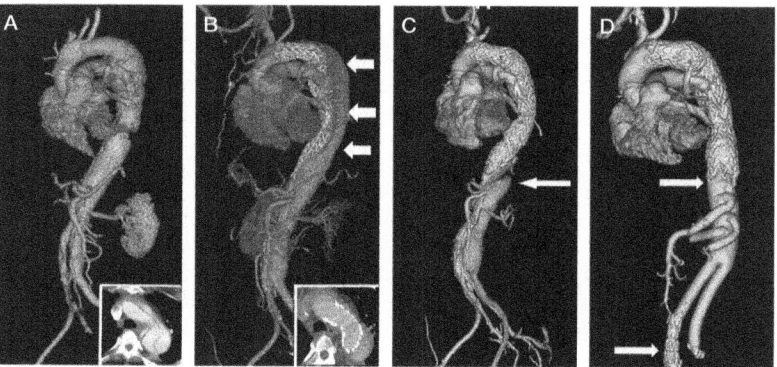

Figure 36-3. *A*, Secondary treatment failure in a patient with a prior aortic valve replacement (AVR) deemed high-risk for thoracic aortic replacement for his CTBAD. *B*, Persistent false lumen flow is shown by the three large arrows. *C*, Despite eventual thrombosis of the thoracic component of the dissection, there was aneurysmal degeneration of the visceral segment. *D*, At open conversion with visceral debranching, the existing TEVAR and the iliac limb of a prior EVAR were used for the proximal and distal anastomosis.

dissection and renal malperfusion who underwent TEVAR and renal artery stenting.[15] Their patient would be considered a secondary treatment failure in our series, due to the need for distal extension and iliac stenting to seal other entry points causing persistent false lumen flow. Despite the need for a second intervention, their patient had a successful repair out to 57 months post-op.

Given the emergent nature of these clinical scenarios, we believe that emergent TEVAR in Marfan patients presenting in this manner is a reasonable alternative to open therapy. Although these patients often require future interventions, the secondary interventions are generally elective in nature and have not been complicated by the endovascular procedure in our experience.

ANASTOMOTIC DISRUPTION

Our series included a patient who underwent TEVAR for acute postoperative disruption of the distal aortic anastomosis. The disruption was successfully sealed, but the patient had a prolonged and complicated ICU course secondary to profound shock resulting from the anastomotic disruption, and died at postoperative day 30 with multiorgan system failure. No other case reports are available for endograft use in a case such as this, and this is certainly, and thankfully, an unusual clinical circumstance. Given the emergent nature and the likelihood of mortality from a repeat open procedure, we feel that an endovascular method is a reasonable alternative to emergent open reintervention in a clinical scenario such as this.

PSEUDOANEURYSM

Two patients in our series underwent endograft placement for pseudoaneurysms at the descending thoracic aorta associated with previous open repair. One patient underwent TEVAR after five prior open aortic operations with a successful result and no further interventions. The second patient had a history of four previous aortic operations before undergoing TEVAR for an anastomotic pseudoaneurysm. The initial TEVAR led to a successful exclusion of the aneurysm, but continued follow-up demonstrated further degeneration of the more distal thoracic aorta (secondary failure) leading to a visceral debranching and a second TEVAR. Unfortunately, this patient succumbed to multisystem organ failure after complications from this repair.

Other case reports detail successful repair of anastomotic pseudoaneurysms (Baril et al.[13] and Fleck et al.[9]) including one of an ascending aortic pseudoaneurysm (Roux et al.[8]). Certainly, if the proximal or distal landing zone of the endovascular device is within Dacron, there is likely to be successful seal and fixation at that end of the endovascular treatment zone. The area in question is the native aorta that is either already dissected or at risk for future dissection or aneurysm. This portion of the aorta in a patient with a proximal pseudoaneurysm is often effectively similar to a patient with a chronic dissection, which constitutes the largest group of patients in our series. The results of TEVAR in Marfan patients with chronic type B dissection are outlined separately below.

CHRONIC TYPE B DISSECTION WITH ANEURYSMAL DEGENERATION

The majority of the available literature regarding TEVAR in Marfan patients involves the elective treatment of chronic type B aortic dissection (CTBAD) with aneurysmal degeneration. This is perhaps the most controversial group of patients given the elective nature and the uncertainty of the durability of repair. Eleven of the sixteen patients in our study (51 of the 66 included in Table 36-1) underwent endograft placement for this indication. Not surprisingly, this is the group with the highest proportion of primary treatment failures, which were predominantly due to persistent false lumen flow and further aneurysmal enlargement of the stented aorta.

Treating chronic dissections with an endovascular approach and landing in dissected aorta inherently violates one of the basic premises of endovascular therapy for aneurysms, which is the importance of proximal and distal seal. Despite this issue, abating flow into the false lumen and inducing thrombosis can often lead to favorable aortic remodeling in patients with aneurysms associated with chronic dissection. Because the mode of failure for these patients is largely the result of persistent false lumen flow, our current practice is to cover the majority of the dissected aorta to the level of the celiac artery. The negative impact of this approach may be a higher rate of spinal cord ischemia, but we do not have enough patients to determine if this is more than a theoretical concern.

We recently published our series of TEVAR for chronic dissection[19] as well as an analysis of our secondary interventions after TEVAR.[20] In those studies, we reported that secondary interventions in dissection patients are not uncommon, even outside of the CTD population. Despite this, we are able to obtain successful therapy in the majority of patients, and most repeat interventions in the CTBAD population are elective in nature. When patients do require a subsequent open intervention, we are generally able to either explant the graft, or utilize the graft in the open repair. Furthermore, we found in our analysis that these repeat interventions do not affect survival when compared to patients who do not need further interventions, so it does not appear that we are negatively impacting the patients in the long term by using an endovascular-first approach. While these results from our general CTBAD population may not be entirely applicable to the Marfan patients, they appear to have similar results in our small series.

CONCLUSIONS

Marfan patients often present therapeutic dilemmas due to previous open operations, complex aortic anatomy, and comorbid conditions in combination with lifelong risk of aortic degeneration. The advent of endovascular therapies has provided an attractive alternative to open operation, but the durability of the repairs in is question, especially in patients with CTDs. While endovascular therapy is certainly not successful for all patients with Marfan syndrome, we have demonstrated that these procedures can be efficacious for select patients in both the emergent and elective setting.

Notably, elective endovascular treatment of patients with CTBAD and aneurysm has not been evaluated by a clinical trial, and is not approved by the FDA with the existing devices on the market. Thus, much of what is known about this patient population can only be obtained by single center experiences, and practitioners should be critical of these data before this practice is widely adopted. In our experience at the University of Florida, we have demonstrated that patients with CTBAD can be successfully treated with TEVAR, but a high rate of reintervention to maintain a successful repair or treat contiguous or distant disease should be expected. Given the small numbers, we are uncertain if the results from our non-CTD patients can be applied to the Marfan population, but our results to date have been similar.

Given the frequent need for reintervention after TEVAR in Marfan patients, the selected treatment should take into account each patient's geographic ability and willingness to follow-up as they should after their intervention, and a more frequent rate of follow-up imaging than usual after TEVAR may be required. Furthermore, we believe that treatment of patients with aortic disease related to CTDs should be undertaken in large volume centers to ensure proper postoperative care and follow-up, and that a multidisciplinary approach is imperative to good outcomes. Finally, any attempt at an endovascular intervention should not delay, complicate, or preclude treatment with an open operation, which remains the standard of care in these patients.

REFERENCES

1. Bentall H, De Bono A. A technique for complete replacement of the ascending aorta. *Thorax.* July 1968;23(4):338–339.
2. Silverman DI, Burton KJ, Gray J, et al. Life expectancy in the Marfan syndrome. *Am J Cardiol.* January 15, 1995;75(2):157–160.
3. Gott VL, Greene PS, Alejo DE, et al. Replacement of the aortic root in patients with Marfan's syndrome. *N Engl J Med.* April 29, 1999;340(17):1307–1313.
4. Mingke D, Dresler C, Pethig K, et al. Surgical treatment of Marfan patients with aneurysms and dissection of the proximal aorta. *J Cardiovasc Surg (Torino).* February 1998;39(1):65–74.
5. Akin I, Kische S, Rehders TC, et al. Current role of endovascular therapy in Marfan patients with previous aortic surgery. *Vasc Health Risk Manag.* 2008;4(1):59–66.
6. Svensson LG, Kouchoukos NT, Miller DC, et al. Expert consensus document on the treatment of descending thoracic aortic disease using endovascular stent-grafts. *Ann Thorac Surg.* January 2008;85(1 Suppl):S1–S41.
7. Zaman MJ, Carre V, Parvin S, et al. Endovascular stent repair for a dissecting thoracoabdominal aneurysm is feasible in the setting of a district general hospital: a multidisciplinary approach. *Heart.* August 2002;88(2):E4.
8. Roux D, Brouchet L, Rousseau H, et al. Treatment of a fistula at the distal anastomosis after Bentall operation with endoluminal covered stent. *Ann Thorac Surg.* December 2002;74(6):2189–2190.
9. Fleck TM, Hutschala D, Tschernich H, et al. Stent graft placement of the thoracoabdominal aorta in a patient with Marfan syndrome. *J Thorac Cardiovasc Surg.* June 2003;125(6):1541–1543.
10. Ince H, Rehders TC, Petzsch M, et al. Stent-grafts in patients with marfan syndrome. *J Endovasc Ther.* February 2005;12(1):82–88.
11. Dong Xu S, Zhong Li Z, Huang FJ, et al. Treating aortic dissection and penetrating aortic ulcer with stent graft: thirty cases. *Ann Thorac Surg.* September 2005;80(3):864–868.
12. Botta L, Russo V, Grigioni F, et al. Unusual rapid evolution of type B aortic dissection in a marfan patient following heart transplantation: successful endovascular treatment. *Eur J Vasc Endovasc Surg.* October 2006;32(4):358–360.
13. Baril DT, Carroccio A, Palchik E, et al. Endovascular treatment of complicated aortic aneurysms in patients with underlying arteriopathies. *Ann Vasc Surg.* July 2006;20(4):464–471.

14. Marcheix B, Rousseau H, Bongard V, et al. Stent grafting of dissected descending aorta in patients with Marfan's syndrome: mid-term results. *JACC Cardiovasc Interv*. December 2008;1(6):673–680.
15. Geisbusch P, Kotelis D, von Tengg-Kobligk H, et al. Thoracic aortic endografting in patients with connective tissue diseases. *J Endovasc Ther*. April 2008;15(2):144–149.
16. Waterman AL, Feezor RJ, Lee WA, et al. Endovascular treatment of acute and chronic aortic pathology in patients with Marfan syndrome. *J Vasc Surg*. May 2012;55(5):1234–1240; discussion 1240–1241.
17. Eid-Lidt G, Gaspar J, Melendez-Ramirez G, et al. Endovascular treatment of type B dissection in patients with marfan syndrome: mid-term outcomes and aortic remodeling. *Catheter Cardiovasc Interv*. April 10, 2013.
18. Gelpi G, Mazzaccaro D, Romagnoni C, et al. Hybrid endovascular treatment of an aortic root and thoracoabdominal aneurysm in a high-risk patient with marfan syndrome. *Vasc Endovasc Surg*. May 2013;47(4):300–303.
19. Scali ST, Feezor RJ, Chang CK, et al. Efficacy of thoracic endovascular stent repair for chronic type B aortic dissection with aneurysmal degeneration. *J Vasc Surg*. July 2013;58(1):10–17 e11.
20. Scali ST, Beck AW, Butler K, et al. Secondary Aortic Intervention after Thoracic Endovascular Aortic Repair: Incidence, Outcomes, and Pathologic Specific Implications for Surveillance. Presented at the *Society for Clinical Vascular Surgery Annual Meeting*, Miami, FL, March 15, 2013. Submitted for publication.

37

Distribution and Mortality of Wartime Vascular Injuries in Afghanistan and Iraq

Todd E. Rasmussen, MD and Nigel Tai, MS

INTRODUCTION

Epidemiology is defined as the study of the distribution and determinants of health-related states or events in human populations, and the application of this study to the prevention and control of health problems. The global burden and impact of trauma as an agent of death and disability is increasingly well characterized. However, while the prevalence and incidence of individual vascular injury patterns have been reported in single institution studies, the more broad epidemiological study of vascular trauma is relatively understudied. Possible reasons for this include the different causes of vascular trauma, the heterogeneity of associated injuries, injury often associated with in which vascular trauma, the direct and indirect consequences of vascular injury to other body systems, and the unsuitability of modern trauma scoring methodologies to capture the effects of vascular injury on patient outcome.

Nonetheless, as a leading cause of hemorrhage-related mortality and extremity amputation, understanding the historic and contemporary epidemiology of vascular trauma is important. With respect to trauma, recognizing the populations at risk forms the foundation for targeting of hospital resource and provider education, in essence informing the design of trauma and vascular care systems. Additionally, better description of mechanisms, case-mix and demography empowers comparison of properly stratified outcomes following vascular injury, whether used to assess performance within or between institutions, or to track outcomes. Case-mix and other epidemiological data are used to inform quality improvement initiatives, to construct fair reimbursement schedules for treating hospitals, to understand the impact of external socioeconomic realities, to influence the design and assessment of preventative public health interventions, and to inform wider health and social policy. In essence, if clinicians who are to treat vascular trauma are to anticipate injury patterns, track changes and put in place effective programs to prevent or mitigate the effects, then the study of injury distribution is an essential function of practice. The objective of this chapter is to outline the general circumstances, incidence, and population effects of vascular trauma, as viewed from the epidemiological perspective. This endeavor will be taken with a focus on combat injury encountered in the wars in Iraq and Afghanistan but will also include reference to civilian trauma for important context.

CATEGORIES OF VASCULAR TRAUMA

Attempting to compare and contrast vascular injury epidemiology is hampered by the variable nature of trauma and the multiple and interrelated factors that determine outcome (such as concomitant injuries to soft tissue, bony, and neurological structures). This difficulty is made more significant by the lack of uniformity among investigators as to appropriate injury descriptors, outcome metrics, and follow-up periods. Most studies in both the military and civilian domains offer descriptions of cohorts comprising specific vascular regions (extremities) or anatomical areas (e.g., crural vessels)—this provides detail at the expense of full epidemiologic perspective. Rates of vascular trauma are conflicted by use of different definitions of population-at-risk, invoking different denominators and inflating or deflating prevalence accordingly. Outcomes are defined differently and with varying degrees of accuracy. For instance, mortality rates may be built upon definitions such as death while an inpatient, ignoring those who expire prior to reaching hospital.

Reported vascular injury distribution is dependent upon data and countries with mature trauma systems where accurate data collection is mandated offer a more fruitful if narrow perspective on injury rates and causes. Similarly, while wartime populations often have higher vascular injury rates than peace-time cohorts, the presence of detailed injury data (with accurate description of the denominator populations) is directly related to whether a trauma systems approach to injury data collection is deployed by the military medical services. It is fair to say that countries without a trauma systems approach to injury management, whether in their military or civilian populations, are usually unable to describe the effect of vascular trauma in populations-at-risk. Since most developing countries fall into such categories, it is correct to assume that the global burden of vascular trauma is unknown.

Vascular trauma may be broadly categorized according to mechanism of injury (iatrogenic, blunt, penetrating, blast, combination injuries), anatomical site of injury (further subdivided in to compressible and noncompressible hemorrhage), and by wider contextual circumstances (military, civilian). Each of these domains may be further stratified, with military injury being subdivided by patient status (combatant, noncombatant) and category of conflict (civil war, counter-insurgency warfare, maneuver warfare, etc.). Civilian injuries may be similarly contextualized by local circumstances (such as urban or rural trauma). For the purposes of this chapter, the context will be considered under two broad conditions concerning the injurious mechanism: vascular injury caused during military conflict (whether among interstate, intrastate, or nonstate actors) and that which occurs in the context of civilian circumstances.

VASCULAR TRAUMA AND MILITARY CONFLICT

Vascular injury that occurred in World War I (WWI), World War II (WWII), Korea, and Vietnam can be conceived as a product of industrial war waged between nation states. Warfare over the past two decades has lost many of the characteristics that defined previous engagements; the term *War amongst the people* has gained credibility as the ability of nations to employ force with utility has declined. This refers to the modern reality in which "the people in the streets and houses and fields – all the people, anywhere – are the battlefield." Military engagements can take place anywhere, with civilians around, against civilians, in defense of civilians. Civilians are the targets, objectives to be won, as much as an opposing force. As such, vascular trauma inflicted by high-energy military ballistic projectiles and purpose-built or improvised blast weaponry can affect two populations at risk: combatants and noncombatant (civilians).

VASCULAR TRAUMA IN COMBAT TROOPS

Contemporary data confirm that exsanguination is the major cause of death in wounded soldiers and that the prevalence of vascular trauma seems to have changed markedly over the past century.[1-3] Estimates from allied surgeons in WWI suggested overall vascular trauma rates of 0.4% to 1.3%.[4] De Bakey characterized vascular injury burden in WWII as affecting 0.96% of all patients and for the Korean and Vietnam wars the rate of vascular injury was judged to be higher at 2%–3%.[5-9]

Coalition militaries engaged in modern combat operations in Afghanistan (2001) and Iraq (2003–2011) have invested substantially in detailed trauma registries in order to capture injury data. Such data bases have been used to characterize miscellaneous injury patterns so that force protection (body armor, vehicle design) and treatment protocols can be continually updated and aligned to contemporary trauma archetypes. Interestingly, present rates of wartime vascular trauma confirm a much higher prevalence than in the previously mentioned campaigns.[3,10,11]

In a comprehensive study summarizing recent US military experience, White and colleagues analyzed vascular cases entered into the United States Joint Theater Trauma Registry (JTTR) from 2002 to 2009.[3] Defining the denominator as battle-related injuries sufficiently severe to prevent return to duty in the combat theater, the specific incidence of vascular injury (defined as the *total incidence injury*) was found to be 12% (1570 of 13,076 cases). The incidence of injuries requiring an operation (defined as the *operative incidence*) was found to be 9% (1212 of 13,076 cases). The analysis looked for differences in vascular injury incidence between troops deployed to Iraq and Afghanistan, and found significantly different rates of 12.5% and 9%, respectively. Peak rates of injury in either theater differed with combat tempo, accounting for 15% of all injuries in 2004 (Iraq) and 11% in 2009 (Afghanistan). Other differences included causative mechanism, with blast accounting for 74% and 67% of injuries in Iraq and Afghanistan (overall contribution 73%). There was no difference in the anatomical distribution of the injuries, nor the *died of wounds* (DOW) rate (6.4%) between theaters. Wounds were principally sustained to the extremities (79%), torso (12%), and cervical regions (8%). In the torso, the most commonly injured vessels were the iliacs (3.8%) followed by the aorta (2.9%) and subclavian arteries (2.3%), followed by injuries to the inferior vena cava (1.4%). In the neck, 109 carotid injuries accounted for 7% of injuries.

In the study by White and colleagues, it was noted that the vascular injury burden borne by the extremities in Iraq and Afghanistan was remarkably similar to that noted by DeBakey in WWII, although the higher contemporary rate of cervical and aortic injury was attributed to increased survivability and far shortened medivac times.[3] Overall, the authors concluded that the rate of vascular injury in these wars was five times that previously reported from Vietnam and Korea. Interestingly, this estimation of incidence also ran higher than that reported from early analyses of around 4%–5% published from US military hospitals in Iraq.[10,12] However, it is important to note that these early reports from the wars in Afghanistan and Iraq did not include nonoperated cases and were generally confined to descriptions of vascular cases identified *in-theater*. When the analysis includes such cases the overall rate of vascular incidence rises. For instance, by determining rates among patients repatriated back to the continental United States and screened for unrecognized vascular injury or that presenting in a delayed fashion, Fox and colleagues described a prevalence of 7%.[13]

The marked increase in rates of wartime vascular injury recorded by these contemporary authors, as opposed to that documented by previous generations, is striking. The reasons for this finding are unconfirmed. As well as increased wound survivability, other reasons may include: (a) the very high rate of blast-related injury etiology in these campaigns, (b) overestimation of the population-at-risk in earlier reports (thus inflating the denominator), and (c) more accurate capture of "minor" nonoperated vascular wounds (adding to the numerator in the current studies).

In a similar but smaller British study, Stannard and colleagues scrutinized the records of 1203 UK servicemen injured through enemy action between 2003 and 2008.[11] Unlike the US JTTR, the British JTTR dataset also included patients who were *killed in action* (KIA), that is who died prior to reaching a medical treatment facility. Characterization of injury was made from clinical data and from *postmortem* examinations conducted by the UK Coroner system. It was determined that 110 (9%) of this cohort sustained injuries to named vessels, of which more than two-thirds had extremity vascular injuries. Blast wounds accounted for 54% and 76% of patients sustaining torso-cervical and extremity wounds respectively. Some 66 of the 110 died before any surgical intervention could be undertaken, indicating the highly lethal nature of vascular wounding patterns. In particular, no patient with a combination of vascular injuries affecting more than one body region (torso, extremity, cervical) survived to an operation.[11] A further defining difference in wound pattern observed between patients surviving to operation (versus those who did not) was presence or absence of a torso vascular injury, with none of those sustaining an injury to a named vessel in the abdomen or thorax undergoing operative intervention. Cervical vascular injuries also proved highly lethal, with 13 of 17 patients succumbing. On the other hand, of 76 patients with extremity vascular injuries, 37 survived to surgery with one postoperative death. Interventions on 38 limbs included 19 damage control procedures (15 primary amputations, 4 vessel ligations in a group characterized by a median mangled extremity score of 9) and 19 definitive limb revascularization procedures (11 interposition vein grafts, 8 direct repairs), with a limb salvage (primary assisted patency) rate of 84%. This UK group concluded that while favorable limb salvage rates are achievable in casualties able to withstand revascularization, torso vascular injury is usually not amenable to successful surgical intervention.[11]

LOCAL NATIONAL POPULATIONS INJURED IN WARTIME ENVIRONMENT

Few studies have examined the burden of vascular injury in civilians during times of war. The registries of military trauma systems may be biased toward data collection among their own troops, or in such cases where information is captured, there is usually no data on outcomes due to lack of follow-up in war-afflicted societies. In a first of its kind study, Clouse and colleagues recorded that 30% and 24% of all vascular casualties treated at a Level III (major trauma center equivalent) US facility in Iraq were either civilian or local national combat forces.[10,14] Extremity vascular injuries were more prevalent in US forces compared with the local population (81% versus 70%), whereas vascular injury to the torso was less common in US forces (4% versus 13%). Cervical vascular injury occurred with similar prevalence in the military and host national populations (14% versus 17%). The authors hypothesized that the lack of protective body armor and the more liberal use tourniquets by US forces was responsible for these observations. Specifically, that body armor protected against torso vascular injury and tourniquets increased the survivability and therefore documentation of military troops with extremity vascular trauma. Interestingly, vascular injuries were noted to be overrepresented in the local nationals; although 40% of those admitted to the facility were of Iraqi origin, they made up to 51% of the vascular injury cohort.

Several lessons can be taken from this unique clinical study. Foremost, deployed military hospitals are traditionally configured and resourced for the care of their own nation's soldiers, so understanding this additional burden associated with caring for a local national population of injured civilians, insurgents, and even military is important. In a supplementary report from Peck and colleagues at the Air Force Theater Hospital in Balad, Iraq, it was determined that the incidence of vascular trauma amongst 4323 locals was 4.4%.[14] In this study, the authors focused on extremity injuries, which affected 70% of vascular casualties, and observed that the median length of stay from presentation to definitive wound closure was 11 days. Host national casualties underwent a median of three operations during this period in order to manage associated soft tissue and orthopedic injuries and achieve definitive wound management. Notably, the age range in this study of host national patients injured during a wartime scenario was 4–68 years and included 12 pediatric vascular injuries.[14] Mortality among this cohort of civilians was 1.5% with complications occurring in 14% of patients. The early limb salvage rate in those with extremity vascular injury was 95% but longer term follow-up was not possible among this host national population.

This experience from the US military corroborates earlier reports from wartime scenarios. Sfeir and colleagues described a population of 366 lower-limb extremity wounded vascular cases, sustained by a mixed population of combatant and non-combatants during the Lebanese civil war over a 16-year period ending in 1990.[15] Two-thirds of patients in this experience were injured from firearms (i.e., gunshot wounds). Distribution of the lower extremity vascular injuries included 118 popliteal injuries, 252 femoral injuries, and 16 tibial level vessel injuries. The mortality in this cohort was 2.3% all of which occurred in those with injuries in the femoral distribution. The amputation rate among the patients in the Sfeir study was 6% and highest (12%) for those sustaining popliteal vascular injury. Similar to the more contemporary reports, the authors attributed failure of limb salvage to physiologic instability (i.e., shock), delay in extremity vascular repair (i.e., six or more hours of ischemia), and the presence of long bone fracture.

CIVILIAN POPULATION VASCULAR TRAUMA

The impact of vascular trauma in the civilian setting is largely unknown in societies without recourse to large population datasets. Even in the United States, which is served by the National Trauma Data Bank® (NTDB®) (a national registry administered by the American College of Surgeons, receiving data from more than 900 trauma facilities), large scale studies are few. In 2010, Demetriades and colleagues attempted to characterize the nature of vascular trauma in 22,089 patients, including children, drawn from a trauma population of more than 1.8 million case files recorded in the NTDB®.[16] Accepting the almost inevitable reporting bias that accompanies analysis of such retrospective data, it was determined that the overall incidence of vascular injury during the study period (2002–2006) was 1.6%. Four-fifths of the injured were male and the average age was 34 years. Half of the patients (51%) sustained a penetrating mechanism; the top four mechanisms of injury were motor vehicle collisions, firearms, stab wounds, and falls. Just under a quarter of patients presented in hemorrhagic shock and over half had an Injury Severity Score of more than 15.[16] Abdominal and chest injuries accounted for more than 25% and 24% of the trauma burden respectively, with arm and leg injuries contributing 26% and 18%. Adult mortality among those with vascular trauma was 23% and vessels associated with the highest rates of amputation were the axillary (upper limb amputation rate of 6%) and popliteal arteries (lower limb amputation rate of 15%). This impressive dataset summarized the national burden of vascular injury but provided limited or only indirect information on the regional or local patterns of injury required to prepare individual surgeons and facilities for workload and case-mix.[16]

URBAN POPULATIONS

Inner-city populations in countries such as the United States and South Africa have been characterized as having high rates of interpersonal violence; much of it mediated by low-energy handgun or bladed weaponry. South Africa has a homicide rate of 32 per 100,000 whereas the United States figure is 4.8 per 100,000 and that in the United Kingdom is 1.7 per 10,000. However, there is regional variation in violence rates even within societies where violent injury is common. For instance, in South Africa, the numbers of homicides within a region is a function of population size and also rates of crime within that population, with Limpopo (a rural region, population 5.5 million) experiencing 762 murders in 2009–2010, and Gauteng (an urban region of 8.8 million, including Johannesburg) experiencing 3444 murders over the same time frame. Similarly, the murder rate in urban areas of United States cities is approximately twice that of suburban and rural areas.

Of course, the relationship between urbanicity, concentration, and population homicide rates is not universal. Australia has an overall murder rate of 1.2 per 100,000, yet the homicide rate in the sparsely populated Northern Territories is 3.96 per 100,000, compared to 0.8 in Victoria State. The degree to which national and urban murder statistics translate to violent vascular injury is difficult to quantify. However, it is unsurprising to note that the majority of classic reports detailing the burden, type, and outcomes from vascular trauma come from urban institutions serving inner city and economically disadvantaged populations. As described previously, population-wide data garnered from the NTDB® suggest the contemporary overall prevalence of vascular injury in civilian patients is 1.6% whereas in urban areas the rate been quoted as 2.3% in a New York Level I Trauma Centre and 3.4% in a Level II center in El Paso, Texas.[17,18] These reports characterize the "at risk demographic" to be a young, male population and demonstrate that the mortality in those with vascular trauma is approximately twice that of patients without this injury pattern. Not surprisingly, penetrating mechanisms of injury seem to be overrepresented in patients with vascular injury. The El Paso authors reported that of patients with vascular injury, 40% had a penetrating mechanism whereas only 10% of those with nonvascular trauma were injured in such a manner.[18]

The largest US single center study of vascular trauma was published in 1988 and emanated from Houston.[19] This report typifies the experience of many large inner-city urban centers and was undertaken with the aim of deriving epidemiologic conclusions that would guide trauma center and health logisticians. The study encompassed a 30-year period, describing 5760 cardiovascular injuries in 4459 patients. The authors of this study set themselves the task of accounting for the entire vascular injury cohort, rather than restricting themselves to specific vessels, utilizing multiple corroborative documentary sources rather than a single registry. The study confirmed that the burden of vascular trauma in the city was being borne by young men (86% male gender of average age 30 years), 90% of whom had been injured by firearms (gunshot 52%; shotgun 7%) or knives (31%).[19] The study confirmed that the wounding pattern in civilian circumstances, even where ballistic penetrating injury is the norm, does not follow that seen in wartime. Torso and neck injuries accounted for two-thirds of all injuries, while lower extremity injuries (including the groin) comprised only 20%. Indeed, whereas very few soldiers with injuries to the large vessels of the abdomen are seen by military surgeons, trauma to the abdominal vasculature accounted for 34% of the vascular injury cohort seen in Houston, a fact attributed to the maturation of the city's Emergency Medical Services.[19]

Trends in epidemiologic factors including changes in the local population, changes in local crime patterns (noting the increased burden of trauma that accompanied criminal narcotic activity), and provision of healthcare infrastructure were carefully described. The authors of the Houston report noted a sixfold surge in vascular trauma, with 163 and 1069 injured patients in the first and last respectively five years of the study. As this study did not detail the denominator data (total number of trauma patients treated for each time period), it was not possible to assess for trends in the proportion of patients with vascular trauma. Furthermore, trauma scores, physiology, and crude outcome measures such as mortality were not provided, thereby limiting characterization of case-mix and reducing the utility of this impressive dataset for the purposes of comparison. Despite these drawbacks, this classic paper serves as template for other investigators seeking to describe vascular trauma epidemiology among their communities.[19]

Urban metical centers in South Africa have reported large series of vascular injuries focusing on individual vessels and body regions though the overall burden of vascular trauma among the population is less clear in these studies.[20] In Australia, Sydney and Perth have reported vascular trauma rates of 1%–1.8% with penetrating mechanisms contributing up to 42% of cases.[21] Reports from individual centers in the United Kingdom emphasize the relative rarity of noniatrogenic vascular trauma in the general and university hospital setting alike, however the rates of vascular trauma among certain inner city populations may approach those seen in North America centers.[22] In 2011, a six-year study in the lead trauma center for London determined that 256 patients (4.4%) out of 5823 trauma admissions sustained vascular injury (Personal

Communication August 2013, Mr Zane Perkins, Royal London Hospital). Penetrating trauma led to 135 (53%) vascular injuries while the remainder of injuries resulted from blunt trauma.[22]

In the London experience, patients with blunt mechanism vascular injury were more severely injured than patients with penetrating injury (median ISS of 29 versus 11, respectively), had greater mortality (26% versus 10%, respectively), and higher limb amputation rates (12% versus 0%, respectively).[23] These differences remained when comparing injuries in each anatomical zone. Patients with blunt vascular trauma were twice as likely to require a massive blood transfusion (47% versus 27%) and had a fivefold longer hospital length of stay (median 35 versus 7 days) compared to patients with penetrating injury. Recent development of a national trauma registry and trauma systems approach in the United Kingdom's National Health Service (NHS) will allow better plotting of the impact of vascular trauma, especially with regard to inner city "hot-spots."

RURAL POPULATIONS

The large reports on vascular trauma are mostly from urban centers, but nonurban and rural populations have discrete injury profiles and patients who have unique requirements, particularly regarding timely access to care. Endeavors by North American researchers studying trauma systems serving rural populations have shed light on injury patterns in these more isolated settings. In 1982, Koivunen et al. reviewed 89 patients from the state of Missouri, a third of whose injuries were farm-related, and found that the delay between injury and arrival at a trauma center averaged 3.4 hours. A total of 82% of injuries involved extremities and 35% were ligated with an amputation and mortality rate of 16% and 6%, respectively. The complication rate associated with vascular repair in this series was 12%. The authors noted that the majority of complications and all deaths and amputations were in patients suffering trauma from farm, industrial, and motor vehicle accidents.[24]

Twelve years later, the same group looked at the influence of time-to-treatment on outcome in 210 patients from mostly rural areas, noting a time period of six hours prior to the introduction of a helicopter retrieval service and four hours afterwards. Amputation rates decreased from 18% to 7% during these two periods supporting the notion of expedited time to care for patients with vascular trauma. In the largest North American civilian series to date, Oller examined 1148 vascular injuries in 978 patients reported from eight trauma centers in a largely rural state. In this study, 80% of patients were transferred from lower levels of care at smaller more peripheral facilities. Over the time course of the study, vascular trauma accounted for 3.7% of all trauma cases entered in the registry. The amputation rate was 1.3% among those with extremity injuries, which accounted for 47% of the total cohort. The authors of this study reached similar conclusions to the Missouri cohort with respect to rural vascular injury in that the patients were older, had a higher incidence of blunt mechanisms, longer duration of hospital admission, and higher mortality (14%). Oller and colleagues argued that for optimum care, trauma services serving rural patients with vascular injuries must configure to enable prompt identification, resuscitation, and early transport of patients to major trauma centers for definitive care.[25]

VASCULAR TRAUMA AND PATIENT AGE

The rate and effect of vascular trauma in pediatric and elderly populations is important. Pediatric vascular trauma is a rare phenomenon but has potential for long-term functional consequences. Any therapy, surgical or nonoperative, requires the surgeon to take into account the developmental needs of the child. Vascular injury in the older population occurs in the context of native atherosclerotic occlusive disease and physiologically less resilient patients.

A number of studies have revealed that the rate of vascular injury is very low in pediatric trauma cases regardless of age used to define the pediatric population. Penetrating trauma in the pediatric populations is a common mechanism and, as in adult vascular trauma, is overrepresented as a cause of vascular compared to non-vascular injury. For instance, in Klinker et al.'s 12-year study of 106 vascular injuries among 9108 patients aged 18 and under, treated at a children's hospital, 1.1% of all trauma admissions had vascular injury.[26] In this study, the prevalence for those with blunt injury was 0.4% whereas that with penetrating injury was 4.5%. Notably, there were as many wounds caused by glass injury as there were gunshots (24 in each case). The authors noted on the burden of extremity vascular trauma with an amputation rate of 10.7% (most from mangled extremities secondary to train or lawn mower accidents), the overall mortality rate of almost 10% (frequently associated with head injury), and the paucity of thoracic aortic injury in this cohort.

Barmparas and colleagues' analysis of pediatric vascular injury among 251,787 US patients in the NTDB® supports findings from previous studies. In this report, pediatric cases, defined as 15 years or younger, were compared to the adult vascular trauma cohort. The prevalence of pediatric vascular injury was 0.6% compared to the rate 1.6% in the adult group. Pediatric patients had lower ISS with a high but less frequent incidence of penetrating injury (42% vs. 51%).

There were also differences in the distribution of vascular injury between the pediatric and adult cohorts in the Barmparas study. Pediatric patients sustained more blunt and penetrating upper extremity vascular injuries but less penetrating chest and abdominal vascular injuries than adults. Interestingly, the upper extremity bore the brunt of pediatric vascular injury with brachial vessel trauma occurring in 13% of patients and forearm vascular injuries occurring in 22% of the group. The incidence of blunt thoracic aortic injury was much lower in children involving only 9% of pediatric patients with blunt vascular injury compared to 26% of adults with blunt mechanism. Mortality was also lower in the pediatric compared to the adult cohort (13.2% vs. 23.2%, respectively), a difference that persisted even after correcting for differences in ISS, Glasgow Coma Score (GCS) and mechanism. There was no difference in the frequency of amputation between the adult and pediatric cohorts with lower extremity vascular injury (8% vs. 9%, respectively). The authors drew attention to the fact that, despite the survival advantage observed in pediatric patients, the rate of penetrating injury was sobering, and that a fifth of children who had been shot died from their injury.

There have been fewer studies of the epidemiology of vascular injury in geriatric patients. In 2011, a study from the NTDB® based on the same population dataset utilized by Demetriades's group for their pediatric study was reported.[27] This study characterized vascular trauma in patients over the age of 64 and revealed an incidence of 0.7% compared to 2% in the younger (16 to 64 year old) cohort. The older cohort had a lower prevalence of male gender (61% vs. 82%) and penetrating injury (16% vs. 54%)

but a higher ISS (27 vs. 21) compared to the younger group. Notably, the thoracic aorta, the most commonly injured vessel in those suffering blunt trauma, was more frequently injured in the elderly than in the younger cohort (38.9% vs. 24.2%, respectively).

Other differences in injury distribution among the elderly included a higher rate of penetrating neck and arm injury and more blunt chest and abdominal vascular injuries in the older (greater than 64 years old) cohort. The authors of this report described a linear increase in thoracic aorta injuries with increasing age and a corresponding decrease in injuries to the forearm vessels and femoro-popliteal axis.[27] Interestingly, no significant difference in amputation rates was described between the older (2%) and younger (3%) cohorts in terms of overall, upper limb, or lower limb vascular injuries. The younger patient cohort was more likely to undergo fasciotomy than the older group (10% vs. 3%, respectively) although the authors were unable to account for this. Mortality in the older cohort was double that in the younger group (44% vs. 22%). Being over 64 years old was associated with an odds ratio of death of 4 after adjusting for gender, ISS, low GCS, presence of shock, mechanism of injury, and body region of injury. Unsurprisingly, older patients also had a longer ICU stay although their overall length of hospital stay (10 days) did not differ from the younger group.

IATROGENIC VASCULAR TRAUMA

Many surgeons encounter vascular injury not as a result of accident or criminal assault but due to misadventures during an open operation or endovascular access or instrumentation. These injuries typically occur in older patients with comorbidities undergoing treatment of chronic or age-related cardiovascular disease. In this context, iatrogenic trauma may be the chief cause of vascular injury in peaceful countries where percutaneous cardiac, neurological, and endovascular therapies are established. One European review of the burden of iatrogenic vascular trauma estimated an incidence of 35%–42%. However, even in underdeveloped countries iatrogenic trauma may account for a significant proportion of the vascular injury workload. In Sweden, where repairs for vascular trauma constitute 1.3% of all emergency and elective vascular workloads, a review of national vascular registry data revealed that iatrogenic etiology accounted for 48% of vascular injuries, with penetrating and blunt trauma accounting for 29% and 23%, respectively.[28]

The most commonly injured vessel in these reports is the right femoral artery, which is consistent with a complication from endovascular access. The authors of one study found that the incidence of iatrogenic vascular trauma had increased 150% between 1993 and 2004 due to the increased use of endovascular procedures. As expected, patients with iatrogenic vascular trauma are older, with median age of near 70 and have a higher incidence of comorbid conditions such as cardiac disease and renal dysfunction. Mortality of patients suffering iatrogenic vascular injury is approximately double that of patients affected by noniatrogenic trauma (4.9% vs. 2.5%). Two small but recent studies from provincial and tertiary referral centers in England reported that 71% and 73% of vascular injuries were iatrogenic underscoring the common nature of this phenomenon. Both studies found poorer outcomes in patients with iatrogenic vascular trauma compared to those with noniatrogenic causes with patients undergoing noncardiac, peripheral interventions fairing the worst.

VASCULAR TRAUMA, LIFESTYLE, AND SOCIOECONOMIC FACTORS

Several investigators have focused on one type of vascular injury pattern in order to investigate the effect of other epidemiological factors on outcome. For example, some have examined the emerging problem of obesity on the outcome of vascular injury in polytrauma patients.[29] Simmons and colleagues studied 115 patients with lower extremity vascular injuries over a five-year period ending in 2005 and dichotomized the group by a Body Mass Index (BMI) of 31 or more. Interestingly this group found that in general, obese patients exhibited no difference in amputation rate or mortality, although a BMI of greater than 40 was associated with a poorer overall outcome.

In North America, poverty and race are recognized to influence outcome from trauma.[30] It is unclear to what extent these factors are intrinsic drivers of outcome, and to what extent they represent summary descriptors of multiple competing and compounding subfactors. To answer this, Crandall sought a more homogeneous trauma grouping and examined the fate of patients with lower extremity vascular injury to investigate the impact of race and insurance status. Using an NTDB population of 4928 patients, the authors found that those who were of Latino, African American, Asian American, or Native American origin had a higher Odds Ratio of death (1.45), as did the uninsured cohort (1.62). The African American and Latino cohorts made up 51% and 19% of penetrating vascular patients, but these groups only contributed 12% and 10% to the blunt injury cohort. When outcomes were stratified by mechanism of injury, no difference was found with respect to mortality in bluntly injured patients, whatever their insurance status or race. Patients injured by penetrating mechanisms who were uninsured had worse mortality, but race only trended toward statistical significance in the prediction models studied. The authors concluded that by focusing on one injury pattern, they had observed a lessening of the compounding effect of injury heterogeneity. This study pointed out that genotypic differences in response to penetrating injuries, provider factors, and poor capability of injury measurements to describe the effect of penetrating injury may all contribute to the observed differences.

Certainly, it is doubtful that current trauma scoring systems capture the effect of vascular trauma on populations. This is unsurprising given the low frequency of vascular trauma within the reference populations used to construct the index models that these systems employ to empower prediction. Loh and colleagues explored this issue in a small series of 50 patients with vascular trauma, matched to an injury severity score of 25, against 50 nonvascular trauma patients. Predicted mortality in the vascular injury group was estimated to be 14%, 4%, 15%, and 19% by injury severity score (ISS), revised trauma score (RTS), acute physiology and chronic health evaluation II (APACHE II), and trauma injury severity score (TRISS), respectively. The actual mortality of the cohort was 24%. The authors concluded that these scoring systems were better at predicting mortality in patients without vascular injury and concluded that conventional trauma scoring systems underestimate the impact of vascular trauma on mortality.

SUMMARY

The distribution of vascular trauma and its contribution to morbidity and mortality is relatively well understood within some populations, notably within coalition forces having fought in the wars in Afghanistan and Iraq. In this wartime population, the prevalence of vascular injury is 12% and higher than that reported from the Korean and Vietnam wars. The level of characterization of vascular injury distribution and its effect on morbidity and mortality is lower, and in most cases absent, in civilian populations where data injury is not collected and analyzed. Although the incidence and prevalence of vascular trauma is not well investigated, where data are available, the prevalence is lower in civilian than in trauma cohorts. Civilian vascular trauma also has a different distribution with proportionally more torso vascular trauma compared to more extremity injuries in coalition forces injured in combat. Iatrogenic trauma is increasing in prevalence as endovascular techniques become more widely accepted and employed. If vascular and trauma surgeons are to tackle the consequences of vascular injury in a holistic manner, then understanding the local circumstances of the epidemiology is key to better targeting of surgical endeavor, hospital resource, and preventative measures. Good data acquisition and analysis in local, regional, and national populations-at-risk underwrites good epidemiology and must be considered when planning for and implementing trauma systems responsible for patients with vascular injury.

REFERENCES

1. Holcomb JB, McMullin NR, Pearse L, et al. Causes of death in U.S. Special Operations Forces in the global war on terrorism 2001–2004. *Ann Surg*. 2007;245:996–991.
2. Kelly JF, Ritenour AE, McLaughlin DF, et al. Injury severity and causes of death from Operation Iraqi Freedom and Operation Enduring Freedom: 2003–2004 versus 2006. *J Trauma*. 2008;64:S21–S26.
3. White JM, Stannard A, Burkhardt GE, et al. The epidemiology of vascular injury in the Wars in Iraq and Afghanistan. *Ann Surg*. 2011;253:1184–1189.
4. Bowlby A, Wallace C. The development of British surgery at the front. *Br Med J*. 1917;1:705–721.
5. DeBakey ME, Simeone FA. Battle injuries of the arteries in World War II: an analysis of 2471 cases. *Ann Surg*. 1946;123:534–579.
6. Hughes CW. The primary repair of wounds of major arteries: an analysis of experience in Korea in 1953. *Ann Surg*. 1955;141:297–303.
7. Hughes CW. Arterial repair during the Korean War. *Ann Surg*. 1958;147:555–561.
8. Rich NM, Hughes CW. Vietnam vascular registry: a preliminary report. *Surgery*. 1969;65:218–226.
9. Rich NM, Baugh JH, Hughes CW. Acute arterial injuries in Vietnam: 1,000 cases. *J Trauma*. 1970;10:359–369.
10. Clouse WD, Rasmussen TE, Peck MA, et al. In-theater management of vascular injury: 2 years of the Balad vascular registry. *J Am Coll Surg*. 2007;204:625–632.
11. Stannard A, Brown K, Benson C, et al. Outcome after vascular trauma in a deployed military trauma system. *Br J Surg*. 2011;98:228–234.
12. Sohn VY, Arthurs ZM, Herbert GS, et al. Demographics, treatment, and early outcomes in penetrating vascular combat trauma. *Arch Surg*. 2008;143:783–787.
13. Fox CJ, Gillespie DL, O'Donnell SD, et al. Contemporary management of wartime vascular trauma. *J Vasc Surg*. 2005;41:638–644.
14. Peck M, Clouse D, Cox M, et al. The complete management of extremity vascular injury in a local population: a wartime report from the 332nd Expeditionary Medical Group/Air Force Theater Hospital, Balad Air Base. *J Vasc Surg*. 2007;45:1197–1205.
15. Sfeir RE, Khoury GS, Kenaan MK. Vascular trauma to the lower extremity: the Lebanese war experience. *Cardiovasc Surg*. 1995;3:653–657.

16. Barmparas G, Inaba K, Talving P, et al. Pediatric vs adult vascular trauma: a National Trauma Databank review. *J Pediatr Surg.* 2010;45:1404–1412.
17. Loh S, Rockman C, Chung C, et al. Existing trauma and critical care scoring systems underestimate mortality among vascular trauma patients. *J Vasc Surg.* 2011;53:359–366.
18. Galindo RM, Workman CR. Vascular trauma at a military level II trauma center. *Current Surgery.* 2000;57:615–618.
19. Mattox KL, Feliciano DV, Burch J, et al. Five thousand seven hundred sixty cardiovascular injuries in 4459 patients: epidemiologic evolution 1958 to 1987. *Ann Surg.* 1989;209:698–705.
20. Bowley D, Degiannis E, Goosen J, Boffard K. Penetrating trauma in Johannesburg, South Africa. *Surg Clin North Am.* 2002;82:221–235.
21. Sugrue M, Caldwell E, D'Amours S, et al. Vascular injury in Australia. *Surg Clin North Am.* 2002;82:211–219.
22. Magee TR, Collin J, Hands LJ, et al. A ten year audit of surgery for vascular trauma in a British teaching hospital. *Eur J Vasc Endovasc Surg.* 1996;12:424–427.
23. Stannard A, Brohi K, Tai N. Vascular injury in the United Kingdom. *Perspect Vasc Surg Endovasc Ther.* 2011;23:27–33.
24. Koivunen D, Nichols WK, Silver D. Vascular trauma in a rural population. *Surgery.* 1982;91:723–727.
25. Oller D, Rutledge R, Thomas C, et al. Vascular injuries in a rural state: a review of 978 patients from a state trauma registry. *J Trauma.* 1992;32:740–746.
26. Klinkner DB, Arca MJ, Lewis BD, et al. Pediatric vascular injuries: patterns of injury, morbidity, and mortality. *J Pediatr Surg.* January, 2007;42(1):178–182; discussion 182–183.
27. Konstantinidis A, Inaba K, Dubose J, et al. Vascular trauma in geriatric patients: a national trauma databank review. *J Trauma.* October, 2011;71(4):909–916.
28. Rudström H, Bergqvist D, Ogren M, Björck M. Iatrogenic vascular injuries in Sweden. A nationwide study 1987–2005. *Eur J Vasc Endovasc Surg.* 2008;35:131–138.
29. Brown CV, Neville AL, Rhee P, et al. The impact of obesity on the outcomes of 1153 critically injured blunt trauma patients. *J Trauma.* 2005;59:1041–1052.
30. Rosen H, Saleh F, Lipsitz S, et al. Downwardly mobile: the accidental cost of being uninsured. *Arch Surg.* 2009;144:1006–1011.

38

Endovascular Management of Vascular Malformations: New Insights and Results

Robert L. Vogelzang, MD

Much has been written about the classification and treatment of vascular malformations over the past several decades. These extraordinarily complex and diverse lesions largely thwarted attempts at effective surgical therapy for many years but have received considerable attention over the past several decades. The modern management of congenital malformations has been positively impacted by the development and refinement of endovascular therapy and advances in imaging, and as a result we have a much better understanding of the anatomy, morphology, and architecture of these rare lesions. Classification schemes based on imaging have also allowed better patient selection; as a result most physicians believe that endovascular methods should be the primary method of treatment. Despite these advances, the optimal methods for treating these congenital lesions are not yet defined.[1,2] This is not to say that significant progress has not been made; unequivocally, it has. In this brief contribution, we will highlight two major advances made in the treatment of vascular malformations. First, we will discuss our conclusion (as exemplified by our personal experience) that ethanol embolotherapy is a proven and effective method of treating most vascular malformations. Second, we will illustrate our experience with a dramatic technical development in endovascular therapy of arteriovenous malformations (AVMs) that allows certain types to be cured, often in a single treatment.

EMBOLIZATION OF VASCULAR MALFORMATIONS WITH ETHANOL: THE NORTHWESTERN EXPERIENCE

We began to treat vascular malformations over 30 years ago and attempted surgical extirpation and a variety of embolization techniques for both high-flow AVMs and low-flow (venous and lymphatic) lesions. Many of these attempts failed because we did not fully understand the lesions or the extent of the abnormality given the relatively limited nature of imaging and our use of agents that were largely ineffective. For example, we believed (incorrectly as it turned out) that purely mechanical occlusive agents such as particulates and coils should be used in both AVMs and venous malformations. This was incorrect, recurrences and outright failures were depressingly common.

Beginning in the late 1980s, inspired by the seminal work and clinical experiences of Yakes, we began to explore the use of ethanol for the treatment of vascular malformations.[3-5] We found this path to be difficult sledding; ethanol was very toxic and produced significant tissue damage when injected incorrectly or in inappropriate doses and at times we were profoundly discouraged. However, despite the difficulties associated with using ethanol, we believed that the agent was worth continuing to work with because we saw dramatic resolution and cures in many low-flow lesions and marked improvement in many AVMs. We persisted in our efforts and developed better methods and gained greater understanding how to properly use this remarkably powerful, caustic sclerosing agent. As a result, we now believe that effective treatment *must* destroy or damage the primitive vascular endothelium in the nidus of these lesions; any treatment that does not do this will not be effective. The essential structural and functional element of any vascular malformation is the nidus. Understanding both the precise anatomy and location of the nidus is critical, since embolization with ethanol demands precise deposition of an appropriate dose of the agent in/at the nidus to avoid nontarget embolization. In our opinion and for the majority of lesions (with the exception of one type of AVM), only ethanol can destroy these cells and precipitate vascular thrombosis, occlusion, and elimination of the nidus.

Recently, we undertook a retrospective analysis of our experience with ethanol embolization of vascular malformations in order to assess the long-term efficacy of this treatment at a single center. Over 12 years, 46 patients with venous malformations (31) and AVMs (15) were treated with ethanol embolization. Clinical and imaging follow-up was performed in all. A total of 102 treatments were given with an average volume of ethanol of 8.8 mL (range 1–35 mL). Twelve patients had additional treatment with metallic coils in certain types of AVMs. All procedures were performed under general anesthesia.

Overall results showed that 24 of 46 or 52% were cured and exhibited no symptoms after treatment. About 12 patients (26%) were improved, 6 patients (13%) had no change, and 4 patients (8.6%) had worsening of symptoms and failed treatment. There were similar rates of success in both AVMs and VMs; 48% of VMs and 60% of AVM patients were cured. Overall, 77% of patients with venous malformations and 80% of AVMs were cured or improved. We found that imaging follow-up correlated very closely with clinical symptoms. (Figs. 38-1–38-4) All patients who had both failures and successes were associated with either positive results and disappearance of lesion on imaging or negative results and lack of response on imaging. There was no difference in outcomes over a wide number of variables including lesion type, location, age, gender, lesion size, and number of treatments.

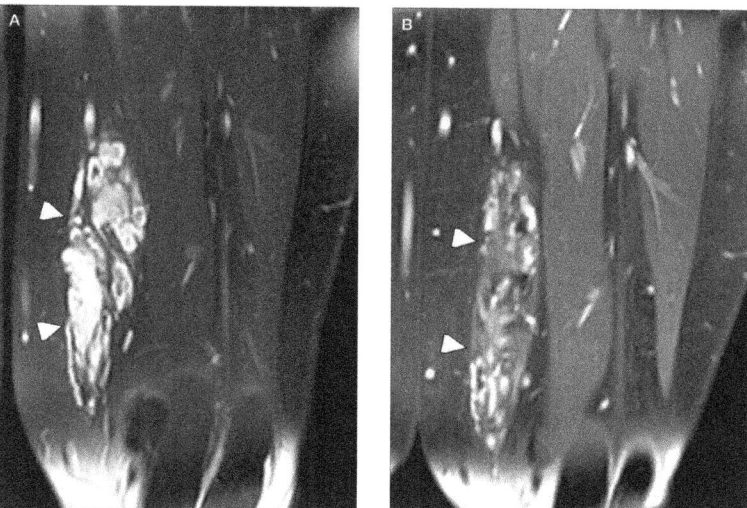

Figure 38-1. Large painful venous malformation of thigh before (*A*) and one year after (*B*) ethanol embolization. Note marked decrease in signal intensity and size. Patient was asymptomatic.

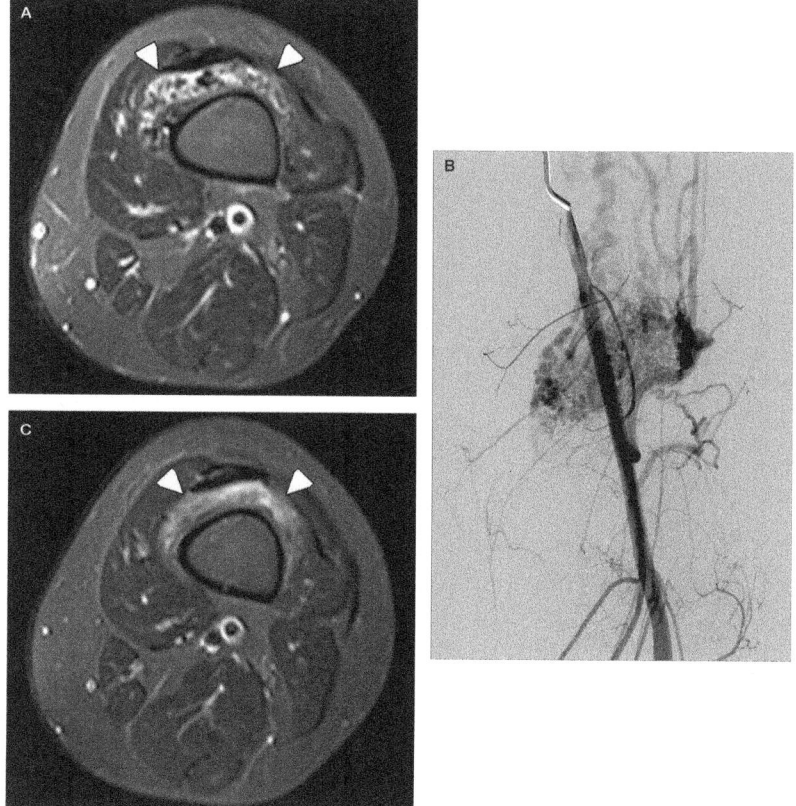

Figure 38-2. MR correlation with symptom resolution following treatment of suprapatellar AVM producing pain and swelling. Pretreatment (*A*), pretreatment angiogram (*B*), and MR 18 months posttreatment (*C*) showing decrease in flow voids and residual edema; patient was asymptomatic.

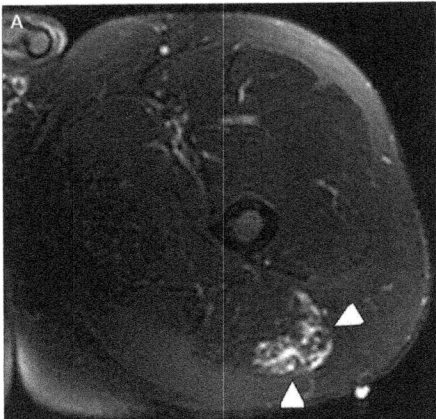
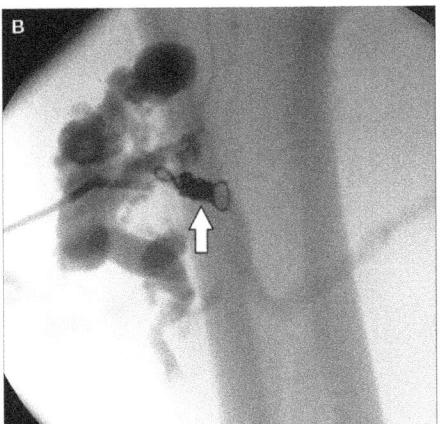
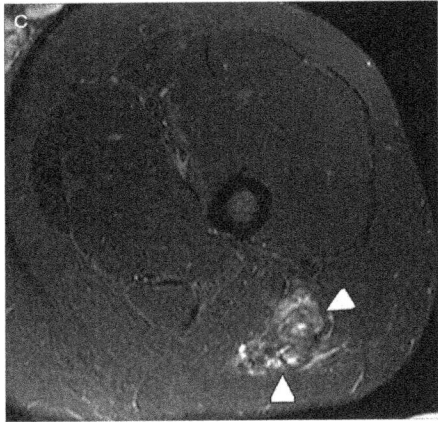

Figure 38-3. Treatment failure with persistent MR-positive findings. Painful thigh venous malformation before (*A*) and after (*C*) treatment showing continued signal intensity. Pain was not resolved. Embolization with coil (*B* arrow) in outflow vein. Patient underwent resection of the lesion.

The complication rate in this patient group was 24% which was in the expected range consistent with other reports. Minor complications occurred in six or 13% of individuals and major complications in five patients. The major complications were permanent ulnar neuropathy, digital amputation in a patient with a hand AVM, calf compartment syndrome requiring fasciotomy, skin necrosis requiring escharectomy, and severe gluteal pain and sciatic neuropathy that resolved in four to six weeks.[6] Obviously, these complications emphasize the obvious point that ethanol is powerful and toxic. In the wrong (inexperienced) hands it can do enormous damage. We believe that it should only be used at medical centers and by physicians who see these lesions and patients regularly. Ethanol should *not* be used by physicians who only see an occasional malformation. Ethanol is also well known to produce intense pulmonary vasospasm, hemodynamic collapse, and death after a bolus administration during embolization. Shin et al. discovered that limiting boluses to no more than 7–8 mL (for an average patient) eliminates this problem and we now rigorously adhere to that guidance.[7]

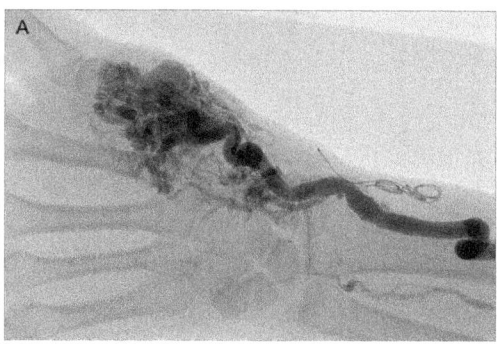
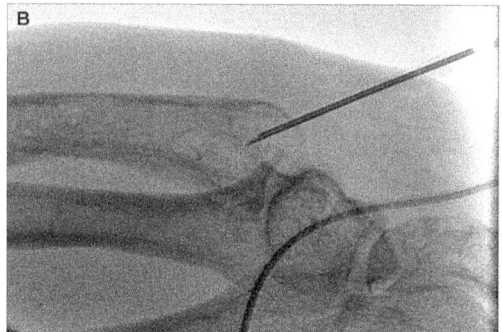
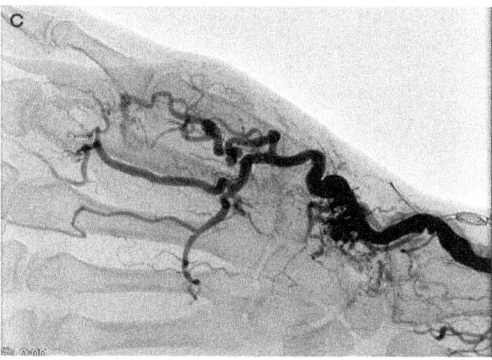

Figure 38-4. Hand AVM before (A) treatment. B, shows direct puncture of intraosseous lesion of proximal metacarpal that was treated with ethanol. Follow-up angiogram in asymptomatic patient at one year showing minimal residual hypervascularity, but no shunting.

Our experience mirrors that of other groups, all of whom have had excellent outcomes with the use of ethanol as a principal treatment agent.[2,4,5,8–11] We conclude that ethanol embolization when appropriately performed by an experienced operator produces excellent outcomes in most vascular malformations. We believe that it is the agent of choice if the goal of treatment is to make a positive impact on these symptomatic lesions.[6]

CURATIVE TRANSVENOUS COIL/ETHANOL EMBOLIZATION OF TYPE I AND II AVMS: A MAJOR ADVANCE IN AVM THERAPY

As we previously stated, understanding the nidus is critical to effective treatment. In AVMs, the nidus is essentially a conglomeration of arteriovenous connections of varying sizes and types but deciphering the nature and location of the nidus on an angiographic sequence can be a daunting challenge. In order to assist physicians in identifying and locating the nidus, various classification schemes to describe and categorize the diversity of AVMs have been proposed over the years. In 1993, Houdart et al. devised a classification scheme that divided intracranial AVMs into three types based on the nidus.[12] This useful scheme was modified by Cho et al. in 2006 for use in body and extremity AVMs that were classified into four types: type I with 1–3 separate arteries shunting to a single draining vein, type II with multiple arterioles shunting into a single draining vein. The specific anatomy of types I and II is that of a single dominant outflow vein. Type III AVMs have multiple shunts between arterioles and venues, with this type further subdivided into IIIa and IIIb[13] (Fig. 38-5).

Cho et al. found that type II (there were no type I lesions in their study) lesions were completely cured in 85% of patients generally by direct puncture and the use of ethanol and/or coils. They were not the first group to attack these lesions via the venous outflow component; Yakes as well as Jackson et al. also reported high cure rates for similar AVMs.[14,15] More recently, Park and his colleagues reviewed 176 patients with AVMs which they treated; 39 AVMs were type I or II. In these patients, the authors stated that the likelihood of cure was very high.[8]

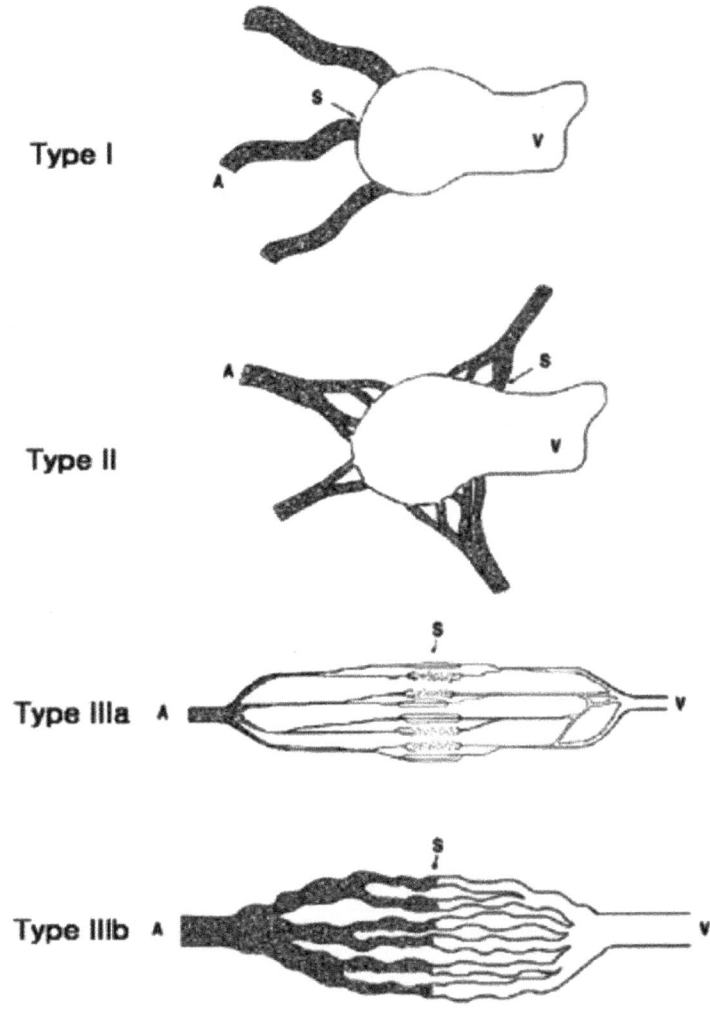

Figure 38-5. Classification of AVMs per Houdart et al. as modified by Park et al. Type I and type II AVMs have three or more arteries shunting to a single vein. Type IIIa AVMs have multiple nondilated fine arteriovenous fistulae and type IIIb lesions has multiple hypertrophied and dilated A-V fistulas that appear as a complex vascular network. (From Park et al., 2012. Used with permission.)

These observations prompted us and others to begin to look for this anatomy and to target the venous outflow sac or component whenever it was seen. The results have been dramatic; once such favorable anatomy is identified, the venous outflow is targeted and (generally) directly punctured and packed with embolization coils and treated with ethanol until flow ceases. We have discovered that many high-flow AVMs can be treated via the transvenous route in a simple method that produces outstanding results and very low complication rates. Our experience reported earlier confirmed the effectiveness of the transvenous approach; all our cures of AVMs were in types I and II.[6] This route affords a measure of safety and simplicity that has not been previously available.

The basic principles of this method include the following:

1. Identification of a proper and suitable AVM. This includes AVMs in which the largest outflow component is a large vein itself, or one in which there is a dominant outflow vein.
2. The use of direct puncture and "packing" of the venous outflow structure with coils; catheterization of the venous outflow is sometimes necessary.
3. Occasional need to control the residual malformation with the use of small amounts of ethanol introduced only into the coil pack.

The results of these interventions have been remarkable; many AVMs including extensive large and lesions that previously were felt to be impossible to treat have been *cured* in one or two stages. We recently reviewed our results of these interventions in pelvic AVMs and compared the results of treatment before and after the introduction of the method (Figures 38-6 to 38-8).

Between 1999 and 2010, 12 patients with pelvic AVMs underwent arterial embolization with 100% ethanol and/or transvenous (transcatheter or direct puncture) coil embolization under general anesthesia. In the first five patients, the pelvic AVM was partially devascularized with multiple staged arterial treatments with ethanol followed later by definitive, apparently curative coil embolization. After observing the benefits of the transvenous approach in our initial five patients, transvenous coil embolization alone was used in the final seven cases. Patients underwent follow-up pelvic angiography at various intervals after treatment to assess for recurrence.

The first five patients in our series had a total of 25 (range 2–8) transarterial ethanol embolizations followed later by a single transcatheter or direct puncture transvenous embolization session with coils. Of the seven subsequent patients, six had only single-stage transvenous embolization; one patient required three transvenous coil embolizations for a massive intraosseous pelvic AVM. None of the transarterial ethanol treatments resulted in cure on follow-up arteriography, but there was reduction in overall AVM flow. Conversely, all 12 patients had immediate complete cessation of AVM shunting and flow after transvenous coil embolization and this curative effect persisted on follow-up angiography in the 11/12 patients who were studied at an average of 10.6 months after final embolization. One patient had clinical and CT follow-up with no recurrence. There was one complication in the transarterial ethanol group, skin necrosis that resolved with conservative wound care.[16]

In conclusion, the treatment of vascular malformations has seen considerable advancement in the past two decades. Better imaging, greater understanding of the morphology and classification of lesions, improved techniques have all combined to give real hope to patients with vascular malformations.

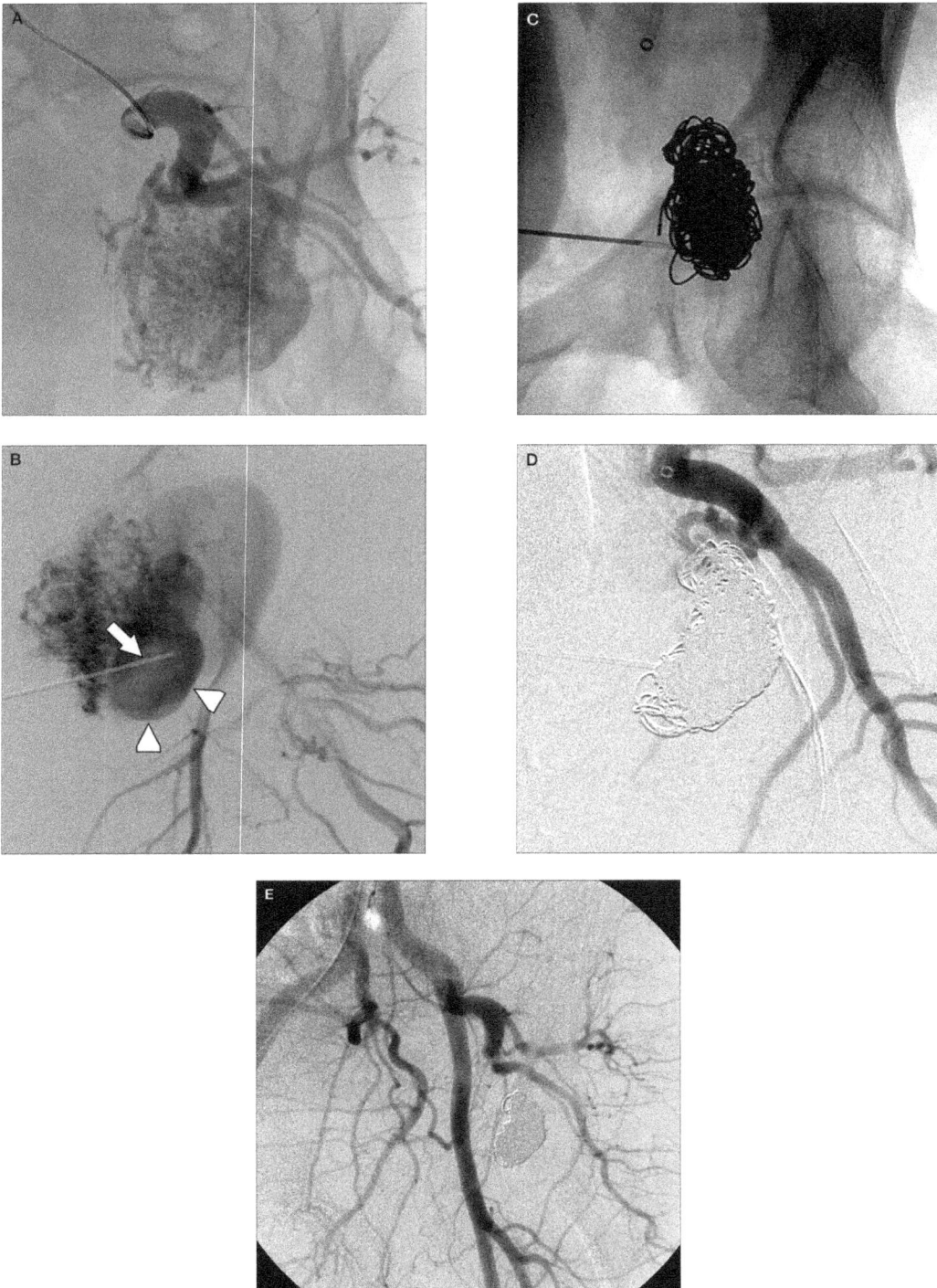

Figure 38-6. Single stage cure of type II pelvic AVM by coil embolization of venous outflow. Pretreatment angiogram (*A*) showing shunting into single vein outflow. (*B*) shows direct needle puncture (arrow) of single-outflow venous sac (arrowheads) with packing by coils (*C*). Immediate postembolization angiogram (*D*) and one year follow-up angiogram (*E*) with no AVM.

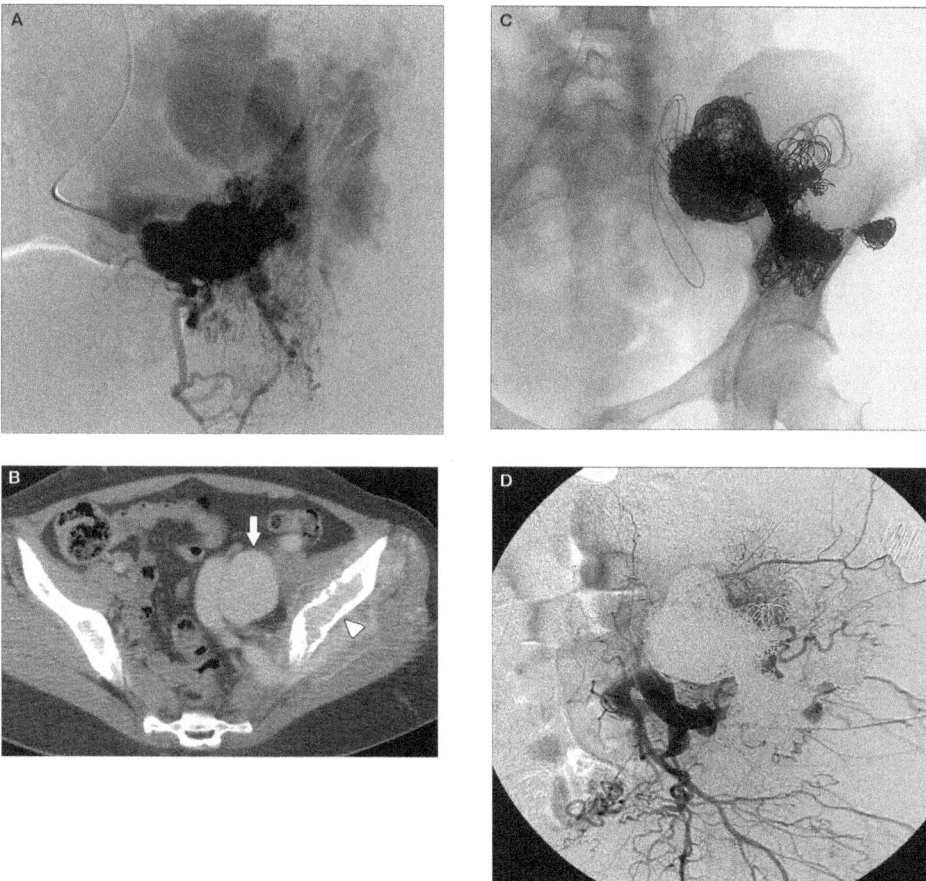

Figure 38-7. Multistage coil and ethanol embolization of massive type II intraosseous pelvic AVM (*A*) causing lytic destruction of iliac wing on CT (*B* arrowhead). Note hugely dilated outflow vein; this was one of the targets of coil embolization along with bone lesion (*C*). Follow-up at one year showing disappearance of AVM with patient now asymptomatic.

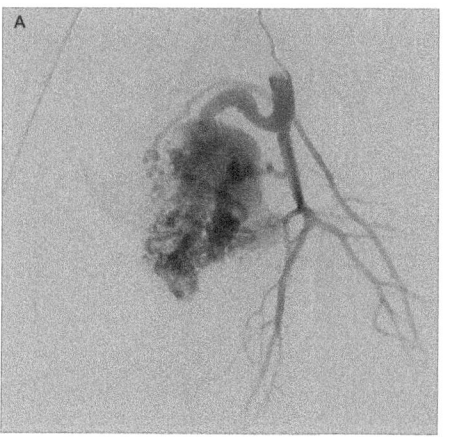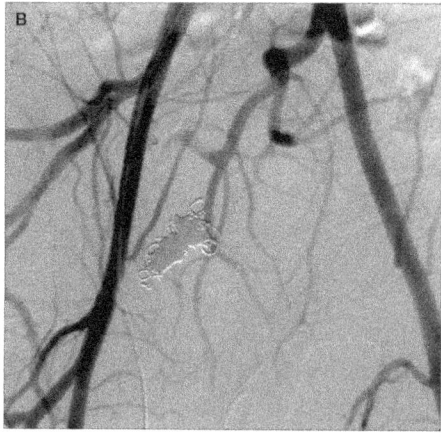

Figure 38-8. Single stage coil embolization and cure of type II pelvic AVM, before (*A*) and two years after (*B*) coil embolization.

REFERENCES

1. Gloviczki P, Duncan A, Kalra M, et al. Vascular malformations: an update. *Perspect Vasc Surg Endovasc Ther.* 2009;21:133–148.
2. Do YS, Yakes WF, Shin SW, et al. Ethanol embolization of arteriovenous malformations: interim results. *Radiology.* 2005;235:674–682.
3. Yakes WF, Rossi P, Odink H. How I do it. Arteriovenous malformation management. *Cardiovasc Intervent Radiol.* 1996;19:65–71.
4. Yakes WF. Endovascular management of high-flow arteriovenous malformations. *Semin Intervent Radiol.* 2004;21:49–58.
5. Yakes WF, Luethke JM, Merland JJ, et al. Ethanol embolization of arteriovenous fistulas: a primary mode of therapy. *J Vasc Interv Radiol.* 1990;1:89–96.
6. Vogelzang RL, Atassi R, Vouche M, et al. Ethanol embolotherapy of vascular malformations: clinical outcomes at a single center. *J Vasc Interv Radiol.* 2013, In Press.
7. Shin BS, Do YS, Cho HS, et al. Effects of repeat bolus ethanol injections on cardiopulmonary hemodynamic changes during embolotherapy of arteriovenous malformations of the extremities. *J Vasc Interv Radiol.* 2010;21:81–89.
8. Park KB, Do YS, Kim DI, et al. Predictive factors for response of peripheral arteriovenous malformations to embolization therapy: analysis of clinical data and imaging findings. *J Vasc Interv Radiol.* 2012;23:1478–1486.
9. Do YS, Park KB, Park HS, et al. Extremity arteriovenous malformations involving the bone: therapeutic outcomes of ethanol embolotherapy. *J Vasc Interv Radiol.* 2010;21:807–816.
10. Doppman JL, Pevsner P. Embolization of arteriovenous malformations by direct percutaneous puncture. *AJR Am J Roentgenol.* 1983;140:773–778.
11. Do YS, Kim YW, Park KB, et al. Endovascular treatment combined with emboloscleorotherapy for pelvic arteriovenous malformations. *J Vasc Surg.* 2012;55:465–471.
12. Houdart E, Gobin YP, Casasco A, et al. A proposed angiographic classification of intracranial arteriovenous fistulae and malformations. *Neuroradiology.* 1993;35:381–385.
13. Cho SK, Do YS, Shin SW, et al. Arteriovenous malformations of the body and extremities: analysis of therapeutic outcomes and approaches according to a modified angiographic classification. *J Endovasc Ther.* 2006;13:527–538.
14. Yakes WF. Ethanol embolotherapy management of pelvic arteriovenous malformation. (abstract) *J Vasc Inter Radiol.* 2010;21(2):S77.
15. Jackson JE, Mansfield AO, Alison DJ. Treatment of high-flow vascular malformations by venous embolization aided by flow occlusion techniques. *Cardiovasc Intervent Radiol.* 1996;19:323–328.
16. Vogelzang RL, Yakes WF. Pelvic AVMs: Curative Transvenous Coil Embolization in 12 Patients. International Society For The Study Of Vascular Anomalies Annual Meeting 2012 (abstract).

39

Advanced Techniques for Retrieval of Difficult Inferior Vena Cava Filters

Sharon C. Kiang, MD and Brian G. DeRubertis, MD

INTRODUCTION

Inferior vena cava (IVC) filter have shown to be safe and effective in the prevention or reduction of pulmonary embolism (PE) in patients whom have contraindications to anti-coagulation or whom have failed anticoagulation therapy.[1-3] Early IVC filters included permanently implantable devices such as the Bird's Nest (Cook Medical, Bloomington, IN), the Vena Tech (B. Braun Interventional Systems, Inc., Bethlehem, PA), the Simon Nitinol (Bard Peripheral Vascular Inc., Tempe, AZ), and the Greenfield (Boston Scientific Corporation, Natick, MA) filters.[4,5]

However, the risks associated with long-term placements of these devices including symptomatic IVC thrombosis and the development and propagation of deep venous thrombosis[6,7] have led to the development of retrievable IVC filters. In the past decade, the placement of percutaneously implantable IVC filters has skyrocketed, during which time, these devices have been found to have low complication rates and excellent efficacy in the prevention of PE.[8,9]

The surveillance and subsequent retrieval of temporary IVC filters have been complicated by this device being placed by multiple medical specialists (vascular surgeons, critical care specialists, and trauma surgeons), leading to a diverse patient population without a centralized monitoring and surveillance system for timely retrieval. This has led to patients with temporary IVC filters returning for retrieval after the recommended indwelling time, which requires advanced complex IVC retrieval techniques outside of standard techniques.

This chapter will emphasize the advanced techniques for IVC filter retrieval. In addition, it will emphasize the pitfalls of long indwelling filters.

IVC FILTER RETRIEVAL DECREASES LONG-TERM COMPLICATIONS

Although the benefits for temporary IVC filter placement has been well accepted, the long-term benefits of filter dwelling are not as well advertised. A randomized study showed a lower rate of PE at 12 days in patients with IVC filter placement compared to those without but showed no difference in PE or survival rate at two years, suggesting that there is benefit to using retrievable filters while preventing long-term complications.[10]

The long-term complications of IVC filters are diverse, ranging from technical difficulties at the time of placement to formation of thrombus to incorporation of the filter in the caval wall. IVC filters can migrate (3%–69%) and cause caval perforation (9%–24%), thrombosis (6%–30%), total caval occlusion (4%–30%), and insertion site thrombosis.[7,11,12] Furthermore, recent reports have increasingly documented higher rates of recurrent deep venous thromboembolism and subsequent development of post-thrombotic syndrome (5%–70%).[11–13] These complications emphasize the need for filter retrieval once caval interruption is no longer necessary.

OBSTACLES IN THE RETRIEVAL OF TEMPORARY IVC FILTER

It is estimated that 259,000 temporary IVC filters were placed in 2012 but a literature review of large single institutions estimated that only 20%–34% of these temporary filters were retrieved.[14–16] The reasons for such poor retrieval rates are multifactorial. The most common reason for retained filter placement is due to patients being lost to follow-up. This is especially true for the trauma population, where there is a high rate of temporary filter placement due to this population's high rate of multisystemic injuries while also being in a demographic that is known to have low follow-up rates. It is estimated that 91.5% of temporary filters placed in the trauma population are retained as permanent filters.[16] Strategies to improve filter retrieval have included filter registries to track filters and initiatives to remove filters before discharge from hospitals. Furthermore, initiatives for patient education providing information on filters and estimated dates for retrieval have also begun, so patients may participate in this process.

Technical failure for filter retrieval has been shown to increase with longer dwell times of the filters. Although manufacturer's data shows that some filters maybe safely removed after 300 dwell days, a review of a large level I trauma center noted increased retrieval failure rates at 85 days.[16] The reasons for increased failure after longer dwell times are due to multiple reasons. Filter thrombosis, strut integration into caval wall, and limitations in familiarity with advanced retrieval techniques are just a few reasons for failure of retrieval. Overall, attention should be focused on increasing filter retrieval rates.

STANDARD IVC FILTER RETRIEVAL METHOD

The success of filter retrieval depends on filter dwell time, filter strut penetration of endothelialization with the caval wall, and IVC wall and hook relationship. It has been shown in the literature that dwell time remains one of the most important factors for retrieval. This has prompted the FDA to issue a Safety Alert on IVC filters in 2010 urging all physicians

TABLE 39-1. CURRENTLY AVAILABLE RETRIEVABLE IVC FILTERS

Filter	Manufacturer	Material	Design	Retrieval Approach	Retrieval Window in Initial Clinical Trials (Days)
ALN Optional	ALN	Stainless steel	Conical with centering legs	IJ	6–722
Option	Argon Medical	Nitinol	Conical	IJ	1–175
Eclipse	Bard Peripheral	Nitinol	Conical with centering struts	IJ	5–300
Celect	Cook Medical	Conichrome	Conical with centering struts	IJ	7–466
Tulip	Cook Medical	Conichrome	Conical	IJ	2–20
Optease	Cordis Corporation	Nitinol	Hexagonal double basket	IJ.Femoral	3–48

responsible for patients with IVC filters to have these devices removed as soon as mechanical protection from PE is no longer necessary.[17]

The retrieval guidelines for each filter are consistent with that determined by the device's premarket clinical trials (Table 39-1) although it has been shown that retrieval is still possible outside of these guidelines. Several filters have been identified as having open indications for retrieval (G2 Eclipse, Bard Peripheral Vascular, Inc; ALN Implants Chirurgicaux, Ghisonaccia, France) with limitations on its retrievability window.

For standard retrieval of an uncomplicated temporary IVC filter, most filters follow a similar protocol using retrieval kits designed for that specific filter. Under local or conscious sedation, the right-sided internal jugular vein is punctured under duplex visualization. A 5 Fr sheath is then introduced. A pigtail catheter is then placed over a guidewire to the level of the caval confluence and a diagnostic venogram is then performed. If there is less than 25% of thrombus incorporation into the filter and there is patent caval venous flow proximal to the filter, then the filter can be removed.

The actual removal of the filter requires that a stiff guidewire be placed distal to the filter. The retrieval kit sheath (9–11 Fr) is then passed over the wire to just below the filter into the infrarenal IVC. An endo-snare catheter or retrieval cone is then used to engage the hook or the retrieval hub at the top of the filter device. Once engaged, gentle traction is applied to the snare as the retrieval device is coaxially placed over the filter to collapse the struts, thus disengaging them from the caval wall. The filter is then extracted through the internal jugular and completion venography is performed through the sheath.

FILTER COMPLICATIONS: WHEN THE STANDARD FILTER RETRIEVAL TECHNIQUE FAILS

When filters cannot be retrieved through standard technique, investigations into possible filter complications need to be initiated. Filter complications are frequently discovered incidentally on radiographic examinations,[18] but their significance remains largely unknown and underappreciated among interpreting radiologists, referring clinicians, and patients themselves unless the findings are severe.[19] Filter tilt (with or without retrieval hook incorporation into the caval wall), endothelialization of filter struts, filter fracture, or filter penetration should be investigated before more aggressive attempts at filter retrieval are begun.

Advanced complicated techniques to retrieve these complicated filters are difficult and often fall out of the manufacturer's published protocols. Large multi-institutional data documenting success or pitfalls for advanced techniques are lacking. The mechanism of complications associated with embedded, fractured, and penetrating filters remains poorly understood, and the alternative retrieval methods used to manage these complications, along with resultant clinical outcomes, have not been adequately assessed in prospective studies. Future prospective studies to establish safe and effective techniques will be needed in the future to ensure that all patients can have safe and effective filter retrieval.

When attempting complex filter retrieval, the use of certain advanced retrieval techniques may be associated with increased risks of complications, including access site injuries secondary to increased sheath sizes required, intra-procedural caval thrombosis or vasospasm, and the potential for caval injury and hemorrhage. These risks need to be discussed with patients. For those patients who prefer to retain filters rather than accept these risks, the possibility for complex filter complications including erosion, fractures, and organ penetration as future complications need to be disclosed to the patient.

TILTED AND ADHERENT FILTERS: COMPLEX FILTER RETRIEVAL TECHNIQUES

There are two main reasons why filter cannot be retrieved through standard technique: (1) inability to grasp the proximal filter hook or hub secondary to filter tilt and (2) dense adherence of either the filter hub or struts into the cava wall.

Centering Techniques for the Tilted Filter

Some of the filters available in the United States and Europe (G2 Eclipse, Bard Peripheral Vascular Inc.; Celect, Cook Medical) have centering legs that help prevent filter tilt although all filters have some degree of tilt in which the filter hook lies against the caval wall allowing endothelialization and/or incorporation of the hook (Fig. 39-1), which prevents engagement of the hook by standard techniques. In the literature, it is estimated that as many as 20%–40% of filters cannot be removed by using standard methods[20] because they have become firmly embedded along the vessel wall.

The goal of centering techniques is to return the proximal filter hook into the center of the cava, allowing it to be engaged by retrieval devices. One technique employs a 0.035 steerable guidewire that is directed from the right internal jugular vein, down the side of the embedded hook down through a sheath at the right common femoral vein (Fig. 39-2A). Applying traction on the guidewire on both the internal jugular and right femoral sides, the filter can be "straightened" so that the hook returns to the center of the cava.

If guidewire traction fails, an angioplasty balloon can be placed between the cava and the embedded portion of the cava (Fig. 39-2A, B). Gentle inflation of the balloon

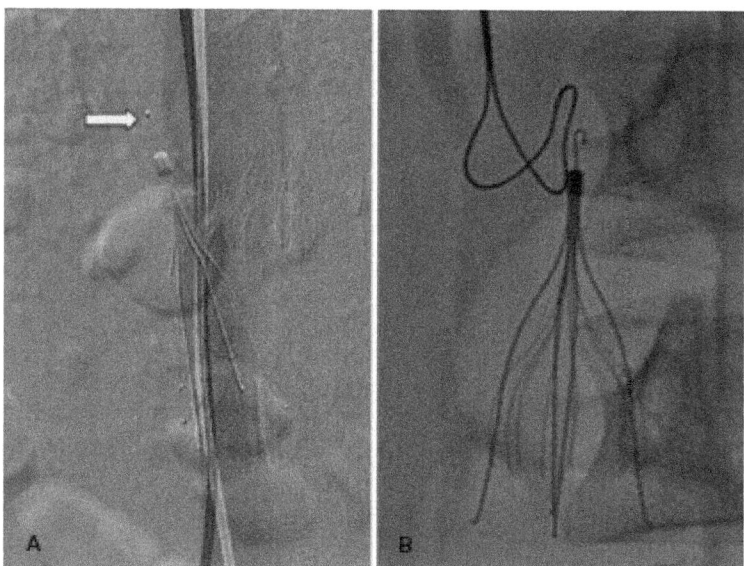

Figure 39-1. *A,* Tilting of the filter hook can lead to the hook being embedded in the caval wall (yellow arrow) due to the overgrowth of intimal hyperplastic tissue over the hook. *B,* Cine image of a snare being unable to engage the hook of the filter due to hyperplastic tissue covering the hook. Reprnted with permission from DeRubertis.[21]

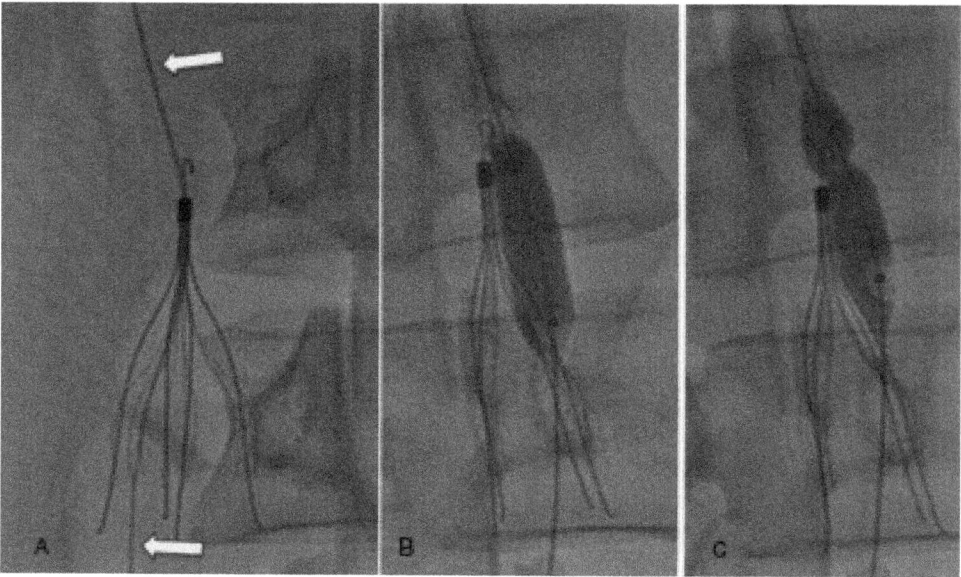

Figure 39-2. *A,* Right internal jugular to right femoral vein wire access (yellow arrows) can be used to center the filter within the cava, allowing the snare to capture the filter hook easily. *B,* Inflation of a balloon between the filter and the caval wall can disrupt the intimal hyperplastic tissue that covers the retrieval hook, thus allowing the hook to be centered. *C,* Intimal hyperplastic tissue around the hook causes a waste in the balloon during inflation.

can disrupt the intimal hyperplasic tissue from the filter hook with further inflation "pushing" the hook toward the center of the cava. To further straighten the filter, endoscopic forceps (rigid bronchoscopy forceps and endomyocardial biopsy forceps) can be used to grasp the underside of the filter from a femoral approach to straighten the filter.

Snare-Over Technique

An additional method to center the filter is to pass the snare over the guidewire technique (Fig. 39-3A, B). In this case, the guidewire acts as a "rail" so that the snare opens directly above the hook in an "in-line" fashion.

Another method to utilize snare is to help develop a guidewire loop technique. The sheath at the right internal jugular is upsized to a 12 or 14 Fr sheath. A 0.035 stiff angled Glidewire (Terumo Interventional Systems, Inc, Somerset, NJ) is passed between the struts of the filter into the infrarenal cava (Fig. 39-4A). A 5 Fr vena cava filter (VCF) catheter (Cook Medical) is then passed over the wire and reformed below the filter to that the distal end of the VCF points cephalad. The Glidewire is then passed through the VCF in a cephalad direction (Fig. 39-4B, C). The snare is then passed through the sheath separately and used to capture the floppy part of the Glidewire to guide it back out of the sheath so that both ends of the Glidewire are coming through the internal jugular sheath.[21]

The VCF is removed and the snare is then reloaded onto both ends of the Glidewire down to the hook of the filter. With tension on both ends of the Glidewire, the snare is then used to grasp the hook of the filter. Once engaged, the Glidewire is removed and the sheath is passed over the filter in a coaxial manner to collapse the filter for removal (Fig. 39-4D, E).

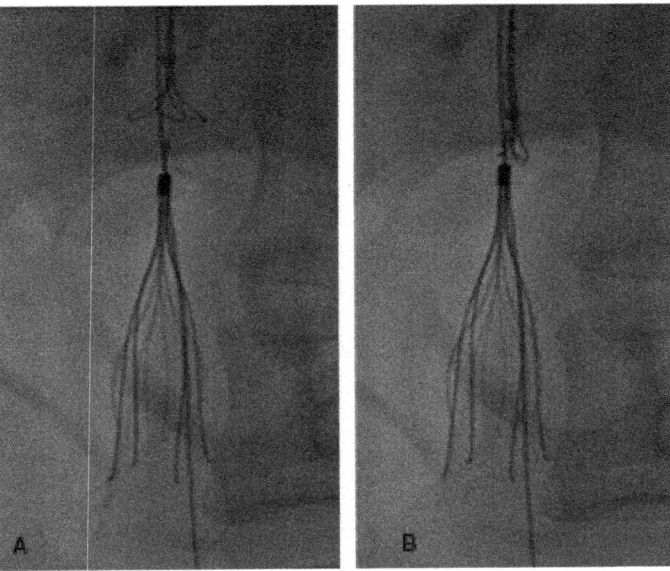

Figure 39-3. In the snare-over-guidewire technique, the guidewire adjacent to the retrieval hook is backloaded through the snare, A, and the snare catheter is then advanced over the guidewire to guide the snare loop around the retrieval hook, B.

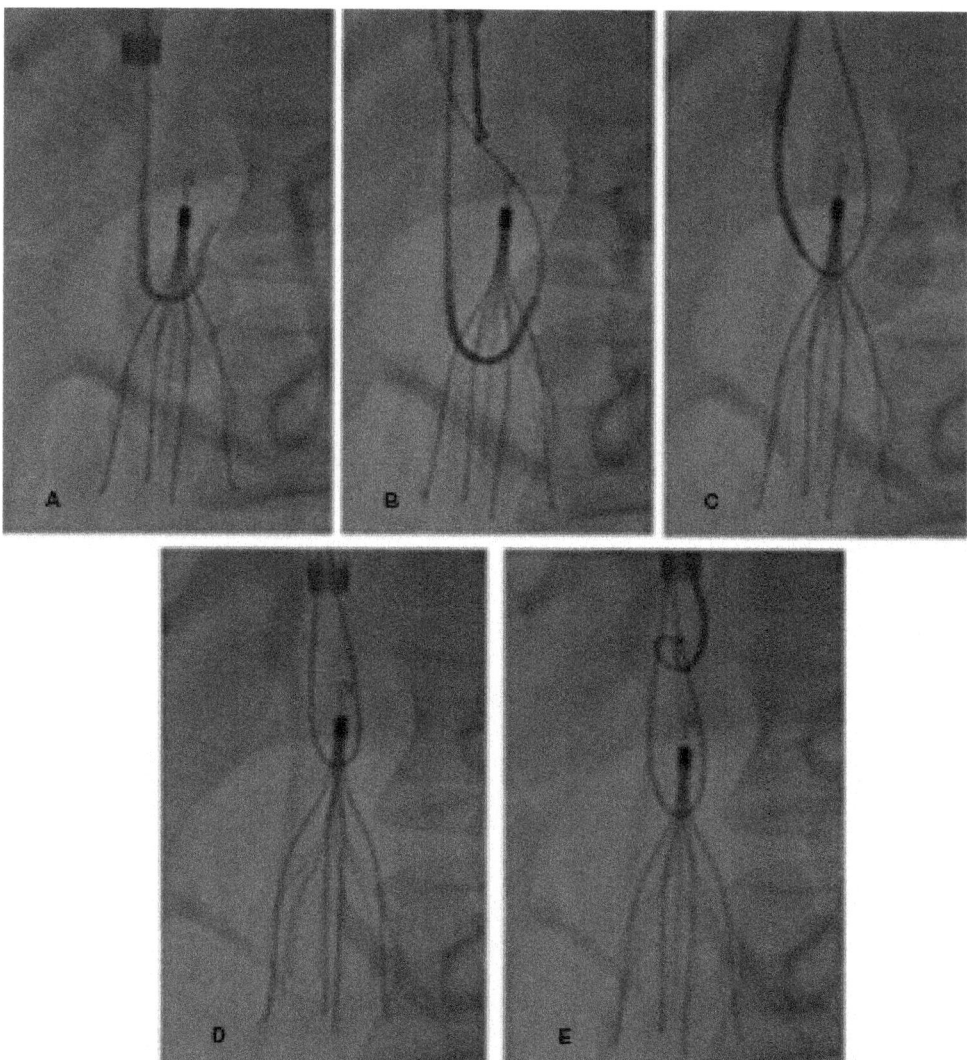

Figure 39-4. The snare-over-loop technique uses a curved catheter placed between the struts of the filter, *A*, to create a guidewire loop, which is then snared, *B* and *C*, and brought out of the cephalad internal jugular sheath. Traction applied to this guidewire loop, *D*, then allows for centering of the filter and can be used to guide a snare down to and around the retrieval hook, *E*.

COAXIAL DOUBLE-SHEATH DISSECTION FOR THE EMBEDDED FILTER

Other than tilt, densely adherent endothelial tissue can trap the filter so that it cannot be removed with the usual amount of force. Embedded filter removal is a technically demanding procedure that must be performed meticulously to minimize damage to the underlying vein. Analysis of the adherent tissue harvested has noted a predominance of neointimal hyperplasia or fibrosis in 96% of the analyzed specimens with no evidence of venous intima.[22] In these instances, the use of two coaxial sheaths to promote a gentle twisting motion can help dissect the hyperplastic tissue off the filter struts. A 10 Fr, 55-cm sheath placed coaxially within a 14 Fr, 45-cm Performer sheath (Cook Medical) can be used (Fig. 39-5A–D).[21]

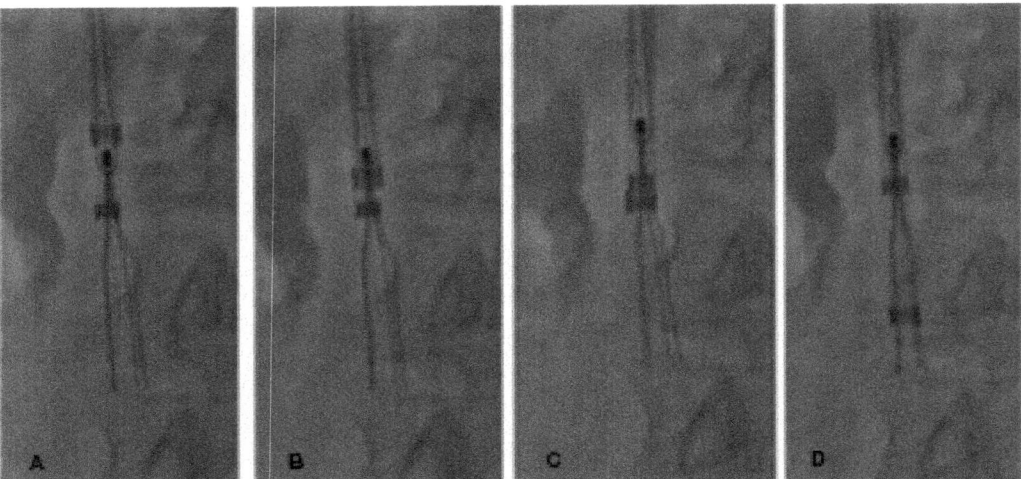

Figure 39-5. The double-sheath dissection technique utilizes a coaxial sheath configuration in which the two sheaths are manipulated simultaneously in a twisting and to-and-fro motion to dissect the attachments between the filter and the caval wall.

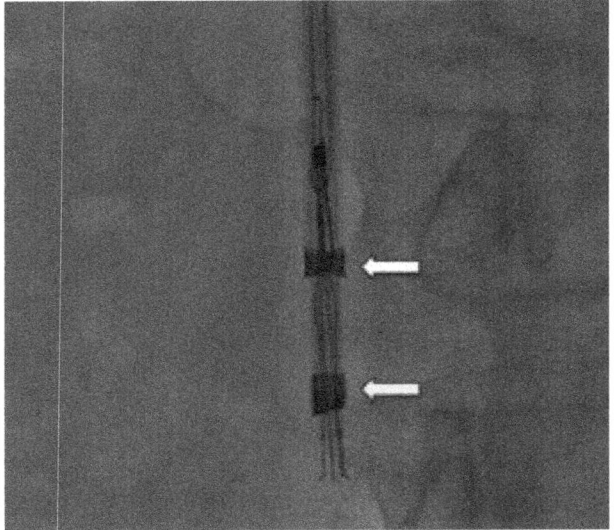

Figure 39-6. Laser-assisted filter retrieval uses a coaxial sheath system, including a 12-Fr SLS II sheath (yellow arrow) through a 14 Fr Performer sheath (white arrow). This method uses the double-sheath dissection technique and the effects of laser photoablation of the overlying intimal hyperplastic tissue.

LASER-ASSISTED DOUBLE SHEATH DISSECTION FOR THE EMBEDDED FILTER

Advancement of IVC filter retrieval has included the adaptation of pacemaker lead extraction laser sheaths to cut through the hyperplastic tissue surrounding a completely embedded filter. The CVX-300 excimer XeCl laser system (Spectranetics Corporation,

Colorado Springs, CO) utilizes a coaxial sheath system by passing a 12 Fr, 50-cm laser cannula (SLS II laser sheath, Spectranetics Corporation, 60 mL/mm^2) through a 14 Fr, 45-cm Performer sheath (Fig. 39-6). At the same time, a 6 Fr, 23-cm Brite-Tip sheath (Cordis Corporation, Bridgewater, NJ) is inserted into the end of the laser sheath for hemostasis.[23]

The retrieval hook of the filter is snared while the outer sheath is advanced over the filter. The laser sheath is then activated for two to five seconds as it is slowly advanced over the filter. The intimal hyperplastic tissue is then photoablated around the struts.[23] Once the struts are freed, the filter is then collapsed into the sheath and removed.

CONCLUSION

The use of temporary IVC filters remains an important method to prevent PE in patients intolerant or refractory of anticoagulation. The increased use of these devices demand a method of surveillance and efficacy of retrieval as the complications of long-term filter presence are recognized. Ongoing development and investigation into aggressive techniques for complex filter retrieval in conjunction with increased filter retrieval awareness will aid in preventing long-term filter complications.

REFERENCES

1. Ferris EJ, McCowan TC, Carver DK, McFarland DR. Percutaneous inferior vena cava filters: follow-up of seven designs in 320 patients. *Radiology*. 1993;188:851–856.
2. Greenfield LJ, Proctor MC. Twenty year clinical experience with the Greenfield filter. *Cardiovasc Surg*. 1995;3:199–205.
3. Athanasoulis CA, Kaufman JA, Halpern EF, et al. Inferior vena cava filters: review of a 26-year experience. *Radiology*. 2000;216:54–66.
4. Zhu X, Tam MD, Bartholomew J, et al. Retrievability and device related complication of the G2 filter: a retrospective study of 139 filter retrievals. *J Vasc Interv Radiol*. 2011;22:806–812.
5. Arabi M, Wilatt JM, Shield JJ, et al. Retrievability of optional vena cava filters with caudal migration and caval penetration: report of three cases. *J Vasc Interv Radiol*. 2010;21:923–926.
6. Blebea J, Wilson R, Waybill P, et al. Deep venous thrombosis after percutaneous insertion of vena cava filters. *J Vasc Surg*. 1999;30:821–829.
7. Crochet DP, Stora O, Ferry D, et al. Vena-Tech-LGM filter: long-term results of a prospective study. *Radiology*. 1993;188:857–860.
8. Millward SF, Olivia VL, Bell SD, et al. Gunther Tulip retrievable vena cava filter: results from the registry of the Canadian Interventional Radiology Association. *J Vasc Interv Radiol*. 2001;12:1053–1058.
9. Grande WJ, Trerotola SO, Reilly PM, et al. Experience with the recovery filter as a retrievable inferior vena cava filter. *J Vasc Interv Radiol*. 2005;16:1189–1193.
10. Decousus H, Leizorovicz A, Parent F, et al. A clinical trial of vena cava filters in the prevention of pulmonary embolism in patients with proximal deep-vein thrombosis. *N Engl J Med*. 1998;338:409–416.
11. Imberti D, Ageno W, Carpenedo M. Retrievable vena cava filters: a review. *Curr Opin Hematol*. 2006;13:351–356.
12. Mohan CR, Hoballah JJ, Sharp WJ, et al. Comparative efficacy and complications of vena cava filters. *J Vasc Surg*. 1995;21:235–245.

13. PREPIC Study Group. Eight-year follow up of patients with permanent vena cava filters in the preventative of pulmonary embolism: the PREPIC (Prevention du Risque d'Embolie Pulmonaire par Interruption Cave) randomized study. *Circulation.* 2005;112:416–422.

14. Karmy-Jones R, Jurkovich GJ, Velmahos GC, et al. Practice patterns and outcomes of retrievable vena cava filters in trauma patients: an AAST multicenter study. *J Trauma.* 2007;62:17–24.

15. Johnson ON 3rd, Gillespie DL, Aidinian G, et al. The use of retrievable inferior vena cava filters in severely injured military trauma patients. *J Vasc Surg.* 2009;49:410–416.

16. Sarosiek S, Crowther M, Sloan M. Indications, complications and management of inferior vena cava filters. *JAMA.* 2013;173(7):513–517.

17. U.S. Food and Drug Administration. Removing retrievable inferior vena cava filters: initial communication. August 9, 2010. http://www.fda.gov/MedicalDevices/Safety/AlertsandNotices/ucm221676.htm. Accessed October, 2012.

18. Zhou D, Spain J, Moon E, et al. Retrospective review of 120 Celect inferior vena cava filter retrievals: experience at a single institution. *J Vasc Interv Radiol.* 2012;23:1557–1563.

19. Tam MD, Spain J, Lieber M, et al. Fracture and distant migration of the Bard Recovery filter: a retrospective review of 363 implantations for potentially life-threatening complications. *J Vasc Interv Radiol.* 2012;23:199–205.

20. Ray CE, Mitchell E, Zipser S, et al. Outcomes with retrievable inferior vena cava filters: a multicenter study. *J Vasc Interv Radiol.* 2006;17:1595–1604.

21. DeRubertis BG. Advanced IVC filter retrieval techniques. *Endovascular Today.* November, 2012:69–73.

22. Kuo WT, Robertson SW, Odegaard JI, Hofmann LV. Complex retrieval of fractured, embedded, and penetrating inferior vena cava filters: a prospective study with histologic and electron microscopic analysis. *J Vasc Interv Radiol.* 2013;24(5):622–630.

23. Kuo WT, Tong RT, Hwang GL, et al. High-risk retrieval of adherent and chronically implanted IVC filters: techniques for removal and management of thrombotic complications. *J Vasc Interv Radiol.* 2009;20:1548–1556.

40

Congenital Malformations of the Inferior Vena Cava

Mila H. Ju, MD; Ashley K. Vavra, MD; Hari R. Kumar, MD; and William H. Pearce, MD

Congenital malformations of the inferior vena cava (IVC) are uncommon. Generally, the anomalies are discovered as incidental findings or are found in association with deep venous thrombosis (DVT) of the lower extremities. Anomalies of the IVC present problems for both open vascular surgery and endovascular procedures. Exposure of the aorta is difficult with a left-sided IVC, retroaortic renal veins, and duplication of the vena cava. Abnormalities of the IVC are also problematic for the placement of IVC filters and access for cardiac electrophysiologists. This chapter will review the etiology of common abnormalities of the IVC and the limited literature related to the surgical and endovascular treatment for these abnormalities.

EMBRYOLOGY AND CLASSIFICATION

The formation of the IVC is a complex process. It occurs between the sixth and eighth weeks of gestation.[1-3] The vena cava is formed from three paired embryotic veins. These veins are the posterior cardinal veins, subcardinal veins, and supracardinal veins. The vena cava is composed of four segments: the hepatic, suprarenal, renal, and infrarenal. Table 40-1 describes the embryotic origins of each segment. While no specific event in the embryogenesis of the IVC can be identified, there are clear associations between the renal agenesis and other cardiovascular abnormalities associated with congenital abnormalities of the IVC. Anomalies of the IVC are found in 0.6%–2.0% of patients with cardiovascular defects compared with 0.3% of the population with no cardiovascular defects.[2] Agenesis of either kidney has been identified in association with vena cava abnormalities.[4] Congenital heart diseases associated with IVC anomalies include dextrocardia, septal defects, transposition of the great vessels, pulmonary artery stenosis, and a common atrium. In addition, there appears to be a genetic distribution in that, in one family, multiple individuals were affected with both IVC anomalies and multiple congenital defects.[5]

TABLE 40-1. EMBRYOLOGIC ORIGINS OF THE IVC

IVC Segment	Origin
Hepatic	Vitelline vein
Suprarenal	Right subcardinal vein
Renal	Right supra subcardinal and postsubcardinal anastomosis
Infrarenal	Right supracardinal vein
Azygos system	Supracardinal veins

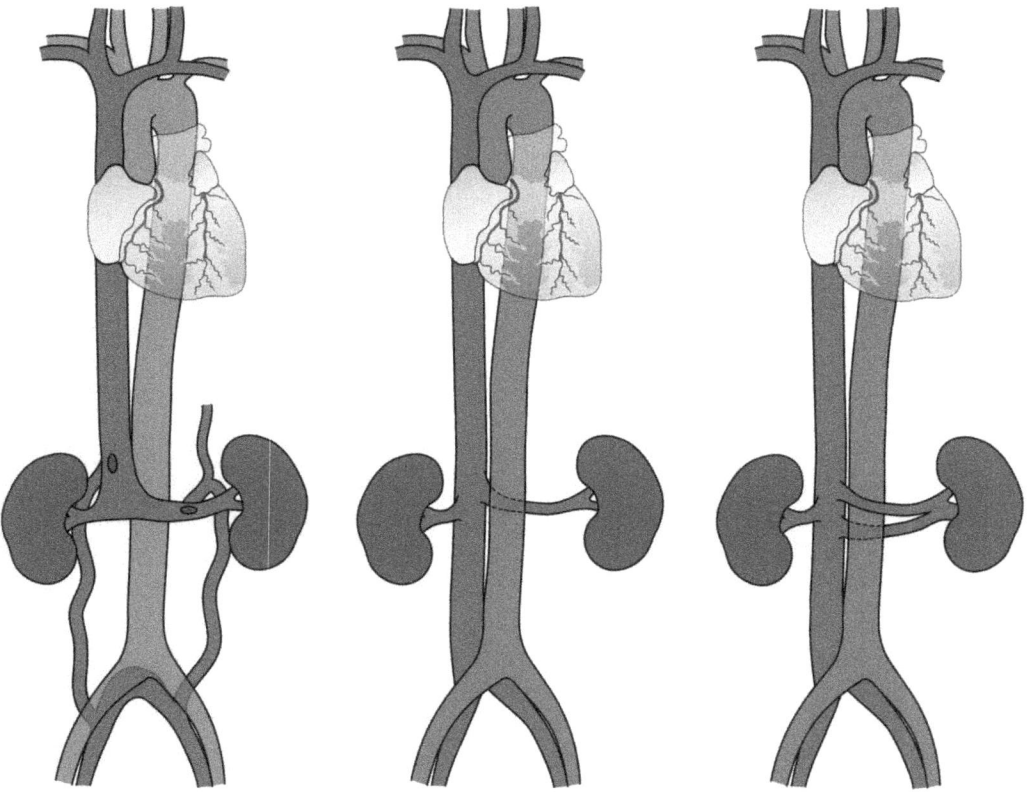

Figure 40-1. Absent subrenal segment of IVC.

Figure 40-2. Retroaortic left renal vein.

Figure 40-3. Circumaortic venous ring.

Fourteen different abnormalities are possible within the embryologic scheme of development of the IVC. Eleven of these conditions have been described clinically (Figs. 40-1–40-11). However, it is debated whether agenesis of the IVC is even possible.[6–8] According to Ramanathan, "embryologic dysgenesis of the right supracardinal vein has been cited as a possible mechanism (for agenesis of the IVC). However, this does not explain the failure of the post-cardinal veins to persist. A single embryologic event does not fully explain infrarenal absence."[6]

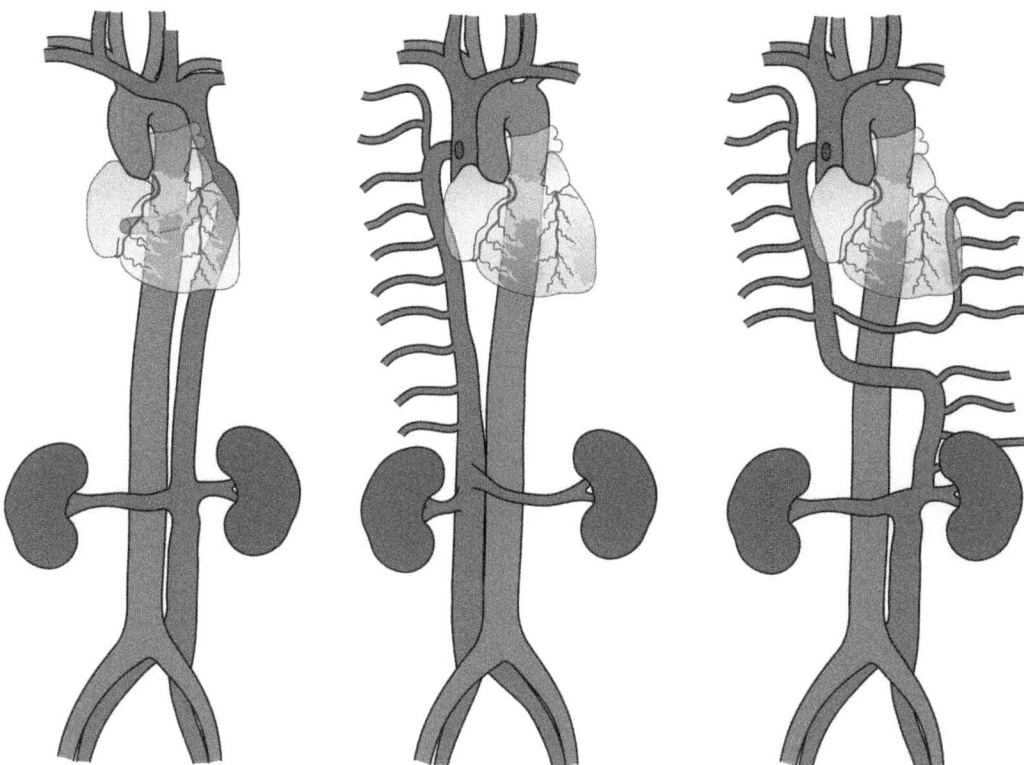

Figure 40-4. Left-sided vena cava.

Figure 40-5. Azygos continuation of IVC.

Figure 40-6. Left IVC with hemiazygos continuation.

According to Ramanathan and others, it has been suggested that the absence of the IVC is the result of perinatal thrombosis. Ramanathan cites the case of a 12-year-old who presented with a painful swollen leg. As an infant, within 24 hours of delivery, this same child was found to have thrombosis of the IVC.[6] Thus, it is possible that a perinatal event has resulted in loss of the IVC and may explain why many patients who have this finding have been successfully treated with endovascular techniques (see section on "Surgical and Endovascular Treatment").

CLINICAL PRESENTATION

The clinical presentation of patients with anomalies of the IVC is varied.[9–11] While it is estimated that a small percentage of the population has these abnormalities, the exact incidence is far from known. Frequently, congenital anomalies of the IVC are discovered as incidental findings on CT scans for other reasons; therefore, the true incidence of anomalies of the IVC may never be known. However, it is clear that anomalies of the IVC are associated with DVT.[12–14] Ruggeri was one of the first to emphasize the association of IVC abnormalities as a risk factor for idiopathic DVT. He reported four cases of agenesis

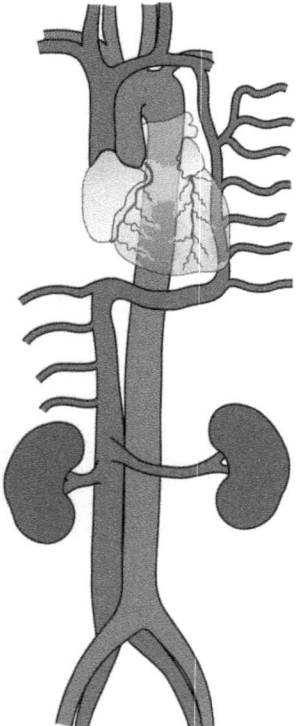

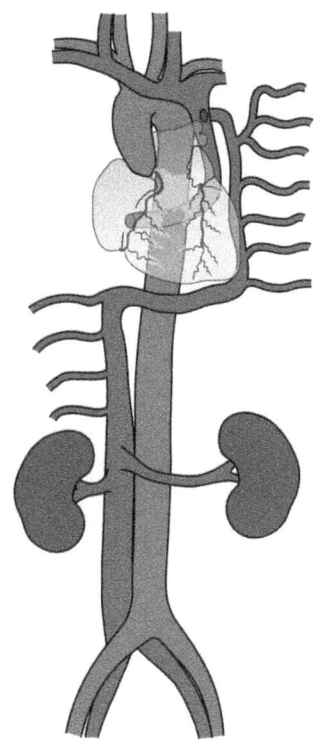

Figure 40-7. Azygos continuation of IVC with left SVC (version 1).

Figure 40-8. Azygos continuation of IVC with left SVC (version 2).

of the IVC with associated lower extremity DVT. None of his patients had thrombophilia and he estimated the percentage of DVT associated with absence of the IVC was 5.3%.[15] In a review of 97 patients with thrombotic occlusion of the iliac veins, five (5.2%) of the patients had an anomaly of the IVC.[16] These patients were significantly younger than the other patients, with a mean age of 25 (±6 years). In another review by Gayer, nine patients with DVT were found to have abnormalities of the IVC.[17] In this study, the patients had absence of the suprarenal vena cava, three had absence of the infrarenal vena cava, and one patient had a double vena cava with a ring and absence of the suprarenal vena cava. These patients presented with DVT in both legs more than 50% of the time. The patients, in addition to the abnormality of the IVC, also had genetic abnormalities of thrombophilia or a precipitating cause. Seven of the nine patients had genetic markers of thrombophilia. In the remaining two patients, additional risk factors included dehydration and hormonal therapy. Thus, while it is likely the stasis created by the abnormal IVC is a risk factor, there must be an associated condition that leads to the development of DVT. Any young patient who presents with bilateral, unprovoked clots of the lower extremities should be evaluated for abnormalities of the IVC.

Chronic venous insufficiency also has been reported in patients with anomalies of the IVC.[10,18] De Maeseneer reported on 35 patients with AIVC with a follow-up ranging from 0 to 28 years.[10] The diagnosis of agenesis of the vena cava was made in these patients at the mean age of 26 years. In longitudinal follow-up, unilateral or

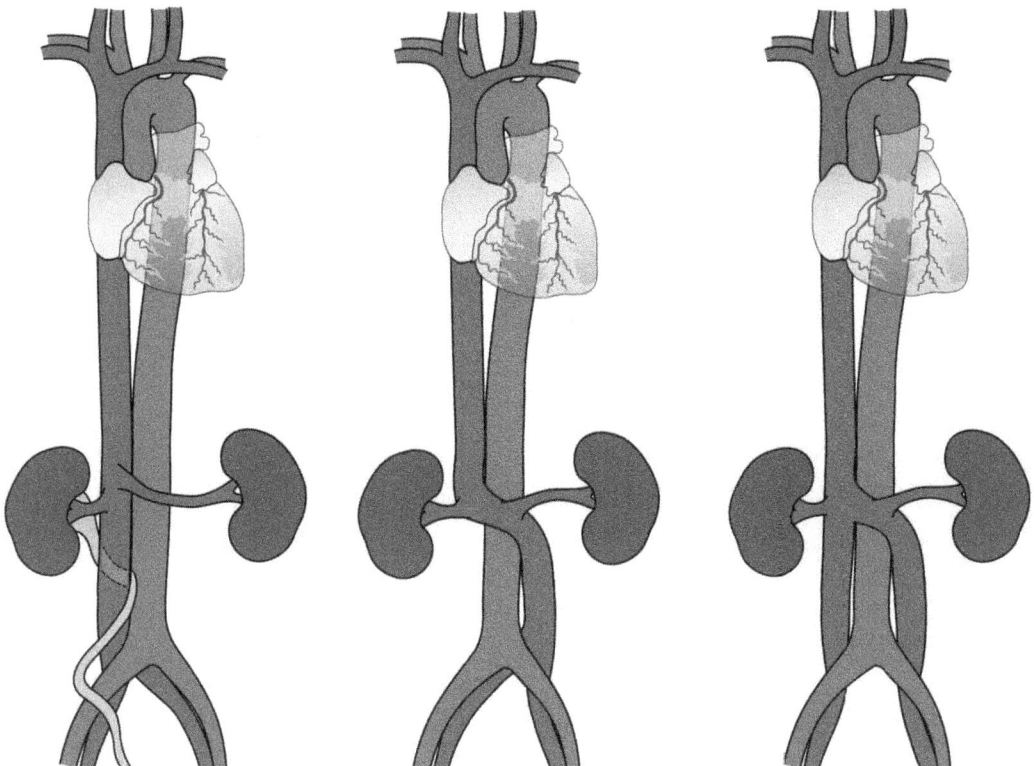

Figure 40-9. Retrocaval ureter.   **Figure 40-10.** Left IVC.   **Figure 40-11.** Double IVC.

bilateral ulcerations had occurred in 11 of 35 patients (31%). Forty-nine percent of the patients had a C4–C6 CEAP (C̲linical severity/E̲tiology/A̲natomy/P̲athophysiology) classification. Thrombophilia was present in 46% of patients. However, it is unclear from this article whether venous valvular reflux is from a congenital absence of the venous valves or is secondary to recurrent episodes of DVT.

DESCRIBED ANOMALIES OF THE IVC

As mentioned earlier, there are 14 different possible abnormalities of the IVC. To date, only 11 have been described. Many of the more common types are discussed in this chapter.

The most common anomaly of the IVC occurs with the number and location of the renal veins. (Figs. 40-2 and 40-3) Circumaortic renal veins occur in perhaps as many as 8.7% (Fig. 40-12A, B). When this occurs, the anterior left renal vein drains the adrenal gland while the posterior drains the left gonadal vein. In many radiographic studies, retroaortic renal veins occur in at least 2% of the population.

A left-sided IVC results from regression of the right supracardinal vein (Figs. 40-4 and 40-10). Its estimated incidence is between 0.2% and 0.5%. A duplicated IVC also is uncommon and occurs in 0.2%–3% of patients (Figs. 40-11 and 40-13A, B). With both

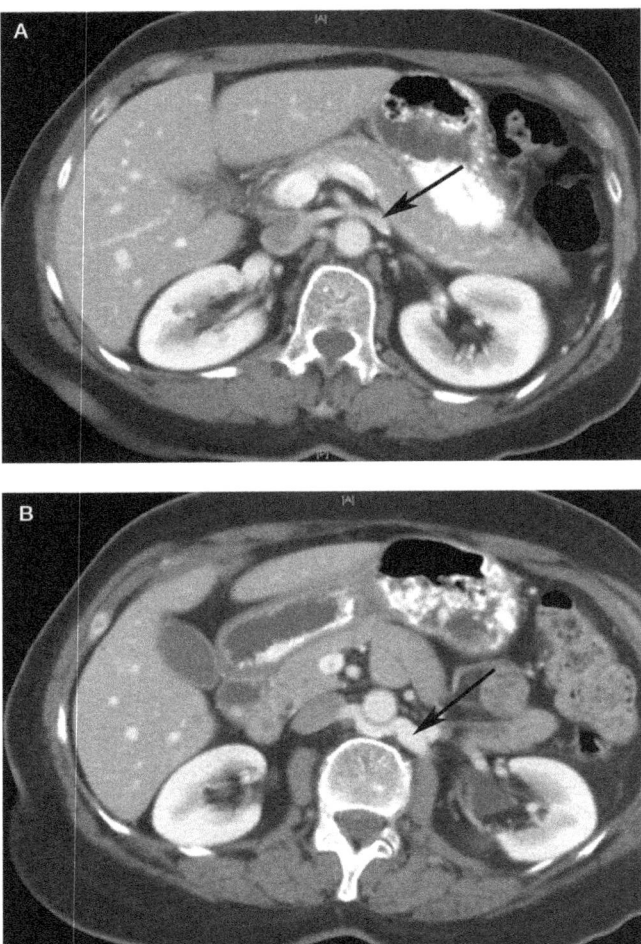

Figure 40-12. *A*, Circumaortic renal veins—anterior. *B*, Circumaortic renal veins—posterior.

the duplicated IVC and the left-sided IVC, the left renal vein is the major conduit for the blood passing from the left side of the body to the right side. A very infrequent occurrence is a left-sided vena cava with the development of a *right* May–Thurner syndrome. In this abnormality, the left iliac artery crosses the right iliac vein, producing symptoms opposite to that of a standard description of a May–Thurner syndrome (Fig. 40-14).

Another common abnormality is the absence of the hepatic IVC, which is commonly called the azygos continuation of the IVC[19,20] (Figs. 40-5–40-8 and 40-15A–C). In this condition, there is atrophy of the right subcardinal vein. This occurs in 0.6% of patients. It often is detected as an abnormality of the azygos system during a chest CT evaluation. Here, the venous drainage from the liver empties directly into the atrium, while flow from the rest of the body is through the azygos system to enter into the superior vena cava. This abnormality is commonly associated with other cardiovascular abnormalities.

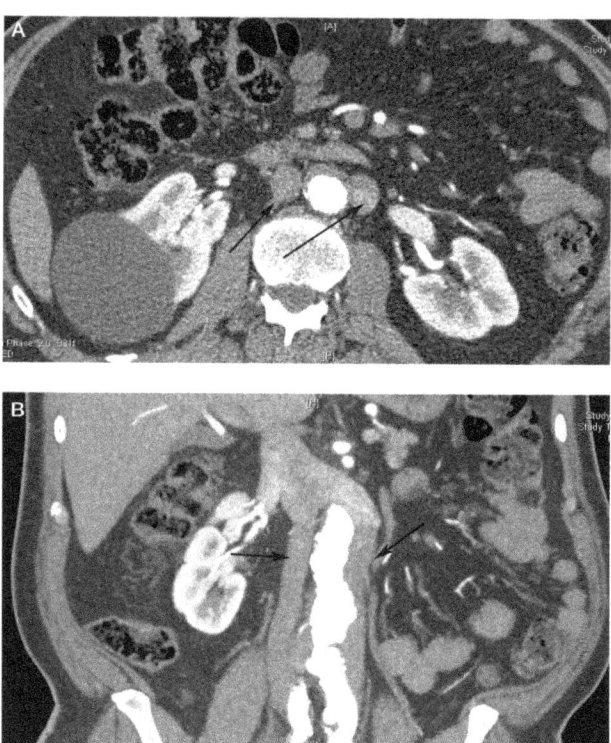

Figure 40-13. *A*, Transaxial view of duplicated IVC. *B*, Coronal view of duplicated IVC.

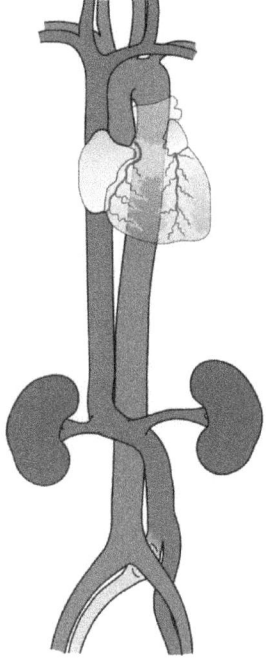

Figure 40-14. Right-sided May–Thurner syndrome.

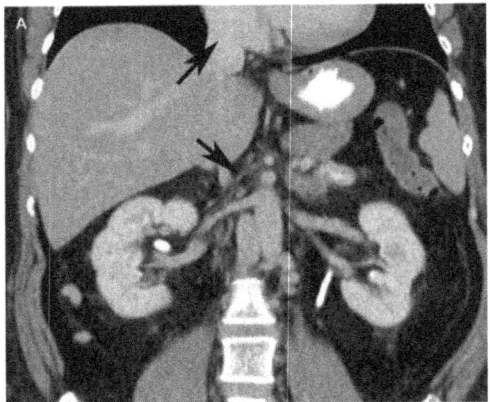
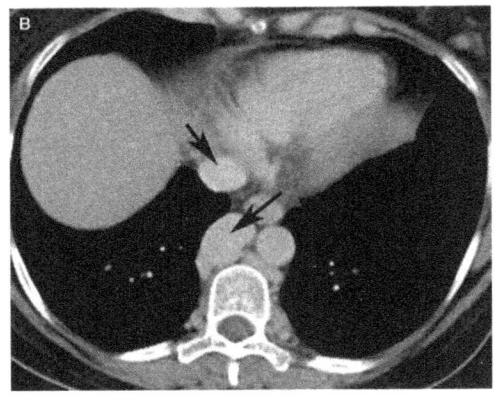
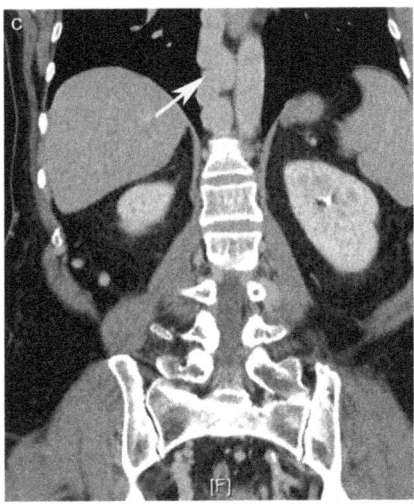

Figure 40-15. *A,* Atretic suprarenal vena cava. *B,* Azygos continuation with separate venous drainage from the liver. *C,* Azygos continuation.

VASCULAR SURGICAL IMPLICATIONS AND TREATMENTS

Anomalies of the IVC present several problems for the vascular surgeon. The first is the direct surgical and endovascular complications associated with these abnormalities. Aljabri and associates describes the incidence of major venous and renal abnormalities related to aortoiliac surgery. In their study, they found a retroaortic left renal vein, a circumaortic left renal vein, a left-sided IVC, a duplicated IVC, and preaortic confluence of the iliac veins.[21] During open surgery, these abnormalities are particularly problematic when repairing abdominal aortic aneurysms or performing aortoiliac reconstructive surgery. Preoperative knowledge of these anomalies is important to avoid any potential injury to these structures. Before the onset of routine use of CT scans, aortic exposure required identification of the left renal vein before clamping.[22] Even with viewing a normal anterior left renal vein, occasional injuries would occur to an unrecognized retroaortic vein (circumaortic renal veins). Such injuries were often associated with substantial hemorrhage.

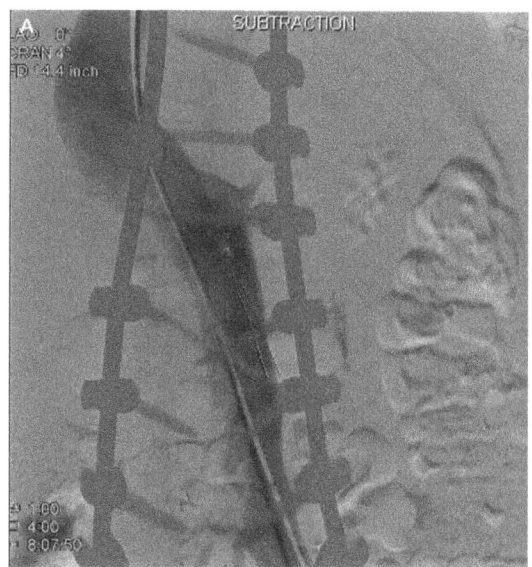
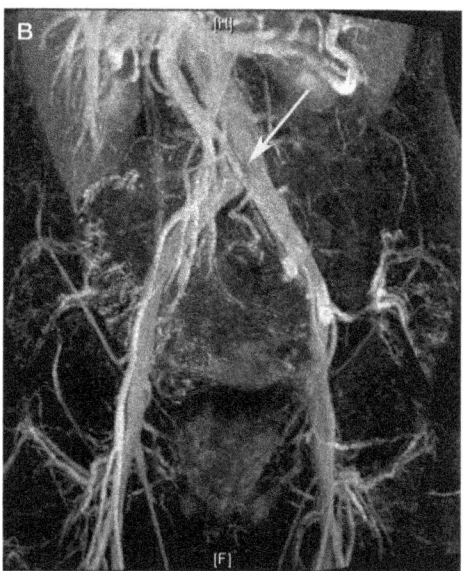

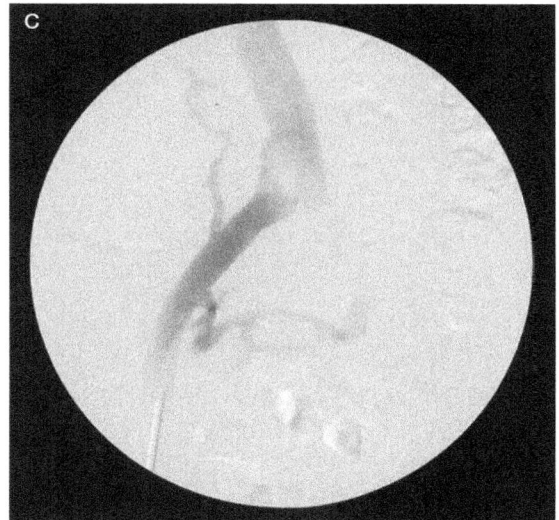

Figure 40-16. *A*, IVC filter placement in patient with right-sided May–Thurner syndrome. *B*, MRV demonstrating right sided vena cava with right iliac vein stenosis by left iliac artery. *C*, Venagram of right iliac vein demonstrating obstruction by left iliac artery.

The main problem of IVC abnormalities associated with endovascular therapy is with the placement of IVC filters (Fig. 40-16A). The most common problem is an unrecognized duplicated IVC, in which a filter was placed only on one side, leaving the patient unprotected against pulmonary embolism. This situation may be difficult to avoid but is best recognized when the left renal vein is much larger than one would expect. In addition, we have encountered several other abnormalities that have made placement of IVC filters difficult. One was a patient with a loop, which was identified by intraoperative venacavography. The second was the patient described earlier, in which there appeared to be a right-sided May–Thurner syndrome, which was not discovered until the patient had undergone further imaging (Fig. 40-16A–C). The abnormalities also become important to the cardiologist who is performing right-sided heart catheterizations and ablations. The anomalies associated with the suprarenal cava, that is, the azygos continuation, may prevent the operator from reaching the heart from the femoral veins.

SURGICAL AND ENDOVASCULAR TREATMENT

There is only scattered literature that discusses the role of either surgery or endovascular repair of IVC anomalies. There are a number of case reports describing surgical intervention for venous disease of the lower extremities. The largest of these studies was by Sagban who described a single-center experience with 15 cases.[23] These patients presented with a history of DVT and 14 of the patients had evidence of thrombophilia. The surgical indications included acute thrombosis, post-thrombotic syndrome, and bleeding from a venous aneurysm. The surgical treatment was varied and was commonly associated with replacement of the IVC with or without thrombectomy. A thoracoabdominal bypass was performed in two patients. Thoracoabdominal incisions were used on a majority of patients along with a temporary arteriovenous fistula. There is no operative mortality and primary patency was 53%. Unfortunately, there is no change in the CEAP classification in follow-up. In a case report, Dougherty described a 41-year-old male with a history of severe venous stasis disease and absence of the IVC. A prosthetic bypass graft was performed from external iliac to the intrathoracic azygos vein. The patient had symptomatic relief for at least 30 months follow-up.[18]

Reports of the endovascular treatment of anomalies of the IVC are uncommon. However, we have treated two patients recently who presented with DVT and IVC occlusion. These patients underwent thrombolysis and were found to have atretic hypoplastic IVCs (Fig. 40-17A–D). Both of these patients were treated with stenting of both the iliac system and the IVC. The follow-up is short (less than two years), but both patients have had relief of their symptoms. The patients are maintained on long-term anticoagulation. This treatment is only possible if the catheters can be placed across the atretic segment. In addition, we have had a patient who presented with bilateral iliac vein aneurysms, an atretic intrahepatic vena cava, and lower extremity thrombosis. The caval abnormality was not treated.

COMMENTS

In general, abnormalities of the IVC are rare. When they do occur, they present problems for both open vascular surgery and endovascular procedures. The embryology of the IVC is a complex process. Numerous combinations and permutations of abnormalities of the vena cava may occur. The abnormalities of the vena cava are easily detected on CTA or MRA. In most instances, congenital abnormalities of the IVC are found as incidental findings or in association with DVT. Most of the patients who present with DVT associated with vena cava abnormalities are young and have bilateral disease. In addition, many of the patients have associated thrombophilia or precipitating factors such as dehydration or trauma. The treatment in these patients is varied. In general, the treatment is limited to those patients with debilitating symptoms. Vena cava reconstruction may be surgical or endovascular. The therapy is tailored to the patient's specific complaints and anatomy. The reported results of both

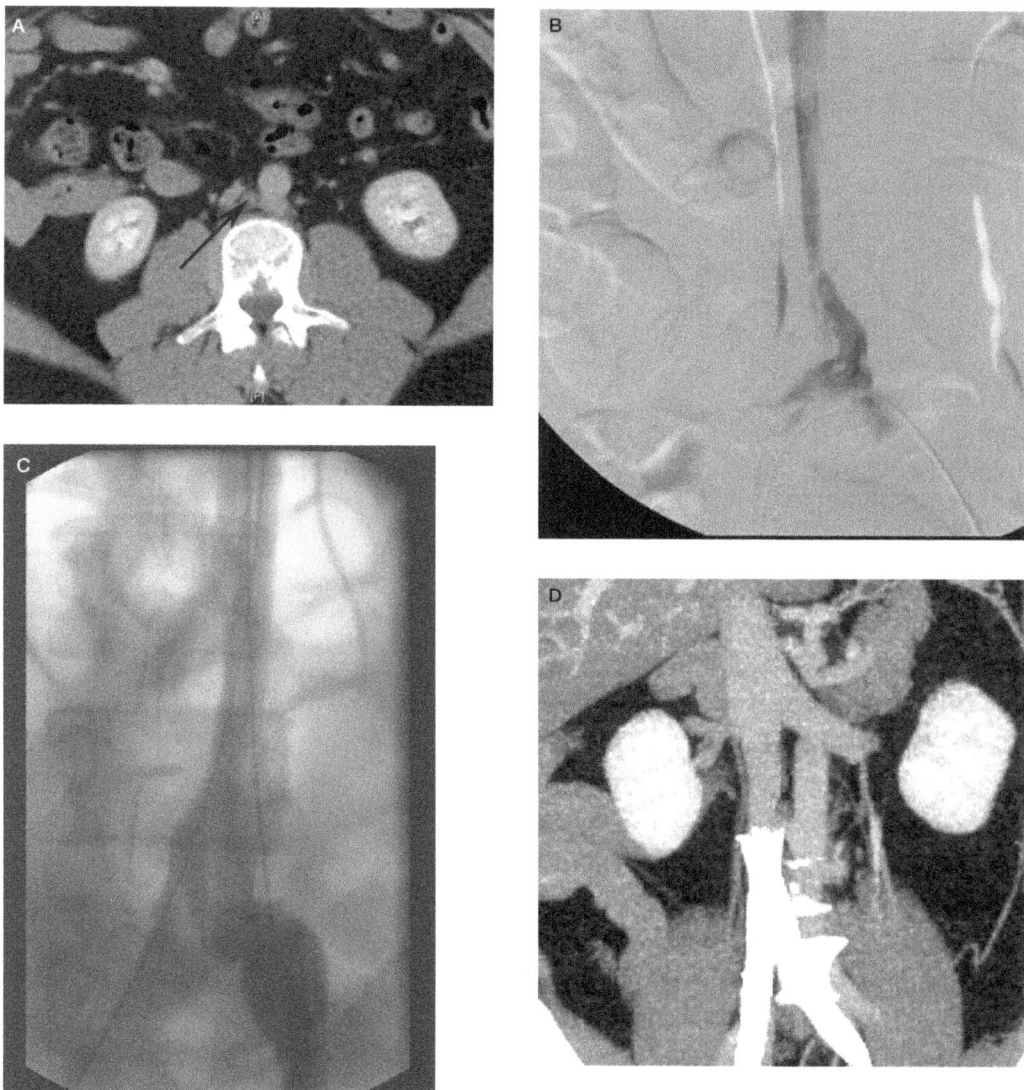

Figure 40-17. *A*, CT scan showing atretic IVC. *B*, Venagram demonstrating the atretic vena cava. *C*, Vena cava following angioplasty. *D*, IVC following angioplasty and stenting.

open and endovascular surgery appear to be satisfactory. Unfortunately, the venous disease associated with these abnormalities seems to be unimproved by caval reconstruction.

REFERENCES

1. Phillips E. Embryology, normal anatomy, and anomalies. In: Ferris EJ, Hipona FA, Kahn PC, et al, eds. *Venography of the Inferior Vena Cava and Its Branches.* Baltimore, MD: Williams & Wilkins; 1969:1–32.
2. Bass JE, Redwine MD, Kramer LA, et al. Spectrum of congenital anomalies of the inferior vena cava: cross-sectional imaging findings. *Radiographics.* 2000;20:639–652.

3. Minniti S, Visentini S, Procacci C. Congenital anomalies of the venae cavae: embryological origin, imaging features and report of three new variants. *Eur Radiol.* 2002;12:2040–2055.
4. Gayer G, Zissin R, Strauss S, Hertz M. IVC anomalies and right renal aplasia detected on CT: a possible link? *Abdom Imaging.* 2003;28:395–399.
5. Obernosterer A, Aschauer M, Mitterhammer H, Lipp RW. Congenital familial vascular anomalies: a study of patients with an anomalous inferior vena cava, and of their first-degree relatives. *Angiology.* 2004;55:73–77.
6. Ramanathan T, Hughes TM, Richardson AJ. Perinatal inferior vena cava thrombosis and absence of the infrarenal inferior vena cava. *J Vasc Surg.* 2001;33:1097–1099.
7. Iqbal J, Nagaraju E. Congenital absence of inferior vena cava and thrombosis: a case report. *J Med Case Rep.* 2008;2:46.
8. Lambert M, Marboeuf P, Midulla M, et al. Inferior vena cava agenesis and deep vein thrombosis: 10 patients and review of the literature. *Vasc Med.* 2010;15:451–459.
9. Gil RJ, Pérez AM, Arias JB, et al. Agenesis of the inferior vena cava associated with lower extremities and pelvic venous thrombosis. *J Vasc Surg.* 2006;44:1114–1116.
10. De Maeseneer MGR, Hertoghs M, Lauwers K, et al. Chronic venous insufficiency in patients with absence of the inferior vena cava. *J Vasc Surg Venous Lymphat Disord.* 2013;1:39–44.
11. Baeshko AA, Zhuk HV, Ulezko EA, et al. Congenital anomalies of the inferior vena cava and the clinical manifestations. *Eur J Vasc Endovasc Surg.* 2007;14:8–13.
12. Chee YL, Culligan DJ, Watson HG. Inferior vena cava malformation as a risk factor for deep venous thrombosis in the young. *Br J Haematol.* 2001;114:878–880.
13. Sarlon G, Bartoli MA, Muller C, et al. Congenital anomalies of inferior vena cava in young patients with iliac deep venous thrombosis. *Ann Vasc Surg.* 2011;25:265.e5–265.e8.
14. Takehara N, Hasebe N, Enomoto S, et al. Multiple and recurrent systemic thrombotic events associated with congenital anomaly of inferior vena cava. *J Thromb Thrombolysis.* 2005;19:101–103.
15. Ruggeri M, Tosetto A, Castaman G, Rodeghiero F. Congenital absence of the inferior vena cava: a rare risk factor for idiopathic deep-vein thrombosis. *Lancet.* 2001;357:441.
16. Obernosterer A, Aschauer M, Schnedl W, Lipp RW. Anomalies of the inferior vena cava in patients with iliac venous thrombosis. *Ann Intern Med.* 2002;136:37–41.
17. Gayer G, Luboshitz J, Hertz M, et al. Congenital anomalies of the inferior vena cava revealed on CT in patients with deep vein thrombosis. *AJR Am J Roentgenol.* 2003;180:729–732.
18. Dougherty MJ, Calligaro KD, DeLaurentis DA. Congenitally absent inferior vena cava presenting in adulthood with venous stasis and ulceration: a surgically treated case. *J Vasc Surg.* 1996;23:141–146.
19. Anderson RC, Adams P Jr, Burke B. Anomalous inferior vena cava with azygos continuation (infrahepatic interruption of the inferior vena cava). Report of 15 new cases. *J Pediatr.* 1961;59:370–383.
20. Brodelius A, Johannson BW, Sievers J. Anomalous inferior vena cava with azygous and hemiazygous continuation. *Acta Paediatr.* 1962;51:331–336.
21. Aljabri B, MacDonald PS, Satin R, et al. Incidence of major venous and renal anomalies relevant to aortoiliac surgery as demonstrated by computed tomography. *Ann Vasc Surg.* 2001;15:615–618.
22. Karkos CD, Bruce IA, Thomson GJ, Lambert ME. Retroaortic left renal vein and its implications in abdominal aortic surgery. *Ann Vasc Surg.* 2001;15:703–708.
23. Sagban TA, Grotemeyer D, Balzer KM, et al. Surgical treatment for agenesis of the vena cava: a single-centre experience in 15 cases. *Eur J Vasc Endovasc Surg.* 2010;40:241–245.

Abdominal Aortic Diseases

41

Final results of the Open Versus Endovascular Repair (OVER) Trial for AAA

Frank A. Lederle, MD

BACKGROUND

Randomized trials have shown that endovascular repair reduces perioperative mortality compared with the standard open procedure, but in the British Endovascular Aneurysm Repair Trial 1 (EVAR-1) and the Dutch Randomized Endovascular Aneurysm Management (DREAM) trial, this advantage was lost within two years due to excess late deaths in the endovascular groups. In the earlier report of the more recent OVER Trial, excess late deaths were not observed in the endovascular group at two years.

METHODS

Eligible patients had abdominal aortic aneurysm (AAA) for which repair was planned and that had (1) a maximum diameter of at least 5.0 cm, or (2) a maximum diameter of at least 4.5 cm plus rapid enlargement or saccular morphology, or (3) an associated iliac aneurysm ≥3.0 cm. Patients had to be a candidate for both procedures and meet the manufacturer's indications for the endovascular system that might be used. Patients were randomized to endovascular repair with any FDA-approved system or to open repair.

RESULTS

We randomized 881 patients at 42 Veterans Affairs medical centers between October 2002 and April 2007. Patients were followed for up to nine years (mean 5.2 years) and as of the end of the study in October 2011 vital status was confirmed for all patients.[1] Randomized

467

patients had a mean age of 70 years, 99% were male, and 43% had an AAA smaller than 5.5 cm. More than 95% completed the assigned repair. For the primary outcome of all-cause mortality, 146 deaths occurred in each group, hazard ratio (HR) 0.97, 95% CI 0.77, 1.22, $P = 0.81$. The previously reported reduction in perioperative mortality with endovascular repair was sustained at two years (HR 0.63, CI 0.40–0.98, $P = 0.04$) and three years (HR 0.72, CI 0.51, 1.00, $P = 0.05$), but not thereafter. Ten aneurysm-related deaths occurred in the endovascular repair group (2.3%) compared with 16 (3.7%) in the open repair group ($P = 0.22$). Six aneurysm ruptures were confirmed in the endovascular group compared with none in the open group ($P = 0.03$). A significant interaction was observed between age and treatment ($P < 0.006$), such that for patients less than age 70, survival was better in the endovascular group, whereas for those more than age 70, it tended to be better in the open group.

CONCLUSIONS

Endovascular and open repair resulted in similar long-term survival. The perioperative survival advantage of endovascular repair was sustained for several years, but rupture after endovascular repair remains a concern. Endovascular repair led to better long-term survival in younger patients, but not in the older patients for whom benefit was most expected.

REFERENCE

1. Lederle FA, Freischlag JA, Kyriakides TC, et al. Long-term comparison of endovascular and open repair of abdominal aortic aneurysm. *N Engl J Med*. 2012;367:1988–1997. http://www.nejm.org/doi/full/10.1056/NEJMoa1207481#t=article

42

Outcomes of Percutaneous Treatment of Type II Endoleaks

Abdulhameed Aziz, MD and Patrick J. Geraghty, MD

INTRODUCTION

Since its 1991 introduction, endovascular aneurysm repair (EVAR) has progressed through multiple device iterations and has become the dominant repair modality for infrarenal abdominal aneurysms. It is thus notable that despite the broad acceptance of EVAR within the vascular surgical community, management of type II endoleaks (T2EL) remains a contentious issue. Some experts advocate routine presurgical or intra-procedural maneuvers to diminish the overall occurrence of endoleaks, whereas most practitioners prefer to address T2EL only when accompanied by concerning features, such as sac expansion. Concerns regarding the cost of T2EL surveillance and risk of subsequent treatment have even led to the development of EVAR devices specifically designed to mitigate T2EL formation, such as the Nellix™ system (currently undergoing clinical evaluation in the United States).

The reasons for lack of treatment consensus include our knowledge deficit regarding the natural history of specific endoleak presentations, the failure of the vascular community to organize multicenter studies of this relatively uncommon phenomenon, and the belated recognition that T2EL frequently persist or recur following initial intervention. We still struggle to definitively answer the most simple and direct questions regarding T2EL: Are we able to accurately diagnose them? Are some or all T2EL benign? Does concomitant sac growth pose greater risk, and if so, at what amount of growth? Are the risks of intervention justified?[1] In this chapter, we offer a focused look at several of these issues and suggest a treatment algorithm based on currently available data. As the foregoing caveats imply, this algorithm is likely to change as our knowledge base improves and further outcomes data accrue.

IS T2EL IN THE ABSENCE OF SAC GROWTH A BENIGN PHENOMENON?

Careful interpretation of outcomes data is required to avoid an overly aggressive use of interventionsinthe treatment of T2EL. If one looks at the outcomes of "unfractionated" T2EL, some degree of aneurysm sac growth will usually be noted, raising the question as to whether all T2EL merit reintervention. The simple answer, based on current literature, is no. As we will address in greater detail, careful angiography will show that a substantial share of these troublesome T2EL are in fact occult type I or III endoleaks.[2,3] Endoleak duration also appears to negatively influence EVAR outcomes, as persistent and recurrent T2EL have been shown to pose the highest risk of sac growth and need for reintervention.[4–6] Aneurysm rupture attributed to T2EL is quite uncommon, although several such cases were reported by the Massachusetts General Hospital group. Of these four cases, one occurred on EVAR postoperative day two, suggesting that procedural manipulation was the most likely cause of wall disruption, and a second rupture occurred following implantation of a surgeon-customized graft.[6]

Our group published an early experience with management of T2EL in 2004.[7] We analyzed 486 consecutive infrarenal EVAR, with a mean follow-up of approximately 22 months. T2EL were detected in 90 (18.5%) of patients. The endoleaks persisted beyond six months in 35 (7.2%), yet only five of those patients (1% of the total) showed aneurysm sac growth of >5 mm. Those five patients underwent percutaneous intervention with apparent procedural success. No aneurysm rupture occurred in the study group. Thus, our policy has been to recommend a selective approach to intervention for T2EL, with primary focus assigned to persistent T2EL demonstrating sac growth of >5 mm, an approach recently echoed by El Batti and coworkers.[5]

THE IMPORTANCE OF ANGIOGRAPHIC ASSESSMENT

The past several years have seen a critical reappraisal of the results of endoleak intervention. While recurrence rates are disappointingly high in many series, these retrospective studies have nonetheless matured our approach to T2EL management. An excellent example of this process is the recognition that diagnostic arteriography, through the transfemoral or translumbar approach, reveals an unexpectedly high incidence of occult type I or type III endoleaks. In the authors' review of their institutional experience with percutaneous intervention for T2EL accompanied by aneurysm sac growth, 9 of 42 (21%) of patients undergoing arteriography were discovered to have occult type I (5/42) or type III (4/42) endoleaks. These individuals subsequently underwent definitive endovascular intervention.[2] Investigators at the University of Chicago similarly detected type I or type III endoleaks on arteriography in 4/25 (16%) of patients selected for treatment of purported T2EL with sac growth, and a further 5/25 (20%) were later reclassified as type III endoleaks on delayed CT scanning.[8]

MIDTERM AND LONG-TERM RESULTS OF PERCUTANEOUS INTERVENTION FOR T2EL WITH SAC GROWTH

Success following percutaneous intervention for T2EL with sac growth can be measured by any of several standards, including freedom from aneurysm rupture/aneurysm-related mortality, freedom from continued sac growth/reintervention, or freedom from endoleak persistence/recurrence. The latter measure is notably difficult to achieve, due to the tendency of T2EL to persist or recur despite presumed ablation at the time of intervention. In the Washington University in St. Louis experience using transfemoral and translumbar coil and/or glue embolization, follow-up to a mean of 23 months after intervention showed a sobering 72% rate of persistent and/or recurrent T2EL on blinded independent review of CT imaging. Similarly, investigators at the University of Chicago demonstrated persistent or recurrent T2EL in 4/16 (25%) of patients at 28 months of follow-up, and the Columbia/Cornell groupnoted a 24% rate of ongoing endoleak at 3.5 years postintervention, even though the majority of patients underwent secondary procedures in an attempt to achieve ablation.[3,8] El Abatti and coworkers from France achieved successful outcome for T2EL intervention (defined as cessation of endoleak and stable sac diameter) in only 7 of 40 (22%) patients treated with coil embolization or surgical vessel clipping.[5] Finally, in the Cleveland Clinic experience, 95 patients underwent T2EL intervention for sac growth and were followed out to five years. Although Sarac et al. did not provide data regarding the persistence or recurrence of endoleak, 24% required repeat intervention, and 56% experienced continued aneurysm growth of >5 mm.[9]

The modest success achieved at these tertiary centers highlights the complex nature of T2EL ablation. In some respects, these endoleaks mimic the behavior of complex arteriovenous malformations, in that multiple feeding vessels are common, and endoleak nidus obliteration appears to be of value in achieving sustained success. As noted by Baum et al. in 2002, embolization of a solitary feeding vessel (in this instance, the inferior mesenteric artery [IMA]) led to endoleak recurrence in 80% of patients.[10] It seems likely that durable ablation requires both nidus obliteration and embolization/clipping of most, if not all, feeding vessels. Although case reports have described the potential for complications with T2EL intervention, including spinal cord ischemia and inadvertent caval embolus formation,[11,12] more aggressive deployment of polymerizing embolic agents can achieve both nidus and feeding branch ablation. In particular, the use of Onyx® (ev3, Irvine, CA) has been recently championed by Abularrage and Bosiers.[11,13] This ethylene vinyl alcohol copolymer is dissolved in dimethylsulfoxide and suspended micronized tantalum powder. Among the reported advantages of Onyx are predictable polymerization times and lack of adhesion to the delivery catheter. These features permit deliberate and complete obliteration of the nidus, with intentional extension of the polymerizing mixture into the feeding vessels. Cannulation of the endoleak flow channel is a requisite for success in these procedures, and refinements such as the triaxial technique described by Shimohira and coworkers may prove useful in that endeavor.[14]

PROPHYLACTIC MEASURES: CAN T2EL BE PREVENTED?

The desirability of T2EL avoidance is by now quite clear. As noted above, the incidence of T2EL accompanied by sac growth is fairly small, and no convincing analysis has yet been provided that would justify universal prophylactic measures from a risk/benefit or even acost-effectiveness standpoint. Nonetheless, several investigators have provided intriguing data on T2EL prophylaxis, and one device manufacturer (Nellix, Endologix Inc., Irvine, CA) has received marketing approval within the European Economic Area (CE Mark) for an EVAR device that is designed to ablate extra-luminal aneurysm sac dead space.

The Mount Sinai group found that routine preoperative embolization of a patent IMA decreased the incidence of postoperative T2EL and the need for subsequent intervention. However, T2EL incidence post-IMA embolization remained fairly high in this series at 34%. In addition, 10 of 108 patients in the study group required readmission for abdominal pain and endoscopy to rule out ischemic colitis, and a single patient died from complicated ischemic colitis following IMA embolization.[15]

TABLE 42-1. SUGGESTED MANAGEMENT ALGORITHM FOR TYPE 2 ENDOLEAK AFTER EVAR

Type II endoleak documented on post-EVAR surveillance

Sac diameter decreases, remains stable, or shows <5 mm increase in comparison to initial post-EVAR study

Sac diameter shows >5 mm increase in comparison to initial post-EVAR study

Continue routine surveillance program

Hypertension treatment, statin therapy, discontinue antithrombotic medications if possible

Treat type I and/or type III endoleak with endovascular or open surgical intervention

Diagnostic angiography to rule out occult type I or type III endoleak

- transfemoral and/or translumbar approach, depending on local expertise
- may be combined with simultaneous intervention, particularly if translumbar access utilized

Targeted type II endoleak intervention

- Ablate all inflow/outflow vessels
- Embolize/ablate nidus (dead space)

Continued growth with persistent or recurrent type II endoleak:

- Repeat intervention targeted to visualized feeding vessels; consider use of alternate modalities (e.g., laparoscopic clipping)
- Consider open conversion

Continue routine surveillance program

Continued growth without visualized endoleak:

- Consider endograft relining
- Consider peritoneal windowing
- Consider open conversion if landing zone integrity is threatened

Stable or decreasing aneurysm sac size, regardless of endoleak recurrence

Using a different approach that they refer to as aneurysm sac "thrombization," Ronsivalle and coworkers undertook embolization of the aneurysm sac with fibrin glue (± embolization coils) at the time of initial EVAR. A total of 180 patients were followed to 26 months after EVAR + sac thrombization, with T2EL incidence of only 2.2%.[16] More extensive study of this technique is warranted, given its potential for cost-effective reduction of T2EL reintervention and related complications.

SUMMARY AND CURRENT TREATMENT ALGORITHM

The accompanying algorithm (Table 42-1) details our current approach to the management of T2EL following EVAR. As previously noted, diagnostic arteriography may unmask occult type I and type III endoleaks, making this an indispensable feature in the management of T2EL with aneurysm growth. The use of a 5-mm growth cutoff is admittedly subjective, but commonly utilized within the available literature. If the T2EL should recur, there is a paucity of data to guide subsequent reintervention. In selected cases, we have found alternate techniques (e.g., laparoscopic clipping of proximal lumbar inflow vessels) to be complementary, particularly when the initial intervention may have diminished the possibility of reintervention through the same route.

Although there is broad consensus regarding the need for intervention in the setting of persistent T2EL accompanied by aneurysm sac growth, the outcome data presented here clearly indicate the need for improvement in our interventional strategies, as endoleak persistence and recurrence are frequent and vexing occurrences. It is hoped that further refinement of available techniques, as well as addition of novel therapies, will soon permit definitive, single-setting interventions that yield durable endoleak ablation.

REFERENCES

1. Karthikesalingam A, Thrumurthy SG, Jackson D, et al. Current evidence is insufficient to define an optimal threshold for intervention in isolated type II endoleak after endovascular aneurysm repair. *J Endovasc Ther*. 2012;19(2):200–208.
2. Aziz A, Menias CO, Sanchez LA, et al. Outcomes of percutaneous endovascular intervention for type II endoleak with aneurysm expansion. *J Vasc Surg*. 2012;55(5):1263–1267.
3. Gallagher KA, Ravin RA, Meltzer A J, et al. Midterm outcomes after treatment of type II endoleaks associated with aneurysm sac expansion. *J Endovasc Ther*. 2012;19(2):182–192.
4. Chang RW, Goodney P, Tucker LY, et al. Ten-year results of endovascular abdominal aortic aneurysm repair from a large multicenter registry. *J Vasc Surg*. 2013.doi: 10.1016/j.jvs.2013.01.051.
5. El Batti S, Cochennec F, Roudot-Thoraval F, Becquemin, JP. Type II endoleaks after endovascular repair of abdominal aortic aneurysm are not always a benign condition. *J Vasc Surg*. 2013;57(5):1291–1297.
6. Jones JE, Atkins MD, Brewster DC, et al. Persistent type 2 endoleak after endovascular repair of abdominal aortic aneurysm is associated with adverse late outcomes. *J Vasc Surg*. 2007;46(1):1–8.
7. Steinmetz E, Rubin BG, Sanchez LA, et al. Type II endoleak after endovascular abdominal aortic aneurysm repair: a conservative approach with selective intervention is safe and cost-effective. *J Vasc Surg*. 2004;39(2):306–313.

8. Funaki B, Birouti N, Zangan SM, et al. Evaluation and treatment of suspected type II endoleaks in patients with enlarging abdominal aortic aneurysms. *J Vasc Interv Radiol.* 2012;23(7):866–872;quiz 872.

9. Sarac TP, Gibbons C, Vargas L, et al. Long-term follow-up of type II endoleak embolization reveals the need for close surveillance. *J Vasc Surg.* 2012;55(1):33–40.

10. Baum RA, Carpenter JP, Golden MA, et al. Treatment of type 2 endoleaks after endovascular repair of abdominal aortic aneurysms: comparison of transarterial and translumbar techniques. *J Vasc Surg.* 2002;35(1):23–29.

11. Bosiers MJ, Schwindt A, Donas KP, Torsello G. Midterm results of the transarterial use of Onyx in the treatment of persisting type II endoleaks after EVAR. *J Cardiovasc Surg.* (Torino), Apr05, 2013;54(4):469–475.[EPUB ahead of print]

12. Ioannou CV, Tsetis DK, Kardoulas DG, et al. Spinal cord ischemia after endovascular embolization of a type II endoleak following endovascular aneurysm repair. *Ann Vasc Surg.* 2012;26(6):860 e1–860 e7.

13. Abularrage CJ, Patel VI, Conrad MF, et al. Improved results using Onyx glue for the treatment of persistent type 2 endoleak after endovascular aneurysm repair. *J Vasc Surg.* 2012;56(3):630–636.

14. Shimohira M, Hashizume T, Suzuki Y, et al. Triaxial system for embolization of type II endoleak after endovascular aneurysm repair. *J Endovasc Ther.* 2013;20(2):200–204.

15. Ward TJ, Cohen S, Fischman AM, Kim, et al. Preoperative inferior mesenteric artery embolization before endovascular aneurysm repair: decreased incidence of type II endoleak and aneurysm sac enlargement with 24-month follow-up. *J Vasc Interv Radiol.* 2013;24(1):49–55.

16. Ronsivalle S, Faresin F, Franz F, et al. Aneurysm sac "thrombization" and stabilization in EVAR: a technique to reduce the risk of type II endoleak. *J Endovasc Ther.* 2010;17(4):517–524.

43

Predictors of AAA Sac Enlargement after Endovascular Aortic Aneurysm Repair

Patrick Thompson, BS and Andres Schanzer, MD

The modern open surgical management of abdominal aortic aneurysms (AAA) has changed little since its inception in the 1950s. Endoaneurysmorrhaphy, first described by Rudolph Matas in 1888, involved ligating the branches of an aneurysm from within the aneurysm sac. Approximately 25 years later at the beginning of the 20th century, Alexis Carrel received the Nobel Prize for demonstrating the feasibility of suture repair of arteries and perfecting an anastomotic technique to join two vessels. With these techniques established, an AAA could be repaired by anastomosis of a synthetic conduit to the aorta just proximal and distal to the AAA thereby preserving antegrade blood flow.[1] Dubost was the first to marry these two techniques in 1952 with the first report of a successful open AAA repair with homograft replacement.[2] Aside from the development of various different types of conduit materials, open AAA repair has remained largely unchanged through to the present day.

The most dramatic shift in the surgical management of AAA occurred in 1991 when Juan Parodi reported the first endovascular abdominal aortic aneurysm repair (EVAR).[3] This transformative moment marks the beginning of minimally invasive AAA repair as an alternative to open surgical repair. While the elective management of AAA had traditionally depended solely on open surgical repair,[4,5] these recent developments in catheter-based, endovascular techniques led to a substantial increase in the proportion of AAAs managed electively using EVAR. Currently, over 70% of elective AAA repairs in the United States are performed with EVAR.[6]

There are three large prospective randomized controlled trials that have compared outcomes after elective open AAA repair to those after EVAR (Table 43-1).[7-9] In general, the findings across all three studies have been concordant and can be summarized as follows: (1) the perioperative morbidity and mortality is significantly lower after EVAR repair than after open repair of AAA, (2) the short-term survival

TABLE 43-1. SUMMARY OF THE RESULTS FROM THE RANDOMIZED CONTROLLED TRIALS AND THE MEDICARE PROPENSITY-SCORE-MATCHED COMPARISON OF EVAR WITH OPEN ABDOMINAL AORTIC ANEURYSM REPAIR

Trial	Study Arm (n)	Short-Term Mortality[a]	Long-Term Mortality[b]
The United Kingdom Endovascular Aneurysm Repair 1 Trial (EVAR 1 Trial)[7]	EVAR (626)	1.8% at 30 days	23.1% at 4 years
	Open AAA (626)	4.3% at 30 days	22.3% at 4 years
The Dutch Randomized Endovascular Aneurysm Management Trial (DREAM Trial)[8]	EVAR (173)	1.2% at 30 days	31.1% at 6 years
	Open AAA (178)	4.6% at 30 days	30.1% at 6 years
Outcomes Following Endovascular vs. Open Repair of Abdominal Aortic Aneurysm: A Randomized Trial (OVER Trial)[9]	EVAR (444)	0.5% at 30 days	7.0% at 2 years
	Open AAA (437)	3.0% at 30 days	9.8% at 2 years

Abbreviations: AAA, abdominal aortic aneurysm; EVAR, endovascular aortic aneurysm repair.
[a]$P < .05$ for each comparison in each trial.
[b]P = nonsignificant for each comparison in each trial.

advantage of EVAR diminishes during long-term follow-up such that if patients survive beyond approximately two years, the long-term survival of patients is similar for both groups, and (3) although the reintervention rate after EVAR is higher than after open repair, most of these reinterventions are performed with catheter-based techniques, albeit at overall higher costs.

While each study shows that EVAR confers a substantial early survival benefit, this benefit is lost in every trial at different points of long-term follow-up. Despite being the subject of numerous studies, consensus around a satisfactory explanation for this conundrum has not emerged. Possible explanations include poor compliance with follow-up resulting from patients not fully understanding the critical importance of lifetime surveillance, device fatigue and subsequent failure, persistence of an elevated inflammatory state associated with the presence of an intact aneurysm leading to cardiovascular events, and device failures due to treatment of unfavorable anatomy outside of the specified instructions for use.

Rates of AAA sac enlargement after EVAR are not negligible. Dr. Makaroun and colleagues demonstrated, in a large University Series, the rate of aortic sac enlargement after EVAR to be 21% at five years.[10] In another recent study, even in patients treated for a type II endoleak in whom surveillance detected AAA sac enlargement, 55% continued to show expansion greater than 5 mm by five years after treatment.[11]

To interpret appropriately the studies that compare outcomes after EVAR and open AAA repair, it is important to understand the context in which they were obtained. The clinical trials for regulatory approval and postmarketing analyses, as well as the randomized controlled trials that compared EVAR to open AAA repair, have included only patients in whom the specific anatomic requirements defined in the device Instruction for Use (IFU) were met.[9,12-15] Studies utilizing national databases have also been limited in that these studies lack access to preoperative and postoperative aortic and iliac artery anatomic measurements and therefore have been unable to assess whether devices were used in accordance with published IFU or whether adherence to IFU affected the rate of device failure and thereby clinical outcomes.[6,16] Thus, the proportion of patients and the outcomes of patients who undergo EVAR that had anatomy outside of the device IFU are largely undocumented with respect to both short- and long-term mortality and complication rates, with the exception of a small number of single-center reports.[17–19]

The issue of adherence to the specific anatomic requirements defined in the device IFU is of paramount importance when considering the long-term results of the EVAR trial mentioned above.[7] The late follow-up of this cohort demonstrated that the early survival advantage of patients undergoing EVAR disappeared with time, and that a significant proportion of late deaths after EVAR were due to aneurysm rupture (27 AAA ruptures in the EVAR group; five within 30 days of surgery and 22 after that).[7] Although the exact mechanism was not determined for each patient that died due to aortic rupture after endovascular repair in the EVAR study, the authors thought that the early aortic ruptures were preventable had a CT scan been done before discharge.[20] The cases of late aortic rupture and death were found to be closely linked to aortic aneurysm sac enlargement.[20] Since aortic rupture has been shown to be an important cause of late death in highly selected patient populations within clinical trials, it is reasonable to hypothesize that commercial use of EVAR devices in patients who did not meet device IFU could result in a higher rate of postoperative aortic sac enlargement and thereby put such patients at higher risk of aortic rupture.

To address the rate of compliance with IFU, we conducted a study using data from a large, multicenter cohort CT scan database, to determine the degree of compliance with IFU anatomic guidelines for EVAR, to examine changes in compliance with the IFU over the last decade, and to determine the relationship between baseline aortic and iliac artery anatomic characteristics and incidence of aortic aneurysm sac enlargement after EVAR.[21] The primary limitation of this study was that although the number of patients studied was large, no clinical characteristics of the patients were available and the generalizability of this population to patients undergoing EVAR in the United States could not be established. Similarly, no information was available about which, if any, interventions were performed in response to the findings of a CT scan.

Patients undergoing EVAR between January 1, 1999, and December 31, 2008, were assembled from a medical imaging repository at M2S, Incorporated (West Lebanon, NH). Utilizing standardized algorithms, M2S creates three-dimensional (3D) computer models from computed tomography (CT) images of aortic aneurysms. In addition to serving as the core imaging lab for several large aneurysm management trials,[22–24] M2S also provides these services to both private and academic hospitals throughout the world. For purposes of this study, M2S provided de-identified data on all patients in their prospectively acquired database who underwent a CT scan before EVAR and had at least one CT scan post-EVAR between 1999 and 2008 in the United States. Using these criteria, 10,228 patients in the United States who underwent EVAR for AAA repair between 1999 and 2008 were identified.

This study demonstrated that in this cohort of patients, the incidence of AAA sac enlargement post-EVAR was 41% at five years, a rate that increased over the time period of the study. When all EVAR-treated patients were classified according to IFU criteria, 5983 (58.5%) patients were outside of compliance with the most conservative device IFU available on the market, and 3178 (31.1%) patients were outside of the most liberal IFU available on the U.S. market (Fig. 43-1). Liberalization of the anatomic

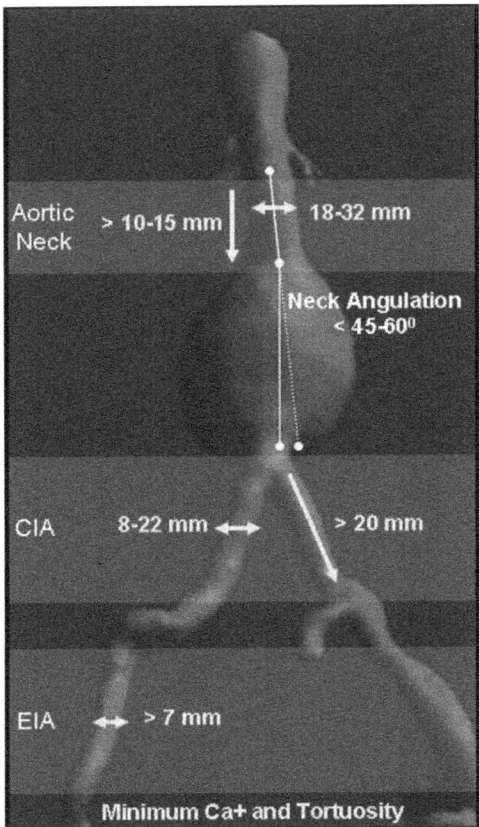

Figure 43-1. The aortic and iliac arterial anatomy boundary conditions defined by the "Instructions for Use" that are packaged with each FDA-approved commercial endovascular aortic device.

characteristics deemed suitable for EVAR has occurred and several of these factors, including aortic neck diameter, aortic neck angle, and common iliac artery diameter, were independently associated with aortic aneurysm sac enlargement (Table 43-2). These observations raise the question as to whether such liberalization is justified using current endovascular device designs.

This analysis of M2S data was meant to be a starting point for a critical conversation in the evolving field of endovascular aneurysm repair, rather than a conclusion. It has now been established unambiguously that the risk of late rupture after EVAR is higher than initially believed.[20] A consensus exists that the primary anatomic determinant of late AAA rupture after EVAR is aortic sac enlargement.[20,25] It is likely that the rate of aortic sac enlargement after EVAR will be dependent on the specific patient population and endovascular device studied. For example, the recent study mentioned above by Dr. Makaroun found the rate of aortic sac enlargement after EVAR to be 21% at five years[10]; although less than the 41% found in this study, this rate of late aortic sac enlargement is still far higher than previously documented. Based on this analysis of patients undergoing EVAR in the M2S database, patients undergoing EVAR outside industry-recommended guidelines occurs frequently and this practice increases the risk of late aortic sac enlargement.

TABLE 43-2. SIGNIFICANT INDEPENDENT PREDICTORS FOR AORTIC ANEURYSM SAC ENLARGEMENT IDENTIFIED ON MULTIVARIABLE COX PROPORTIONAL HAZARDS ANALYSIS

Covariates	Hazard Ratio (95% CI)	P-Value
Age (years)		
<60	Reference	
60–69	0.80 (0.60–1.05)	.11
70–79	0.87 (0.67–1.14)	.31
≥80	1.32 (1.03–1.75)	.05
Female	0.96 (0.82–1.13)	.64
AAA diameter		
Maximum AAA diameter ≥55 mm	0.97 (0.86–1.10)	.62
Aortic neck length		
Length >15 mm		
Length 10–15 mm	0.87 (0.71–1.07)	.19
Length <10 mm	0.94 (0.77–1.15)	.53
Aortic neck diameter		
Diameter at lowest renal artery <28 mm		
Diameter at lowest renal artery 28–32 mm	1.80 (1.44–2.23)	<.0001
Diameter at lowest renal artery >32 mm	2.07 (1.46–2.92)	<.0001
Conical neck	1.17 (0.97–1.42)	.10
Aortic neck angle		
Aortic neck angle <45°		
Aortic neck angle 45–60°	1.04 (0.90–1.21)	.58
Aortic neck angle >60°	1.96 (1.63–2.37)	<.0001
Iliac diameter		
Both common iliac arteries <20 mm		
Only one common iliac arteries >20 mm	1.46 (1.21–1.76)	<.0001
Both common iliac arteries >20 mm	1.31 (0.99–1.74)	.06
Endoleak during follow-up	2.70 (2.40–3.04)	<.0001

Undoubtedly, EVAR represents a tremendous advance in the treatment of AAA and has provided significant benefit to many patients. However, if the widespread application of this technique continues to grow in patients with unfavorable anatomy, these benefits will be offset by increased rates of treatment failure, costly reinterventions, and the potential for late aneurysm rupture. In this context, we are reminded that the high rate of technical feasibility and the outstanding short-term results after EVAR are only meaningful to patients if its ability to protect them against death from AAA rupture is durable over the long term.

A prospective EVAR registry that incorporates an independent imaging registry is necessary to define more precisely the specific aortic and iliac artery anatomic characteristics suitable for EVAR with currently available commercial devices. In patients with anatomy proven to be disadvantaged for currently available commercial devices, endovascular technologies need to evolve so that these anatomic challenges can be treated more effectively. While the next generation EVAR devices, the branched and fenestrated endovascular grafts available at some select sites in trials,[26–28] do provide a means to treat patients with anatomy unfavorable for standard EVAR, these devices are still limited by complexity, requirement for large doses of radiation, prolonged procedure times, expense, and availability. Finally, it is imperative that vascular surgery training programs remain committed to maintain the technical skills of their trainees to perform open surgical repair of AAA that do not have anatomy amenable to endovascular repair. Creative training solutions that incorporate realistic simulation with tactile feedback may be necessary as the number of open aortic cases continues to decline.

In summary, over the past two decades, vascular surgeons have successfully introduced and embraced a new, minimally invasive approach to the treatment of AAA. Countless patients have benefitted from EVAR and it should be noted that in an exceptionally brief span of time, vascular surgeons have developed and implemented the necessary skill set required to provide EVAR to patients safely, with extremely low perioperative mortality. We now find ourselves at a critical moment that requires a rigorous assessment of the advantages and disadvantages of EVAR, as it has become the mainstay for AAA treatment. Device development with a focus on durability to prevent late AAA sac enlargement and rupture is an imperative. While next generation EVAR devices, such as the highly promising branched and fenestrated solutions currently undergoing investigation will expand the anatomic boundary conditions suitable for successful EVAR, current technology makes careful patient selection critical. Caution should be exercised when patients selected for EVAR do not meet device instructions for use and, most importantly, each patient and treating physician must commit to lifelong follow-up incorporating careful endograft imaging surveillance.

REFERENCES

1. Creech O, Jr. Endo-aneurysmorrhaphy and treatment of aortic aneurysm. *Ann Surg.* 1966;164:935–946.
2. Dubost C, Allary M, Oeconomos N. Resection of an aneurysm of the abdominal aorta: reestablishment of the continuity by a preserved human arterial graft, with result after five months. *AMA Arch Surg.* 1952;64:405–408.
3. Parodi JC, Palmaz JC, Barone HD. Transfemoral intraluminal graft implantation for abdominal aortic aneurysms. *Ann Vasc Surg.* 1991;5:491–499.
4. Lederle FA, Wilson SE, Johnson GR, et al. Immediate repair compared with surveillance of small abdominal aortic aneurysms. *N Engl J Med.* 2002;346:1437–1444.
5. Mortality results for randomised controlled trial of early elective surgery or ultrasonographic surveillance for small abdominal aortic aneurysms. The UK small aneurysm trial participants. *Lancet.* 1998;352:1649–1655.
6. Schwarze ML, Shen Y, Hemmerich J, Dale W. Age-related trends in utilization and outcome of open and endovascular repair for abdominal aortic aneurysm in the united states, 2001–2006. *J Vasc Surg.* 2009;50:722–729 e722.
7. Greenhalgh RM, Brown LC, Powell JT, et al. Endovascular versus open repair of abdominal aortic aneurysm. *N Engl J Med.* 2012;362:1863–1871.
8. De Bruin JL, Baas AF, Buth J, et al. Long-term outcome of open or endovascular repair of abdominal aortic aneurysm. *N Engl J Med.* 2010;362:1881–1889.
9. Lederle FA, Freischlag JA, Kyriakides TC, et al. Outcomes following endovascular vs open repair of abdominal aortic aneurysm: a randomized trial. *JAMA.* 2009;302:1535–1542.

10. Hogg ME, Morasch MD, Park T, et al. Long-term sac behavior after endovascular abdominal aortic aneurysm repair with the excluder low-permeability endoprosthesis. *J Vasc Surg.* 2011;53:1178–1183.
11. Sarac TP, Gibbons C, Vargas L, et al. Long-term follow-up of type ii endoleak embolization reveals the need for close surveillance. *J Vasc Surg.* 2012;55:33–40.
12. Prinssen M, Verhoeven EL, Buth J, et al. A randomized trial comparing conventional and endovascular repair of abdominal aortic aneurysms. *N Engl J Med.* 2004;351:1607–1618.
13. EVAR trial participants. Endovascular aneurysm repair versus open repair in patients with abdominal aortic aneurysm (EVAR trial 1): randomised controlled trial. *Lancet.* 2005;365:2179–2186.
14. Matsumura JS, Brewster DC, Makaroun MS, Naftel DC. A multicenter controlled clinical trial of open versus endovascular treatment of abdominal aortic aneurysm. *J Vasc Surg.* 2003;37:262–271.
15. Greenberg RK, Chuter TA, Sternbergh WC, 3rd, Fearnot NE. Zenith AAA endovascular graft: intermediate-term results of the US multicenter trial. *J Vasc Surg.* 2004;39:1209–1218.
16. Schermerhorn ML, O'Malley AJ, Jhaveri A, et al. Endovascular vs. open repair of abdominal aortic aneurysms in the medicare population. *N Engl J Med.* 2008;358:464–474.
17. Fulton JJ, Farber MA, Sanchez LA, et al. Effect of challenging neck anatomy on mid-term migration rates in aneurx endografts. *J Vasc Surg.* 2006;44:932–937; discussion 937.
18. Abbruzzese TA, Kwolek CJ, Brewster DC, et al. Outcomes following endovascular abdominal aortic aneurysm repair (EVAR): an anatomic and device-specific analysis. *J Vasc Surg.* 2008;48:19–28.
19. Greenberg RK, Clair D, Srivastava S, et al. Should patients with challenging anatomy be offered endovascular aneurysm repair? *J Vasc Surg.* 2003;38:990–996.
20. Wyss TR, Brown LC, Powell JT, Greenhalgh RM. Rate and predictability of graft rupture after endovascular and open abdominal aortic aneurysm repair: data from the EVAR trials. *Ann Surg.* 2010;252:805–812.
21. Schanzer A, Greenberg RK, Hevelone N, et al. Predictors of abdominal aortic aneurysm sac enlargement after endovascular repair. *Circulation.* 2011;123:2848–2855.
22. Wang GJ, Carpenter JP. The powerlink system for endovascular abdominal aortic aneurysm repair: six-year results. *J Vasc Surg.* 2008;48:535–545.
23. Deaton DH, Mehta M, Kasirajan K, et al. The phase i multicenter trial (staple-1) of the aptus endovascular repair system: results at 6 months and 1 year. *J Vasc Surg.* 2009;49:851–857; discussion 857–858.
24. Jordan WD Jr, Moore WM Jr, Melton JG, et al. Secure fixation following EVAR with the powerlink XL system in wide aortic necks: results of a prospective, multicenter trial. *J Vasc Surg.* 2009;50:979–986.
25. Mertens J, Houthoofd S, Daenens K, et al. Long-term results after endovascular abdominal aortic aneurysm repair using the Cook Zenith endograft. *J Vasc Surg.* 2011;54:48–57 e42.
26. Greenberg RK, Qureshi M. Fenestrated and branched devices in the pipeline. *J Vasc Surg.* 2010;52(4 suppl):15S–21S.
27. Chuter T, Greenberg RK. Standardized off-the-shelf components for multibranched endovascular repair of thoracoabdominal aortic aneurysms. *Perspect Vasc Surg Endovasc Ther.* 2011;23:195–201.
28. Greenberg RK, Sternbergh WC, 3rd, Makaroun M, et al. Intermediate results of a United States multicenter trial of fenestrated endograft repair for juxtarenal abdominal aortic aneurysms. *J Vasc Surg.* 2009;50:730–737 e731.

44

Inflammatory Aneurysms: Repair Open or with EVAR?

William M. Stone, MD and Grant T. Fankhauser, MD

INTRODUCTION

In 1935 James reported the findings of an inflammatory aneurysm in a patient with ureteral obstruction from a retroperitoneal inflammatory process.[1] The patient was also noted to have a large abdominal aortic aneurysm, but the correlation of inflammation and aneurysm formation had not been previously reported. In 1955 Garrett and Schumacker[2] reported the case of a 13 cm abdominal aortic aneurysm presenting with fibrosis and retroperitoneal inflammation. The patient also had ureteral obstruction related to a dense inflammatory process in the retroperitoneum. The first series of inflammatory aneurysms was reported in 1972 when Walker et al. reported a series of 19 patients who had abdominal aortic aneurysms and retroperitoneal fibrosis.[3] They were the first to coin the term "inflammatory aneurysms." Approximately 3%–10% of abdominal aortic aneurysms are now characterized by abnormal inflammation surrounding the aneurysm.[4] This finding is classically described as a white, glistening fibrotic surface with a thickened aneurysmal wall. The inflammatory process frequently involves neighboring structures such as the ureters, vena cava, or duodenum. Between 15% and 30% of patients with this inflammatory aneurysm have entrapment of the ureters with resultant hydronephrosis. This reaction leads to significant adhesion formation within the retroperitoneum and increases the morbidity of open surgical intervention.

Histologically, the tissues of inflammatory abdominal aortic aneurysms (IAAAs) demonstrate elastic and muscular fibers of the aortic media that have been replaced by fibrosis. Inflammatory cells such as plasma cells and lymphocytes are also present.[5] Clinically, these patients present with symptoms of abdominal pain radiating to the back; fatigue and weight loss are not uncommon. Frequently noted is an elevated erythrocyte sedimentation rate. The key to diagnosis is the degree of retroperitoneal fibrosis. Imaging with computed tomography (CT) has been the primary means for establishing the diagnosis preoperatively. Historically the diagnosis was often not made until the time of open surgical repair, but the diagnosis is made more frequently now before surgery with more routine axial imaging.

The fibrotic changes seen in patients with inflammatory aneurysms present an increased risk of morbidity during open surgery. This surgical challenge has been reported numerous times in the literature with suggestions of higher morbidity, higher mortality, longer operating time, and increased need for transfusions.[6] Because of these risks, it has been theorized that endovascular repair (EVAR) could offer an advantage in the treatment these aneurysms. There are conflicting reports with opinions on the advantages and the disadvantages of treating IAAA with EVAR.[7–10]

The prevailing management of patients with IAAA is still surgical, either open or endovascular. While there may be emerging theories of medical treatment, the mainstay of therapy remains intervention. While it is attractive to consider EVAR in an effort to avoid complications documented in open surgical repair, little long-term data exist that validates its efficacy. In particular, although case reports suggest decreased inflammation and the resolution of ureteral obstruction, there are few series to suggest that this reliably occurs after EVAR for inflammatory aneurysms.

OPEN REPAIR

While IAAA can be approached through a midline incision, many surgeons elect to utilize a retroperitoneal approach. This affords direct access to the aorta while minimizing the manipulation of fibrotic intraperitoneal tissues. Preoperative ureteral stent placement is a common strategy for ureteral identification when there is extensive inflammation. In addition, these stents may be left in place until resolution of the inflammatory process occurs to help correct ureteral obstruction. Encountering an unanticipated inflammatory aneurysm is becoming less common with the increased use of preoperative axial imaging such as CT. Inflammatory aneurysms are often unanticipated in those patients presenting with rupture since preoperative imaging is often not obtained.

The morbidity of open repair of IAAA most frequently involves injury to adjacent structures. The inflammatory process obscures normal tissue planes and leads to more bleeding than with normal tissue. This subsequently leads to injury of surrounding structures and thus increases the risk of complications. Several authors have reported high complication rates and as many as 25% of patients require suprarenal aortic cross clamp for adequate repair. These are compelling reasons to attempt EVAR.

ENDOVASCULAR REPAIR

Avoiding an inflamed, fibrotic retroperitoneum is the driving force behind the desire to repair IAAA endovascularly. Aneurysms that are anatomically suitable are tempting to treat with a stent graft, but there has been debate as to whether the inflammatory process will regress after repair. Some surgeons believe that the inflammation might persist despite aneurysm exclusion and eventual open repair could be necessary. However, several series now suggests that there is resolution of this inflammation and that EVAR should be the first line of therapy.

PUBLISHED REPORTS ON ENDOVASCULAR REPAIR OF INFLAMMATORY ANEURYSMS

The outcomes of open surgery for the management of inflammatory aneurysms are noted with an increased complication rate compared to noninflammatory aneurysms. In one large series it was demonstrated that operative mortality increased threefold when comparing inflammatory to noninflammatory aneurysms.[6] In addition, there is a significant increase in major morbidity between open surgery for inflammatory aneurysms compared to noninflammatory aneurysms.[11] In the early years of vascular surgery, extensive retroperitoneal adhesiolysis was routinely performed.[12] This practice led to major complications including enterotomies and duodenal injury. Furthermore, there was a significant rate of ureteral injury due to this extensive dissection. In order to decrease the perioperative complications, it was suggested in the late 1970s to avoid extensive adhesiolysis in an inflamed retroperitoneum.[13]

In light of the morbidity and mortality from open repair of IAAA, the option of endovascular aneurysm is intuitively appealing. However, the benefit from endovascular intervention is still unproven. Does the endovascular approach reduce not only the risk of aneurysmal rupture but also the long-term risk of periaortic fibrosis? Not only are the ureters potentially involved in the inflammatory process, but the duodenum and kidneys may be involved as well. Certain groups, such as the one from Liverpool,[14] would suggest that EVAR is not suitable for IAAA due to the persistence of perianeurysmal fibrosis after endograft placement. Other publications, such as the meta-analysis from the EUROSTAR and other meta-analyses, offer mixed results.[8–10,15]

The technical success of EVAR in our institution was 100%. All of the aneurysms undergoing attempt at EVAR were treated successfully. Aneurysm size was significantly reduced postoperatively in this group of patients. The amount of periaortic fibrosis was significantly reduced in six of seven patients who underwent postoperative imaging. One of those seven patients demonstrated stable inflammation on follow-up. Aneurysm sac shrinkage was present in seven of nine patients. The remaining two patients had no change in the size of the aneurysm. There were no endoleaks identified in any patient undergoing EVAR during periprocedural imaging or during long term follow-up.

In a series involving nine patients from Modena, Italy, the long-term results of EVAR are discussed.[16] They reported good survival rates with follow-up as long as 60 months. Technical success was achieved in a significant number with low mortality. Aneurysm sac shrinkage occurred in 89% of patients. There was no aneurysm rupture or aneurysm-related death. A 55% reduction in the inflammatory process was seen by measuring the thickness of the periaortic fibrosis in this group of patients. This finding is similar to our results of the Mayo Clinic series (Table 44-1).

One of the most extensive series of EVAR for IAAA to date would be the report from the EUROSTAR database.[8] This study compares the results of IAAAs versus noninflammatory aortic aneurysms managed with EVAR. This series includes 52 patients with IAAA, which represents 1.4% of the EUROSTAR data. All patients had the diagnosis of inflammatory aneurysm made by CT imaging. The mean age of patients with inflammatory aneurysms was approximately six years younger than noninflammatory aneurysms. There were other significant differences found in this series and identified by other large series of inflammatory aneurysms. These include the prevalence of smoking was significantly greater in patients with inflammatory aneurysms and

TABLE 44-1. PREOPERATIVE AGE AND ANEURYSM SIZE

Age(years)	EVAR	Open	Total	
N	10	59	69	
Mean (SD)	72.2 (8.02)	66.2 (10.43)	67.1 (10.29)	
SEM	2.54	1.36	1.24	(*p*=0.09)
Median	71.5	68.0	68.0	
Range	(62.0–82.0)	(23.0–83.0)	(23.0–83.0)	
Preoperative size (cm)				
N	10	56	66	
Mean (SD)	5.9 (1.24)	6.3 (1.57)	6.2 (1.52)	
SEM	0.39	0.21	0.18	(*p*=0.51)
Median	6.0	6.0	6.0	
Range	(4.0–8.3)	(3.4–11.3)	(3.4–11.3)	

the prevalence of hypertension was significantly lower. Also, cardiac and pulmonary disease is less common in patients with inflammatory aneurysms compared to those with noninflammatory aneurysms. This may be due to the younger age of patients with inflammatory aneurysms. Operating time for EVAR in inflammatory aneurysms compared to noninflammatory aneurysms was not significantly different. There was a significant increase in the rate of limb stenosis or occlusion in patients with inflammatory aneurysms. This problem may be related to the severe inflammatory reaction surrounding the aneurysm. However, this finding was not found in our series but may be related to the type of endograft used. Overall, the morbidity and mortality were not significantly different between inflammatory and noninflammatory aneurysms. Minor complications such as access-site infections were likewise not statistically different.

The EUROSTAR data also provide results for long-term outcomes.[8] It is interesting to note that there was no significant difference in the rate of endoleaks when comparing EVAR for IAAA versus those undergoing EVAR for a noninflammatory aortic aneurysm. Additionally, there was no difference in device migration, kinking, or thrombosis. There was also no difference in aneurysm shrinkage between the two groups. What was significantly different was the decline in renal function in the IAAA group. If patients were followed long-term, renal function deteriorated in 27% of all IAAA patients. The effect of EVAR on the amount of inflammatory fibrosis is less clear. EVAR demonstrated a significant reduction in the amount of inflammation in only half of the patients.

The results published by Puchner et al. from Vienna parallel the results of the EUROSTAR data.[10] This meta-analysis of the treatment of inflammatory aortic aneurysms by EVAR had a mean follow-up of 18 months. The results are quite similar to both ours and the EUROSTAR data. Periaortic fibrosis was reduced by approximately 51% in this group; in 42% there was no significant change in periaortic fibrosis; and in 7% there was an increase in the periaortic fibrosis postoperatively. In this series, in comparison with our reported results, there was a large male predominance, similar to the EUROSTAR, with 98% of the patients being male. In another large meta-analysis, Paravastu and coworkers presented a review of open versus EVAR for IAAA.[14] They again demonstrated a significantly higher mortality rate with open repair (6.2% versus 2.4%). They suggest that there is no significant difference in open versus EVAR on the resolution of the inflammatory process. Patients demonstrating significant reduction in fibrosis included 73% in the open group versus 65% with use of EVAR (p=ns). In the open group hydronephrosis and hydroureter were improved in 69% of the patients, whereas only 38% in the EVAR group shower improvement (p=0.01). In addition, the hydronephrosis or hydroureter progressively worsened in 9% in the open group versus 21% of the patients in the EVAR group. However, the all-cause one-year mortality was significantly greater in the open group versus the EVAR group (p=0.01).

RECENT EXPERIENCE

We recently performed a retrospective review on all patients with the diagnosis of IAAA undergoing repair from January 1, 1999, through July 31, 2011, in the Mayo Clinic System. This included all patients from Mayo Clinic in Rochester, MN, Phoenix, AZ, and Jacksonville, FL. The diagnosis of IAAA was made by the operating surgeon at the time of intervention in those patients undergoing open repair and was dependent on the clinical judgment of the vascular surgeon. In patients undergoing EVAR the diagnosis of IAAA was made by radiologic interpretation of computerized tomography. Excluded from review were those patients who had inflammation noted on radiographic imaging but were not deemed by the surgeon to have a true inflammatory aneurysm at the time of surgery. Also excluded were those patients with infectious etiologies.

OVERALL RESULTS

During the 12-year study period, 69 patients underwent intervention for repair of IAAA and were included for review (Table 44-2). During the same time period approximately 3500 noninflammatory AAA were repaired. The mean age of patients undergoing intervention for IAAA was 67.1 years (range 23–83 years) including 53 males (77%) and 16 (23%) females. The majority of patients experienced symptoms of pain (36/69, 52%). Four patients (5.6%) presented with ruptured IAAA. Ureteral involvement in the inflammatory process by CT imaging was seen in 23 patients (32.3%), and 21 of the 23 (91.3%) underwent preoperative ureteral stent placement. Mean preoperative aneurysm size in the overall group was 6.2 cm in maximum diameter (range 3.4–11.3cm) and did not include the rind. Follow-up ranged from 1 to 144 months with a mean of 41.1 months. Eighteen patients (25.7%) were lost to follow-up. There was one postoperative death (1.4%) in a patient undergoing open repair for a ruptured suprarenal IAAA.

TABLE 44-2. CURRENT RESULTS AND COMPARISON TO PUBLISHED DATA

	Coppi et al.[16]	Lange et al.[8]	Mayo Clinic
IAAA treated with EVAR	9	52	10
Aneurysm-related deaths	0	1 (1.8%)	0
Patients with decreased periaortic inflammation post-op	78%	—	86%
Patients with decreased aneurysm size post-op	89%	87%	70%

RESULTS OF OPEN REPAIR

Fifty nine of the 69 patients (85.5%) with IAAA underwent conventional open aneurysm repair during the study period. Three patients (5.0%) presented with ruptured aneurysm. Ureteral involvement with inflammation was present in 21 (34.4%), and preoperative ureteral stent placement was performed in 19 of these patients. Four patients (6.7%) were administered perioperative steroids for treatment of comorbid conditions but not for resolution of the inflammatory process. Supra renal aortic cross clamping was required for repair in 36 (61%) of these patients to attain adequate control of the aorta.

Preoperative mean aneurysm size was 6.3 cm (range 3.4–11.3 cm). A midline abdominal incision was performed in 52 patients (88%), a retroperitoneal approach was utilized in 6 patients (10%), and bilateral subcostal incision was performed in 1 patient (1.6%). Twenty-two major postoperative complications occurred in these 59 patients (37.9%) undergoing open repair. These complications included renal insufficiency in five patients (8.3%) needing postoperative dialysis. Ischemic colitis was present in two patients (3.3%), but no patient required colonic resection. Postoperative ureteral obstruction requiring intervention occurred in three patients (4.9%). There was one death (1.6%) in the 30-day postoperative period in a patient presenting with a ruptured suprarenal IAAA. There were no aneurysm-related deaths identified during follow-up.

Mean follow-up was 42.6 months (median 29.0) with a range of 1 to 144 months. 17 patients (28.3%) were lost during the follow-up period. Of 42 patients (71.1%) who had postoperative imaging, all had resolution of the aneurysm sac. Hydronephrosis was found to resolve in 7/12 patients (58.3%).

RESULTS OF ENDOVASCULAR REPAIR

There were 10 patients (14%) who underwent EVAR for management of their IAAA during the study period. The mean age was 72.2 years. Preoperatively, eight patients (80%) experienced abdominal pain and, one of these (10%) presented with a ruptured aneurysm. Two patients (20%) had ureteral involvement in the inflammatory process and one of those required pre-procedural stenting. Preoperative mean aneurysm size was 5.9 cm (range 4.0–8.3 cm).

Postoperative aneurysm size decreased in seven patients (70%), with two patients (20%) showing no change in aneurysm size and one patient lost during the follow-up period. Mean follow-up was 33.6 months. Postoperative mean aneurysm size was 4.73 cm. The mean change in size was a decrease of 1.12 cm. Of all patients with postoperative imaging, there was a mean decrease in aneurysm size of 17.8% (range 57.6%–0%). The inflammatory rind preoperatively measured 5.4 mm in mean thickness in patients with IAAA undergoing EVAR. Postoperatively, the mean size of inflammatory rind was 2.7 mm. One patient had increase in the size of the inflammatory rind but had no change in the size of the aneurysm sac. All other patients had decrease in the size of the inflammatory rind. Mean decrease in the thickness of the inflammatory rind was 50.8% (range 92.1%–0%). Postoperative abdominal pain was resolved in six of seven patients (85.7%) following EVAR.

Two patients (20%) developed atrial fibrillation postoperatively, but there were no other significant complications reported. No patient required subsequent intervention for repair of the aneurysm, and no endoleaks were identified in follow-up. There was no perioperative mortality and no patient died of aneurysm-related causes during the follow-up period.

ARGUMENTS AGAINST EVAR

Endovascular aortic aneurysm repair in itself produces inflammation in the aorta. This reaction is not as immediate a response as in open repair; however, over time it may be significant.[17] It has been hypothesized that this increase in inflammation may be due to reaction to the Dacron in the endograft, however, similar results have been demonstrated in grafts using PTFE. The possibility that EVAR generates its own inflammatory reaction adds to the skepticism that EVAR will promote the resolution of inflammation in IAAA. This skepticism is unfounded based on our results in which inflammation improved in all cases of EVAR.

Numerous reports demonstrate, similar to our present series, that EVAR for inflammatory aneurysm successfully reduces the size of the aortic aneurysm in a majority of patients. It also reduces the amount of periaortic fibrosis but not to the extent that open aneurysm repair does. EVAR outcomes are achieved with a lower morbidity and one-year mortality. The Achilles heel of EVAR for IAAAs revolves around renal and ureter involvement. The improvements in hydroureter and hydronephrosis are inferior with EVAR compared to open repair. We hypothesize that this difference in renal improvement may be related to the fact that the periaortic fibrosis resolves at a slower rate compared to open repair. On the basis of our results and results in literature, one would suggest that EVAR is appropriate treatment for inflammatory aortic aneurysms where there is no renal or ureter involvement in the inflammation. It may also be successful treatment for a proportion of patients with renal or ureter involvement if they are poor open surgical risks.

CONCLUSIONS

EVAR is an effective treatment for inflammatory aneurysms, but there may be less resolution of the inflammatory process. Follow-up imaging in necessary to monitor the involvement of the ureters and resolution of any hydronephrosis. Further intervention may be necessary after EVAR repair. Open surgical repair is always an option. The suitability of the patient for a major operation must be balanced with the possibility that EVAR may not resolve all the inflammatory process.

REFERENCES

1. James TGI. Uremia due to aneurysm of the abdominal aorta. *Br J Urol*. 1935;7:157.
2. Schumacker HB Jr, Garrett R. Obstructive uropathy from abdominal aortic aneurysm. *Surg Gynecol Obstetr*. 955;100:758–761.
3. Walker DI, Bloor K, Williams G, Gillie I. Inflammatory aneurysms of the abdominal aorta. *Br J Surg*. 1972;59:609–614.

4. Sueyoshi E, Sakamoto I, Uetani M. Endovascular repair of inflammatory abdominal aortic aneurysm: serial changes of periaortic fibrosis demonstrated by CT. *Abdom Imaging*. 2009;34:523–526.

5. van Bommel EF, van der Veer SJ, Hendriksz TR, Bleumink GS. Persistent chronic peri-aortitis ('inflammatory aneurysm') after abdominal aortic aneurysm repair: systematic review of the literature. *Vasc Med*. 2008;13:293–303.

6. Pennell RC, Hollier LH, Lie JT, et al. Inflammatory abdominal aortic aneurysms: a thirty-year review. *J Vasc Surg*. 1985;2:859–869.

7. Hechelhammer L, Wildermuth S, Lachat ML, Pfammatter T. Endovascular repair of inflammatory abdominal aneurysm: a retrospective analysis of CT follow-up. *J Vasc Intervent Radiol. JVIR*. 2005;16:737–741.

8. Lange C, Hobo R, Leurs LJ, et al. Results of endovascular repair of inflammatory abdominal aortic aneurysms. A report from the EUROSTAR database. *Eur J Vasc Endovasc Surg*. 2005;29:363–370.

9. Hinchliffe RJ, Macierewicz JA, Hopkinson BR. Endovascular repair of inflammatory abdominal aortic aneurysms. *J Endovasc Ther*. 2002;9:277–281.

10. Puchner S, Bucek RA, Rand T, et al. Endovascular therapy of inflammatory aortic aneurysms: a meta-analysis. *J Endovasc Ther*. 2005;12:560–567.

11. Sultan S, Duffy S, Madhavan P, et al. Fifteen-year experience of transperitoneal management of inflammatory abdominal aortic aneurysms. *Eur J Vasc Endovasc Surg*. 1999;18:510–514.

12. Ruppert V, Verrel F, Kellner W, et al. Endovascular repair of inflammatory abdominal aortic aneurysms: a valuable alternative?—Case report and review of literature. *Ann Vasc Surg*. 2004;18:357–360.

13. Goldstone J, Malone JM, Moore WS. Inflammatory aneurysms of the abdominal aorta. *Surgery*. 1978;83:425–430.

14. Vallabhaneni SR, McWilliams RG, Anbarasu A, et al. Perianeurysmal fibrosis: a relative contra-indication to endovascular repair. *Eur J Vasc Endovasc Surg*. 2001;22:535–541.

15. Paravastu SC, Ghosh J, Murray D, et al. A systematic review of open versus endovascular repair of inflammatory abdominal aortic aneurysms. *Eur J Vasc Endovasc Surg*. 2009;38:291–297.

16. Coppi G, Rametta F, Aiello S, et al. Inflammatory abdominal aortic aneurysm endovascular repair into the long-term follow-up. *Ann Vasc Surg*. 2010;24:1053–1059.

17. Abdelhamid MF, Davies RS, Adam DJ, et al. Changes in thrombin generation, fibrinolysis, platelet and endothelial cell activity, and inflammation following endovascular abdominal aortic aneurysm repair. *J Vasc Surg*. 2012;55:41–46.

45

Blunt Abdominal Aortic Injury

Sherene Shalhub, MD, MPH and
Megan Brenner, MD, MS

BACKGROUND/INCIDENCE/EPIDEMIOLOGY

Blunt abdominal aortic injury (BAAI) remains one of the most challenging injuries. Many patients die of hemorrhage before hospital arrival and those who survive to the hospital can be hemodynamically unstable due to hemorrhage and associated injuries.[1,2] The reported incidence of BAAI is less than 1% of all blunt trauma–associated injuries, Since 1996, 117 cases of have been reported as case reports or case series with motor vehicle crashes being the predominant mechanism. Table 45-1 summarizes the demographics and associated injuries of 100 cases reported with sufficient detail for data extrapolation.

ANATOMY/PHYSIOLOGY

The abdominal aorta is a retroperitoneal structure tethered to the spinal column, the peritoneum, and abdominal viscera. In a motor vehicle crash, injury occurs due to compressive forces associated with deceleration resulting in direct and indirect biomechanical forces that stretch the aortic wall and compress the aorta against a high-pressure column of blood. This has been described as a "seat belt aorta."[3] These direct and indirect forces lead to intimal tears, pseudoaneurysm, rupture, or thrombosis. The most common location is inferior to the renal arteries as shown in Table 45-1. Other mechanisms include long distance falls from heights, direct compression of the aorta, and penetrating injuries.

Depending on the magnitude of the traumatic forces, BAAI presents as a spectrum of disease. This includes minimal aortic injury (MAI),[4] intimal flaps or dissection, and free rupture of the aorta (Fig. 45-1). Rupture of the aortic wall can also be due to branch vessel avulsion.[1] BAAI can be complicated by thrombosis and acute arterial insufficiency. Injuries involving the adventitia can cause pseudoaneurysm formation as shown in Figure 45-1C. Since 1996, the most commonly reported type of BAAI were intimal tears/flaps (41%) followed by pseudoaneurysms (29%).[5]

TABLE 45-1. A SUMMARY OF THE CLINICAL PRESENTATION, ASSOCIATED INJURIES, AND LOCATION OF ABDOMINAL AORTIC INJURY OF 100 BLUNT ABDOMINAL AORTIC INJURY CASES REPORTED SINCE 1996

	N = 100 (Values Are Also %)
Median age (range)	30 years (1–89)
Male	70
Hypotensive on admission (<90 mm Hg)	34
Cardiac arrest in route, ED or OR	14
Abdominal wall ecchymosis (Seat belt sign)	34
Associated injuries	
Retroperitoneal hematoma	50
Small bowel injury	38
Spine fracture	32
Mesenteric hematoma/laceration	26
Solid organ injury	25
Colon injury	22
Lower extremity ischemia	17
Pelvic fracture	16
Pneumothorax/hemothorax	13
Traumatic brain injury	11
Rib fractures	10
Abdominal wall degloving	9
IVC injury	8
Location on aorta	
Diaphragmatic hiatus to SMA	8
SMA to RA	6
Infrarenal	86

Abbreviations: ED, emergency department; OR, operating room; RA, renal artery; SMA, superior mesenteric artery.

CLINICAL ASSESSMENT

The initial presentation of BAAI is variable and dependent on presence of free rupture of the aortic wall, branch vessel avulsion, or concomitant inferior vena cava injury.[1] These cases present with hemodynamic instability due to hemorrhagic shock. In a recent BAAI series, 75% of these cases had cardiac arrest in the emergency department and 38% required an emergency department thoracotomy.[5]

In the hemodynamically stable patient, abdominal wall ecchymosis due to seat belt injury can be seen in one-third of cases and should raise the index of suspicion for associated hollow viscous and aortic injuries. Tamponade is usually associated with retroperitoneal hematoma and may allow a temporary period of hemodynamic

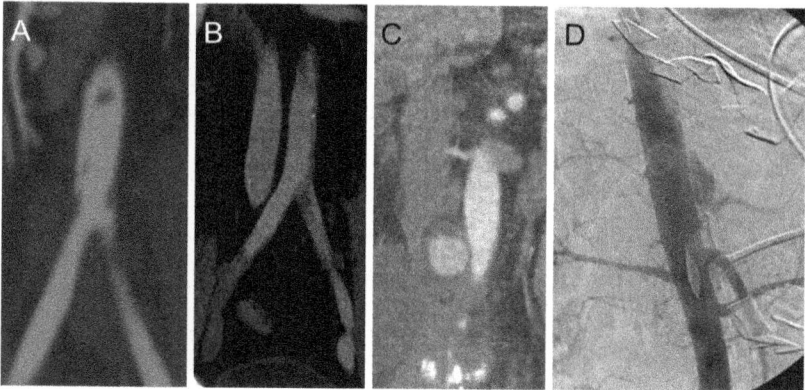

Figure 45-1. Examples of blunt abdominal aortic injuries. *A,* Coronal computed tomography (CT) image demonstrating two infrarenal intimal tears measuring less than 1 cm each between the inferior mesenteric artery and aortic bifurcation. This case was managed nonoperatively with resolution of the intimal tears on follow-up imaging. *B,* Coronal CT image demonstrating a large intimal flap extending from the renal arteries to the iliac arteries with thrombosis of the right common lilac artery. This injury was repaired by endovascular stent graft placement. *C,* Coronal CT image demonstrating an infrarenal pseudoaneurysm found incidentally two weeks post–blunt trauma. This injury was repaired by endovascular stent graft placement. *D,* An aortogram demonstrating active extravasation at the site of avulsed celiac artery. This was treated by endovascular cuff placement.

stability. Further diagnostic testing such as CT scan may then be obtained, which can provide critical information in further determining treatment strategies for these complex injuries. Concomitant limb ischemia may be present due to intimal flaps complicated by thrombosis and acute arterial insufficiency, thus it is imperative to assess the peripheral vasculature for involvement of limb ischemia during the initial assessment.

DIAGNOSTIC TESTING

Proceeding to further diagnostic testing is dependent on the findings of the primary survey. In the case of the hemodynamically stable patient, a CT arteriogram (CTA) is the initial diagnostic modality of choice, allowing for rapid evaluation of the aortic anatomy and high degree of sensitivity in the detection of abdominal injuries.[6,7] Intravenous contrast is an important step in the protocol that allows even the most minor injuries to be seen. Based on aortic contour abnormalities seen on CTA, the aortic injuries can be classified[5] as follows:

Intimal tear/minimal aortic injury (MAI): absence of aortic external contour abnormality and intimal defect and/or thrombus of <10 mm in length or width
Large intimal flap (LIF): absence of aortic external contour abnormality and intimal defect and/or thrombus of ≥10 mm in length or width
Pseudoaneurysm: external aortic contour abnormality and contained rupture
Rupture: external aortic contour abnormality with free contrast extravasation or hemoperitoneum found upon laparotomy

INTRAVASCULAR ULTRASOUND

Intravascular ultrasound (IVUS) is an endovascular imaging tool that may play a significant role in the diagnosis of vascular injury in the future. Developed in the 1960s by Born for two-dimensional imaging of coronary vessels, the IVUS takes the concept of ultrasound and applies it to a "view from the inside" approach. The IVUS is the most sophisticated diagnostic tool available as it is the only modality able to visualize all three arterial layers simultaneously. It allows measurement of lumen diameter to accurately size stent grafts, examine wall thickness, lesion shape, size, and type, as well as visualizing blood flow with the color-flow mode.

IVUS can be used for diagnostic purposes by its ability to determine chronic variants from acute injuries, rule out injuries deemed indeterminate by other modalities, and determine candidates for endovascular therapy.[8] A comparison of CT, angiography, and IVUS studies in blunt traumatic aortic injury reported an unmatched sensitivity and specificity (100%) of the IVUS compared to all other modalities.[4] During treatment of vascular injury, the IVUS can give accurate measurements for sizing and placement of stent grafts as well as confirm apposition and absence of endoleak (potentially decreasing contrast exposure). The IVUS may be used as a screening tool, for follow-up of minor injuries, or in lieu of CTA or angiogram when contrast is contraindicated. Its use in the diagnosis and management of BAAI is unproven; however, it is an attractive option in the multitrauma patient, given its capabilities to provide useful information without potential renal toxicity.

MANAGEMENT

The management of BAAI is evolving with the advances in trauma evaluation and endovascular intervention and is tailored to the type of BAAI.[9,10] Utilizing a CTA as the initial diagnostic modality of choice in hemodynamically stable patients has resulted in increasingly frequent detection of otherwise clinically occult aortic injuries such as minimal aortic injuries (MAI).[4,11–13] Moreover, reports of endovascular stent grafts placement for BAAI are increasing in frequency signaling a paradigm shift in management.

NONOPERATIVE MANAGEMENT

Two of the largest series of BAAI in the literature suggest that based on radiologic findings, a reasonable proportion of patients may be managed nonoperatively. A series from the University of Washington identified 28 individuals with BAAI over a 14-year period.[5] BAAI presented as MAI (21%), LIF (39%), pseudoaneurysm (11%), and free rupture (29%). Nonoperative management with blood pressure control using β-blockers coupled with antiplatelet therapy and close follow-up was utilized in 32% of the cases, all MAI, and uncomplicated LIF. This was successful as the injury remained stable or resolved on follow-up. Another series from the University of Maryland identified 17 BAAI patients over an 11-year period.[12] MAI was seen in 52% of the cases, all managed nonoperatively without complications except in one case which progressed to a pseudoaneurysm within eight months.

In general, cases of BAAI with MAI and uncomplicated LIF can be managed nonoperatively with blood pressure control using β-blockers, if tolerated, antiplatelet therapy with aspirin (81 mg daily), and close follow-up with repeat CTA. The natural history in these cases appears to be a decrease in size and resolution[4,5,11,14]; however, long-term surveillance is required to document complete resolution or stability, as even MAI can progress to a more complex lesion.[12] For the more extensive injuries such as pseudoaneurysms or LIF complicated by thrombosis or acute arterial insufficiency, operative repair is warranted. The timing of repair is dependent on the patient's hemodynamic status and the presence of acute limb ischemia.

OPEN REPAIR

Initial management is determined by the hemodynamic state of the patient in addition to results of the Focused Assessment with Sonography for Trauma (FAST) scan. During the primary survey of the injured patient, the FAST scan detects free fluid in the abdomen. If positive in the hemodynamically unstable patient, prompt exploratory laparotomy is warranted.

Perioperative considerations include a wide prep from the sternal notch to upper anterior thighs. This allows access to the anterior thorax should a thoracic injury be identified or if vascular control through the thorax is needed. Distally preparing the upper anterior thighs allows for saphenous vein harvest should vascular reconstruction be necessary. If associated bowel injury is suspected, broad spectrum antibiotic should be administered before incision.

A midline laparotomy incision can be made rapidly and allows exposure of all zones of the abdomen. Initial inspection identifies areas of ongoing hemorrhage, contained hematoma, or evidence of bowel ischemia.[15] Further exposure is guided by the location of the associated hematoma, which may be supramesocolic or inframesocolic and indicates aortic injury until proven otherwise. In the case of a supramesocolic hematoma, proximal control of the aorta can be obtained at the diaphragmatic hiatus. The supraceliac aorta is exposed by opening the gastrohepatic ligament, lateral retraction of the left lobe of the liver, and caudal retraction of the stomach. The esophagus is mobilized laterally, its location facilitated by the presence of a nasogastric or orogastric tube. Aortic control can be achieved manually with compression or by vascular clamp placement. Full exposure of the supraceliac aorta and its branches is achieved with left medial visceral rotation (the Mattox maneuver). For an inframesocolic hematoma, exposure is obtained in a transperitoneal fashion similar to that of an infrarenal aneurysm: caudal retraction of the transverse colon, retraction of the small intestine to the right, and cephalad mobilization of the third and fourth portions of the duodenum. The proximal extent of this exposure is the left renal vein that can be divided if necessary between clamps for more cephalad access to the aorta. Proximal control of the aorta can be obtained immediately below the renal arteries or at the diaphragm.[16]

Repair of the aorta is determined by extent of injury and presence of gross contamination from hollow injury. In cases of aortic tears, multiple injuries can be connected and closed in linear fashion using polypropylene suture, Dacron patch aortoplasty, or Dacron graft interposition depending on the size of the tear.[16] In cases of intimal flaps complicated by thrombosis and acute arterial insufficiency, repair is accomplished with thrombectomy and tacking sutures of the intimal flap or Dacron graft interposition if the damage to the intima is substantial. Pseudoaneurysms usually require excision with primary end-to-end anastomosis or interposition grafting.

In cases in which damage control laparotomy is needed, shunts such as chest tubes and endotracheal tubes can be used to establish temporary control, in a damage control fashion until hypothermia, coagulopathy, and acidosis are corrected.

Severe contamination from hollow viscus injury can place the aortic grafts at risk of infection. Thus ligation of the injured aorta with extra-anatomic bypass, such as axillobifemoral bypass, may be required. Endovascular repair of the aortic injury may be considered as discussed in the following section.

ENDOVASCULAR REPAIR

Management of BAAI has been extrapolated from experience with blunt thoracic aortic injuries (BTAI). The 1st and 2nd American Association for the Surgery of Trauma (AAST) BTAI trials, endovascular management significantly reduced the mortality of BTAI from 31% to 13% within a decade.[9,10] In comparison to BTAI, there are few studies to guide BAAI management. In a recent review of the National Trauma Data Bank of 436 patients with BAAI from 180 centers, 90% were managed nonperatively. Of those who underwent operative repair, 69% underwent endovascular repair, with the remainder undergoing open aortic repair and two extra-anatomic bypasses.[17] A recent series of BAAI demonstrated that 60% of lesions were limited to the intima, and the rates of nonoperative and endovascular management were 32% and 21%, respectively.[5] These studies suggest that BAAI management may be evolving similar to changes in BTAI.[10,13,18,19]

The use of endovascular stent graft placement in cases of BAAI offers an attractive alternative to open repair because of less invasive nature of the intervention in patients with isolated aortic injuries as well as those with multisystem trauma. Endovascular repair offers a practical solution for the cases associated with severe gross contamination of the abdomen from hollow viscus injury. Thus, placement of the trauma patient on a radiolucent table allows for the utilization of endovascular interventions should they become needed. With the endovascular approach in mind, the abdominal aorta zones of injury can be classified based on feasibility of endovascular approach[5] as follows (Fig. 45-2):

Zone I injuries occur from diaphragmatic hiatus to the superior mesenteric artery (SMA)
Zone II injuries include the SMA and the renal arteries
Zone III injuries are from the inferior aspect of the renal arteries to the aortic bifurcation

Zone I and III injuries are amenable to endovascular repair whereas Zone II lesions are not amenable to endovascular repair without fenestration for the SMA and renal arteries.

Although the durability of these repairs is yet to be proven, these interventions can be used as a stabilizing measure for critically ill patients and a bridge to open elective definitive repair in the future. Clearly long-term follow-up is required in these cases.

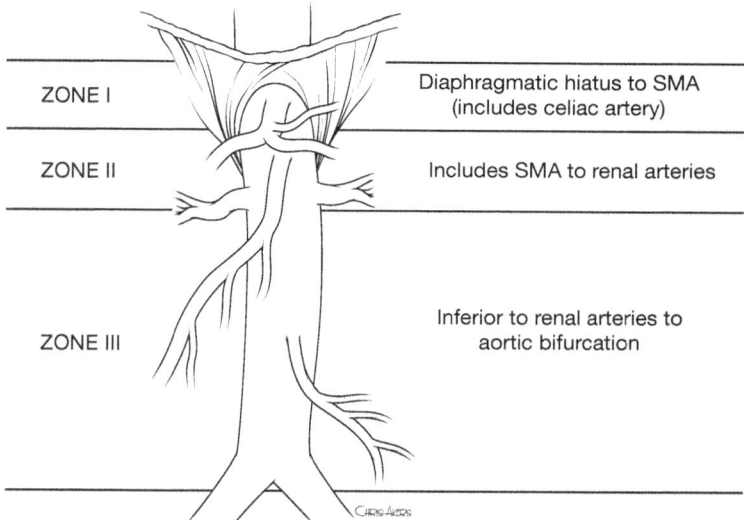

Figure 45-2. Classification of the abdominal aorta zones of injury based on feasibility of endovascular approach. Zone I and III injuries are amenable to endovascular repair whereas Zone II lesions are not amenable to endovascular repair without fenestration for the SMA and renal arteries.

RESUSCITATIVE ENDOVASCULAR BALLOON OCCLUSION OF THE AORTA (REBOA)

The most common cause of death from aortic trauma remains noncompressible hemorrhagic shock compounded by ongoing coagulopathy, thus early proximal control of the aorta is a life-saving maneuver.[1,5,20,21]

Classically, this is obtained through a resuscitative anterolateral thoracotomy for which outcomes remain poor.[22] The placement intra-aortic occlusion balloon (IAOB) in the descending thoracic aorta through transfemoral access offers expeditious proximal aortic occlusion and hemorrhage control. Once this is in place, the patient can be stabilized before entering the abdomen, and further angiographic imaging can be obtained, thus facilitating a decision for endovascular versus open repair of injury. This technique has been described in cases of ruptured abdominal aortic aneurysms and more recently described as an adjunct for control of exsanguinating hemorrhage.[23,24] The first contemporary case series using resuscitative endovascular balloon occlusion of the aorta (REBOA) by acute care surgeons in trauma patients suggests that REBOA may improve outcomes from non-compressible torso hemorrhage.[25] The ongoing AAST multi-institutional Aortic Occlusion for Resuscitation in Trauma and Acute Care Surgery (AORTA) trial will help determine the utility of REBOA in cases of hemorrhage from abdominal sources including the abdominal aorta.

THE HYBRID TRAUMA OPERATING ROOM

The prevailing model in many trauma hospitals is an operating room without angiographic capabilities and a separate interventional radiology suite. This arrangement can lead to delayed delivery of definitive treatment to a patient who requires multiple, concurrent,

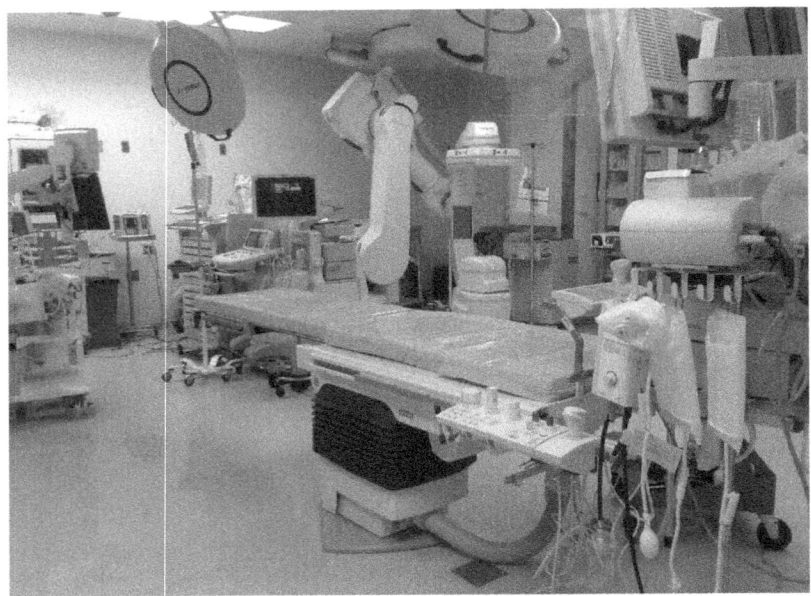

Figure 45-3. Trauma Hybrid Operating Room at RA Cowley Shock Trauma Center, University of Maryland, Baltimore. Angiography capability is provided by Siemens Zeego system whose C-arm is advanced into the operating field when needed and returns to its stored position away from the table during open procedures.

and urgent procedures such as a patient sustaining an aortic injury and hollow viscus injury or more commonly a patient requiring pelvic arterial embolization and an abdominal exploration. The basic principle of the hybrid operating room is the coupling of a standard operating room with angiographic imaging capabilities (Fig. 45-3). An operating room equipped with a radiolucent table, C-arm, monitors, and equipment for both endovascular and open procedures could potentially offer significant benefit to the injured patient. The ability to perform multiple procedures almost simultaneously such as exploratory laparotomy and an intraoperative arteriogram without change in location or delay provides rapid assessment and expeditious care of the trauma patient.

MORTALITY

The overall reported mortality for BAAI ranges from 32% to 78%.[1,5,11,20,21] The mortality varies by the type of aortic injury. In the cases of MAI, uncomplicated LIF, and pseudoaneurysms, the mortality is 11% based on recent literature review, while mortality from free aortic rupture is 100%.[5] Most deaths occur during the initial operative exploration and are attributed to uncontrolled hemorrhage and associated injuries. The second leading cause of death is attributed to complications of malperfusion.[20]

SUMMARY

Abdominal aortic injury is rare and is associated with high morbidity and mortality. High index of suspicion with expeditious diagnosis and repair is lifesaving. CTA is the preferred method of diagnosis in the hemodynamically stable patient. MAI and uncomplicated LIF can be managed medically with close follow-up. Complicated LIF, pseudoaneurysms, and ruptures mandate operative repair by open or endovascular repair. Adjuncts to diagnosis such as the IVUS should be further investigated. Damage control techniques such as REBOA and the use of a hybrid operating room have the potential to improve survival in patients with BAAI. Data from prospective registries are warranted.

REFERENCES

1. Deree J, Shenvi E, Fortlage D, et al. Patient factors and operating room resuscitation predict mortality in traumatic abdominal aortic injury: a 20-year analysis. *J Vasc Surg.* 2007;45:493–497.
2. Asensio JA, Chahwan S, Hanpeter D, et al. Operative management and outcome of 302 abdominal vascular injuries. *Am J Surg.* 2000;180:528–533.
3. Dajee H, Richardson IW, Iype MO. Seat belt aorta: acute dissection and thrombosis of the abdominal aorta. *Surgery.* 1979;85:263–267.
4. Malhotra AK, Fabian TC, Croce MA, et al. Minimal aortic injury: a lesion associated with advancing diagnostic techniques. *J Trauma.* 2001;51:1042–1048.
5. Shalhub S, Starnes BW, Tran NT, et al. Blunt abdominal aortic injury. *J Vasc Surg.* 2012;55:1277–1285.
6. Nguyen D, Platon A, Shanmuganathan K, et al. Evaluation of a single-pass continuous whole-body 16-MDCT protocol for patients with polytrauma. *AJR Am J Roentgenol.* 2009;192:3–10.
7. Mellnick VM, McDowell C, Lubner M, et al. CT features of blunt abdominal aortic injury. *Emerg Radiol.* 2012;19:301–307.
8. Azizzadeh A, Valdes J, Miller CC III, et al. The utility of intravascular ultrasound compared to angiography in the diagnosis of blunt traumatic aortic injury. *J Vasc Surg.* 2011;53:608–614.
9. Fabian TC, Richardson JD, Croce MA, et al. Prospective study of blunt aortic injury: Multicenter Trial of the American Association for the Surgery of Trauma. *J Trauma.* 1997;42:374–380.
10. Demetriades D, Velmahos GC, Scalea TM, et al. Operative repair or endovascular stent graft in blunt traumatic thoracic aortic injuries: results of an American Association for the Surgery of Trauma Multicenter Study. *J Trauma.* 2008;64:561–570.
11. Paul JS, Webb TP, Aprahamian C, Weigelt JA. Intraabdominal vascular injury: are we getting any better? *J Trauma.* 2010;69:1393–1397.
12. Harris DG, Drucker CB, Brenner ML, et al. Patterns and management of blunt abdominal aortic injury. *Ann Vasc Surg.* 2013;27(8):1074–1080. [Epub June 20, 2013].
13. Neschis DG, Scalea TM, Flinn WR, Griffith BP. Blunt aortic injury. *N Engl J Med.* 2008;359:1708–1716.
14. Aladham F, Sundaram B, Williams DM, Quint LE. Traumatic aortic injury: computerized tomographic findings at presentation and after conservative therapy. *J Comput Assist Tomogr.* 2010;34:388–394.
15. Goaley TJ, Dente CJ, Feliciano DV. Torso vascular trauma at an urban level I trauma center. *Perspect Vasc Surg Endovasc Ther.* 2006;18:102–112.
16. Wall MJ, Jr., Tsai PI, Gilani R, Mattox KL. Open and endovascular approaches to aortic trauma. *Tex Heart Inst J.* 2010;37:675–677.
17. de Mestral C, Dueck AD, Gomez D, et al. Associated injuries, management, and outcomes of blunt abdominal aortic injury. *J Vasc Surg.* 2012;56:656–660.
18. Azizzadeh A, Keyhani K, Miller CC, III., et al. Blunt traumatic aortic injury: initial experience with endovascular repair. *J Vasc Surg.* 2009;49:1403–1408.
19. Starnes BW, Lundgren RS, Gunn M, et al. A new classification scheme for treating blunt aortic injury. *J Vasc Surg.* 2012;55:47–54.

20. Roth SM, Wheeler JR, Gregory RT, et al. Blunt injury of the abdominal aorta: a review. *J Trauma*. 1997;42:748–755.

21. Burkhart HM, Gomez GA, Jacobson LE, et al. Fatal blunt aortic injuries: a review of 242 autopsy cases. *J Trauma*. 2001;50:113–115.

22. Burlew CC, Moore EE, Moore FA, et al. Western Trauma Association critical decisions in trauma: resuscitative thoracotomy. *J Trauma Acute Care Surg*. 2012;73:1359–1363.

23. Stannard A, Eliason JL, Rasmussen TE. Resuscitative endovascular balloon occlusion of the aorta (REBOA) as an adjunct for hemorrhagic shock. *J Trauma*. 2011;71:1869–1872.

24. Morrison JJ, Percival TJ, Markov NP, et al. Aortic balloon occlusion is effective in controlling pelvic hemorrhage. *J Surg Res*. 2012;177:341–347.

25. Brenner ML, Moore LJ, DuBose JJ, et al. A clinical series of resuscitative endovascular balloon occlusion of the aorta for hemorrhage control and resuscitation. *J Trauma Acute Care Surg*. 2013;75(3):506–511.

Thoracic/ Thoracoabdominal Diseases

46

Chronic Thoracic Dissection: Outcomes of Open Repair

Mark F. Conrad, MD, MMSc

INTRODUCTION

Unlike the abdominal aorta, wherein degenerative aneurysm and some element of aortoiliac occlusive disease are the pathologies of concern, the thoracic aorta is potentially involved with a spectrum of pathologies whose management involves the breath of cardiovascular specialists. Certain of these pathologies such as uncomplicated acute type B aortic dissections are typically managed primarily or exclusively with medical therapies. However, as a type B aortic dissection becomes chronic, patients are at risk of aortic degeneration and subsequent aneurysmal dilation of the outer wall of the false lumen, with an unpredictable temporal sequence.[1]

Aneurysms that simultaneously involve the thoracic and abdominal aorta, and/ or those aneurysms including the visceral aortic segment are referred to as thoracoabdominal aortic aneurysms (TAA). Such aneurysms are uncommon when compared to isolated infrarenal aneurysm, comprising no more than 2%–5% of the total spectrum of degenerative aortic aneurysm. TAA are classified according to the extent of aortic involvement with the now familiar Crawford classification (Fig. 46-1). TAA extent I and II require resection of the entire descending thoracic aorta and are therefore accompanied by increased risk of perioperative complications including spinal cord ischemia. While a majority of TAA are degenerative in nature and occur in association with hypertension, smoking, and frequently with evidence of vascular disease in other territories, up to 20% of TAA are the sequelae of chronic aortic dissection.

It has been estimated that more than 50% of patients with chronic type B dissections develop a TAA that ruptures or requires TAA resection within four years of their initial presentation.[2,3] Under such conditions, operative repair is typically more complex than in patients with degenerative aneurysms leading to longer cross-clamp times and increased renal and spinal cord ischemia. Indeed, in Crawford's sentinel report of 605 patients, chronic dissection was associated with a significantly higher risk of

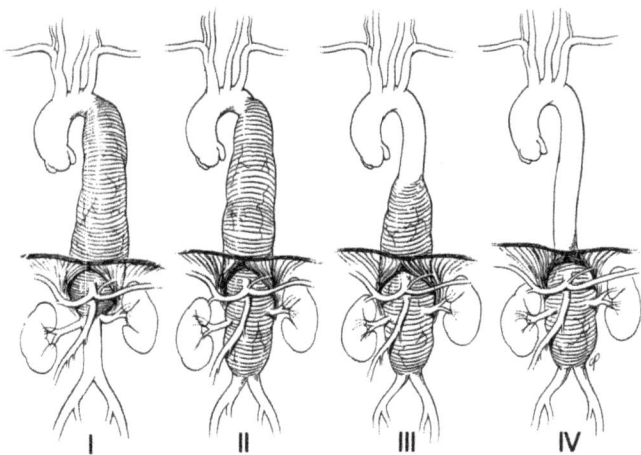

Figure 46-1. Crawford classification of the extent of thoracoabdominal aortic aneurysms.

paraplegia than patients with degenerative aneurysms (30.4% vs. 7.4%, $p < 0.0001$)[4] and, a subsequent review of the world's literature 10 years later also identified chronic dissection as a predictor of increased spinal cord ischemic risk.[4]

The modern era in the surgical management of TAA began with a simplified operative approach to these lesions that involved the reconstruction of the aneurysmal aorta with direct anastomoses of the aortic origin of visceral and intercostal vessels to the main Dacron graft (Fig. 46-2). The addition of intraprocedural adjuncts such as distal aortic perfusion through atrial-femoral bypass,[5] epidural cooling,[6] and the monitoring of motor-evoked potentials (MEPs)[7] has improved the expected paraplegia rates after repair of type I–III TAA especially in patients with aneurysms secondary to chronic dissection. In several recent series that have applied these adjuncts to TAA repair, dissection was no longer identified as a predictor of adverse outcomes on multivariate analysis.[8,9] Indeed, when Svensson presented an update of the Crawford experience (now including 1509 patients), chronic dissection was only significant on univariate analysis and was eliminated from the multivariate model because it was not an independent predictor of spinal cord ischemia.[10]

This chapter reviews the current techniques for open repair of TAA with emphasis on issues specific to patients with chronic dissection. Protective adjuncts will be discussed as well as the indications and rational for their use. Contemporary outcomes will be presented showing how these adjuncts have improved operative mortality and postoperative spinal cord ischemia.

PRINCIPALS OF TREATMENT

The general approach to the repair of thoracoabdominal aneurysms is depicted in Figure 46-2. A clamp and sew technique (Fig. 46-2A) with adjuncts such as regional hypothermic protection of the spinal cord and kidneys can be used in the majority of patients with type III and IV TAA while distal perfusion with atrial-femoral bypass (Fig. 46-2B) is used for more complex patients and those with type I and II TAA.

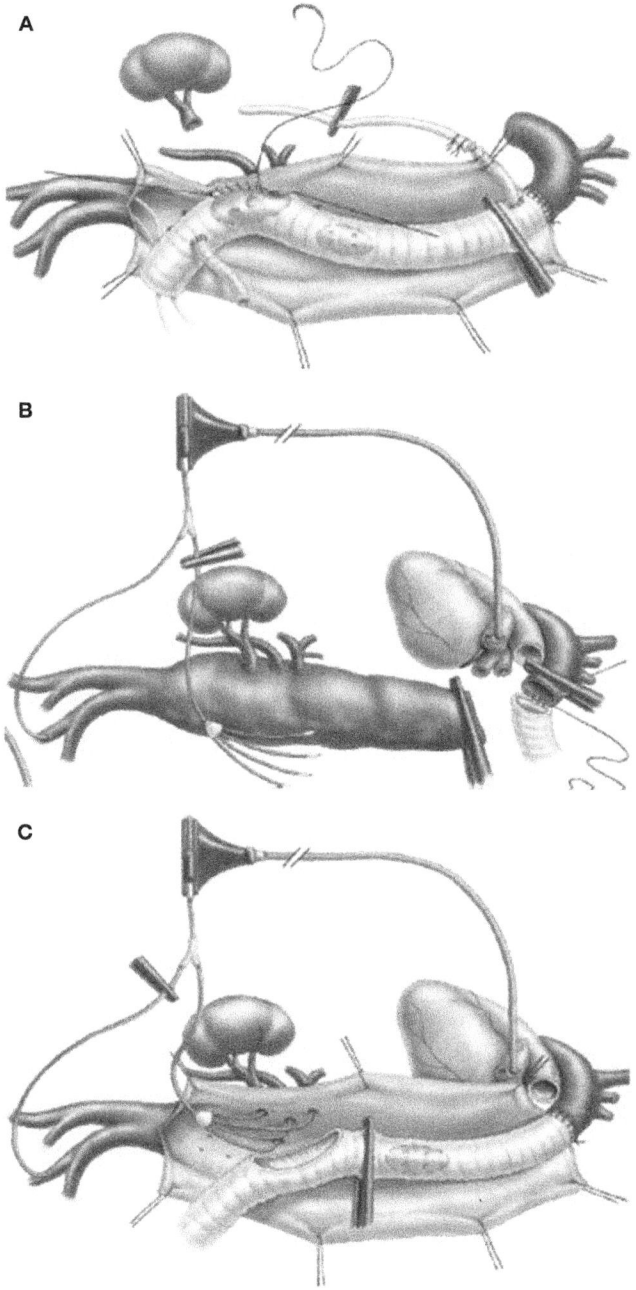

Figure 46-2. Approaches to operative conduct of thoracoabdominal aneurysm repair. (*A*) Our modified clamp and sew technique with inline mesenteric shunting after proximal anastomosis completion, providing pulsatile arterial flow that can be inserted into either the celiac axis (as depicted) or the superior mesenteric artery (SMA), and cold renal perfusion into both kidneys. Critical intercostal vessels are reconstructed (dotted line), and a single inclusion button anastomosis for reconstruction of celiac, superior mesenteric, and right renal arteries is possible in the majority of cases. The left renal artery is reconstructed with a side-arm graft. (*B*) Repair with atriofemoral bypass and sequential aortic clamping. Two clamps are placed proximally to initially allow proximal anastomosis completion with retrograde, transfemoral aortovisceral perfusion. (*C*) Subsequently, the distal clamp is moved caudad to allow critical intercostals reconstruction while renovisceral perfusion is provided by "octopus" catheters.

Clamp and Sew

The clamp and sew technique allows for the provision of regional hypothermic protection to the section of the spinal cord that is at greatest risk of ischemic injury during the procedure. An iced saline solution is infused epidurally during cross-clamping providing moderate (25°C–27°C) hypothermic protection to the spinal cord. In addition, a bolus (250 cc) of renal preservation fluid (4°C lactated ringers with 25 g of Mannitol/liter and 1 g methyl prednisolone per liter) is infused directly into the ostia of each renal artery after the aorta is opened. This is followed by a continuous drip of the same delivered through 6 Fr perfusion balloon-tipped catheters. The initial bolus results in a decline of renal parenchymal temperature to 15°C, and the subsequent continuous infusion maintains the renal core temperature around 25°C as measured by direct temperature probes in the renal cortex.

Another adjunct in the clamp and sew approach involves inline mesenteric shunting aimed at blunting the profound metabolic and hemodynamic disturbances that occur after restoration of blood flow to the mesenteric circulation. As depicted in Figure 46-2A, a 10 mm Dacron sidearm graft is sewn to the main aortic graft so as to be located just beyond the region of the proximal anastomosis. A 20–24 F arterial perfusion cannula is attached to the sidearm graft and immediately after completion of the proximal anastomosis; pro-grade pulsatile perfusion can be established into either the celiac axis or superior mesenteric artery (SMA) to minimize visceral ischemic time and its potential contribution to coagulopathic bleeding. In our experience, pulsatile arterial perfusion can thus be re-established to the mesenteric circulation within 25 minutes of the initial placement of the aortic clamp.

Distal Aortic Perfusion With Motor-Evoked Potentials

A desire to further reduce spinal cord ischemic complications led to a recent shift in our operative approach to applying distal aortic perfusion through left atrial femoral bypass with intraoperative MEP monitoring to dynamically assess spinal cord ischemia during repair of type I and II TAA.[7,9] This practice was driven by recent demonstration of the concept of the collateral network of the spinal cord with a dominant contribution from the pelvic (hypogastric arteries) circulation below the proximal clamp where intraoperative support of the cord's collateral network could be achieved with distal aortic perfusion.[11,12] The addition of MEP monitoring affords the surgeon objective criteria for selective intercostal artery revascularization, thus replacing the subjective or routine posture toward intercostal vessel reimplantation.

TECHNICAL COMPONENTS

Because the majority of TAA secondary to chronic dissection are repaired using distal aortic perfusion in our practice, TAA repair with atriofemoral bypass (rather than the clamp and sew method) will be the main focus of this section. Irrespective of individual preferences concerning the technical conduct of the operation, the key to operative success remains the provision of broad, continuous exposure of the entire left posterolateral aspect of the thoracoabdominal aorta. The patient is positioned on the table in the right lateral decubitus position. The location and extent of the thoracic portion of the incision is determined by the proximal extent of the aneurysm as the posterior portion of a standard posterolateral thoracotomy incision is only necessary for type I and type II aneurysms (Fig. 46-3). We keep the thoracic portion of the incision low and have found that the fifth or sixth interspace with posterior division of the sixth or seventh ribs provides adequate exposure for even the more proximal aneurysms. The costal margin is divided at the level of the sixth interspace and a self-retaining retractor system is placed to ensure continuous exposure of the entire operative field. A thoracoabdominal incision at the eighth interspace will usually provide adequate exposure for a type IV aneurysm, and a double lumen tube for deflation of the left lung is generally not necessary in these cases. The abdominal portion of the incision is not extended to the midline; rather, it is kept well lateral on the abdominal wall along the border of the rectus sheath. The advantage of this approach is that it allows the visceral contents to lay within the abdominal cavity thus decreasing evaporative fluid and heat losses. The abdominal portion of the incision is transperitoneal allowing direct inspection and assessment of the visceral circulation when the case is completed.

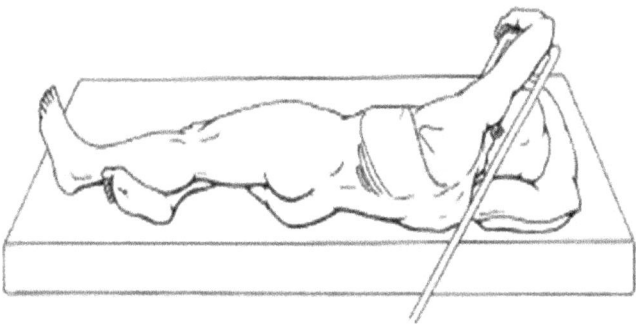

Figure 46-3. Positioning of patient for the thoracoabdominal approach.

Exposure of the left posterolateral aspect of the abdominal aorta is obtained by entering the plane posterior to the spleen, left kidney, and left colon. The abdominal contents are then reflected to the patient's right and the left ureter is identified and preserved under laparotomy pads. The retroperitoneal fatty and lymphatic tissues overlying the aorta are transected with electrocautery and the large posterior branch of the left renal vein that courses across the aorta is identified and divided. Located topographically close to this vein is the left renal artery. Once identified, this is dissected back toward its origin on the aorta, which serves as a suitable point to initiate the cephalad and caudal division of the retroperitoneal tissues over the aorta inferiorly and division of the median arcuate ligament and diaphragmatic crura superiorly.

There are several methods by which the incision in the diaphragm may be managed. The quickest and simplest method that affords excellent exposure is direct radial division of the diaphragm from underneath the costal margin to the aortic hiatus. This approach, however, will irrevocably paralyze the left hemidiaphragm and ultimately contribute to postoperative respiratory embarrassment. A second approach involves the circumferential division of the diaphragm through its muscular portion leaving a few centimeters attached laterally to the chest wall. There is benefit to preserving the phrenic innervation to the left hemidiaphragm by dividing only a portion lateral to the phrenic nerve insertion and then taking down the muscular fibers of the aortic hiatus. A large Penrose drain can be passed around the diaphragm pedicle and used to retract superiorly and inferiorly as needed during the reconstruction. We have applied this method liberally, particularly in patients with evidence of preoperative pulmonary compromise. After deflation of the left lung, the thoracic component of the dissection is typically straightforward. Electrocautery is used to divide the mediastinal pleura over the aneurysm and proximal aorta. For type I and type II aneurysms, proximal control of the aorta in the region of the left subclavian artery origin is necessary. Further mobility of the vagus nerve is gained by dividing it distal to the origin of the left recurrent nerve, which should be identified and preserved. Should more proximal control be necessary, the ligamentum arteriosum is divided on the underside of the aortic arch. Care must be taken to keep the dissection directly on the aortic arch to avoid injuring the left main pulmonary artery. In patients with chronic dissection, the prior inflammation from the dissecting process makes exposure in this area difficult, and care must be taken to avoid injury to surrounding structures that may be adherent to the aortic arch. The aorta is surrounded with a vessel tape on either side of the left subclavian artery depending on the proximal extent of the aneurysm. Blunt dissection on the posterior aspect of the aorta is used to clear sufficient normal aorta to allow placement of the cross clamp while maintaining adequate length of aorta for an accurate proximal aortic anastomosis. External control of the left subclavian artery is desirable but not mandatory as intraluminal balloon control can be obtained if the aortic clamp is placed proximal to the left subclavian artery. The celiac and SMA are controlled externally as this controls back bleeding, makes the vessels easy to identify during repair, and facilitates subsequent visceral Doppler interrogation (Fig. 46-4).

Sequential clamp sites are selected along the aorta to allow for distal perfusion during the proximal work on the aorta. Typically, these are located just below the location of the proximal anastomosis, above the visceral vessels and below the renal arteries. The first clamp site allows continuous perfusion to the visceral vessels and spinal

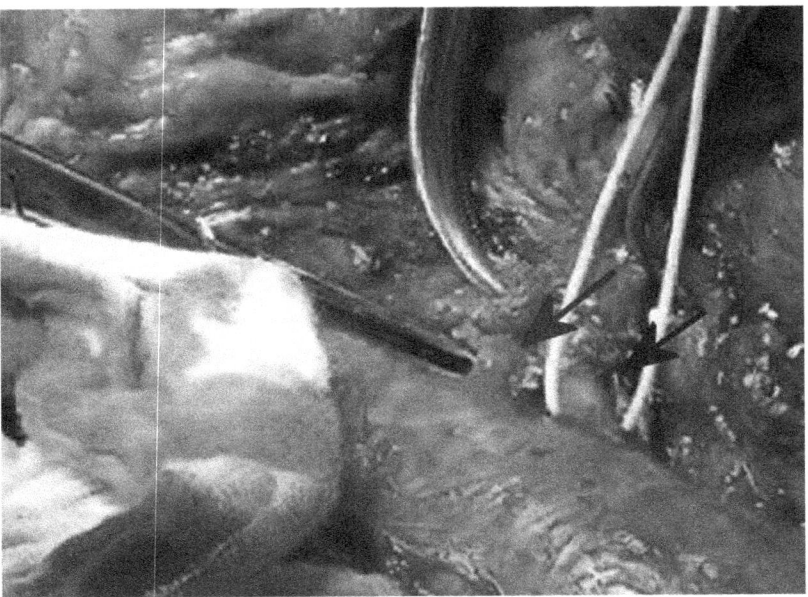

Figure 46-4. Dissection of the visceral vessels. The right arrow is pointing to the celiac trunk and the left arrow points to the SMA.

cord during creation of the proximal anastomosis. The second maintains visceral perfusion while the intercostals are evaluated and controlled, and the third perfuses the pelvis while the visceral button is being sewn.

Next, the aortic prosthesis is prepared by attaching a 6 mm polytetrafluoroethylene (PTFE) side-arm graft that will serve as the conduit for left renal artery reconstruction. For most aneurysms, a Dacron graft is the preferred conduit. However, a PTFE conduit is used to repair mycotic aneurysms because of its decreased susceptibility to infection.

Distal aortic perfusion is initiated by cannulating the left atrium through the left inferior pulmonary vein. A purse string is sewn in the vein before cannulation to prevent bleeding after the cannula is removed. The inferior pulmonary vein must be dissected completely free of surrounding tissue so that it does tear when the suture is tied down after decannulation. Access is obtained in one of the femoral arteries (usually the left for convenience) through a cutdown, and a cannula is placed over a wire into the distal aorta. It is important that this cannula is in the true lumen in dissection patients and the best side for access can usually be gleaned from preoperative imaging. An arterial line is placed in the opposite groin to monitor mean arterial pressures during the cross clamp. Once the circuit is established, flows are titrated to keep a mean arterial pressure of 60 mmHg. This can be adjusted throughout the case to maintain adequate perfusion to the spinal cord.

At this point, the surgeon begins the clamping sequence in close cooperation with the anesthesiologist and perfusionist. The two proximal clamps are placed, and the aorta is transected between them. Unlike the abdominal aorta where the posterior wall is often left intact, the proximal thoracic aorta should be completely transected and freed of surrounding tissue to avoid injury to the esophagus. If a dissection flap is encountered at the level of the anastomosis, a fenestration can be made by cutting the flap back to the clamp above the suture line so that both luminae flow freely into the graft. The proximal anastomosis is created with a 3-0 or 4-0 prolene suture with a small needle to minimize trauma to the aorta. We usually use a line of felt pledget to ensure that the anastomosis does not leak. If there is bleeding after the proximal clamp is removed, re-clamp before attempting repair as sewing on a pressurized aorta in the face of a dissection will only bring misery.

Once the proximal anastomosis is complete and hemostatic, a clamp is placed above the visceral vessels and the remainder of the thoracic aorta is opened. The dissection flap is often stiff and fibrotic and will need to be transected to view the intercostal arteries. Unlike degenerative aneurysmal disease wherein luminal thrombus has led to occlusion of many of the intercostal arteries, patients with chronic dissections often maintain patency of most if not all of the intercostal vessels. Once the entire descending thoracic aorta is exposed in a patient on atrial femoral bypass, the intercostal vessel orifices usually back-bleed profusely and the proximal vessels are quickly oversewn. The intercostal arteries in the critical T_9 to L_1 aortic segment are evaluated for potential reimplantation into the main body of the graft. These vessels are controlled with intraluminal balloons to prevent further bleeding and the negative "sump" effect on net spinal cord perfusion caused by exposure of these orifices to atmospheric pressure. MEPs are performed during this phase of the procedure. Any deterioration in MEP should prompt either an increase in the stimulus intensity or an increase in distal perfusion pressures. A sudden drop in MEP amplitude (occurring within 2–10 minutes) or a sustained progressive drop (within 10–40 minutes) of >75% from baseline should be considered significant and a complete loss of the MEPs is associated with a high incidence of postoperative paraplegia. If the MEPs remain stable, the occlusion balloons are left in place and attention is turned to the visceral segment.

The clamp is moved below the renal arteries. The left renal artery is transected and infused with 300 cc renal cold solution followed by a continuous drip at gravity. The aneurysm is opened in the abdomen, atherothrombotic debris is evacuated, and the intimal flap is excised. Visceral and renal artery reconstruction is carried out next. Orificial endarterectomy should be performed when significant occlusive lesions of the right renal and superior mesenteric arteries exist. This involves incising the diseased intima and media and developing a proper endarterectomy plane that can be verified by noting the pinkish color of the inner adventitia. In cases where aortic endarterectomy is required, the superior mesenteric and celiac arteries should be dissected sufficiently to facilitate countertraction from the external side of the vessel. This, however, is not possible with the right renal artery. In the event that the calcified end of the obstructing plaque does not feather nicely, sharp excision under direct vision is the best way to end the endarterectomy plane. The most common method of visceral and renal artery reconstruction, in our experience, is a single inclusion button that encompasses the origins of the celiac, superior mesenteric, and right renal arteries (Fig. 46-5). If the aneurysm is excessively large in the visceral aortic segment, the wide separation of the visceral/renal ostia may necessitate individual inclusion button anastomoses for each vessel. Alternatively, the SMA and right renal artery can be re-implanted as a single inclusion while reconstruction of the celiac trunk is deferred until later. The aortic graft is placed under tension, and an elliptical side island is excised from the main aortic graft. This ellipse usually begins on the lateral aspect of the graft and spirals posteriorly in the region of the right renal artery reconstruction. With the graft under tension, it is possible to complete the posterior portion of the anastomosis using single bites of the suture passing through both the aorta and the Dacron graft. Suture bites are taken close to the origin of the visceral vessels to avoid leaving excess aneurysmal aortic wall. As the posterior aspect of this suture line continues around the inferior border of the right renal artery, care is taken to insure that it is not compromised by generous suture bites as they pass outside of the aorta (Fig. 46-5). It is important to identify the course of the right renal artery to avoid renal artery occlusion in circumstances where the right renal artery drapes over a large infrarenal component of the aneurysm. A 6 mm short balloon expandable stent can be placed in the right renal artery to ensure that it is not compromised by the suture line (Fig. 46-5). Just before completion of this suture line, backbleeding and patency of the celiac, superior mesenteric, and right renal arteries are verified, and the inline mesenteric shunt is clamped and removed. A single flush of the proximal aortic cross-clamp is performed to ensure that no clot or debris has built up in the graft.

Reconstruction of the left renal artery is now accomplished with a separate side-arm graft of 6 mm PTFE. This provides a direct deliberate anastomosis in end-to-end fashion while allowing flexibility to deal with the spectrum of occlusive lesions, multiple renal arteries, and other wrinkles that may be encountered. It is important to orient this side-arm graft so that it will not kink when the left renal artery is returned to its anatomic position. Some surgeons advocate the use of a single inclusion button that contains the renal arteries and the visceral vessels. This often requires the inclusion of too great an area of the native, aneurysmal aorta unless the aneurysm is small in the visceral artery segment. A single, pristine left renal artery and orifice may be directly re-implanted and the clamp is then advanced to a position inferior to the origin of the left renal artery graft prior to completing the distal aortic anastomosis.

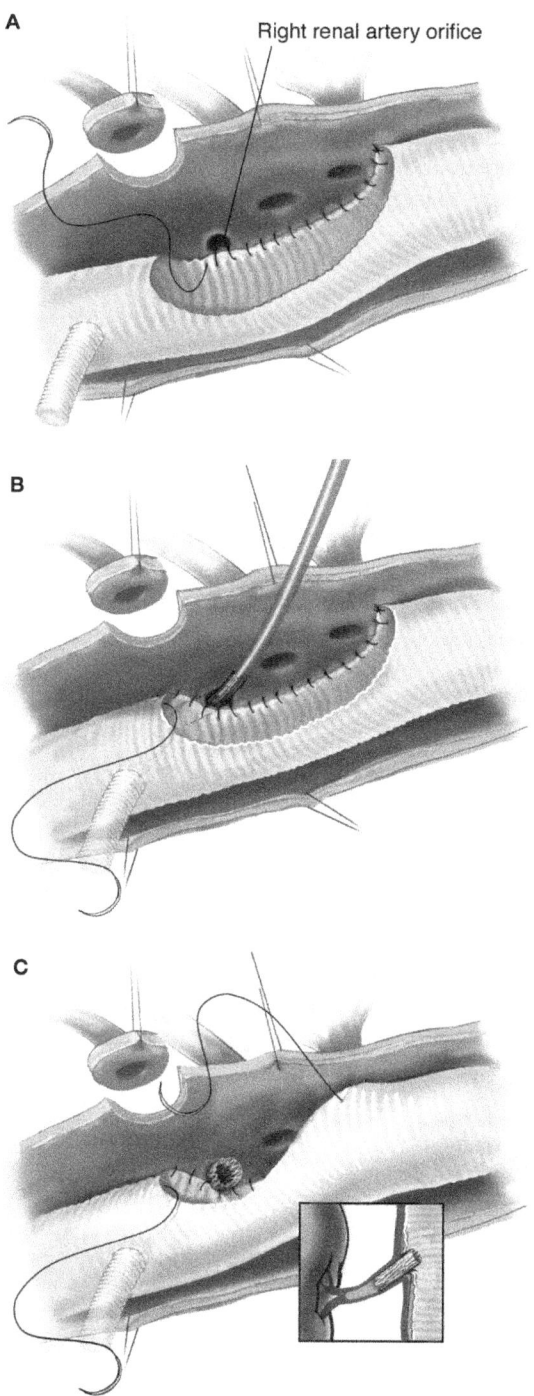

Figure 46-5. Management of the visceral aortic segment. (*A*) The inclusion button back wall is sewn first with the distal stitches placed in the origin of the right renal artery. (*B*) As the anastomosis continues away from the renal artery, a balloon expanding stent is placed in the renal artery under direct vision to prevent compromise to the lumen. (*C*) The stent has been successfully deployed and the proximal portion of the anastomosis is completed.

At this point, distal aortic perfusion is stopped and the cannulas are removed. The suture on the pulmonary vein is tied down with a pledget. The common femoral artery is repaired under direct vision. We make every effort to perform a tube graft reconstruction to the aortic bifurcation unless there is gross aneurysmal disease of the proximal common iliac arteries. If the dissection extends into the iliac arteries, it is important to identify the true and false lumenae. The false lumen is obliterated with suture, and the anastomosis is performed to the true lumen. If the intimal flap is stiff and the true lumen is unclear, the flap can be excised beyond the anastomosis for double barrel flow to the legs, but this can lead to further aneurysmal degeneration of the iliac arteries in the future. After reestablishment of flow to the lower extremities and verification of adequate lower extremity perfusion by intraoperative pulse volume recordings, Doppler signals in the left renal, celiac, and superior mesenteric vessels are checked in addition to palpation of the SMA pulse in the root of the mesentery.

Then next step of the operation is re-evaluation of the intercostal vessels. If the MEP were stable throughout the case, the balloons can be removed and the vessels oversewn. We have found that re-implantation of the intercostals is rarely necessary with this approach. If the decision is made to reconstruct the intercostal vessels, this can be accomplished through an inclusion button anastomosis. Intercostal arteries in the region of a proximal or distal aortic anastomosis can be reconstructed using a long beveled suture line (Fig. 46-6). Other methods of intercostal vessel re-anastomosis include the attachment of additional short side-arm grafts to the main aortic graft or, in cases where vessel origin is rotated superiorly and to the patient's left side, implantation to the main aortic graft using Carrel patches of aorta that contain the intercostal vessels may be feasible (Fig. 46-6).

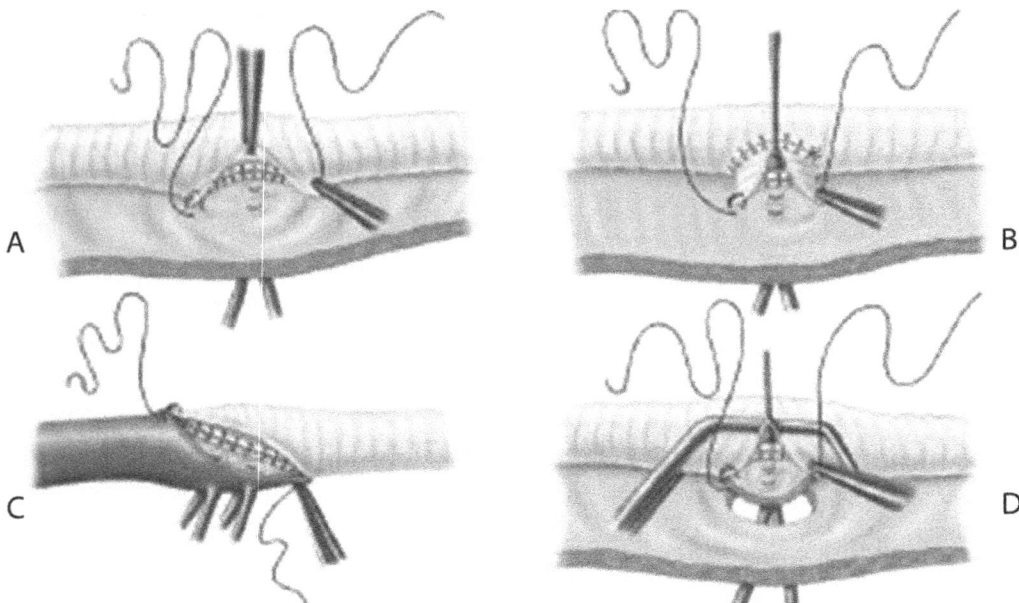

Figure 46-6. Methods of management of critical intercostals arteries. (A) Inclusion button anastomosis. (B) Separate sidearm graft. (C) Beveled anastomosis preservation when possible. (D) Carrel patch mobilization and direct reimplantation into the graft.

Hemostasis will usually be adequate at this point but infusions of platelets and fresh frozen plasma are typically increased at this point in the operation when a final check for surgical hemorrhage is made. Careful inspection of the inferior aspect of the aneurysm sac in both the chest and the abdomen is necessary to detect back-bleeding lumbar and/or intercostal vessels that can be a source of significant postoperative hemorrhage. The redundant aneurysm sac is then sutured securely over the aortic prosthesis in the abdomen and the chest. The left kidney is returned to its anatomic position and perinephric fat suffices to provide adequate coverage of the aortic graft in the region of the visceral aortic segment. Before closure, renal artery reconstructions are interrogated with a Doppler one final time. Closure of extensive incisions typically takes close to an hour, and two teams are utilized.

RESULTS OF TREATMENT

We recently reviewed our results with repair of type I–III TAA using DAP and MEP monitoring in which 37% of the patients had aneurysms secondary to chronic dissection. The perioperative mortality was 2% and the total paraplegia rate was 0%.[13] When we compared patients who undergo TAA for chronic dissection to those with degenerative aneurysms, there was no difference in the 30-day mortality or paraplegia rates between the two cohorts.[14] This is despite the fact that patients with chronic dissection had a higher preoperative risk profile than those with degenerative aneurysms as they were more likely to present in an emergent/urgent fashion, to have a connective tissue disorder, and to be Crawford type I and II TAA.

A study from the Cleveland Clinic of patients treated during the same time period as Crawford's original series reported a paraplegia rate of 35% in the 16 patients with dissection. This was not significantly different from the overall 21% incidence of paraplegia in the series but likely would have been if the study was powered adequately.[15] Safi et al. reported a contemporary series of TAA repair of which 27% had chronic dissection. Their overall neurologic deficit rate was 4.3% with no difference between the two groups (3.6% dissection vs. 4.5% degenerative, $p = 0.58$).[9] Another report detailed 660 patients undergoing TAA repair (21% dissection), and again there was no difference in spinal cord ischemia between the two cohorts (2.9% dissection vs. 5.5% degenerative).[8]

Historically, we have used the clamp and sew technique with epidural cooling for spinal cord protection in most TAA repairs with atrial-femoral bypass being reserved for patients in whom a complex proximal repair is anticipated.[6] Indeed, 22% of our chronic dissection patients in our historic series were treated with this adjunct. Others have championed an aggressive application of atrial-femoral bypass, with contemporary series of TAA for chronic dissection reporting the use of distal perfusion in 40%–80% of patients.[8,9] Jacobs et al. reported a spinal cord ischemia rate of 4% in a series of 118 patients with type I and II TAA treated with distal perfusion.[16] We have recently adopted a similar posture of the regular application of atrial-femoral bypass with monitoring of MEPs for patients with Crawford type I and II aneurysms regardless of etiology with initial favorable results.[13]

The best way to manage patent intercostal arteries, especially those in the critical region between T8-L1, remains controversial. Historically, the majority opinion (and consistent with our practice) has been an aggressive posture toward intercostal reconstruction in the T8-L1 segment.[5,6,8] Previously, we correlated sacrifice of intercostal vessels therein with an increased risk of SCI.[17] Yet this technical operative adjunct has both a weak evidence base to support its use and, at least in most iterations, is a largely "blind" maneuver (i.e., the surgeon genuinely has no data as to the necessity of such intercostal re-implant). A recent large series of TAA repair reported re-implantation of intercostal arteries in 58% of their cohort (80% of type I and II repairs) and found the SCI rate was 5.3% in the group with re-implantation and 13.4% in those that were not re-implanted ($p < 0.025$).[8] However, Svensson noted in a prospective study of intercostal preservation that a majority of separately re-implanted intercostals occlude within the first few hours post-op.[18] The posture toward intercostal reconstruction has changed over time, and a recent review by Acher et al. showed that the addition of intercostal artery revascularization to their other protective adjuncts reduced the SCI risk by 75%.[19] The presence of atrial-femoral bypass can complicate intraoperative decision making as it is common to have vigorous back-bleeding from multiple pairs of intercostal arteries and re-implantation of all vessels would add to the bypass time (and blood turn around) while providing questionable benefit. Because of this, MEPs have been used to predict the need for intercostal reconstruction during atrial-femoral bypass with success.[11,12,16] We now monitor MEPs in all patients with type I–III TAA secondary to chronic dissection. After completing the proximal anastomosis, patent intercostal arteries are identified and occluded with Pruit catheters. We then proceed to create the visceral button, checking MEPs frequently during this time. If the potentials decrease, dominate intercostal arteries are re-implanted through an inclusion button, if not, they are oversewn.[11] This has resulted in the need for few intercostal re-implantations with minimal paraplegia.

Despite various advances in anesthesia and the addition of adjunctive techniques, representative large clinical series, including the most recent publications, indicate that the mortality of elective TAA repair remains essentially unchanged from Crawford's initial 8.9%[4] with most series falling in the 7%–12% range. Indeed, these results represent the "best case" scenario and the "real world" experience is substantially worse. Rigberg et al. evaluated 1010 patients from the California Office of Statewide Health Planning and Development (OSHPD) database and reported a 30-day elective mortality of 19% that increased to 31% at one year.[20] There was also a linear correlation with age at operation so that the one year mortality increased from 18% in patients <60 years old to 40% for patients over 80.[20] Similarly, Cowan et al. reviewed 1542 patients who underwent elective TAA repair across a spectrum of hospitals throughout the United States from the National Inpatient Sample (NIS). The overall mortality for TAA repair was a sobering 22.3% with higher volume surgeons having better outcomes than low volume surgeons.[21] Chronic dissection was not individually evaluated in these reports based on large databases but in multiple contemporary single center series, chronic dissection was not a predictor of 30-day mortality.[8,14,22]

CONCLUSION

Open repair of TAA of chronic dissection origin is complex and requires a thorough knowledge of the underlying pathology to accomplish safely. It is clear that advances in operative technique and the addition of neuroprotective adjunctive measures such as distal aortic perfusion with atrial femoral bypass, regional hypothermia and monitoring of spinal cord perfusion through MEP has improved 30-day outcomes after TAA repair for chronic dissection. The evolution of operative strategy, in particular those protective adjuncts against spinal cord ischemia have played a large role in increasing successful outcomes. However, mortality and paraplegia rates remain significant after this large operation and the ultimate goal is the prevention of aneurysmal degeneration of the false lumen by the promotion of early aortic remodeling in type B dissection.

REFERENCES

1. Sueyoshi E, Sakamoto I, Hayashi K, et al. Growth rate of aortic diameter in patients with type b aortic dissection during the chronic phase. *Circulation.* 2004;110:II256–II261.
2. Juvonen T, Ergin MA, Galla JD, et al. Risk factors for rupture of chronic type b dissections. *J Thorac Cardiovasc Surg.* 1999;117:776–786.
3. Marui A, Mochizuki T, Mitsui N, et al. Toward the best treatment for uncomplicated patients with type b acute aortic dissection: a consideration for sound surgical indication. *Circulation.* 1999;100:II275–II280.
4. Crawford ES, Crawford JL, Safi HJ, et al. Thoracoabdominal aortic aneurysms: preoperative and intraoperative factors determining immediate and long-term results of operations in 605 patients. *J Vasc Surg.* 1986;3:389–404.
5. Safi HJ, Miller CC, 3rd, Huynh TT, et al. Distal aortic perfusion and cerebrospinal fluid drainage for thoracoabdominal and descending thoracic aortic repair: ten years of organ protection. *Ann Surg.* 2003;238:372–380; discussion 380–371.
6. Conrad MF, Crawford RS, Davison JK, Cambria RP. Thoracoabdominal aneurysm repair: a 20-year perspective. *Ann Thorac Surg.* 2007;83:S856–S861; discussion S890–S852.
7. Jacobs MJ, Meylaerts SA, de Haan P, et al. Strategies to prevent neurologic deficit based on motor-evoked potentials in type I and II thoracoabdominal aortic aneurysm repair. *J Vasc Surg.* 1999;29:48–57; discussion 57–49.
8. Coselli JS, LeMaire SA, de Figueiredo LP, Kirby RP. Paraplegia after thoracoabdominal aortic aneurysm repair: is dissection a risk factor? *Ann Thorac Surg.* 1997;63:28–35; discussion 35–26.
9. Safi HJ, Miller CC, 3rd, Estrera AL, et al. Chronic aortic dissection not a risk factor for neurologic deficit in thoracoabdominal aortic aneurysm repair. *Eur J Vasc Endovasc Surg.* 2002;23:244–250.
10. Svensson LG, Crawford ES, Hess KR, et al. Experience with 1509 patients undergoing thoracoabdominal aortic operations. *J Vasc Surg.* 1993;17:357–368; discussion 368–370.
11. Griepp RB, Griepp EB. Spinal cord perfusion and protection during descending thoracic and thoracoabdominal aortic surgery: the collateral network concept. *Ann Thorac Surg.* 2007;83:S865–S869; discussion S890–S862.
12. Jacobs MJ, de Mol BA, Elenbaas T, et al. Spinal cord blood supply in patients with thoracoabdominal aortic aneurysms. *J Vasc Surg.* 2002;35:30–37.
13. Conrad MF, Ergul EA, Patel VI, et al. Evolution of operative strategies in open thoracoabdominal aneurysm repair. *J Vasc Surg.* 2011;53:1195–1201, e1191.
14. Conrad MF, Chung TK, Cambria MR, et al. Effect of chronic dissection on early and late outcomes after descending thoracic and thoracoabdominal aneurysm repair. *J Vasc Surg.* 2011;53:600–607; discussion 607.
15. Cox GS, O'Hara PJ, Hertzer NR, et al. Thoracoabdominal aneurysm repair: a representative experience. *J Vasc Surg.* 1992;15:780–787; discussion 787–788.
16. Jacobs MJ, Mess W, Mochtar B, et al. The value of motor evoked potentials in reducing paraplegia during thoracoabdominal aneurysm repair. *J Vasc Surg.* 2006;43:239–246.
17. Cambria RP, Davison JK, Zannetti S, et al. Clinical experience with epidural cooling for spinal cord protection during thoracic and thoracoabdominal aneurysm repair. *J Vasc Surg.* 1997;25:234–241; discussion 241–233.

18. Svensson LG, Patel V, Robinson MF, et al. Influence of preservation or perfusion of intra-operatively identified spinal cord blood supply on spinal motor evoked potentials and paraplegia after aortic surgery. *J Vasc Surg.* 1991;13:355–365.

19. Acher CW, Wynn MM, Mell MW, et al. A quantitative assessment of the impact of intercostal artery reimplantation on paralysis risk in thoracoabdominal aortic aneurysm repair. *Ann Surg.* 2008;248:529–540.

20. Rigberg DA, McGory ML, Zingmond DS, et al. Thirty-day mortality statistics underestimate the risk of repair of thoracoabdominal aortic aneurysms: a statewide experience. *J Vasc Surg.* 2006;43:217–222; discussion 223.

21. Cowan JA, Jr, Dimick JB, Henke PK, et al. Surgical treatment of intact thoracoabdominal aortic aneurysms in the United States: hospital and surgeon volume-related outcomes. *J Vasc Surg.* 2003;37:1169–1174.

22. Panneton JM, Hollier LH. Dissecting descending thoracic and thoracoabdominal aortic aneurysms: part II. *Ann Vasc Surg.* 1995;9:596–605.

47

Debakey Type III Chronic Dissecting Aneurysms: Outcomes of TEVAR versus Open Thoracoabdominal Aortic Aneurysm Solutions

R. Scott McClure, MD, SM and Joseph E. Bavaria, MD

INTRODUCTION

The impact of endovascular stent grafts on the management of aortic disease is profound. Endovascular stent grafts are now the predominant treatment strategy for degenerative aneurysms of the abdominal aorta, having supplanted open surgical repair.[1] The technology has had an ever-increasing presence in the treatment paradigm for degenerative thoracic and thoracoabdominal aneurysms as well.[2] Experience with endovascular approaches to various other thoracic aortic pathologies has followed,[3] including uncomplicated and complicated aortic dissections, aortic transections, penetrating aortic ulcers, and innumerable other proof of concept case reports scattered throughout the medical literature.

STENT GRAFTS FOR DEGENERATIVE ANEURYSMS OF THE THORACIC AORTA

And though endovascular stent grafts are without question a formidable advance in the management of thoracic aortic disease, to date, despite innumerable studies comparing open surgical repair to thoracic endovascular aortic repair (TEVAR) for degenerative aneurysms of the thoracic aorta, the short-term gains with TEVAR[4,5] are tempered by the more long-term outcomes that caution the overzealous utilization of this technology.[6–9] This

517

cautiousness resides on the basis of futility in elder patients with multiple comorbid conditions and the ineffectiveness of early intervention in patients with aneurysms that have not reached size criteria to otherwise warrant open surgery. Long-term datasets have suggested that any procedure-related survival advantage garnered by the less invasive nature of stent grafts to be rather modest when compared to open surgery in specialized aortic centers in this patient subset.[7–9] Patients unsuitable for open repair, while they may tolerate TEVAR very well, are often too frail to acquire a survival advantage over that which is achieved with medical therapy alone.[6,10] Patient comorbidities, not the degenerative thoracic aneurysm, inevitably determines end of life.

This is not to dismiss TEVAR. Benefits to TEVAR in degenerative aneurysms of the thoracic aorta over open surgery or medical therapy most certainly exist. Delineating which patients are best suited for TEVAR, however, is a pervasive challenge that at present remains unsolved.

STENT GRAFTS FOR ACUTE COMPLICATED DEBAKEY III AORTIC DISSECTIONS

In contrast to degenerative thoracic aneurysms, where the patient population to attain the most utility from TEVAR remains somewhat obscure, the beneficial effects of stent grafts to treat patients with acute complicated Debakey III aortic dissections is becoming more and more convincing.[11,12] Often presenting in emergent or extreme conditions with either aortic rupture or true lumen collapse and malperfusion syndromes, stent graft deployment across the intimal tear site to restore perfusion to the true lumen and promote aortic remodeling becomes a lifesaving procedure in this critically ill population. Several observational studies have shown a reduced mortality with TEVAR in comparison to surgery or medical therapy in these patients.[11–13] Although a randomized trial has never materialized, the general consensus within the aortic community is that TEVAR has become the preferred therapeutic option for acute complicated Debakey III aortic dissections.[13,14]

STENT GRAFTS FOR DEBAKEY III CHRONIC DISSECTING ANEURYSMS

In a separate although related aortic process, Debakey III chronic dissecting aneurysms may also prove well suited for TEVAR. Patients who develop a Debakey III dissecting aneurysm have survived the imminent risk to life imposed by an acute aortic dissection but are left with a weakened aortic wall. Subjected to increased wall stress, the dissected aorta becomes susceptible to an accelerated growth rate, persistent aneurysm enlargement, and an inevitable high risk for fatal rupture. Prior to TEVAR, open surgery was the only treatment option for this complex aortic process. Although outcomes with open thoracic and thoracoabdominal surgery to treat chronic dissecting aneurysms have improved overtime, they remain maximally invasive operations that carry an appreciable risk for paraplegia, respiratory failure, renal failure, and mortality.[15–17] The premise for TEVAR to treat Debakey III chronic dissecting aneurysms is that scaffolding across the primary tear site and subsequent distal reentrant tears may promote thrombosis and restriction to the ever-expanding false lumen. In addition, reciprocal improvements to the true lumen dimension in those cases where the true lumen has become significantly compressed may also occur. This remodeling of the aorta, similar to TEVAR for an acute aortic dissection, is thought to protect the patient from further false lumen expansion and fatal aortic wall rupture. However, unlike the pliable lumen present in an acute aortic dissection, a chronically dissected aorta is scarred, nonpliable, and rigid. With this in mind, the theoretically concept to support TEVAR as a viable treatment alternative to open surgery remains controversial in Debakey III chronic dissecting aneurysms, as it remains unclear whether the heavily scarred tissues of a chronically dissected aorta can in fact predictably be remodeled.

THE INSTEAD TRIAL AND AORTIC REMODELING

The INSTEAD trial (Investigation of Stent Grafts in Patients with Type B Aortic Dissection), the only published prospective randomized controlled trial to study the use of endovascular stent grafts in the thoracic aorta, supports the idea that predictable remodeling of the chronically dissected aorta does in fact occur.[18] Whether this remodeling culminates into improved long-term survival remains to be seen.

The INSTEAD trial randomized 140 patients with subacute/ T chronic (>14 days from initial presentation) "uncomplicated" Debakey III aortic dissections to either TEVAR with concomitant optimal medical therapy ($n = 72$) or optimal medical therapy alone ($n = 68$). At two years follow-up, there was no difference in either overall mortality or aorta-related mortality between the two groups.[18] A key finding derived from the study was validation for the current gold standard treatment of uncomplicated Debakey III aortic dissections—medical management focused on anti-impulse therapy and well-controlled blood pressure.

Interestingly, however, despite no appreciable difference in survival at two years, there was a very significant difference in aortic remodeling (with true lumen recovery and thoracic false lumen thrombosis) between the two groups. The TEVAR group showed evidence of aortic remodeling in 91.3% of cases compared to 19.4% of cases in the group of patients receiving medical management alone ($P<0.001$).[18] The clinical impact of this, if any, remains to be seen. Still, it is reasonable to postulate that if TEVAR promoted aortic remodeling in uncomplicated chronic Debakey III aortic dissections prevents or significantly slows aortic wall expansion in comparison to medical therapy, this may impart a survival advantage to TEVAR over a longer duration of follow-up.

More precisely, TEVAR for uncomplicated chronic Debakey III aortic dissections could protect against progressive aneurysm expansion to unsafe dimensions and the inevitable "transition" from an uncomplicated chronic aortic dissection to a complicated chronic Debakey III dissecting aneurysm and the associated rupture risk of this aortic process. The five-year data for the INSTEAD trial will be prudent to our better understanding of TEVARs utility in patients with uncomplicated subacute/chronic Debakey III dissections and the potential survival advantage this technology may impart to patients. For now, optimal medical therapy for an uncomplicated chronic Debakey III aortic dissection remains the preferred initial treatment strategy for all patients suffering from this condition.

THE INSTEAD TRIAL—IMPLICATIONS AND SUPPORT FOR STENT GRAFTING IN DEBAKEY III CHRONIC DISSECTING ANEURYSMS

That the INSTEAD trial was able to show that TEVAR promotes aortic remodeling in the chronically dissected aorta to such a significant degree over medical therapy has two far-reaching implications. The first implication, as discussed above, is that TEVAR may have a role to play in preventative medicine against the development of complicated Debakey III dissecting aneurysms. With placement of stent grafts more aggressively into patients with uncomplicated Debakey III aortic dissections, the occurrence of complicated Debakey III dissecting aneurysms may become less prevalent, as TEVAR remodeling may directly inhibit chronic aneurysm growth from ever occurring.

A second implication is since the chronically dissected aorta has proven to remodel, it legitimizes TEVAR as a potential treatment alternative to open surgery once complicated Debakey III chronic dissecting aneurysms present themselves. As noted earlier in this chapter, the criticism against TEVAR for treating Debakey III chronic dissecting aneurysms was the lack of evidence to support the ability to remodel dissected tissue once it has scarred and become rigid. With clinical trial data to mitigate these concerns, there is a strong platform to support further studies into the use of TEVAR technology for this complex patient population.

To illustrate the significance of this, 20%–50% of uncomplicated Debakey III aortic dissections inevitably present with late complications from distal aortic dissection, primarily due to progressive enlargement of the dissected aorta.[14] Open surgery at specialized aortic centers have produced very good results in properly selected patients and will always have a role to play in this disease process, especially in young patients.[15-17] However, with open thoracoabdominal procedures being so invasive, the comorbid conditions that are present in older patients upon presentation have a drastic impact on operative success, more so than any other cardiovascular procedure. With this, Debakey III chronic dissecting aneurysms are certainly an area where a less invasive TEVAR approach could impart a foreseeable advantage for many patients. Proper TEVAR positioning across the primary tear site and distal reentrant tears of Debakey III dissecting aneurysms may facilitate false lumen thrombosis, prevent further aortic wall expansion, and reduce the risk of fatal rupture without the upfront risks associated with thoracoabdominal surgical repair. It is based on this reasoning that many have embraced the idea of TEVAR in the face of chronic Debakey III dissecting aneurysms, despite the paucity of data available on the topic.

THE PENN EXPERIENCE—OPEN REPAIR AND TEVAR FOR DEBAKEY III CHRONIC DISSECTING ANEURYSMS

The Aortic Surgery Program at the Hospital of the University of Pennsylvania has offered TEVAR in select patients as an alternative to open repair to treat Debakey III chronic dissecting aneurysms for eight years. Between January 2005 and June 2013, 34 patients (~4% of all TEVAR procedures performed during this time period) underwent elective TEVAR for the treatment of Debakey III chronic dissecting aneurysms. Throughout the same time period, 58 patients underwent open surgical repair for the same disease process, for a total of 92 patients having had one or the other intervention.

Methods

The decision to use TEVAR or open surgery was determined by the individual surgeon at the time of presentation and was predicated primarily upon patient anatomy and associated comorbidities.

Noteworthy, when classifying a thoracic aneurysm as a Debakey III chronic dissection, this encompasses two related, although separate, aortic disease entities. The first group consists of those patients with a residual Debakey I aortic dissection after a proximal ascending aortic repair. The second group consists of "de novo" Debakey III dissections that originate distal to the left subclavian artery. Both processes are included in this review. All patients underwent elective open or endovascular repair at least two months after their initial diagnosis of dissection.

The indications for surgery were either (1) a maximum aortic diameter of at least 5.5 cm or (2) an accelerated aortic growth rate of at least 5 mm over a six-month period. All patients had patent false lumens at the time of intervention. Emergent cases for symptoms of impending rupture or known rupture and patients with intramural hematomas were excluded.

The goal at the time of intervention varied depending on the intervention of choice. Open surgery dictated surgical repair and replacement of all aneurysmal aorta. TEVAR on the other hand dictated identification of the primary intimal tear site and all distal fenestrations within the descending thoracic aorta. Stent grafts were oversized 10%–20% in relation to the diameter of the proximal landing zone. Technical success with TEVAR was defined as elimination of antegrade perfusion of the false lumen on completion aortogram. This was achieved in all patients prior to leaving the operating room.

Results

Demographics for both open surgery and TEVAR subsets are listed in Table 47-1. As these are nonrandomized, unmatched cohorts with different anatomical presentations under the greater classification of Debakey III chronic dissecting aneurysms, preoperative characteristics are presented for descriptive purposes only and should not be used to compare these groups. These are most certainly dissimilar patient populations. Patients undergoing open repair were younger. A residual Debakey I dissection was present in 29% of patients having had an open repair versus 35% of patients having had a TEVAR procedure.

Postoperative outcomes for the two subsets are listed in Table 47-2. Hospital mortality was 10% in the open group and 0% in the TEVAR group. Moreover, in the open group, permanent stroke was 3%, permanent paraplegia was 12%, and postoperative dialysis was 10%. No patients in the TEVAR group incurred any of these complications. The mean stay in the intensive care unit was 13 days in the open group compared to 2 days in the TEVAR group. The mean length of hospital stay was 21 days in the open group compared to 7 days in the TEVAR group.

Even with the upfront concession that these are most certainly different patient populations with varied aortic anatomic complexities at presentation, the immediate in-hospital outcomes with TEVAR in what was an older patient subset are difficult to overlook. Clearly, technical success with TEVAR can be accomplished safely with very low morbidity and mortality in this high-risk patient population. However, a technically safe procedure does not necessarily equate to a beneficial procedure. It is not simply a question of whether TEVAR can be performed safely but whether TEVAR

TABLE 47-1. DEMOGRAPHICS FOR DEBAKEY III CHRONIC DISSECTING ANEURYSM PATIENTS UNDERGOING OPEN SURGERY VERSUS TEVAR AT THE UNIVERSITY OF PENNSYLVANIA

	Open Surgery			TEVAR		
	All	Residual Debakey I	De Novo	All	Residual Debakey I	De Novo
N	58	17	41	34	12	22
Age (mean ±SD)	57.3 ± 12	57.6 ± 14	57.1 ± 12	67.3 ± 10	66.0 ± 11	67.3 ± 11
Sex (male)	42 (72%)	12 (71%)	30 (73%)	23 (68%)	8 (67%)	15 (68%)
Hypertension	54 (98%)	16 (94%)	38 (93%)	29 (85%)	11 (92%)	18 (82%)
Prior stroke	9 (16%)	3 (18%)	6 (15%)	4 (12%)	3 (25%)	1 (5%)
Renal failure	9 (16%)	3 (18%)	6 (15%)	1 (3%)	0	1 (5%)
Creatinine (mean)	1.4	1.3	1.1	1.1	0.9	1.1
Dialysis	3 (5%)	1 (6%)	2 (5%)	0	0	0
Smoker	15 (26%)	4 (24%)	11 (27%)	5 (15%)	3 (25%)	2 (9%)
Lung disease (mild or worse)	19 (33%)	5 (29%)	14 (34%)	17 (50%)	7 (58%)	10 (45%)
Diabetic	2 (3%)	0	2 (5%)	4 (12%)	1 (8%)	3 (14%)

Abbreviations: SD, standard deviation; TEVAR, thoracic endovascular aortic repair.

TABLE 47-2. POSTOPERATIVE OUTCOMES FOR DEBAKEY III CHRONIC DISSECTING ANEURYSM PATIENTS UNDERGOING OPEN SURGERY VERSUS TEVAR AT THE UNIVERSITY OF PENNSYLVANIA

	Open Surgery			TEVAR		
	All	Residual Debakey I	De Novo	All	Residual Debakey I	De Novo
N	58	17	41	34	12	22
In-hospital mortality	6 (10%)	1 (6%)	5 (12%)	0	0	0
Stroke	2 (3%)	1 (6%)	1 (2%)	0	0	0
Permanent paraplegia	7 (12%)	0	7 (17%)	0	0	0
Postoperative renal failure	7 (12%)	2 (12%)	5 (12%)	0	0	0
New postoperative dialysis	6 (10%)	1 (6%)	5 (12%)	0	0	0
ICU stay (d), mean (range)	13 (2–71)	9 (2–63)	15 (2–71)	2 (0.6–5)	2 (1–5)	2 (0.6–5)
Ventilator time (h)	160	55	202	7	10	4
Hospital stay (d), mean (range)	21 (2–74)	19 (4–67)	22 (2–74)	7 (3–14)	7 (3–10)	7 (3–14)

Abbreviations: ICU, intensive care unit; TEVAR, thoracic endovascular aortic repair.

truly confers a survival advantage against aortic rupture and aorta-related mortality and overall mortality. Although open surgery continues to expose the patient to an appreciable morbidity and mortality risk, for those who are treated successfully, the treatment is decisive. The problem is eradicated. This is not necessarily the case with TEVAR. Although clinical trial data support the notion that chronically dissected aorta remodels, this does not directly equate to improved survival. Moreover, reinterventions and surveillance are assured to be an integral component to a TEVAR treatment strategy. Data to elucidate the true impact of false lumen thrombosis on late survival in Debakey III dissecting aneurysms is presently unavailable. Long-term outcomes data in these and similar patient subsets at the University of Pennsylvania and other aortic centers are pertinent to discerning the proper penetration that TEVAR should have into the management of this disease process going forward.

Although the currently available follow-up data for TEVAR in Debakey III chronic dissecting aneurysms is in too few patients and for too short a duration for any concrete interpretations, looking ahead, it does give some insights into what to expect from TEVAR as a treatment alternative.

False Lumen Status

Reiterating that which has been noted before, false lumen thrombosis did occur with TEVAR and is presented in Table 47-3. Prior to TEVAR, the thoracic false lumen was patent in all patients (Debakey IIIa chronic dissecting aneurysms and Debakey IIIb chronic dissecting aneurysms), and the abdominal false lumen was patent in all Debakey IIIb patients. Thoracic false lumen thrombosis occurred in all 12 (100%) Debakey IIIa patients and 16 (73%) Debakey IIIb patients. Less satisfying, however, was the persistent patent abdominal false lumen noted in 18 (82%) of 22 Debakey IIIb cases. Moreover, six patients with Debakey IIIb (27%) failed to produce thrombosis altogether in either the thoracic or the abdominal false lumen.

Interpreting these results, Debakey IIIb chronic dissecting aneurysms present a more challenging picture with respect to false lumen thrombosis than Debakey IIIa chronic dissecting aneurysms. Presumably this is due to distal reentrant tears left uncovered at the time of TEVAR and subsequent retrograde perfusion of the false lumen. If complete thrombosis of the false lumen inevitably proves protective in the treatment of Debakey III chronic dissecting aneurysms, the next step will be to delineate the degree of thrombosis necessary to incur benefit. More explicitly, will partial thrombosis of Debakey IIIb chronic dissecting aneurysms have any protective properties, harmful properties, or a negligible impact? Current case series in the literature on the effects of partial thrombosis are mixed with no clear answer one way or the other.

Reinterventions

Although in-hospital mortality and major morbidity were nil in the TEVAR cohort, reinterventions were common. Six (17%) TEVAR patients demonstrated persistent aneurysmal expansion of 1.5 cm or greater during follow-up. Four patients (Debakey IIIa = 1 and Debakey IIIb = 3) developed aneurysmal growth distal to the stent at the level of the celiac artery. A distal TEVAR extension was placed in three of the four patients. The fourth

TABLE 47-3. FALSE LUMEN THROMBOSIS FOR PATIENTS UNDERGOING TEVAR FOR DEBAKEY IIIA AND DEBAKEY IIIB CHRONIC DISSECTING ANEURYSMS

Thrombosis	All (N = 34)				Denovo (n = 22)				Residual Type A (n = 12)			
	Thoracic		Thoracic + Abdominal		Thoracic		Thoracic + Abdominal		Thoracic		Thoracic + Abdominal	
All (N = 34, 22, 12)	28	82%	4	12%	18	82%	2	9%	10	83%	2	17%
Debakey IIIA (N = 12, 8, 4)	12	100%	NA		8	100%	NA		4	100%	NA	
Debakey IIIB (N = 22, 14, 8)	16	73%	4	18%	10	71%	2	14%	6	75%	2	25%

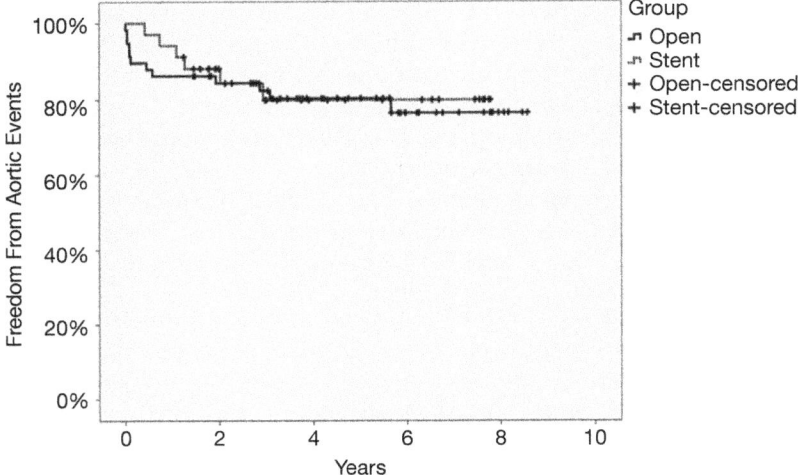

Figure 47-1. Kaplan–Meier survival curves for Debakey III chronic dissecting aneurysms treated with open surgery and TEVAR at the University of Pennsylvania. TEVAR, thoracic endovascular aortic repair.

patient was deemed inoperable at the time of presentation and was treated with optimal medical therapy. The remaining two patients had aneurysmal expansion of the proximal and mid segments of the descending thoracic aorta. Embolization of a type II endoleak from the left subclavian artery was performed in one patient, and the other had a type V endoleak that is being monitored closely with surveillance imaging.

Only four (7%) patients required reintervention in the open surgery group. Two patients underwent subsequent TEVAR. One patient had an intercostal patch leak and the other patient had an aortoenteric fistula. The additional two patients underwent a right hemicolectomy for mesenteric ischemia and a rectus femoris flap for a recurrent groin lymphocele.

Midterm Outcomes

Freedom from combined aortic reintervention, rupture, or aortic-related death at one, three, and five years, respectively, are 94.1%, 79.9%, and 79.9% for TEVAR versus 84.5%, 82.5%, and 80.4% for open repair ($P = 0.90$, mean follow-up 18 months ± 20, range 2–61 months) (Fig. 47-1).

OPEN REPAIR AND TEVAR EXPERIENCE AT OTHER MAJOR AORTIC CENTERS

Open Surgery

Contemporary results for open surgery at other major aortic centers treating Debakey III chronic dissecting aneurysms show similar results to our institution. The Cleveland Clinic reported hospital mortality of 9%, stroke 5%, permanent paraplegia or paraparesis 2%, and renal failure 11% in a cohort of 169 patients undergoing open repair for chronic distal aortic dissections between 2000 and 2008.[16] Almost half of their cohort required a thoracoabdominal repair, and 40% were deemed urgent/emergent cases. Reinterventions were required in 23 patients throughout the study period. Survival at one, two, and five years was 76%, 69%, and 55%, respectively. The Mount Sinai group in New York reported hospital mortality of 10%, stroke 6%, permanent paraplegia 5%, and renal failure 2% in a cohort of 104 patients undergoing open repair for chronic distal aortic dissections between 1994 and 2007.[17] Fifteen patients required reintervention during follow-up. Survival at 1, 5, and 10 years was 78%, 68%, and 59%, respectively.

To review the TEVAR experience is a little more difficult as follow-up with this procedure is limited at the present time. The Duke group has shown similar results to our own experience with this technology. In a cohort of 51 patients between 2005 and 2009, they too had no hospital death, no strokes, and no paraplegia or paresis.[19] At a median follow-up of 27 months, they had 10 deaths and an overall survival of 78% at 5 years. The University of Florida group has also reported their series of 80 patients undergoing TEVAR between 2004 and 2011 for Debakey III chronic aortic dissections.[20] At a median follow-up of 26 months, although hospital mortality was low at 2.5%, the overall neurologic event rate was 17%. Permanent paraplegia was 6% and stroke was 8%. A reintervention was required in 29% of the cohort with 16% occurring within the previously treated aortic segment. Survival at one and five years was 89% and 70%, respectively. A recent systematic review of the literature looking specifically at mid-term outcomes for TEVAR in Debakey III chronic aortic dissections through to January 2011 assessed 17 studies with 567 patients.[21] Thirty-day mortality was low at 3.2%, and stroke and paraplegia were less than 1%. With a median length of follow-up of 26 months (range 0.6–97), aorta-related mortality was 4.2% and all-cause mortality was 9.2%. Absolute reintervention rates ranged from 0% to 60%, while the median rate of complete false-lumen thrombosis was 86% (range 39%–100%).

SUMMARY

Chronic dissecting aneurysms of the descending aorta are of a complexity matched by very few other disease processes in cardiovascular medicine. Classically, the only treatment available to absolve patients from these fatal conditions was open thoracic or thoracoabdominal surgical repair. Although surgery remains the definitive solution for these complex problems, the shear amount of surgery required to perform the task can be quite extensive. Many patients faced with Debakey III dissecting aneurysm are unsuitable candidates for open repair. Moreover, even in the most experienced of aortic centers in patients who do have the strength to endure this operation, the risk of morbidity and mortality is not negligible. With the accumulated data from the INSTEAD trial and others to illustrate the ability to remodel dissected aorta beyond the acute phase of injury, in conjunction with the impressive short-term outcomes achieved with TEVAR thus far at select centers, there is certainly justification to explore TEVAR more seriously as a treatment option in Debakey III chronic dissecting aneurysms. A very important unknown that is in need of clarification is the true impact, if any, that TEVAR promoted false lumen thrombosis has on late outcomes. Currently, this answer remains unclear. Longer follow-up of the various datasets is necessary to best contextualize the potential association between false lumen thrombosis and an aorta-related reduction in mortality. This key point will inevitably dictate the utility of TEVAR to treat this disease process.

Still, that there is a role to be played by TEVAR in the management of chronic dissecting aneurysms is absolute. What is important to discern, similar to TEVAR use in degenerative aneurysms, is which patients with dissecting aneurysms are best suited for TEVAR, which is as of yet not well defined.

In an effort to try and define that population, it is presumed that TEVAR is best suited for patients with chronic dissections that are more localized. By focusing TEVAR on more focal dissections, the number of reentrant tears are minimized and the chance of achieving complete thrombosis of the false lumen increases. Patients deemed unsuitable for open repair, yet still maintain a level of social function that ensures TEVAR intervention will not be a futile process will also benefit.

It is pertinent that the aortic community continues to explore TEVAR and its relevance to chronic dissecting aneurysm management, while resisting the temptation to overuse the technology. Both TEVAR and open surgery have their roles to play. Proper patient selection is paramount to success with both treatment alternatives.

REFERENCES

1. Schwarze ML, Shen Y, Hemmerich J, Dale W. Age-related trends in utilization and outcome of open and endovascular repair for abdominal aortic aneurysm in the United States, 2001–2006. *J Vasc Surg*. 2009;50:722–729.
2. Scali ST, Goodney PP, Walsh DB, et al. National trends and regional variation of open and endovascular repair of thoracic and thoracoabdominal aneurysms in contemporary practice. *J Vasc Surg*. 2011;53:1499–1505.
3. Desai ND, Pochettino A, Szeto WY, et al. Thoracic endovascular aortic repair: evolution of therapy, patterns of use, and results in a 10-year experience. *J Thorac Cardiovasc Surg*. 2011;142:587–594.
4. Bavaria JE, Appoo JJ, Makaroun MS, et al. Endovascular stent grafting versus open surgical repair of descending thoracic aortic aneurysms in low-risk patients: a multicenter comparative trial. *J Thorac Cardiovasc Surg*. 2007;133:369–377.
5. Matsumura JS, Cambria RP, Dake MD, et al. International controlled clinical trial of thoracic endovascular aneurysm repair with the Zenith TX2 endovascular graft: 1-year results. *J Vasc Surg*. 2008;47:247–257.
6. Lee WA, Daniels MJ, Beaver TM, et al. Late outcomes of a single-center experience of 400 consecutive thoracic endovascular aortic repairs. *Circulation*. 2011;123:2661–2669.
7. Cheng D, Martin J, Shennib H, et al. Endovascular aortic repair versus open surgical repair for descending thoracic aortic disease: a systematic review and meta-analysis of comparative studies. *J Am Coll Cardiol*. 2010;55:986–1001.
8. Goodney PP, Travis L, Lucas FL, et al. Survival after open versus endovascular thoracic aortic aneurysm repair in an observational study of the Medicare population. *Circulation*. 2011;124:2661–2669.
9. Miller DC. Through the looking glass: the first 20 years of thoracic aortic stent-grafting. *J Thorac Cardiovasc Surg*. 2013;145(suppl 3):S142–S148.
10. Demers P, Miller DC, Mitchell RS, et al. Midterm results of endovascular repair of descending thoracic aortic aneurysms with first-generation stent grafts. *J Thorac Cardiovasc Surg*. 2004;127:664–673.
11. Szeto WY, McGarvey M, Pochettino A, et al. Results of a new surgical paradigm: endovascular repair for acute complicated type B aortic dissection. *Ann Thorac Surg*. 2008;86:87–93.
12. Wilkinson DA, Patel HJ, Williams DM, et al. Early open and endovascular thoracic aortic repair for complicated type B aortic dissection. *Ann Thorac Surg*. 2013;96:23–30.
13. White RA, Miller DC, Criado FJ, et al. Report on the results of thoracic endovascular aortic repair for acute, complicated, type B aortic dissection at 30 days and 1 year from a multidisciplinary subcommittee of the Society for Vascular Surgery Outcomes Committee. *J Vasc Surg*. 2011;53:1082–1090.

14. Svennson LG, Kouchoukos NT, Miller DC, et al. Expert consensus document on the treatment of descending thoracic aortic disease using endovascular stent-grafts. *Ann Thorac Surg.* 2008;85(suppl 1):S1–S41.
15. Leshnower BG, Szeto WY, Pochettino A, et al. Thoracic endografting reduces morbidity and remodels the thoracic aorta in Debakey III aneurysms. *Ann Thorac Surg.* 2012;95:914–921.
16. Pujara AC, Roselli EE, Hernandez AV, et al. Open repair of chronic distal aortic dissection in the endovascular era: implications for disease management. *J Thorac Cardiovasc Surg.* 2012;144:866–873.
17. Zoli S, Etz CD, Roder F, et al. Long-term survival after open repair of chronic distal aortic dissection. *Ann Thorac Surg.* 2010;89:1458–1466.
18. Nienaber CA, Rousseau H, Eggebrecht H, et al. Randomized comparison of strategies for type B aortic dissection. The investigation of stent grafts in aortic dissection (INSTEAD) trial. *Circulation.* 2009;120:2519–2528.
19. Parsa CJ, Williams JB, Bhattacharya SD, et al. Midterm results with thoracic endovascular aortic repair for chronic type B aortic dissection with associated aneurysm. *J Thorac Cardiovasc Surg.* 2011;141:322–327.
20. Scali ST, Feezor RJ, Chang CK, et al. Efficacy of thoracic endovascular stent repair for chronic type B aortic dissection with aneurysmal degeneration. *J Vasc Surg.* 2013;58:10–17.
21. Thrumurthy SG, Karthikesalingam A, Patterson BO, et al. A systematic review of mid-term outcomes of thoracic endovascular repair (TEVAR) of chronic type B aortic dissection. *Eur J Vasc Endovasc Surg.* 2011;42:632–647.

48

Thoracic Endovascular Aortic Repair Complicated by Acute Retrograde Dissection

Judson B. Williams, MD, MHS and G. Chad Hughes, MD

INTRODUCTION

Thoracic endovascular aortic repair (TEVAR) has been increasingly utilized as a treatment option for a variety of aortic pathologies since the first reports of satisfactory results began emerging in the 1990s.[1-3] In March 2005, the Gore TAG thoracic endoprosthesis (W.L. Gore and Associates, Flagstaff, AZ) became the first thoracic endoprosthesis to receive market approval for the treatment of thoracic aortic aneurysm by the Circulatory System Devices Panel of the United States Food and Drug Administration (FDA).[4] In May and June of 2008, the FDA approved two additional thoracic endografts, the Cook Zenith TX2 (Cook Incorporated, Bloomington, IN) and Medtronic Talent (Medtronic Vascular, Santa Rosa, CA) devices, and there are now a total of six FDA-approved thoracic endografts including the Gore C-TAG, Medtronic Valiant, and Bolton Relay (Bolton Medical, Sunrise, FL). Further, the C-TAG and Valiant devices are FDA approved for use in blunt traumatic aortic injury (transection). Although there have been no randomized studies, TEVAR for acute complicated Stanford type B dissection has been found in observational studies to be highly successful in technical implantation and is associated with shorter operating times, reduced blood loss, shorter hospital stay, reduced risk of paraplegia, and lower morbidity and mortality when compared to historical controls as well as contemporaneous open repairs.[5] Prospective clinical trial data to date have been limited to the industry-sponsored Gore C-TAG and Medtronic Valiant trials that have been recently completed. Finally, results are anticipated from the ongoing ADSORB (Acute Uncomplicated Aortic Dissection Type B: Evaluating Stent-Graft Placement or Best Medical Treatment Alone) trial, a prospective randomized trial evaluating the role of TEVAR in uncomplicated dissection currently under way in Europe.[6] Recent population-based studies have indicated that TEVAR trends are mirroring endovascular AAA trends of a decade ago, showing increased endovascular and decreased open repair utilization.[7,8]

Medical device trials, including those leading to FDA approval of TEVAR devices, are typically conducted in tightly monitored environments in specialized medical centers, and postprocedural data is collected for limited periods of time. While such carefully conducted randomized controlled trials provide essential information for determination of safety and efficacy of emerging medical products, the data gathered through randomized controlled trials for transformative technologies such as the TEVAR endoprostheses ultimately serves as prologue to real-world testing of the device by clinicians in everyday practice.[9]

As clinical databases and registries accumulate data, uncommon complications of TEVAR devices are expected to be recognized and characterized, particularly when used for indications outside FDA-specified indications. Accumulating reports have identified retrograde ascending aortic dissection as a potentially lethal complication of TEVAR.[10,11] This chapter will focus on recent evidence from peer-reviewed studies to provide an overview of the incidence, risk factors, etiology, treatment, and outcomes of retrograde ascending aortic dissection (rAAD) as a complication following TEVAR.

INCIDENCE AND RISK FACTORS

The risk of iatrogenic dissection of the ascending aorta after TEVAR has only recently been acknowledged as experience has grown and the clinical applications of TEVAR techniques have expanded.[12] Iatrogenic aortic dissection accounts for approximately 5% of all acute aortic dissections and is a well-known complication of coronary angiography, percutaneous coronary interventions, and open heart surgery. TEVAR has now been added to this list of procedures potentially resulting in iatrogenic dissection, and with increased awareness, forthcoming data is expected. Published reports have identified retrograde ascending aortic dissection (rAAD) as a potential complication of TEVAR for all indications and have estimated the risk of this complication to range between 1.3% and 6.8%.[10,11,13,14]

In one observational study of consecutive U.S. patients undergoing TEVAR from March 2005 through May 2010 at a single high-volume center (Duke University Medical Center, Durham, NC), six cases of rAAD were identified for an overall incidence of 1.9% for rAAD following TEVAR for all indications.[15] Each of the cases was identified in the perioperative period (range 0–6 days), and 30-day/in-hospital mortality was 33%. The rAAD incidence in the Duke series of 3.3%[15] following TEVAR for a dissection indication was consistent with that reported by Dong et al. (2.5%)[11] but lower than that reported by Neuhauser et al. (17.8%).[16]

An important difference between the Duke series[15] and both the European Registry on Endovascular Aortic Repair Complications by Eggebrecht et al.[10] and a Chinese study by Dong et al.[11] is the practice of generally avoiding endograft placement in the native aorta of patients with connective tissue disorders (CTD). The European Registry captured 48 TEVAR cases in Marfan patients (rAAD incidence 8.3%), and 27% (3 of 11) of rAAD cases in the Dong et al. study were patients with the Marfan syndrome.[10,11]

While the rAAD complication was observed following TEVAR with each of the principal devices used in the Duke series, including the Gore TAG, Zenith TX2, and Talent devices, rAAD incidence was observed to be numerically highest with the Talent (4.7%) and Zenith TX2 (3.6%) endografts.[15]

TABLE 48-1. KEY RISK FACTORS FOR RETROGRADE ASCENDING AORTIC DISSECTION FOLLOWING TEVAR

Presence of connective tissue disorder
Ascending aortic diameter >40 mm
Proximal landing zone in native ascending aorta (zone 0)
TEVAR for dissection indication
Endografts utilizing proximal bare springs or barbs for fixation
Excessive balloon molding of the endograft
Excessive stent graft oversizing

Sources: Eggebrecht et al.,[10] Dong et al.,[11] Kpodonu et al.,[14] Williams et al.,[15] Tshomba et al.,[18] Bellos et al.[27]

In a large multi-institutional analysis including 28 centers participating in the European Registry on Endovascular Aortic Repair Complications, Eggebrecht et al. found that 40 of 48 (83%) cases of rAAD following TEVAR occurred when the indication for the procedure was treatment of either acute or chronic descending aortic dissection.[10] Given the typically increased fragility of the aortic wall of patients suffering spontaneous dissection, it is not surprising that investigators have begun discovering a higher incidence of rAAD when treating this pathology. Similarly, in the single-center series from Duke, incidence also appeared higher when performing TEVAR for dissection (3.3%) and also when utilizing native ascending aorta (zone 0) for the proximal landing zone (7.4%).[15] Although Eggebrecht et al. report 16 cases occurring in TEVAR with zone 3 proximal landing zone[10] in the Duke experience, all rAAD cases occurred in the setting of more proximal landing zones (zones 0, 1, or 2). In light of these findings, we replace even the mildly dilated (≥4.0 cm) ascending aorta whenever feasible in patients undergoing zone 0 hybrid arch repair so as to mitigate the risk of retrograde type A dissection. Moreover, the high incidence of retrograde type A dissection may represent a major technical limitation of the zone 0 hybrid arch operation.[16]

In summary, risk factors for rAAD (Table 48-1) have become increasingly defined in the literature, and knowledge of these predisposing factors may help clinicians minimize the incidence of this potentially devastating complication.

ETIOLOGY

The potential etiologies of rAAD following TEVAR may be classified as procedure related (manipulation of wires, sheaths, etc.), device related (proximal fixation, graft oversizing, etc.), and disease progression, although this latter etiology does not necessarily represent true rAAD in all cases and may be due to spontaneous dissection in a patient with pan-aortic disease, especially if the dissection occurs after the index TEVAR procedure.

Excessive radial force from oversizing of the stent graft prosthesis to >20% relative to the diameter of the aorta has been proposed by Kpodonu et al. as a potential causative factor for rAAD following TEVAR.[14] Kpodonu et al. examined only the Gore TAG endoprosthesis and found potentially excessive oversizing of the endograft occurred in three of seven rAAD patients.[14] This did not, by contrast, appear to be a causative factor in the Duke series, with average device oversizing approximately 9% (range 0%–23%) for both those patients with and without rAAD.[15] The work by Kpodonu is supported by other investigators who have found that oversizing of stent grafts >10% results in a higher radial force against the aortic wall, with potential intimal injury and tears occurring if oversizing is >20% of Instructions for Use (IFU) recommendations.[14]

Dynamic interactions between the endoprosthesis and the native aorta may also play a role in rAAD development, particularly in cases with native ascending aorta (zone 0) proximal landing zone. Radial expansion-contraction and translational wall motion are most pronounced for zone 0 aortic endografting.[17,18] Etiology of rAAD in "zone 0" could be referable to both the concomitant arch debranching procedure and the proximal endograft landing zone in the ascending aorta. With regard to debranching-related mechanisms, the risk of aortic side-clamping under pulsatile flow in development of AAD is well known during off-pump coronary artery bypass graft surgery, especially in cases of increased ascending aortic diameter.[19,20] It is unknown whether this risk is increased by the presence of a large anastomosis on the ascending aorta as required for arch debranching. The perils of zone 0 landing are further highlighted by accumulating data to suggest that endograft placement in the native ascending aorta is associated with high rates of retrograde type A dissection and 30-day/in-hospital mortality and should be approached with caution.[21]

Regarding the "endovascular-related" mechanisms, it may be hypothesized that specific endograft characteristics, such as proximal bare springs or hooks, excessive oversizing, or additional balloon dilatation, may theoretically increase the risk of aortic damage and subsequent rAAD. Several groups of investigators have suggested that rAAD may be more common with devices using proximal bare springs, suggesting that this component may confer an increased risk of rAAD.[11,14,22] In the aforementioned European Registry study by Eggebrecht et al., devices with proximal bare springs were used in 27 of 29 (93%) patients suffering TEVAR-related rAAD.[10] Further, 60% of the rAAD cases were classified as induced by the endograft itself, with direct evidence of aortic injury observed during surgery or necropsy in most cases. Other investigators have proposed that balloon dilation of the stent graft may be associated with rAAD following TEVAR.[14,23] Intimal tear could be caused by applying the radial force of balloon angioplasty to devices with proximal bare springs or directly to the aorta itself.

A multitude of aortic-related factors, such as highly angulated aortic arch and inherent fragility of the aortic wall, may also play a role in development of rAAD. As mentioned in the European Registry, 81% of patients who experienced rAAD underwent TEVAR for an aortic dissection indication, the majority of which were acute. The idea that some cases of rAAD following TEVAR are due to disease progression is supported by reports of AAD in patients who have not had any procedure (e.g., optimal medical therapy only for type B aortic dissection) as well as in patients who have undergone conventional open descending aortic replacement.[23,24] With regard to the concept of ascending aortic dissection occurring as a result of disease progression, patients undergoing TEVAR for type B dissection who also have some element of retrograde type A intramural hematoma may be particularly at risk for this phenomenon given the fact that approximately one-third of intramural hematomas will evolve into true dissection in follow-up. This type of dissection of the ascending aorta observed after TEVAR should probably not be classified as a true rAAD, as the dissection is not due to placement of the endograft (Fig. 48-1). Similarly, we have previously observed acute type A dissection in patients status post prior TEVAR in whom the dissection event occurred late (months) after the procedure, and in whom the findings at surgical repair were consistent with spontaneous dissection in that the primary tear was located in the typical location along the greater curve of the ascending

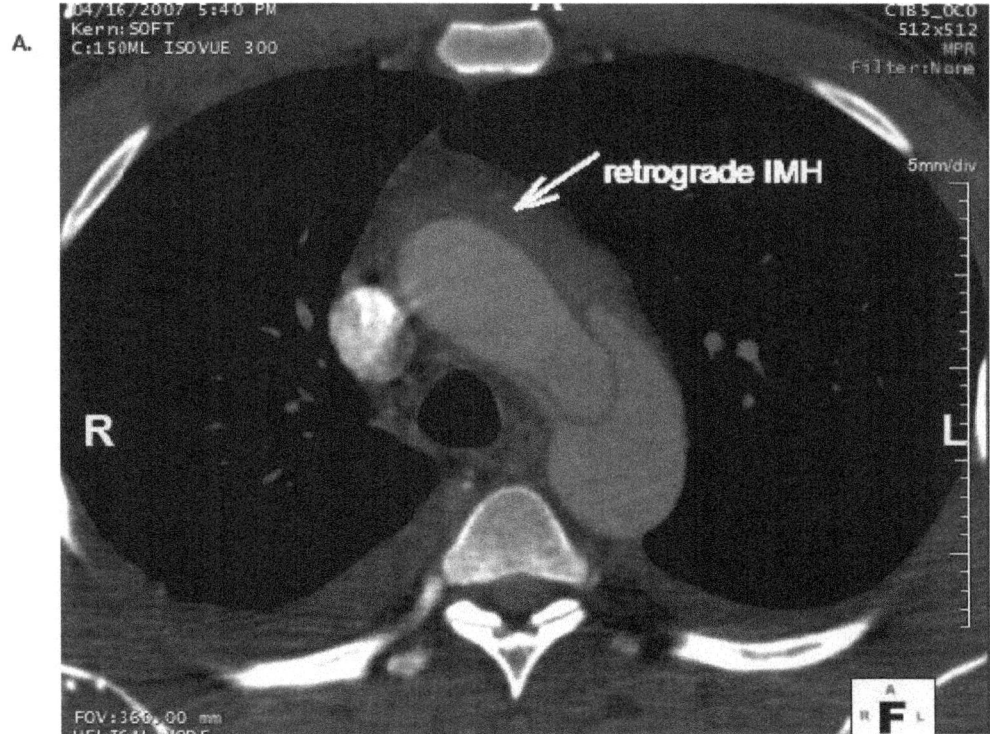

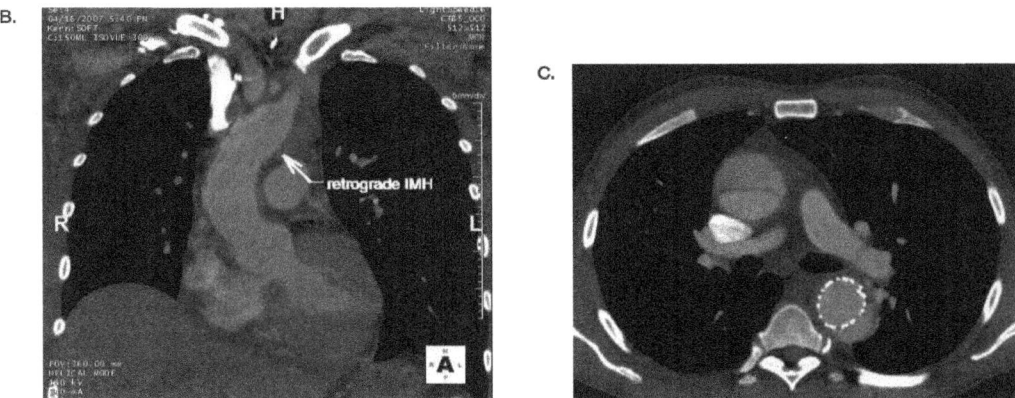

Figure 48-1. Example of patient with acute, complicated type B dissection with associated retrograde type A intramural hematoma component as demonstrated in panels *A* and *B*. The patient underwent TEVAR for his dissection and did well with resolution of his iliofemoral malperfusion syndrome. However, one-month follow-up CTA, *C*, demonstrates that the previously noted ascending aortic intramural hematoma has evolved into a chronic type A dissection for which the patient underwent elective repair. Findings at surgery demonstrated a primary tear in the arch distant from the endograft and not consistent with an endograft-induced etiology.

aorta and not in the region of the endovascular device (Fig. 48-2). We do not consider these cases as true rAAD, as patients with disease of the descending thoracic aorta frequently have a pan-aortopathy due to their underlying aortic risk factors and therefore are at risk for spontaneous dissection as well. Whether a prior TEVAR procedure somehow increases the risk for later spontaneous proximal aortic dissection due to the

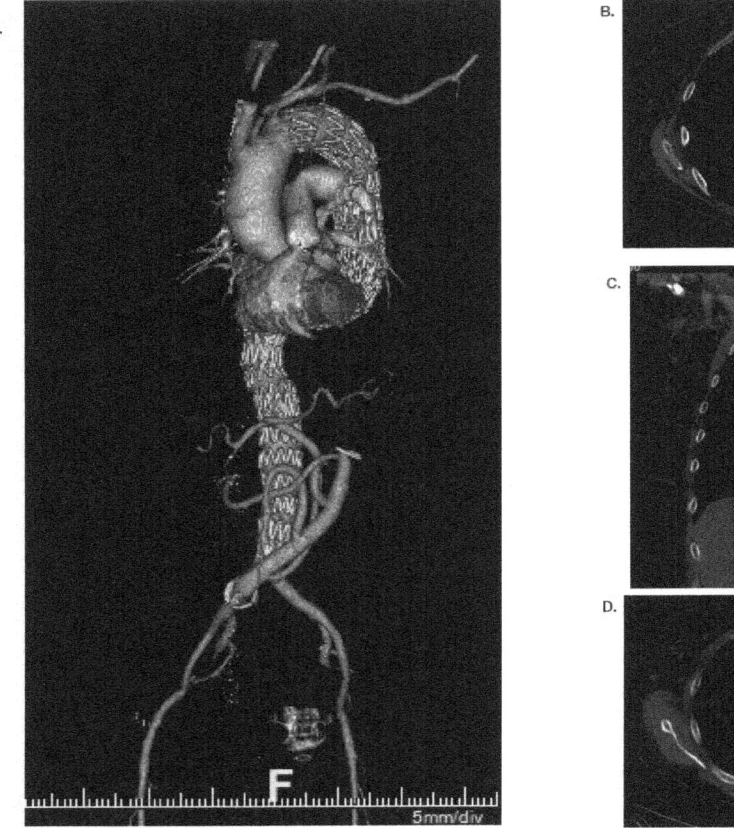

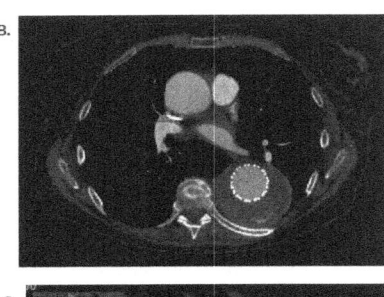

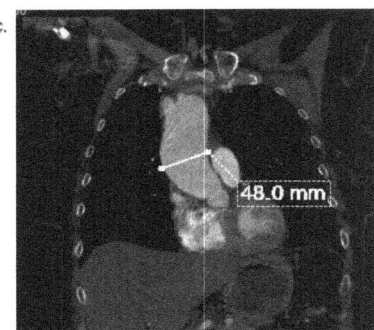

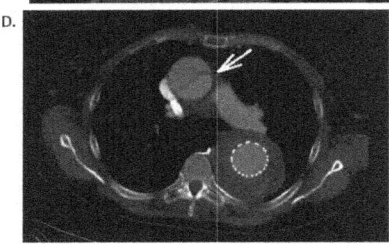

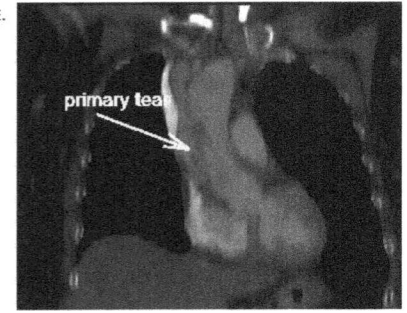

Figure 48-2. *A*, 3D-CTA reconstruction image of 62-year-old female one month status-post hybrid repair of a symptomatic 8.9-cm Extent II thoracoabdominal aortic aneurysm. Note intact ascending aorta. *B*, Axial CTA image from the same scan clearly demonstrating the ascending aorta to be intact and without dissection. *C*, Coronal reconstruction image demonstrating ascending aorta to be moderately dilated to a diameter of 4.8 cm consistent with pan-aortic disease. *D*, Axial CTA image from the same patient five weeks later when she presented with new onset chest pain. Scan demonstrates new type A dissection involving the ascending aorta (arrow). *E*, Coronal reconstruction CTA image demonstrating large primary tear in mid-ascending aorta along the greater curve, which is the typical location for spontaneous ascending dissection. The patient underwent emergent repair including ascending aorta and hemi-arch replacement. Intraoperative findings demonstrated the primary tear in the same location as suggested by the CTA images. Inspection of the aortic arch under deep hypothermic circulatory arrest revealed no tears in the arch with a well-seated proximal endograft, also consistent with spontaneous rather than retrograde ascending aortic dissection in a patient with pan-aortic disease.

increased stiffness of the downstream aorta after endograft placement or micro-injury to the ascending aorta due to catheters or wires used at the time of the procedure is currently unknown and additional investigation in this area is needed.

PREVENTION AND DETECTION

Several strategies should be considered for the prevention and early detection of rAAD following TEVAR. The incidence of rAAD may potentially be reduced by limited device oversizing, avoidance of aggressive postdeployment ballooning, careful patient selection, and avoidance of excessive perioperative hypertension. Knowledge of currently defined risk factors (Table 48-1) is mandatory as well as the fact that the risk of rAAD appears additive when multiple risk factors are present in any given patient.[15]

A significant difference exists between stent grafting for aneurysm versus dissection indications. Utilization of TEVAR technology for treatment of thoracic aortic aneurysm requires the stable fixation of an endoprosthesis to a relatively short proximal and distal landing zone. As opposed to dissection, the aorta for landing is typically more normal in caliber but does require adequate radial force for the stent graft(s) to remain in place. In the treatment of dissection pathology, the entire length of the endoprosthesis typically attaches to the aorta and consequently a lower radial force may be required to achieve stable long-lasting fixation. In cases of dissection, the proximal (occasionally) and in particular the distal landing zones are typically involved in some way by the dissection process, and resistance provided by the aortic wall against the stent graft is reduced. As such, a lower radial force stent graft designed specifically for the treatment of dissection may be beneficial. Moreover, consideration should be given to maximize the ability of stent grafts for dissection to be conformable to the distal arch. Development of less rigid endoprostheses with improved conformability for use in cases of dissection and other high-risk groups may be expected to help reduce the incidence of post-TEVAR rAAD.[22]

Patients with CTD are generally recognized as poor candidates for TEVAR,[23] and placing thoracic endografts in the native aorta of patients with connective tissue disorders should generally be avoided, except possibly in the case of acute complicated type B dissection.[24] CTD patients with previous Dacron graft replacement of segments of the thoracic aorta may be successfully treated with a thoracic endoprosthesis provided there is satisfactory landing zone that does not involve the native aorta.[25] Also, of particular concern with regard to rAAD, one must remain cognizant of stress injury provoked by a passively bent endoprosthesis, which may be more poorly tolerated in the patient with a known CTD. As such, endograft devices without proximal bare springs are recommended when utilizing TEVAR technology for patients with known connective tissue disorders or other risk factors for rAAD.

Excessive oversizing of the stent graft should be avoided in TEVAR. What constitutes excessive oversizing is still a point of discussion, and the relationship between excessive oversizing and the risk of rAAD remains unclear. Oversizing of 10%–15% appears to be adequate for fixation of the endoprosthesis in many large series and oversizing to >20% has been strongly associated with rAAD.[26] In a review and recent retrospective analysis of the literature in the past 10 years, Khoynezhad and White have also cautioned against ballooning outside of the covered portion of the stent graft, which applies balloon pressure directly to the aortic wall.[26]

Careful manipulation of endovascular devices is certainly paramount. Partially deployed stent graft devices should never be advanced. Care should be taken to avoid placement of the end holes of catheters used for contrast power injection directly against the aortic wall (Fig. 48-3). If an endoprosthesis is placed within a proximal landing zone containing some portion of dissected aortic wall, balloon inflation is perilous.

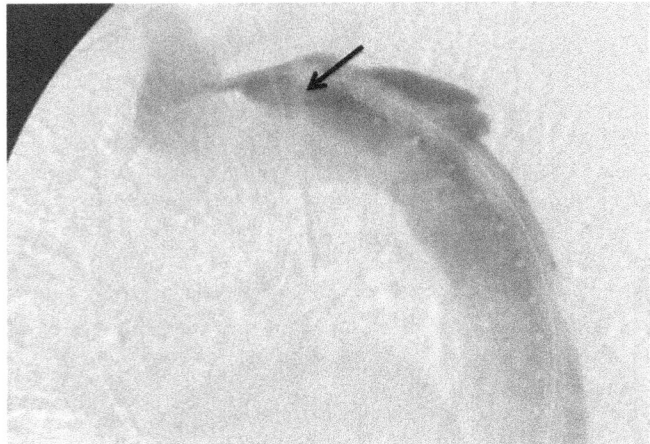

Figure 48-3. Intraoperative aortogram showing acute retrograde type A dissection caused by location of tip of injection pigtail catheter adjacent to the aortic wall (arrow). Angiogram image clearly demonstrates retrograde ascending aortic dissection due to intimal injury caused by the power injection. This was confirmed by intraoperative TEE, and the patient underwent successful open repair after completion of the TEVAR procedure.

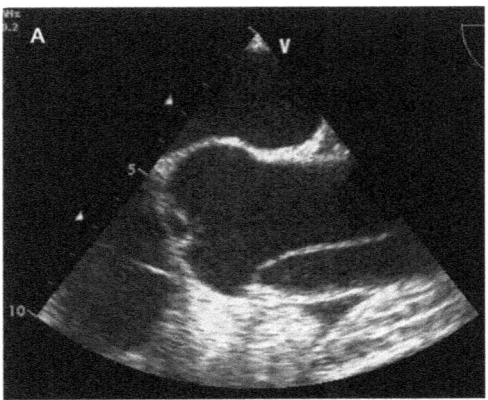

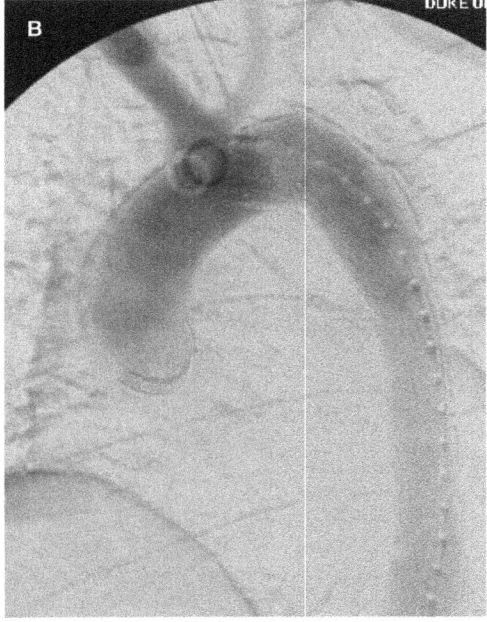

Figure 48-4. *A*, Intraoperative transesophageal echocardiogram (TEE) showing retrograde ascending aortic dissection on a long axis view. *B*, Completion intraoperative angiogram from the same patient did not reveal the presence of the retrograde ascending aortic dissection as seen on the simultaneous TEE, thus highlighting the limitations of angiography alone for the detection of this complication. TEE revealed the complication leading to immediate open repair with proximal aortic replacement.

Transesophageal echocardiography (TEE), completion angiography, and intravascular ultrasound (IVUS) remain important adjuncts for intraoperative detection of rAAD and other complications. Although the role of IVUS in facilitating early detection of rAAD following TEVAR remains somewhat unproven,[27] IVUS is believed by some experts, including ourselves, to have almost 100% diagnostic accuracy.[22] In the Duke series, IVUS was used for detection intraoperatively for two of the six rAAD patients in that study.[15] Completion intraoperative imaging of the ascending aorta with TEE ± IVUS should be considered mandatory following TEVAR as angiography is not entirely reliable in the detection of this complication in our experience (Fig. 48-4).[15] In the follow-up period, computed tomography angiography is the mainstay for diagnosis, although the vast majority of rAADs occur intraoperatively and should therefore be detected at the time of the procedure to allow for early repair and the best chance of a favorable patient outcome.[15]

TREATMENT

Prompt operative intervention, typically with open surgical conversion and graft replacement of the involved ascending thoracic aorta, usually with concurrent hemi-arch replacement, represents the treatment of choice for rAAD complicating TEVAR. Medical management of rAAD has been described for clinically stable asymptomatic patients with expected high mortality with open repair,[28] although we would not recommend this practice unless frank discussions are held with family members regarding the pros and cons, including the risk of rupture, with such an approach. Further, medical management should probably only be utilized for those rAAD discovered beyond the immediate postoperative period, which will be the vast minority of cases in our experience. Medical treatment includes anti-impulse therapy with beta-blockers and afterload reducing agents to maintain heart rate <70 and systolic blood pressure <140 mmHg. In general, retrograde AAD discovered intraoperatively and presumed to be due to the TEVAR procedure mandates' emergent open operation. It is notable that many cases have been discovered even after the patient has achieved hospital discharge, with cases reported as being discovered greater than a year after the procedure. However, it is likely that the vast majority of these late dissections represent missed events, which occurred at the time of surgery, and in which the patient was fortunate enough to survive without intervention.[20] Alternatively, some may represent metachronously developing pathology as outlined above. In the European Registry, 46% of cases occurred within the first 30 days, whereas 31% were noted greater than three months after the TEVAR procedure.[10] Whether these latter cases may be referable to disease progression, as opposed to procedure-related etiologies, is unclear. While the natural history of iatrogenic rAAD is not established, availability of surgeons for open repair of rAAD should be mandatory in any center performing TEVAR given that the optimal treatment appears to be prompt surgical repair.[26,29-31]

CONCLUSIONS

Emerging data indicate that retrograde ascending aortic dissection is a serious complication of TEVAR, which is being utilized as an ever-expanding treatment strategy for a variety of pathologies of the thoracic aorta. This morbid complication warrants careful vigilance for trends with the use of new devices and techniques as well as careful vigilance for individual patients. Thoracic endografting procedures should only be performed by cardiothoracic surgeons or with a cardiothoracic surgeon present and scrubbed for the operation, given that immediate repair due to ascending aortic rupture is occasionally required. Intraoperative TEE ± IVUS assessment of the ascending aorta should be considered standard of care following TEVAR to avoid under-recognition of this often lethal complication in the early perioperative period.[32] Clinical trials testing dissection-specific stent grafts with lower radial force, greater conformability, and elimination of barbs are forthcoming in the United States, and it is hoped that the results of these studies may demonstrate a reduction in the incidence of this complication.

REFERENCES

1. Nienaber C, Fattori R, Lund G, et al. Nonsurgical reconstruction of thoracic aortic dissection by stent-graft placement. *N Engl J Med*. 1999;340:1539–1545.
2. Hughes G, Lee SM, Daneshmand MA, et al. Endovascular repair of descending thoracic aneurysms: results with "on-label" application in the post Food and Drug Administration approval era. *Ann Thorac Surg*. 2010;90(1):83–89.
3. Dake M, Miller DC, Semba CP, et al. Transluminal placement of endovascular stent-grafts for the treatment of descending thoracic aortic aneurysms. *N Engl J Med*. 1994;331(26):1729–1734.
4. Cho J, Haider SE, Makaroun MS. Endovascular therapy of thoracic aneurysms: Gore TAG trial results. *Semin Vasc Surg*. 2006;19(1):1–24.
5. Ulug P, McCaslin JE, Stansby G, Powell JT. Endovascular versus conventional medical treatment for uncomplicated chronic type B aortic dissection. *Cochrane Database Syst Rev*. November 14, 2012;11:CD006512.
6. Brunkwall J, Lammer J, Verhoeven E, Taylor P. ADSORB: a study on the efficacy of endovascular grafting in uncomplicated acute dissection of the descending aorta. *Eur J Vasc Endovasc Surg*. July 2012;44(1):31–36.
7. Walker KL, Shuster JJ, Martin TD, et al. Practice patterns for thoracic aneurysms in the stent graft era: health care system implications. *Ann Thorac Surg*. 2010;90(6):1833–1839.
8. Orandi BJ, Dimick JB, Deeb GM, et al. A population-based analysis of endovascular versus open thoracic aortic aneurysm repair. *J Vasc Surg*. 2009;49(5):1112–1116.
9. Behrman RE, Benner JS, Brown JS, et al. Developing the Sentinel System-a national resource for evidence development. *N Engl J Med*. 2011;364(6):498–499.
10. Eggebrecht H, Thompson M, Rousseau H, et al. European Registry on Endovascular Aortic Repair Complications. Retrograde ascending aortic dissection during or after thoracic aortic stent graft placement: insight from the European Registry on endovascular aortic repair complications. *Circulation*. 2009;120(suppl 11):S276–S281.
11. Dong ZH, Fu WG, Wang YQ, et al. Retrograde type A aortic dissection after endovascular stent graft placement for treatment of type B dissection. *Circulation*. 2009;119(5):735–741.
12. Roberts WC. Aortic dissection: anatomy, consequences, and causes. *Am Heart J*. 1981;101(2):195–214.
13. Neuhauser B, Czermak BV, Fish J, et al. Type A dissection following endovascular thoracic aortic stent-graft repair. *J Endovasc Ther*. 2005;12(1):74–81.
14. Kpodonu J, Preventza O, Ramaiah VG, et al. Retrograde type A dissection after endovascular stenting of the descending thoracic aorta. Is the risk real? *Eur J Cardiothorac Surg*. 2008;33(6):1014–1018.
15. Williams JB, Andersen ND, Bhattacharya SD, et al. Retrograde ascending aortic dissection as an early complication of thoracic endovascular aortic repair. *J Vasc Surg*. May 2012;55(5):1255–1262.

16. Neuhauser B, Greiner A, Jaschke W, et al. Serious complications following endovascular thoracic aortic stent-graft repair for type B dissection. *Eur J Cardiothorac Surg*. 2008;33(1):58–63.

17. Jin S, Oshinski J, Giddens DP. Effects of wall motion and compliance on flow patterns in the ascending aorta. *J Biomech Eng*. 2003;125(3):347–354.

18. Tshomba Y, Bertoglio L, Marone EM, et al. Retrograde type A dissection after endovascular repair of a "zone 0" nondissecting aortic arch aneurysm. *Ann Vasc Surg*. 2010;24(7):952 e1–e7.

19. Chavanon O, Carrier M, Cartier R, et al. Increased incidence of acute ascending aortic dissection with off-pump aortocoronary bypass surgery? *Ann Thorac Surg*. January 2001;71(1):117–121.

20. Williams ML, Sheng S, Gammie JS, et al. Aortic dissection as a complication of cardiac surgery: report from the Society of Thoracic Surgeons database. *Ann Thorac Surg*. December 2010;90(6):1812–1816.

21. Andersen ND, Williams JB, Hanna JM, et al. Results with an algorithmic approach to hybrid repair of the aortic arch. *J Vasc Surg*. March 2013;57(3):655–667;discussion 666–667.

22. Fattori R, Lovato L, Buttazzi K, et al. Extension of dissection in stent-graft treatment of type B aortic dissection: lessons learned from endovascular experience. *J Endovasc Ther*. 2005;12(3):306–311.

23. Waterman AL, Feezor RJ, Lee WA, et al. Endovascular treatment of acute and chronic aortic pathology in patients with Marfan syndrome. *J Vasc Surg*. May 2012;55(5):1234–1240;discussion 1240–1241.

24. Hanna JM, Andersen ND, Ganapathi AM, et al. Five-year results for endovascular repair of acute complicated type B aortic dissection. *J Vasc Surg*. 2013;S0741–5214(13):01280–9.

25. Ganapathi AM, Hanna JM, Andersen ND, et al. Comparison of type I endoleak rates in Dacron versus native aorta landing zones during thoracic endovascular aortic repair. In: Southern Association for Vascular Surgery 37th Annual Meeting, January 23–26, 2013; Paradise Island, Bahamas.

26. Khoynezhad A, White RA. Pathogenesis and management of retrograde type A aortic dissection after thoracic endovascular aortic repair. *Ann Vasc Surg*. March 2013. doi: pii: S0890–5096(13)00039–3.24.

27. Bellos JK, Petrosyan A, Abdulamit T, et al. Retrograde type A aortic dissections after endovascular stent-graft placement for type B dissection. *J Cardiovasc Surg (Torino)*. 2010;51(1):85–93.

28. Lumsden AB, Reardon MJ. Once dissected always dissected! Can stent grafts change the natural history of type B dissections?: a report from the International Registry of Acute Aortic Dissection. *JACC Cardiovasc Interv*. 2008;1(4):403–404.

29. Hagan PG, Nienaber CA, Isselbacher EM, et al. The International Registry of Acute Aortic Dissection (IRAD): new insights into an old disease. *JAMA*, 2000;283(7):897–903.

30. Setacci F, Sirignano P, de Donato G, et al. Acute aortic dissection: natural history and classification. *J Cardiovasc Surg (Torino)*. 2010;51(5):641–646.

31. Luehr M, Etz CD, Lehmkuhl L, et al. Surgical management of delayed retrograde type A aortic dissection following complete supra-aortic de-branching and stent-grafting of the transverse arch. *Eur J Cardiothorac Surg*. April 10, 2013. [Epub ahead of print].

32. Kpodonu J, Ramaiah VG, Diethrich EB. Intravascular ultrasound imaging as applied to the aorta: a new tool for the cardiovascular surgeon. *Ann Thorac Surg*. 2008;86(4):1391–1398.

49

Ascending Repair Combined with Thoracic Endovascular Aortic Repair for Type A Acute Aortic Dissection

William D.T. Kent MD, MSc and S. Chris Malaisrie, MD

INTRODUCTION

Described by Laennec in 1826 as a dissecting aneurysm of the aorta, acute aortic dissection (AAD) has a high rate of mortality. This is particularly true in the case of type A AAD, which has a dismal natural history with death occurring in 80% of patients at two weeks.[1,2] Surgeons are credited with decreasing the lethality of this disease by developing strategies to repair the aorta. Most significant was the invention of the synthetic graft by Debakey and Cooley, which made it possible to replace the ascending aorta.[3] Since then, improvements in surgical repair techniques and ICU care have translated into greater survival through the perioperative period. Repair of type A AAD today, according to the International Registry of Acute Aortic Dissection (IRAD), is associated with a 24% risk of mortality. At centers of excellence in aortic surgery, the risk may be as low as 9%–10%.[4-6] However, over the long term, morbidity and mortality remain substantial. According to several large series, at 10 years after repair, the need for reintervention is between 30% and 50% with an overall mortality rate of approximately 50%.[2,4,7] Given this, repair strategies must evolve to improve results over the long term by decreasing mortality and the need for reintervention. Endovascular techniques may offer the greatest potential to achieve this goal. For chronic thoracic aortic pathology, thoracic endovascular aortic repair (TEVAR) has proven to be a safe, less invasive alternative to open repair. As experience with this technology has grown and stent graft development has progressed, TEVAR has been shown to be applicable in the acute setting as well. For complicated type B AAD, TEVAR is often the treatment of choice, particularly for older patients or those with comorbidities who would be high risk for open repair. Endovascular repair for type A AAD is still evolving and may play an increasingly important role in the future.

THE CONVENTIONAL OPERATION FOR TYPE A
ACUTE AORTIC DISSECTION

First performed in Houston by Dr. Debakey in 1963, the standard strategy for repair of a type A AAD involves replacement of the ascending aorta with an interposition Dacron graft. The conventional cannulation strategy is through a cut-down in the groin to expose the femoral artery and vein for establishment of cardiopulmonary bypass (CPB). Usually effective systemic perfusion is achieved, but it is not unusual to encounter a dissection flap extending into the femoral artery resulting in malperfusion related to dynamic obstruction in the descending thoracic aorta. This can be mitigated by establishing inflow through the axillary artery or the contralateral femoral artery for dual inflow. Although the classical approach is to clamp the distal ascending and resect the dissected tissue of the ascending aorta, as shown in Figure 49-1, the use of hypothermic circulatory arrest (HCA) has become the most common technique since the 1980s. With this technique, the patient is cooled to a systemic temperature of 18°–24° Celsius. The ascending aorta is then opened under HCA to facilitate visualization of the primary intimal tear in the ascending aorta or aortic arch. HCA also facilitates complete resection of the ascending aorta and accurate sewing of the friable dissected aortic tissue in a bloodless field. After completion of the distal anastomosis, systemic flow is reestablished. During rewarming, the proximal anastomosis at the sinotubular junction is performed. As presented in Table 49-1, this achieves the goals of resecting the primary entry tear, correcting acute aortic valve insufficiency and restoring flow in the downstream true lumen.

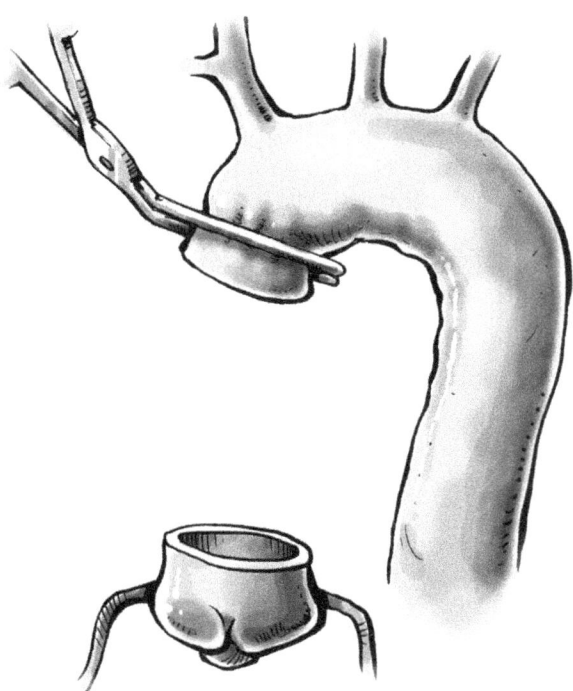

Figure 49-1. Conventional repair of acute type A AAD involving resection of the ascending aorta.

TABLE 49-1. TYPE A ACUTE AORTIC DISSECTION: GOALS OF REPAIR

To resect the dissected ascending aorta, which is at risk of intrapericardial rupture
To eliminate aortic regurgitation by valve resuspension or aortic root replacement
To restore true lumen flow to treat distal malperfusion

ADVANCES IN CONVENTIONAL REPAIR TECHNIQUES

Although the basic principles of repair have remained the same, operative techniques have evolved and this has helped to improve outcomes. The use of cerebral perfusion during HCA was a significant advance. Developed by Ueda in 1990, the original technique using retrograde cerebral perfusion has three advantages: It provides uniform cooling of the brain and lowers the metabolic rate, it flushes out air or debris, and it delivers nutrient rich blood to the brain. More recently, right axillary artery cannulation has been used to provide antegrade cerebral perfusion during HCA. This technique provides more physiologic delivery of oxygenated, nutrient-rich blood, and there is evidence that it is associated with a decreased incidence of stroke and mortality.[8]

Technical advances that have facilitated safe management of the proximal aorta include reliable reconstruction of the dissected aortic root tissue with synthetic material. With preservation of the aortic root, the aortic valve can be resuspended by tacking up the commissures with pledgeted sutures. Surgical adhesives, such as protein hydrogel's, can often be used as an adjunct to this reconstruction with or without Teflon felt.[5] A modified Bentall procedure to replace the aortic root and valve is required in patients with more extensive dissections with severe aortic regurgitation or intrinsically diseased aortic root sinuses. The development of composite mechanical or biologic valve-graft conduits and improved techniques of coronary reconstruction has allowed surgeons to perform these procedures in the setting of AAD with little additional risk.

In some cases, the native valve leaflets are normal despite the presence of a dilated or dissected aortic root. Valve-sparing aortic root replacement (VSARR) procedures allow surgeons to save the native valve while replacing the aortic root.[9] Although VSARR represents a more complicated approach at a time when simple, safe techniques are generally advantageous, it is a viable option for selected patients who are otherwise young and healthy. In this group, VSARR can provide a more durable option than a bioprosthetic valve and has the advantage of not requiring anticoagulation when compared to a mechanical valve. As experience with this operation has grown, there is now evidence that intraoperative mortality with VSARR is equal to that of the modified Bentall procedure and neither technique compromises short-term or midterm survival.[10]

PERIOPERATIVE OUTCOMES

Techniques developed by cardiac surgeons have dramatically reduced the operative mortality of type A AAD. With a mortality rate of 1%–2% per hour without surgical intervention, the achievement of a 10% rate of perioperative mortality at centers specialized in aortic surgery is a noteworthy achievement. Nevertheless, it remains the most high-risk

TABLE 49-2. FACTORS ASSOCIATED WITH INCREASED OPERATIVE MORTALITY

Advanced age (>70)
Shock or cardiac tamponade
Coronary ischemia or infarction
Neurologic deficit
Enlarged aortic root (diameter >44 mm)
Failure to use an open distal anastomosis
Coronary artery bypass grafting
Evidence of distal malperfusion (renal, mesenteric, or limb)

operation commonly performed by cardiac surgeons. The IRAD investigators published the best "real-world" experience from the largest series of consecutive patients that underwent repair of type A AAD at various centers throughout the world. Preoperative risk factors for surgical mortality were assessed and it was determined that age over 70 and a history of aortic valve replacement increased the operative risk. In addition, hypotension, any pulse deficit, and evidence of coronary ischemia and cardiac tamponade were also associated with worse outcomes.[4] Intraoperative factors affecting mortality are often multifactorial and difficult to delineate; however, it is recognized that intraoperative hemorrhage, brain ischemia, and distal malperfusion (manifesting as mesenteric, limb, or renal ischemia) are major drivers of mortality.[11] Technical factors affecting outcome relate to the difficulty of the reconstruction. IRAD data has shown that the presence of an enlarged root (>44 mm), the requirement of coronary artery bypass grafting, and failure to perform an open distal anastomosis are variables associated with mortality.[4] Knowledge of all these factors, as presented in Table 49-2, helps to identify higher risk patients and stimulates evolution of techniques to further improve perioperative outcomes.

Overall survival tends to follow a bimodal pattern. For patients that survive the operative period, the short- to medium-term survival is favorable. A recent series observed that 90% of operative survivors are still alive at one year and 76% are alive at five years post-op.[12] Beyond this point, late morbidity and mortality becomes more significant. This phenomenon may be related to the behavior of the residual dissection flap in the distal aorta.[13] Recently, significant attention has been directed to the associated patent false lumen, which is believed to result in aortic degeneration and aneurysm formation. Aortic enlargement and a reoperation rate as high as 27.5% has been reported.[12–14] Given this, centers of excellence in aortic surgery are now interested in changing the long-term prognosis. Recent advances in technique have focused on inducing thrombosis of the false lumen in an attempt to reduce late aortic complications such as rupture, redissection, reoperation, and death.

THE PATENT FALSE LUMEN AS A DETERMINANT OF LATE OUTCOME

The Stanford classification of dissection labels all dissections involving the ascending aorta as Stanford type A AAD. The Debakey classification, on the other hand, subcategorizes this group into those that are localized to the ascending alone (Debakey type II AAD) and those

TABLE 49-3. CAUSES OF LATE ANEURYSM FORMATION IN THE DISSECTED DESCENDING THORACIC AORTA

Patency of the false lumen

Enlarged descending thoracic aorta (>4 cm)

Large false lumen size

Male gender

that involve the arch and descending thoracic aorta (Debakey type I AAD). Type I AAD represents the large majority of clinical presentations. As previously discussed, perioperative mortality is significant, but those making it through the perioperative period tend to do reasonably well over the short term. Long-term survival, however, is in the range of 50% at 10 years.[14,15] Many of these late deaths have been ascribed to the presence of a residual distal dissection flap with a patent false lumen. Certainly, it is well known that the distal dissected aorta is vulnerable to late aneurysmal dilation and rupture. Conventional reintervention for this has involved open thoracoabdominal procedures, occasionally requiring HCA. In an effort to mitigate the development of late dilation, recent work has been done to define the factors that promote aneurysm formation. As presented in Table 49-3, the presence of a patent false lumen is principal among these and there is evidence that 60%–80% of Debakey type I AAD are associated with this phenomenon.[2] Large false lumen size and evidence of flow on CT angiogram are predictive of late dilation.[16] Griepp and colleagues followed 179 patients with serial CT scans after repair of type A AAD and found that initial aortic size >4 cm, presence of a patent false lumen, and male gender predicted greater growth of the descending aorta.[14] Extrapolation of evidence from literature on type B AAD suggests that partial thrombosis of the false lumen may represent the worst-case scenario associated with the highest likelihood of aneurysm formation.[17] Anatomic features of the dissected aorta most likely predisposing to false lumen patency is the presence of a residual tear that extends into the arch or the presence of reentry tears or fenestrations in the descending aorta. Although it has long been recognized that these residual tears in the distal arch or descending thoracic aorta contribute to complications and poor outcomes over the long term, there has been no good option for addressing them in the acute setting until recently. TEVAR may be an option for sealing these more distal tears and promoting false lumen thrombosis.

HYBRID RECONSTRUCTION TECHNIQUES

Several novel hybrid strategies have recently been introduced that combine classic open repair techniques with TEVAR. Most of these operations involve proximal aortic reconstruction with Dacron performed through a sternotomy combined with TEVAR of the descending thoracic aorta, which can be done at the same time or later. There are two central reasons to address the distal aorta with a stent graft:

1. To treat or prevent distal malperfusion by improving flow in the true lumen
2. To cover reentry tears or fenestrations in the descending thoracic aorta to promote false lumen thrombosis

A recent series compared mortality of patients with preoperative malperfusion syndrome with those without malperfusion and found a perioperative mortality difference of 30% versus 6%, respectively.[18] It is well recognized that malperfusion can be the result of true lumen compression by a pressurized false lumen as is shown in Figure 49-2. TEVAR can successfully expand the true lumen, as shown in Figure 49-3. This can improve downstream perfusion and mitigate the complications of malperfusion. Over the long term, the goal is to facilitate false lumen thrombosis and aortic remodeling, which is evidenced on serial postoperative imaging.[19] Several hybrid techniques have been proposed to achieve this goal.

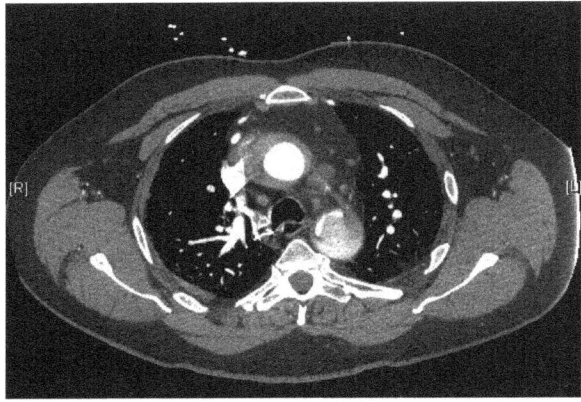

Figure 49-2. Computed tomographic (CT) angiogram showing compression of the true lumen in the descending thoracic aorta.

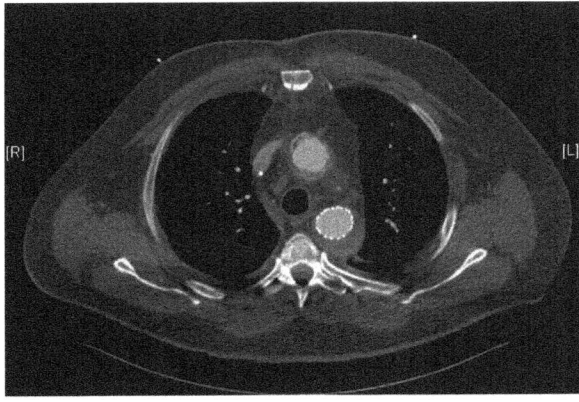

Figure 49-3. CT angiogram showing re-expansion of the true lumen in the descending thoracic aorta after TEVAR.

STRATEGIES FOR HYBRID TYPE A ACUTE AORTIC DISSECTION REPAIR

Hemi-Arch Replacement with Retrograde TEVAR

To accomplish a more complete anatomic reconstruction after type A AAD, particularly with Debakey type I AAD, a technique using a combination of TEVAR of the descending thoracic aorta plus standard proximal reconstruction has been developed. Standard emergency ascending aortic replacement with Dacron is performed first with valve resuspension or aortic root replacement as appropriate. Then, TEVAR is performed after sternal closure in a retrograde approach. An introductory sheath is placed in the femoral artery, and using fluoroscopy and transesophageal echocardiography (TEE), a stiff wire followed by a pigtail catheter is positioned in the true lumen. A stent graft is then deployed with the proximal end situated just distal to the takeoff of the left subclavian artery, as shown in Figure 49-4. Distal procedures such as branch vessel covered stenting or embolization have been reported as adjuncts with this technique. Preoperative CT angiography is used to identify the presence of distal fenestrations or reentry tears and is used to guide the length of stent coverage or determine the need for other distal intervention such as renal artery stenting. Hofferberth and colleagues recently reported on their experience with this approach. Their hybrid series of 19 patients, all of whom underwent Dacron replacement of the ascending aorta with retrograde TEVAR of the descending thoracic aorta, were compared with a group of 18 patients repaired in standard fashion. Outcome analysis demonstrated a significantly reduced incidence of distal malperfusion in those managed

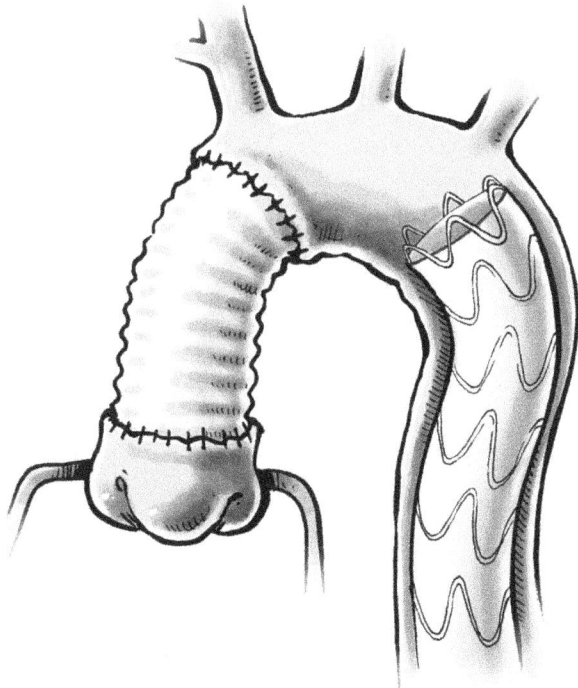

Figure 49-4. Illustration of a completed hybrid reconstruction with vascular graft reconstruction of the ascending aorta and retrograde TEVAR of the descending thoracic aorta.

with the hybrid approach and improved aortic remodeling, substantiated by a higher rate of false lumen thrombosis (80% vs. 9%) and a lower rate of distal aortic reintervention (25% vs. 0%).[20] Although these results are promising, behavior of the stent graft in the distal dissected aorta will determine the efficacy of this strategy over the long term.

Hemi-Arch Replacement with Antegrade TEVAR

This approach also involves standard proximal reconstruction and TEVAR of the descending thoracic aorta; however, it represents a different approach to stent graft deployment and focuses on a more aggressive arch resection. The goal is to resect any reentry tears in the arch and as much dissected tissue as possible by performing an extended hemi-arch replacement under HCA. Then, with the aorta open and before the distal anastomosis is completed, a stent graft is deployed in an antegrade fashion into the true lumen of the descending thoracic aorta under direct vision, as shown in Figure 49-5. The proximal extent of the graft sits just distal to the left subclavian artery takeoff, which leaves a short segment of native aorta between the distal hemi-arch anastomosis and the stent graft. There is evidence to suggest this promotes false lumen thrombosis (Fig. 49-6). In a recent report, 36 stented hybrid repairs were compared with 42 conventional hemi-arch repairs. There was no significant difference in perioperative mortality, and at follow-up, significantly more hybrid patients had obliteration of the distal false lumen (80%) relative to those who had conventional repair (17%). Interestingly, reintervention on the distal aorta was required in both groups with open operation performed in 11% of patients after conventional repair and none after hybrid repair. However, endovascular reintervention for endoleak was

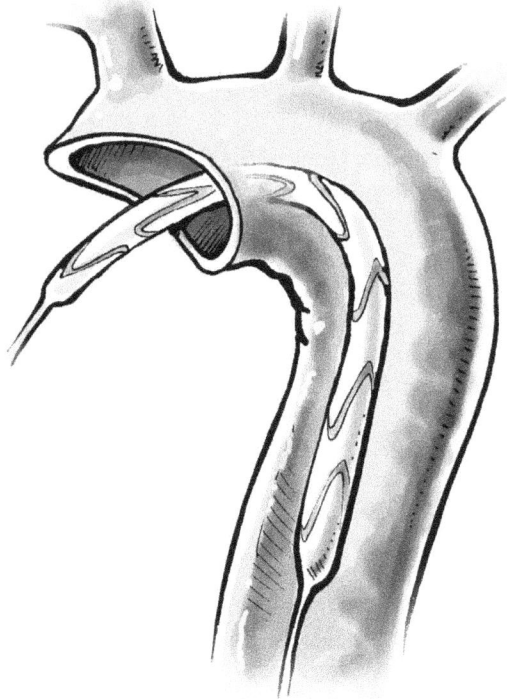

Figure 49-5. Illustration of an alternative strategy of antegrade TEVAR into the true lumen of the open aorta.

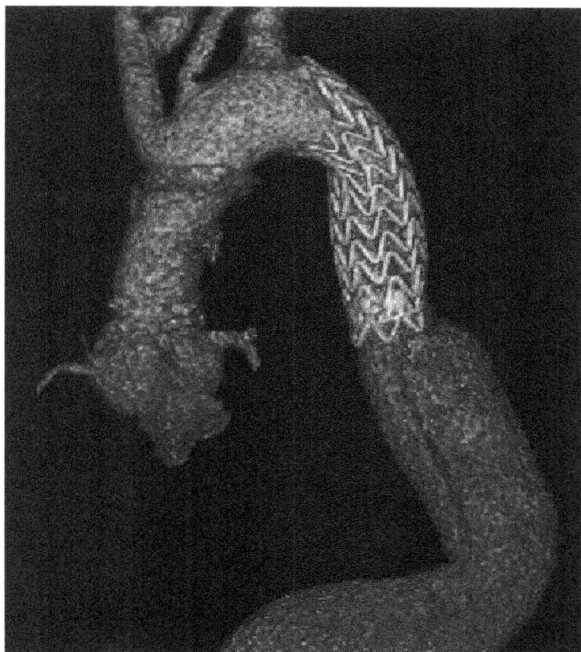

Figure 49-6. Postoperative CT angiogram reconstruction of a patient who underwent extended hemi-arch replacement with antegrade TEVAR of the descending thoracic aorta.

required in 22% of hybrid patients.[15] Therefore, this approach may be more effective at obliterating the false lumen but does appear to require more endovascular reintervention. The higher rate of false lumen thrombosis offers a potential advantage over the long term.

Total Arch Replacement with Elephant Trunk and TEVAR

Although the previously discussed hybrid approaches are more effective at obliterating the patent false lumen in the descending thoracic aorta when compared with standard hemi-arch repair, they leave mid to distal segments of the native transverse arch untreated. Having residual native aorta is a concern because longitudinal studies have shown that the arch is particularly susceptible to late dilation and aneurysm formation after dissection.[2] For this reason, some suggest total arch replacement with elephant trunk is the optimal long-term strategy for managing a Debakey type I AAD.[21,22] This approach can be accomplished as either a single- or two-stage procedure. In both cases, total arch replacement is performed through a sternotomy with antegrade cerebral perfusion during a prolonged period of HCA. An elephant trunk is then left in the proximal descending thoracic aorta as illustrated in Figure 49-7. The presence of an elephant trunk then allows immediate TEVAR inside the Dacron elephant trunk, or alternatively, a stent can be placed in the descending thoracic aorta at a later date if follow-up imaging demonstrates evidence of distal degeneration with aneurysm formation. This seems to be the best approach for a select group of patients with extensive dissections with tears involving the arch or with evidence of arch dilation or aneurysm. For them, the risk of a total arch and elephant trunk creation at the initial operation is significantly less than the risk associated with a standard repair leaving residual native arch tissue that will almost certainly develop a

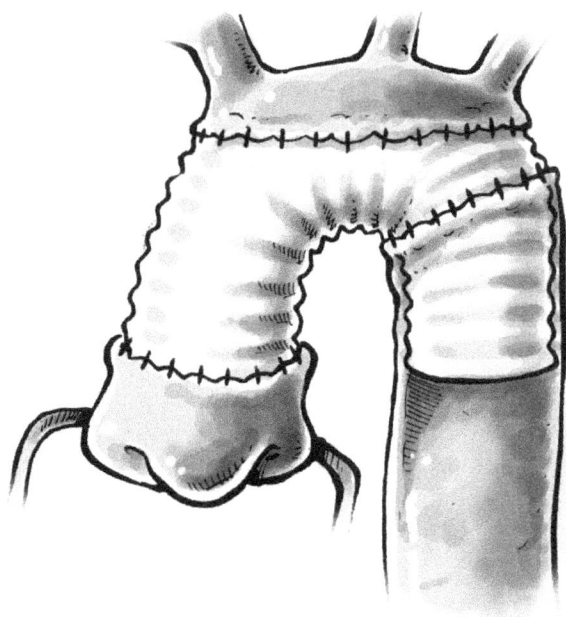

Figure 49-7. Illustration of completed total arch reconstruction with an elephant trunk in the descending thoracic aorta.

pseudoaneurysm, large true aneurysm, or rupture in the future. Furthermore, reports from high volume tertiary care centers have demonstrated that this more extensive procedure can be performed with minimal additional perioperative mortality.[21-23] Although delayed open or endovascular intervention on the descending thoracic aorta can be performed later, in many cases, the false lumen is obliterated at the initial operation. For those with a persistent patent false lumen who develop late complications, a stent graft can be deployed with the proximal landing zone in the Dacron elephant trunk. A key component to the success of this method is careful imaging follow-up, which is required to detect complications of the distal aorta to enable prompt reintervention.

Total Arch Replacement with Hybrid Stent Graft Prosthesis: "Frozen Elephant Trunk" Technique

An alternative approach to achieve total arch replacement with simultaneous stent graft repair of the descending thoracic aorta is to use a hybrid stent graft device. There are several variations of this novel device on the market. The Vascutek Thoraflex™ Hybrid device composed of a covered endovascular stent graft and attached to a 4-branched polyester vascular graft is one example. This product is provided in a short delivery system and is implanted by first introducing the compacted stent portion into the proximal descending thoracic aorta in an antegrade fashion under HCA; the stent is then deployed. The collar, at the interface between the vascular graft and stent, is sewn to the distal aorta and the proximal branched polyester vascular graft is used to replace the arch and ascending aorta, as illustrated in Figure 49-8. Jakob and colleagues followed 29 patients with type A AAD after

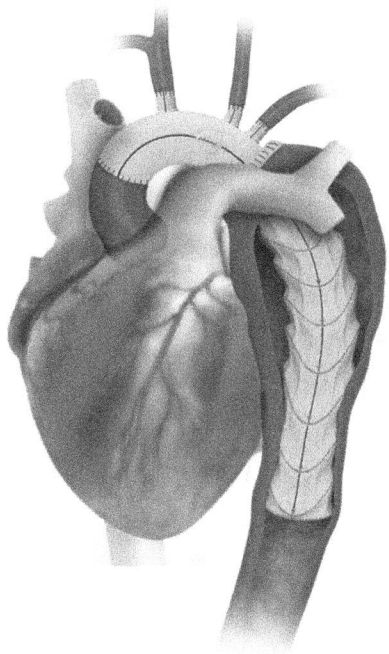

Figure 49-8. Hybrid arch reconstruction with the Vascutek Thoraflex™ Hybrid device, which is composed of a proximal 4-branched vascular graft for total arch replacement and a distal stent-graft for descending thoracic aortic repair. The product has a CE mark and has been commercially available since November 2012.

single-stage repair of the ascending aorta, arch, and proximal descending thoracic aorta with the E-vita® (Jotec, Hechingen, Germany) hybrid stent graft, which is available commercially in Europe but not in North America. Observed perioperative mortality was 10%, there was no incidence of spinal cord ischemia, and false lumen obliteration was observed in 93% of patients immediately after surgery. This finding was maintained at a mean of 19 months of follow-up.[6] Longer follow-up will help to determine whether this composite graft technique sustains thrombosis of the false lumen and whether that will protect patients from late degeneration and aneurysm formation.

Hybrid Aortic Reconstruction with Arch Debranching and Zone 0 TEVAR

Addressing the arch and ascending aorta with TEVAR is the latest frontier for hybrid aortic reconstructive techniques and this entails landing a stent proximally at Zone 0 in the ascending aorta, according to the Ishimaru classification. The techniques of total arch replacement and TEVAR of the descending thoracic aorta all involve total arch replacement with Dacron, which necessitates a prolonged period of HCA. By developing hybrid techniques of total arch repair, the requirement of HCA can be avoided. To date, endovascular approaches to total arch repair have mostly used an arch debranching technique. Zone 0 TEVAR for AAD has been reported by Diethrich and colleagues, who debranched the innominate and left carotid arteries without HCA before using peripheral access to deploy the stent graft.[24] An alternative single-stage approach without HCA to repair the ascending aorta, transverse aortic arch, and proximal descending thoracic aorta with

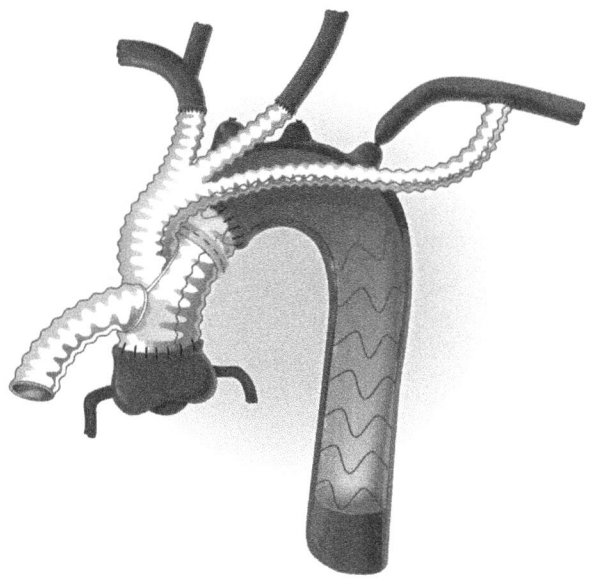

Figure 49-9. Completed hybrid arch reconstruction involving replacement of the ascending aorta with Dacron, arch debranching, and antegrade TEVAR of the descending thoracic aorta.

antegrade TEVAR has recently been described for type A AAD. First, the ascending aorta is replaced without HCA. After arch debranching with a four-limbed graft, a stent is deployed into the true lumen in an antegrade fashion. This approach, as illustrated in Figure 49-9, eliminates the need for HCA and peripheral arterial access for TEVAR.[25] Although these techniques are experimental at present, they represent less invasive strategies than formal total arch replacement and elephant trunk creation and may provide both short- and long-term benefits. Acutely, they may have the potential to decrease bleeding associated with arch reconstruction under deep hypothermia, to decrease the risk of stroke by eliminating long periods of HCA and to treat visceral malperfusion by opening up the true lumen in the descending aorta. Long-term results will determine whether stents designed for more distal locations in the aorta can behave appropriately within the more angulated and mobile arch and ascending aorta.

CONCLUSION

Type A AAD is a disease with a rate of survival that is less than 20% with medical management alone. Operative intervention has an enormous impact on prognosis and results in survival for 80%–90% of patients. A successful repair strategy is focused on three goals: to replace the ascending aorta and prevent rupture into the pericardium, to eliminate aortic regurgitation, and to reestablish true lumen perfusion to correct distal malperfusion. Although achieving these goals has resulted in significant improvements in survival over the short term, the long-term prognosis may be affected by residual dissection in the distal aorta. TEVAR of the descending thoracic aorta has the potential to improve long-term results by covering fenestrations and reentry tears in the distal aorta, eliminating perfusion of the false lumen, and inducing false lumen thrombosis. The resulting aortic remodeling has the potential to reduce long-term reintervention and mortality. In our practice, we elect to use an extended hemi-arch procedure for proximal reconstruction with TEVAR of the descending thoracic aorta in selected cases. This has proven to be a safe strategy with the potential for long-term benefits. As hybrid approaches continue to evolve, there is optimism that new technology may allow safe and effective single-stage total arch replacement and TEVAR of the descending thoracic aorta using a single hybrid stent graft prosthesis (frozen-elephant trunk technique). This would achieve the goals of repair in the acute setting and promote remodeling of the descending thoracic aorta.

REFERENCES

1. Criado FJ. Aortic dissection: a 250-year perspective. *Tex Heart Inst J*. 2011;38(6):694–700.
2. Bonser RS, Ranasinghe AM, Loubani M, et al. Evidence, lack of evidence, controversy and debate in the provision and performance of the surgery of acute type A aortic dissection. *J Am Coll Cardiol*. 2011;58(24):2455–2474.
3. Debakey ME, Cooley DA, Creech O, Jr. Surgical considerations of dissecting aneurysm of the aorta. *Ann Surg*. 1955;142(4):586–612.
4. Rampoldi V, Trimarchi S, Eagle KA, et al. Simple risk models to predict surgical mortality in acute type A aortic dissection: the international registry of acute aortic dissection score. *Ann Thorac Surg*. 2007;83:55–61.
5. Bavaria JE, Pochettino A, Brinster DR, et al. New paradigms and improved results for the surgical treatment of acute type A dissection. *Ann Surg*. 2001;234(3):336–343.
6. Jakob H, Tsagakis K. DeBakey type I dissection: when hybrid stent-grafting is indicated? *J Cardiovasc Surg*. 2010;51:633–640.
7. Tan ME, Morshuis WJ, Dossche KME, et al. Long-term results after 27 years of surgical treatment of acute type A aortic dissection. *Ann Thorac Surg*. 2005;80:523–529.
8. Shihata M, Mittal R, Senthilselvan A, et al. Selective antegrade cerebral perfusion during aortic arch surgery confers survival and neuroprotective advantages. *J Thorac Cardiovasc Surg*. 2011;141:948–952.
9. David T. How I do aortic valve sparing operations to treat aortic root aneurysm. *J Card Surg*. 2011;26:92–99.
10. Subramanian S, Leontyev S, Borger MA, et al. Valve-*sparing root reconstruction* does not compromise survival in acute type A aortic dissection. *Ann Thorac Surg*. 2012;94:1230–1234.
11. Appoo JJ, Pozeg Z. Strategies in the surgical treatment of type A aortic arch dissection. *Ann Cardiothorac Surg*. 2013;2(2):205–11.
12. Zierer A, Voeller R, Hill K, et al. Aortic enlargement and late reoperation after repair of acute type A aortic dissection. *Ann Thorac Surg*. 2007;84:479–487.
13. Gorlitzer M, Weiss G, Meinhart J, et al. Fate of the false lumen after combined surgical and endovascular repair treating Stanford type A aortic dissections. *Ann Thorac Surg*. 2010;89:794–799.
14. Halsted JC, Meier M, Etz C, et al. The fate of the distal aorta after repair of acute type A aortic dissection. *J Thorac Cardiovasc Surg*. 2007;133:127–135.
15. Desai ND, Pochettino A. Distal aortic remodeling using endovascular repair in acute Debakey I aortic dissection. *Semin Thorac Cardiovasc Surg*. 2009;21:387–392.
16. Song JM, Kim SD, Kim JH, et al. Long-term predictors of descending aorta aneurysmal change in patients with aortic dissection. *J Am Coll Cardiol*. 2007;50:799–804.
17. Tsai TT, Evangelista A, Neinaber CA, et al. Partial thrombosis of the false lumen in patients with acute type B aortic dissection. *N Engl J Med*. 2007;357:349–359.
18. Geirsson A, Bavaria JE, Swarr D, et al. Fate of the residual distal and proximal aorta after acute type a dissection repair using *a contemporary* surgical reconstruction algorithm. *Ann Thorac Surg*. 2007;84:1955–1964.

19. Neinaber CA, Rousseau H, Eggebrecht H, et al. Randomized comparison of strategies for type B aortic dissection: the investigation of stent grafts in aortic dissection (INSTEAD) trail. *Circulation.* 2009;120:2519–2528.
20. Hofferberth SC, Newcomb AE, Yii MY, et al. Hybrid proximal surgery plus adjunctive retrograde endovascular repair in acute DeBakey type I dissection: superior outcomes to conventional surgical repair. *J Thorac Cardiovasc Surg.* 2013;145:349–355.
21. Uchida N, Ishihara H, Shibamura H, et al. Midterm results of extensive primary repair of the thoracic aorta by means of total arch replacement with open stent graft placement for an acute type A aortic dissection. *J Thorac Cardiovasc Surg.* 2006;131:862–867.
22. Sun LZ, Qi RD, Zhu JM, et al. Total arch replacement combined with stented elephant trunk implantation: a new "standard" therapy for type A dissection involving repair of the aortic arch? *Circulation.* 2011;123:971–978.
23. LeMaire SA, Price MD, Parenti JL, et al. Early outcomes after aortic arch replacement by using the Y-graft technique. *Ann Thorac Surg.* 2011;91:700–708.
24. Diethrich EB, Ghazoul M, Wheatley GH, et al. Great vessel transposition for antegrade delivery of the TAG endoprosthesis in the proximal aortic arch. *J Endovasc Ther.* 2006;12:583–587.
25. Kent WDT, Herget EJ, Wong JK, et al. Ascending, total arch and descending thoracic aortic repair for acute DeBakey Type I aortic dissection without circulatory arrest. *Ann Thorac Surg.* 2012;94:59–61.

50

Management of Thoracic Stent Graft Collapse

Paul R. Crisostomo, MD and Jae S. Cho, MD

INTRODUCTION

Thoracic endovascular aortic repair (TEVAR) has become a widely disseminated therapy to treat a variety of anatomically suitable descending thoracic aortic pathology. Perceived lower operative mortality, spinal cord ischemia, and cardiopulmonary morbidity compared to open aortic repair have exponentially increased the use of TEVAR worldwide.[1] However, just as any other new technology, it has its own set of complications that need to be addressed and shortcomings that require device modification.

Of the myriad of TEVAR pitfalls including endoleak, migration, and access injury, endograft collapse remains a potentially deadly complication. Thoracic endograft collapse (TEC), also known as device compression or invagination, is the failure of the device to maintain its intended expanded diameter after implantation. Ultimately, TEC can lead to physiologic aortic coarctation, aortic occlusion, malperfusion, and death.[1-4] The purpose of this chapter is to review the risk factors, preventive measures, open and endovascular treatment, and outcomes of TEC after TEVAR.

INCIDENCE

The true incidence of TEC is not entirely clear. The largest recent case series suggest an incidence between 4.4% and 9.3%.[4,5] In contrast, the 2012 Gore Annual Clinical Update reports 196 device compressions after more than 59,000 Gore TAG TEVAR device implants for an incidence of 0.3%.[6] While this may appear rare, it should be noted that Gore TAG collapse occurred more often than migration, stent fracture, and deployment malfunctions combined.[6] In addition to reporting bias, asymptomatic presentations and lack of follow-up in young trauma patients exacerbate the difficulty in determining the true incidence of TEC. TEC is an underappreciated complication with an incidence likely much higher than that reported in the literature.

CAUSES

The most common cause of TEC is inadequate apposition of endograft to the aortic wall secondary to either "bird-beaking" effects (48%) (Fig. 50-1) or excessive oversizing that results in device invagination (20%).[7] Other causes include maldeployment of the endograft, device failure,[8] device undersizing and migration,[6] and progression of aortic disease; TEC has even been reported after cardiopulmonary resuscitation.[9]

In patients with TEC, the most common index indication for TEVAR is blunt traumatic aortic injury (BTAI), 60%–65%, followed by type B dissection, 15%–36%.[4,7,10] Other indications that have resulted in TEC include thoracic aortic aneurysm (TAA), aortic coarctation, aortoesophageal fistula, and intramural hematoma.

The high propensity of TEC in the BTAI subset is due in large part to the small aortic diameter and steeply angulated arches of these young trauma patients. Young BTAI patients have narrow aortic diameters (average of 19.3 mm).[11] Compounded by the lack of smaller size endografts in the early stage of TEVAR, this resulted in excessive oversizing of the endograft (as high 90% has been observed)[12] that can cause device invagination or device infolding. While TEC has occurred in properly oversized endografts, excessive oversizing is a risk factor to the development of TEC. Muhs et al. noted that minimum aortic diameter within the endograft (18.6 ± 1.7 mm vs. 22.4 ± 3.1 mm) predicted TEC.[12] In the Gore report, the mean aortic diameter for trauma patients averaged 19.7 ± 2.7 mm while the implanted device averaged 26.8 mm for an average of 36% oversizing.[6] Jonker et al. observed that the mean oversizing in 60 TEC was 27% compared to 17% in 150 patients without TEC.[7] This is in contrast to Gore TAG Instructions for Use (IFU) that recommends oversizing of 7%–18%.

Another factor that contributes to the high incidence of TEC is the tight aortic arch observed in the young BTAI cohort. An angulated aortic neck makes it difficult for

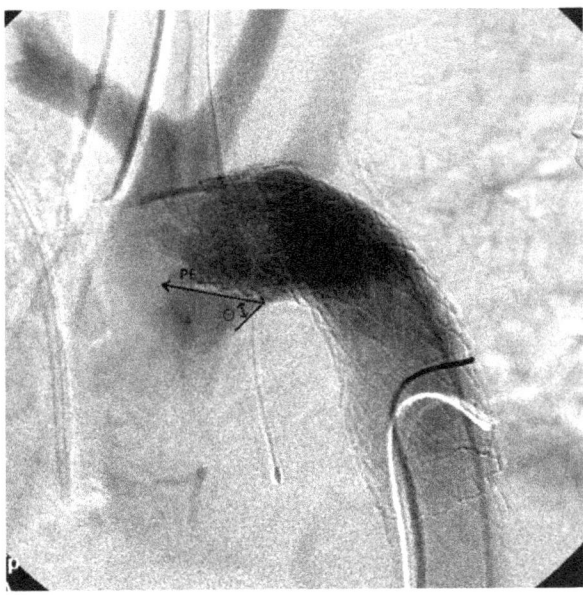

Figure 50-1. Fluoroscopic image of bird beak phenomenon. PE, protrusion extension of stent graft into aortic lumen; Θ, bird-beak angle between endograft and lesser curve of aortic arch.

the first iteration thoracic stent graft to conform to the arch, resulting in a bird-beak. Bird-beak is the malapposition of the proximal stent graft to the aortic wall, with a wedge-shaped gap between the stent graft and the lesser curvature of the aortic arch (Fig. 50-1). While exposing the abluminal surface of the device to the force of the blood flow and causing some loss of seal length, bird-beak, by itself, is a relatively benign condition in most patients. However, Canaud et al. identified four TECs in their series of 285 thoracic endograft implants and found a severely angulated proximal aortic neck (mean angle of 104.5°, range 92°–108°) in all collapsed device patients.[13] Of 64 patients who underwent TEVAR, Ueda et al. recognized that bird-beaking ($n = 28$) and bird beak length was significantly associated with endoleak and TEC (9.3%, $n = 6$).[5]

A computer model utilizing one-way coupled fluid–solid interaction analyses showed that a malapposed endograft generates vortices in the proximal luminal surface close to the angulated aortic arch. A cross section of the endograft (see inset of Fig. 50-2B) revealed that a transmural pressure load difference exists between the abluminal surface and the luminal surface of the malapposed thoracic aortic stent graft that would likely portend TEC. It was noted that protrusion extension (PE) or bird-beak into the aortic lumen and angulation between the stent graft and aortic wall cause increased compression pressure across the stent graft resulting in stent graft diameter reduction, low systolic perfusion pressure, and ultimately TEC.[14] Figure 50-2 summarizes transmural pressure gradient for all examined combinations of PE and

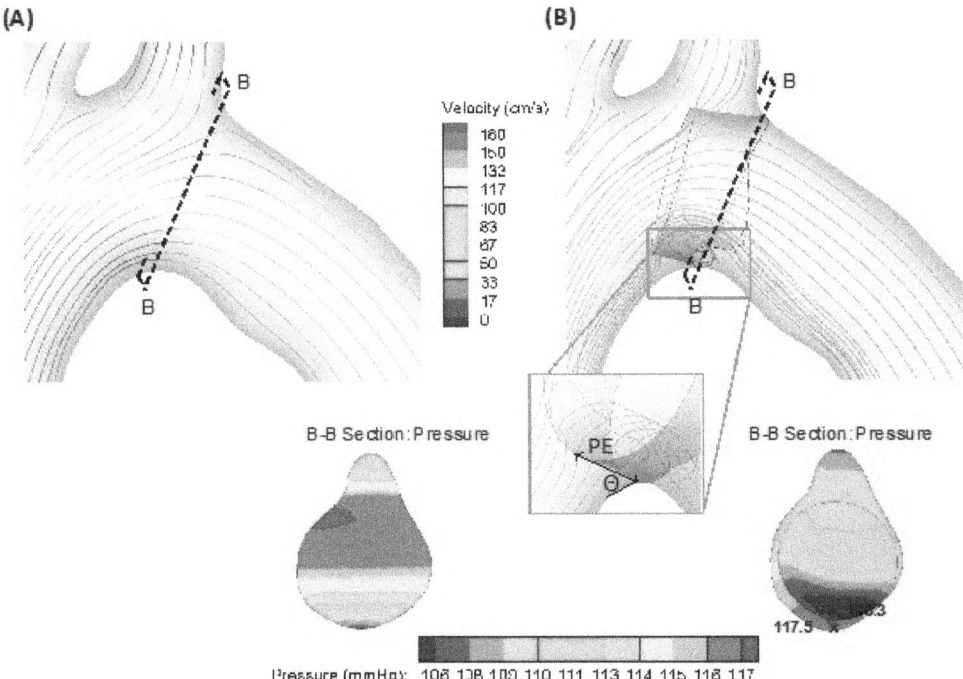

Figure 50-2. Computer model of cross-sectional analysis of aortic pressure. *A*, Aorta, cross section just distal to left subclavian artery. *B*, Aorta after TEVAR placement with bird-beak extension, cross section just distal to left subclavian artery. PE, protrusion extension of stent graft into aortic lumen; Θ, bird-beak angle between endograft and lesser curve of aortic arch; X, measurement of pressure at bird-beak angle. Adapted with permission from Pasta et al.[14]

angulation parameters.[14] Other causes of bird-beaking include devices with low radial force and material fatigue.[4] Angulated aortic neck and the bird-beak configuration are anatomical factors that portend TEC and necessitate closer follow-up intervals.

In the setting of aortic dissection, reentry of the false lumen in the proximal or distal zone of the thoracic aorta uncovered by the endograft can lead to TEC. Following TEVAR for TAA, development of type IA or IB endoleak has been associated with TEC. In other thoracic aortic emergent catastrophes, if an endograft is undersized due to a falsely narrow hypovolemic aorta, a type I endoleak, migration, and subsequent TEC may occur after resuscitation.[6]

DEVICES

Currently, there are four FDA-approved devices that are available for treatment of descending thoracic aorta pathology, but it is unclear whether stent type plays a pivotal role in TEC. Gore was the first thoracic endograft approved by the FDA in 2005 and has been the most popular TEVAR device worldwide. As such, the majority of published TECs occurred with use of the Gore TAG device, but TECs have been reported to occur with Cook Zenith TX2 and other TEVAR devices as well.

In 2008 and again in 2013, with newer, more conformable devices, Canaud et al. compared TEVAR devices from all four manufacturers in a bench top pulsatile flow cadaveric model with varying landing zone angles and oversizing.[15,16] In both studies, the Medtronic Valiant with the greatest radial force remained opposed to the aortic wall at all angles and oversizing. In contrast, the Cook TX2 lost wall apposition at 70° compared to 80° with the Bolton Relay and at 90° with the Gore TAG.[15] Next generation devices still lost device wall apposition, but at improved angles: Cook Zenith TX2 with ProForm and Bolton Relay NBS Plus at 110°, Gore C-TAG at 120°.[16] Oversizing exacerbated this loss of apposition. Not only do next generation devices exhibit greater conformability and radial strength, but they are offered in expanded size ranges to limit oversizing. In 2012, the Gore C-TAG and the Medtronic Valiant endografts received FDA approval for use in BTAI further supporting their use to treat narrow, angled aortic necks that may have caused initial TEC. With their improved design, the Gore C-TAG has had more than 4000 implants and the Medtronic Valiant more than 10,900 implants with no reported TEC.[6,17] Thus, although recent TEVAR design improvements should minimize the incidence of TEC, awareness of thoracic stent graft device limitations especially in emergent patient conditions with limited available stock remains a critical part of planning.

PRESENTATION

A surprising majority of patients with TEC remain asymptomatic. Kasirajan et al. utilized data from the earlier 2008 Gore Annual Clinical Update and revealed that 51% of reported TEC were asymptomatic.[10] Jonker et al. found asymptomatic presentation of TEC in 59% of cases.[7] Tadros et al. also reported a 64% rate of asymptomatic presentation.[4] Symptomatic patients with TEC typically manifested hypertension, back or chest pain, oliguria, claudication, paraplegia, and on physical exam weak or absent femoral pulses. Frequently, symptomatic patients also demonstrated increased risk of mortality. The 2012 Gore Update reports an overall mortality of 7.1% of patients with device compressions.[6] Of the recent review of 60 TECs, Jonker et al. found an overall mortality of 8.3% and in symptomatic patients a mortality of 21.7%.[7] Although variable in presentation, TEC is a potentially deadly complication that warrants attention and treatment.

Just as TEC varies in symptomatic presentation, time to diagnosis varies as well. The majority of TEC (65%) is diagnosed acutely within the first month after implantation.[7] Median time to diagnosis varies from 9 to 15 days in recent large series.[4,7] However, delayed or late presentation, several months or even years from initial TEVAR repair, has been reported.[3] Timing of presentation (acute or chronic) and symptomatic state (asymptomatic or malperfusion) are primary determinants for reintervention.

INTERVENTION

Treatment strategy has not been well established. However, the authors recommend intervention even in asymptomatic patients when TEC is diagnosed based on the following. First, although spontaneous re-expansion of TEC has been reported,[18,19] it is an extremely rare occurrence. Second, untreated asymptomatic collapse may be followed by symptomatic collapse.[3] Third, in the review by Jonker et al., the mortality rate in the untreated TEC group was 38% compared with 3.8% in the treatment group.[7] The management of TEC includes endovascular and open surgical repair.

Endovascular reintervention for TEC is the most practical choice in the acute phase after initial TEVAR deployment. Malperfusion causing hemodynamic lability and ongoing polytrauma comorbidities in acutely ill trauma patients make minimally invasive endovascular repair a first-line modality, even if only to temporize the pathology. The goal of endovascular repair is to increase the radial force at the locus of collapse and improve apposition to the aortic wall. We recommend initial endovascular repair with either balloon mounted stent (e.g., Palmaz stent), high radial force thoracic endograft (e.g., Medtronic Valiant), or relining with next generation TEVAR device with increased radial force and conformability.

Amongst all TEVAR devices, Medtronic Talent and Valiant Captivia devices exhibit the greatest radial force.[15] Multiple reports of Medtronic Talent or Valiant to treat collapse of a different manufacturer have been reported with success. The second generation Gore C-TAG device has been redesigned to have improved flexibility, more generous oversizing windows, and includes both tapered and smaller device diameters that are designed to treat aortas with inner diameters as small as 16 mm. Uniquely, the Gore C-TAG IFU reports safe oversizing of grafts up to 33%; increased Gore C-TAG oversizing results in increased radial force, which could be used to paradoxically treat a TEC due to oversizing from a first generation device. The aforementioned endovascular interventions incorporate increased radial force and/or increased conformability to target many of the causes of initial collapse including bird-beak, lack of wall apposition, and acute arch angle in young patients.

It should be noted, however, that repeat TEVAR with landing zone extension carries several drawbacks. It may increase the risk of retrograde dissection and cerebrovascular events and require debranching or chimney stent grafting. In general, graft extension across the left common carotid artery should be discouraged in young patients who have otherwise normal life expectancy.[20] When it is deemed necessary, open conversion should be strongly considered if the patient is surgically fit. Landing zone extension has had some success but multiple failures manifested as TEVAR recollapse have also been noted with the use of low radial force TEVAR devices.[13] These endovascular options may fail to address some of the initial causes of the TEC including bird-beak, acute aortic angle, and inappropriate device selection.

Placement of a large balloon expandable stent (i.e., the Palmaz stent) without proximal extension into the native aorta is another option. Deployment of a Palmaz stent into the native aorta is not recommended lest a retrograde type A dissection or injury to the aortic arch may occur.[20] Re-expansion with balloon dilation has a high chance of recurrence; it should only be used as a temporizing measure for symptomatic patients when one of aforementioned modalities is not available.

Complete TEC proximally and distally is best managed by open repair with device explantation. TEC most commonly presents as proximal collapse (65.5%) (Figs. 50-3 and 50-4) but complete TEC occurs not infrequently (18.2%).[7] It is reasonable but

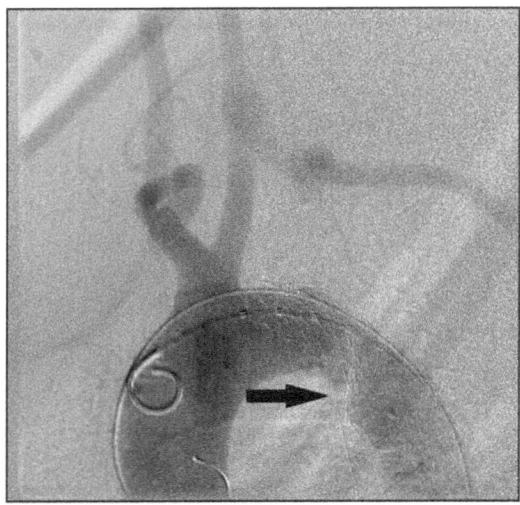

Figure 50-3. Fluoroscopic image of proximal TEVAR collapse. Arrow depicts proximal stent collapse with concomitant bird beak.

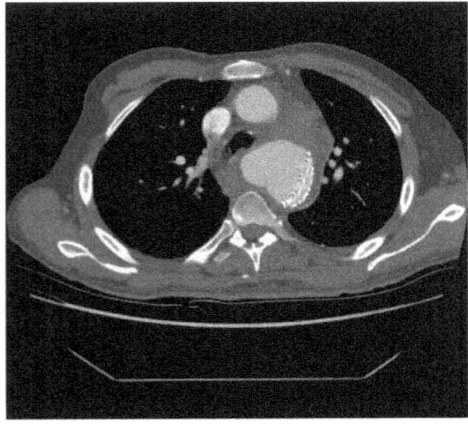

Figure 50-4. Axial computed tomography image of proximal TEVAR collapse.

likely difficult to attempt crossing the complete collapse and follow with endovascular repair. Moreover, explant analysis demonstrated significant material fatigue in patients with total device compression. Thus, we recommend open surgical conversion in the setting of complete endograft collapse. Open surgical options include explantation and aortic prosthetic replacement or axillofemoral bypass. For surgical explantation of thoracic endograft, sternotomy with total extracorporeal circulation, left thoracotomy with/without circulatory arrest and selective antegrade perfusion, and left thoracotomy with/without left heart bypass have been described. Axillobifemoral bypass is an option as either definitive or bridging repair in the hemodynamically unstable, critically ill, or surgically unfit patients. However, in young/healthy patients who have little comorbidity and in those with recurrent collapse, explantation of the collapsed graft and open surgical repair with aortic prosthetic replacement remains the standard.

Late TEC months or years after initial implantation deserves special attention. Jonker found that 25% of TEC reported in the literature was diagnosed after 90 days.[21] Asymptomatic patients could be monitored with close follow-up and serial images as spontaneous resolution of acute and delayed TEC has been reported.[18,19] For symptomatic patients with delayed TEC, endovascular treatment first is preferred, especially when technical aspects of the initial repair can be identified and addressed.

INTERVENTION OUTCOMES

The primary determinant of outcomes appears to be the presence or lack of symptoms. Jonker et al. reported a 21.7% 30-day mortality rate among symptomatic patients, whereas no asymptomatic patients died.[7] Intervention, both endovascular and open, is well tolerated with excellent perioperative outcomes. Greater than 86% success rate of balloon-mounted Palmaz stent to treat TEC indicates this is a feasible option for repair.[10] In cases where a first generation TAG device was used, relining with a newer generation C-TAG achieved a 79% success rate.[10]

Among the compilation of 60 TEC by Jonker et al. who received an intervention, the 30-day mortality was 3.8%, while 38% of patients without treatment expired.[7] Gore update reported 7% mortality following intervention.[10] Death after acute TEC has been attributed to multiorgan failure, cardiac arrest, aortic rupture, and cerebrovascular events. Other major morbidities (15%) tallied included additional endograft placement, bowel resection, embolization, and aortoesophageal fistula.[7]

Open conversion specifically for TEC can be performed safely. In the Gore series, almost 40 open surgical explanations and repairs have been performed with at least an 86% success rate and a mortality rate of 5%.[10] Tadros et al. reported no mortality with open conversion in their series.[4] These results are not inferior to open conversion results for indications not limited to TEC. In a review of the Medtronic Talent Thoracic Registry series, Ehrlich et al. reported a 6.2% mortality rate in 16 open conversions.[22] In a more recent series of 26 patients with delayed conversion to open repair with TEVAR explant for delayed TEVAR complications, Miyahara et al. demonstrated a mortality of 11.5% with stroke, hemorrhage, chylothorax, perioperative myocardial infarction, and acute pulmonary embolism in one patient each.[23]

Long-term outcomes after repair for acute or delayed TEC are not well studied. Jonker et al. reported that with a median follow-up of 6.0 months, three patients suffered deaths related to the collapsed endograft.[7]

CONCLUSION

Despite its inherent limitations, TEVAR remains a fixture of the endovascular surgeon's armamentarium. As we rapidly ascend the TEVAR learning curve and as devices continue to improve, acute TEC in the elective scenario should become a relatively rare event. Nevertheless, emergent situations with limited available thoracic endograft stock remain a setup for increased risk for TEC and require an awareness of the pitfalls and shortcomings to prevent it. Moreover, fenestrated side branch TEVAR likely will require attentiveness to prevent TEC. Delayed TEC presentation may also increase as young patients treated with TEVAR continue to age, necessitating a broad scope of open and endovascular therapy to address it. Further studies are needed to understand and treat these complications as the endovascular future continues to unfold.

REFERENCES

1. Go MR, Barbato JE, Dillavou ED, et al. Thoracic endovascular aortic repair for traumatic aortic transection. *J Vasc Surg.* 2007;46(5):928–933.
2. Go MR, Siegenthaler MP, Rhee RY, et al. Physiologic coarctation of the aorta resulting from proximal protrusion of thoracic aortic stent grafts into the arch. *J Vasc Surg.* 2008;48(4):1007–1011.
3. Shukla AJ, Jeyabalan G, Cho JS. Late collapse of a thoracic endoprosthesis. *J Vasc Surg.* 2011;53(3):798–801.
4. Tadros RO, Lipsitz EC, Chaer RA, et al. A multicenter experience of the management of collapsed thoracic endografts. *J Vasc Surg.* 2011;53(5):1217–1222.
5. Ueda T, Fleischmann D, Dake MD, et al. Incomplete endograft apposition to the aortic arch: bird-beak configuration increases risk of endoleak formation after thoracic endovascular aortic repair. *Radiology.* 2010;255(2):645–652.
6. Gore WL. GORE TAG Thoracic Endoprosthesis Annual Clinical Update 12/5/11, 2012. 2012.
7. Jonker FH, Schlosser FJ, Geirsson A, et al. Endograft collapse after thoracic endovascular aortic repair. *J Endovasc Ther.* 2010;17(6):725–734.
8. Melissano G, Tshomba Y, Civilini E, Chiesa R. Disappointing results with a new commercially available thoracic endograft. *J Vasc Surg.* 2004;39(1):124–130.
9. Rajani RR, Dente CJ, Ball CG, Feliciano DV. Collapse of a thoracic aortic stent graft after cardiopulmonary resuscitation. *Am Surg.* 2009;75(7):626–627.
10. Kasirajan K, Dake MD, Lumsden A, et al. Incidence and outcomes after infolding or collapse of thoracic stent grafts. *J Vasc Surg.* 2012;55(3):652–658; discussion 658.
11. Borsa JJ, Hoffer EK, Karmy-Jones R, et al. Angiographic description of blunt traumatic injuries to the thoracic aorta with specific relevance to endograft repair. *J Endovasc Ther.* 2002;9(suppl 2):II84–II91.
12. Muhs BE, Balm R, White GH, Verhagen HJ. Anatomic factors associated with acute endograft collapse after Gore TAG treatment of thoracic aortic dissection or traumatic rupture. *J Vasc Surg.* 2007;45(4):655–661.
13. Canaud L, Alric P, Desgranges P, et al. Factors favoring stent-graft collapse after thoracic endovascular aortic repair. *J Thorac Cardiovasc Surg.* 2010;139(5):1153–1157.
14. Pasta S, Cho JS, Dur O, et al. Computer modeling for the prediction of thoracic aortic stent graft collapse. *J Vasc Surg.* 2013;57(5):1353–1361.
15. Canaud L, Alric P, Laurent M, et al. Proximal fixation of thoracic stent-grafts as a function of oversizing and increasing aortic arch angulation in human cadaveric aortas. *J Endovasc Ther.* 2008;15(3):326–334.

16. Canaud L, Cathala P, Joyeux F, et al. Improvement in conformability of the latest generation of thoracic stent grafts. *J Vasc Surg*. 2013;57(4):1084–1089.
17. Medtronic. Valiant Thoracic Stent Graft With The Captivia Delivery System 2012 Annual Physician Clinical Update 3/29/2012, 2012. 2012.
18. Costanza M, Sivia P, Amankwah K, Gahtan V. Compression and spontaneous re-expansion of a thoracic endograft placed for acute, traumatic injury of the proximal thoracic aorta. *J Vasc Surg*. 2009;49(3):771–773.
19. Ponton A, Garcia I, Arnaiz E, Bernal JM. Spontaneous re-expansion of a collapsed thoracic endoprosthesis: case report. *J Vasc Surg*. 2008;48(6):1585–1588.
20. Steinbauer MG, Stehr A, Pfister K, et al. Endovascular repair of proximal endograft collapse after treatment for thoracic aortic disease. *J Vasc Surg*. 2006;43(3):609–612.
21. Rodd CD, Desigan S, Hamady MS, et al. Salvage options after stent collapse in the thoracic aorta. *J Vasc Surg*. 2007;46(4):780–785.
22. Ehrlich MP, Nienaber CA, Rousseau H, et al. Short-term conversion to open surgery after endovascular stent-grafting of the thoracic aorta: the Talent thoracic registry. *J Thorac Cardiovasc Surg*. 2008; 135(6):1322–1326.
23. Miyahara S, Nomura Y, Shirasaka T, et al. Early and midterm outcomes of open surgical correction after thoracic endovascular aortic repair. *Ann Thorac Surg*. 2013;95(5):1584–1590.

Index